Clinical Gynecologic Endocrinology and Infertility

SELF ASSESSMENT AND STUDY GUIDE

David B. Seifer
Leon Speroff

Illustration and Page Design by Lisa Million

Clinical Gynecologic Endocrinology and Infertility

SELF ASSESSMENT AND STUDY GUIDE

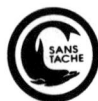

Editor: Charles W. Mitchell
Managing Editor: Marjorie Kidd Keating

Copyright © 1995
Williams & Wilkins
428 East Preston Street
Baltimore, Maryland 21202, USA

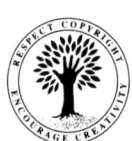

All rights reserved. This book is protected by copyright. No part of this book may be reproduced in any form or by any means including photocopying, or utilized by any information storage and retrieval system without written permission from the copyright owner.

Accurate indications, adverse reactions, and dosage schedules for drugs are provided in this book, but it is possible that they may change. The reader is urged to review the package information data of the manufacturers of the medications mentioned.

Printed in the United States of America

ISBN: 0-683-07901-8

95 96 97 98 99
1 2 3 4 5 6 7 8 9 10

How To Use This Study Guide

The purpose of this study guide is to help you assess and organize the knowledge you gain from reading the Fifth Edition of *Clinical Gynecologic Endocrinology and Infertility*. We have formulated this study guide so that each chapter can serve as your own private tutorial.

Learning objectives are presented at the beginning of each chapter to highlight critical concepts in the textbook *Clinical Gynecologic Endocrinology and Infertility*.

Each chapter contains a short section of pre-study questions (the pre-test). Results with these questions can be compared to results achieved in the larger section of post-study questions (the post-test). We recommend that the post-test section be completed after careful reading of the textbook by Speroff, Glass, and Kase. The answer to each question is linked to a page number, designating the location of the answer in *Clinical Gynecologic Endocrinology and Infertility*.

We hope this study guide makes your learning more effective and enjoyable.

David B. Seifer, M.D.
Providence, Rhode Island

Leon Speroff, M.D.
Portland, Oregon

Contents

How to Use This Study Guide	v
Chapter 1: Molecular Biology for Clinicians	1
Chapter 2: Hormone Biosynthesis, Metabolism, and Mechanism of Action	11
Chapter 3: The Ovary — Embryology and Development	33
Chapter 4: The Uterus	43
Chapter 5: Neuroendocrinology	57
Chapter 6: Regulation of the Menstrual Cycle	77
Chapter 7: Sperm and Egg Transport, Fertilization, and Implantation	97
Chapter 8: The Endocrinology of Pregnancy	107
Chapter 9: Prostaglandins	121
Chapter 10: Normal and Abnormal Sexual Development	131
Chapter 11: Abnormal Puberty and Growth Problems	153
Chapter 12: Amenorrhea	169
Chapter 13: Anovulation and the Polycystic Ovary	187
Chapter 14: Hirsutism	199
Chapter 15: Menstrual Disorders	215
Chapter 16: Dysfunctional Uterine Bleeding	225
Chapter 17: The Breast	235
Chapter 18: Menopause and Postmenopausal Hormone Therapy	247
Chapter 19: Obesity	267
Chapter 20: Reproduction and the Thyroid	277
Chapter 21: Use of Contraception, Sterilization, and Abortion	291
Chapter 22: Oral Contraception	309
Chapter 23: Long-acting Methods of Contraception	325
Chapter 24: The Intrauterine Device (IUD)	335

Chapter 25: Barrier Methods of Contraception	345
Chapter 26: Female Infertility	353
Chapter 27: Recurrent Early Pregnancy Losses	365
Chapter 28: Endometriosis	373
Chapter 29: Male Infertility	387
Chapter 30: Induction of Ovulation	399
Chapter 31: Assisted Reproduction	413
Chapter 32: Ectopic Pregnancy	423
Chapter 33: Clinical Assays	433

1 Molecular Biology for Clinicians

GCAGCCGTATTTCTACTGCGACGAGGAG
GAGAACTT**SPEROFF**CTACCAGCAGCAG
AGCGAGCTGGC**GLASS**AGCCCCGGCGC
CCAGGGATATCTGGAA**KASE**GAAATTCGA
GCTGCTGCCGCCCTGTCCCTAGCCGCG

Learning Objectives

Be able to:

1. Define the basic vocabulary of molecular biology.

2. Discuss the similarities and differences between the techniques of Southern, Northern and Western blot analysis.

3. Understand the principles of polymerase chain reaction, restriction fragment length polymorphisms, cloning.

Pre-Test

A. Instructions: Fill in the blanks

1. The centromere divides the chromosome into two portions, the shorter portion is called the _____ arm and the longer portion is called the _____ arm.

2. RNA differs from DNA, in that it is _____ stranded. Its sugar moiety is _____ and it substitutes _____ for thymine.

B. Instructions: True or False

3. Translation is the synthesis of single-stranded messenger RNA from a double-stranded DNA.

4. c-DNA is the DNA counterpart of all of the messenger RNA isolated from a particular cell or tissue made using reverse transcriptase.

C. Instructions: For the following question choose:

A. if only 1, 2 and 3 are correct
B. if only 1 and 3 are correct
C. if only 2 and 4 are correct
D. if only 4 is correct
E. if all are correct

5. Polymerase chain reaction (PCR)
    1. requires five components which include: a DNA template, oligonucleotide primers, free nucleotides, buffer and Taq polymerase.
    2. may be performed by automatic machinery
    3. can amplify minute amounts of DNA from a single cell
    4. can be useful in prenatal genetic analysis and in preimplantation sexing and diagnosis

Post-Test

A. Instructions: Fill in the blanks

1. Name the technique of transferring DNA from agarose gels onto nitrocellulose filters for the purpose of enabling DNA fragments to be joined with radiolabeled RNA probes: _____.

2. All human somatic cells are _____. There are _____ pairs of autosomes and one pair of sex chromosomes.

3. Only gametes are _____ with 22 autosome chromosomes and _____ sex chromosome.

4. The process of nuclear division in all somatic cells is called _____.

5. _____ is the cell division that forms gametes each with a haploid number of chromosomes.

6. Meiosis has _____ stages and results in the production of _____ haploid cells.

7. In the oocyte, meiosis I is completed after _____ while meiosis II is completed after _____.

8. A gene is composed of a segment of DNA containing the coding codons of nucleotides called _____ and noncoding codons of nucleotides called _____.

B. Instructions: True or False

9. An intron is a segment of a gene that yields a messenger RNA product that codes for a specific product.

10. The enhancer region is the actual area where transcription begins.

11. A few relatively short nucleotide sequences such as the TATA box or CAT box are promoters.

12. Gene expression is composed of transcription of DNA to RNA, RNA processing to produce functional messenger RNA by splicing out extrons, translation of messenger RNA on a ribosome to a peptide chain and protein structural processing to the functioning form.

13. Examples of postranslational processing of proteins include glycosylation of follicle-stimulating hormone and proteolytic cleavage of proopiomelamocortin to ACTH.

14. Southern blot analysis involves denaturing DNA, digestion with restriction enzymes, electrophoresis, transferring from a gel to a membrane and hybridization using specific radiolabeled probes.

15. Western blotting involves electrophoresis to separate codons.

16. In situ hybridization is a technique where DNA or RNA probes are placed directly on a slide of tissue or cells to identify the presence and location of transcript or protein.

17. Polymerase chain reaction (PCR) involves denaturing a single double-stranded DNA followed by annealing primers to its complementary regions then synthesizing a new strand resulting in two new double-stranded DNA.

18. c-DNA contains introns and exons of a gene.

C. Instructions: Match each item with the most appropriate word association

A. Western blot
B. Dot blot
C. PCR
D. RFLP
E. Northern blot
F. Clone
G. Southern blot
H. c-DNA

19. hybridization without electrophoresis
20. hybridization with electrophoresis of RNA
21. DNA primers
22. synthesized from a m-RNA template
23. genetically identical cells
24. hybridization with electrophoresis of proteins

D. Instructions: For each of the following questions choose:

    A. if only 1, 2 and 3 are correct
    B. if only 1 and 3 are correct
    C. if only 2 and 4 are correct
    D. if only 4 is correct
    E. if all are correct

25. Cloning
    1. can be accomplished using a variety of approaches
    2. may involve introducing fragments of DNA into vectors
    3. can use either genomic or complementary DNA
    4. is isolating a gene and making a copy of it

26. Restriction fragment length polymorphisms (RFLPs):
    1. are detectable by Southern blot
    2. are produced by restriction endonucleases
    3. are linked to the disease of interest by chance
    4. are usually deleterious mutations

27. Congenital adrenal hyperplasia
    1. is a sex linked recessive disorder
    2. is a disorder resulting from the absence of an enzyme required for ovarian steroidogenesis
    3. most commonly involves 11-hydroxylase
    4. involves the structural gene for cytochrome P450c 21-hydroxylase located on the short arm of chromosome 6

28. Examples of production of hormones using recombinant technology include
    1. insulin
    2. growth hormone
    3. LH
    4. FSH

29. Transgenic animals
    1. provide models for the study of inherited diseases and tumors
    2. provide a means to carry out experiments in gene therapy
    3. can result from the insertion of a foreign gene into an embryo
    4. can not reproduce

Answers for Chapter 1 — Pre-Test Questions

1. p; q   p.4
The chromosomes vary in size, and all contain a pinched portion called a centromere, which divides the chromosome into two arms, the shorter p arm and the longer q arm.

2. single; ribose; uracil   p.7
DNA consists of two deoxyribose strands in a double helix with the nucleic acids on the inside and the nuclear bases paired by hydrogen bonding, adenine with thymine and cytosine with guanine. RNA differs from DNA in that it is single stranded, its sugar moiety is ribose, and it substitutes uracil for thymine.

3. false   p.13
Transcription is the synthesis of single-stranded messenger RNA from a gene (double-stranded DNA).

4. true   p.22
Complementary DNA cloning focuses on the DNA counterpart of messenger RNA; genomic DNA cloning, using a restriction endonuclease, copies the DNA in genes. Cloning can be also used to make multiple copies of probes or unknown DNA fragments.

5. E   p.21,26
Because the polymerase chain reaction requires alternate heating and cooling, a DNA polymerase resistant to heat is an advantage in that periodic replenishment is not necessary. This problem was solved with the discovery of DNA polymerase (Taq polymerase) in a microorganism (*Thermus aquaticus*) that lives in hot springs and was found in Yellowstone National Park geysers. This high temperature polymerase allows automation of the process.

The technique of polymerase chain reaction has made possible the study of incredibly small amounts of DNA. Most impressive is the amplification of small amounts of degraded DNA from extinct and rare species preserved in museums. DNA from fossils has been amplified and sequenced (e.g., from an 18 million-year-old magnolia plant).

Polymerase chain reaction carried out by automatic machinery allows speedy DNA diagnosis with material amplified from a single cell. This is an important advantage in prenatal genetic analysis and in preimplantation sexing and diagnosis. PCR makes it possible to perform DNA diagnosis from a single cell removed from embryos fertilized in vitro.

Answers to Chapter 1 — Post-Test Questions

1. Southern blot   p.3,19
E.M. Southern of Edinburgh University developed in 1975 the technique to transfer (to blot) DNA from agarose gels onto nitrocellulose filters, enabling DNA fragments to be joined with radiolabeled RNA probes and thus isolated. DNA is first denatured to separate the two strands, then digested by restriction enzymes to produce smaller fragments. The Southern blot method, named after E.M. Southern, determines the fragment sizes. The fragments are separated by electrophoresis. The electrophoresis gel is placed over a thick piece of filter paper with its ends dipped in a high salt solution. A special membrane (nitrocellulose) is placed over the gel and over this is placed a stack of paper towels compressed by a weight. The salt solution rises by wick action into the filter paper; it moves by capillary action through the gel carrying the DNA with it. The DNA is carried to the nitrocellulose membrane to which it binds. The salt solution keeps moving and is absorbed by the paper towels. The nitrocellulose membrane thus creates a replica of the original electrophoresis pattern. The DNA is fixed to the membrane either by high temperature baking or by ultraviolet light. Specific labeled probes than can be introduced for hybridization. **Hybridization** means that a specific probe anneals to its complementary sequence. The fragments with this sequence are then identified by autoradiography.

2. diploid; 22   p.4
Chromosomes are packages of genetic material, consisting of a DNA molecule (which contains many genes) to which are attached large numbers of proteins that maintain chromosome structure and play a role in gene expression. All somatic cells are diploid — 23 pairs of chromosomes.

3. haploid; one   p.4
Human somatic cells contain 46 chromosomes, 22 pairs of autosomes and one pair of sex chromosomes. Only gametes are haploid with 22 autosome chromosomes and one sex chromosome. The two members of any pair of autosomes are homologous, one homologue derived from each parent.

4. mitosis   p.5
All eukaryotes, from yeast to humans, undergo similar cell division and multiplication. The process of nuclear division

in all somatic cells is called mitosis, during which each chromosome divides into two. For normal growth and development, the entire genomic information must be faithfully reproduced in every cell.

5. Meiosis   p.5
Meiosis is the cell division that forms the gametes, each with a haploid number of chromosomes. Meiosis has two purposes: reduction of the chromosome number and recombination to transmit genetic information.

6. two; four   p.5,6
In meiosis I, homologous chromosomes pair and split apart. Meiosis II is similar to mitosis as the already divided chromosomes split and segregate into new cells. The second division follows the first without DNA replication. The end result is the production of 4 haploid cells.

7. ovulation; fertilization   p.6
In the oocyte, meiosis I occurs after ovulation and meiosis II occurs after fertilization. (See figure on page 7 in this Study Guide)

8. exons; introns   p.11
Exon. The segment of a gene that yields a messenger RNA product that codes for a specific protein.
Intron. The segment of a gene not represented in mature RNA and, therefore, noncoding for protein.

9. false   p.12
The introns are not translated into protein products. Only the DNA sequences in the exons (the part that "exits" the nucleus) are transcribed into messenger RNA and then translated into proteins.

10. false   p.12
The area that will initiate DNA action (e.g., DNA binding to the hormone-receptor complex) is called an ***enhancer*** region.

11. true   p.12
The actual area where transcription begins is the ***promoter*** region. Only a few relatively short nucleotide sequences are promoters, such as the T-A-T-A-A sequence, or TATA box, and the C-C-A-A-T sequence, or CAT box. The promoter sites are usually near the start of the coding region of the gene.

12. false   p.13
Gene expression is composed of the following steps: transcription of DNA to RNA, RNA processing to produce functional messenger RNA by splicing out introns, translation of messenger RNA on a ribosome to a peptide chain, and protein structural processing to the functional form. (See figure on page 8 in this Study Guide)

13. true   p.15
The final expression of a gene may not end with the translation process. Further (posttranslational) processing of proteins occurs, such as glycosylation (the gonadotropins) or proteolytic cleavage (conversion of proopiomelanocortin to ACTH).

14. true   p.19
DNA is first denatured to separate the two strands, then digested by restriction enzymes to produce smaller fragments. The Southern blot method, named after E.M. Southern, determines the fragment sizes.

15. false   p.19
Electrophoresis to separate proteins is called ***Western blotting,*** and antibodies are used for the hybridization identification process. Like Northern blotting, Western blotting tests gene expression, not just the presence of a gene.

16. true   p.20
In situ hybridization is the technique where labeled DNA or RNA probes are placed directly on a slide of tissue or cells.

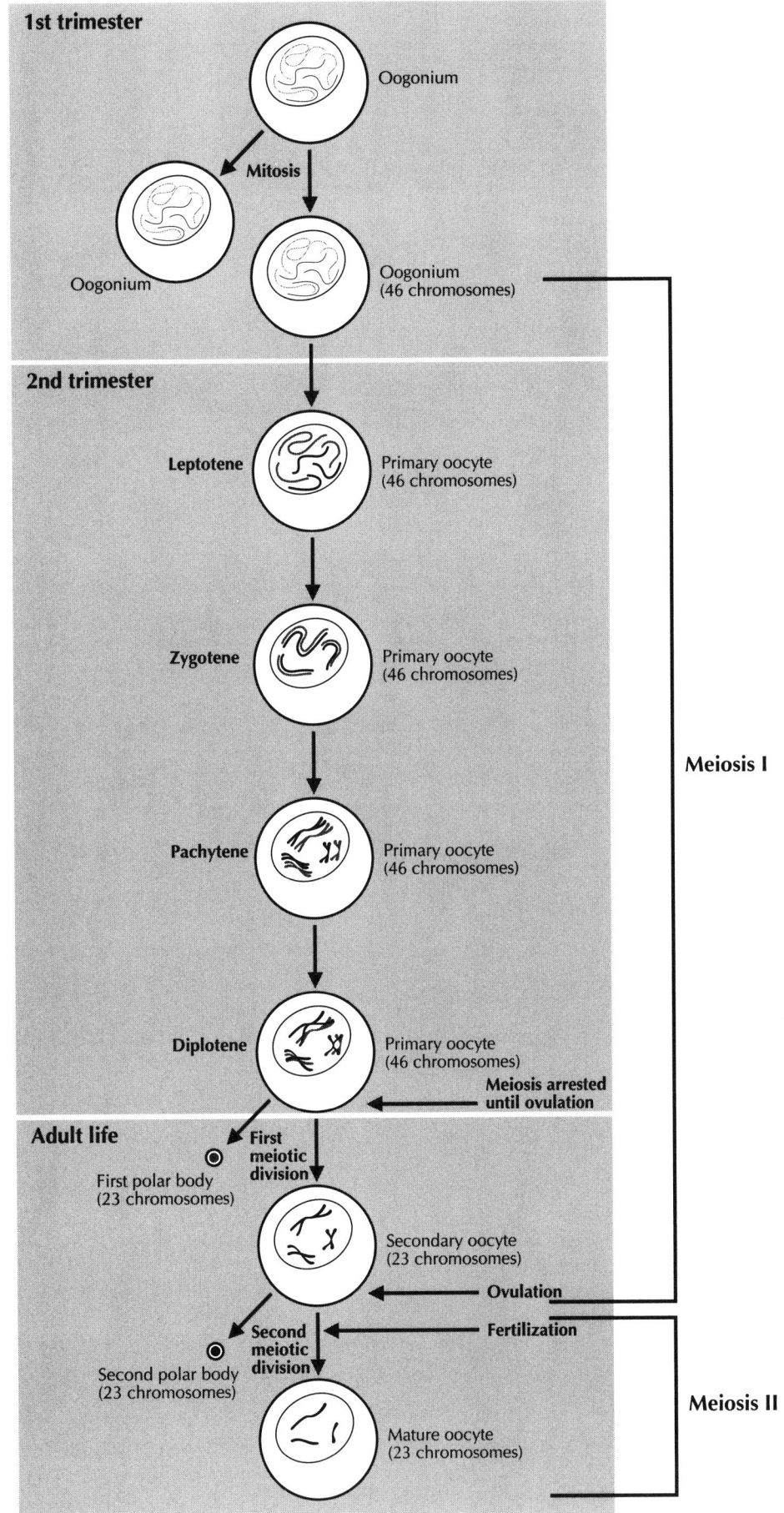

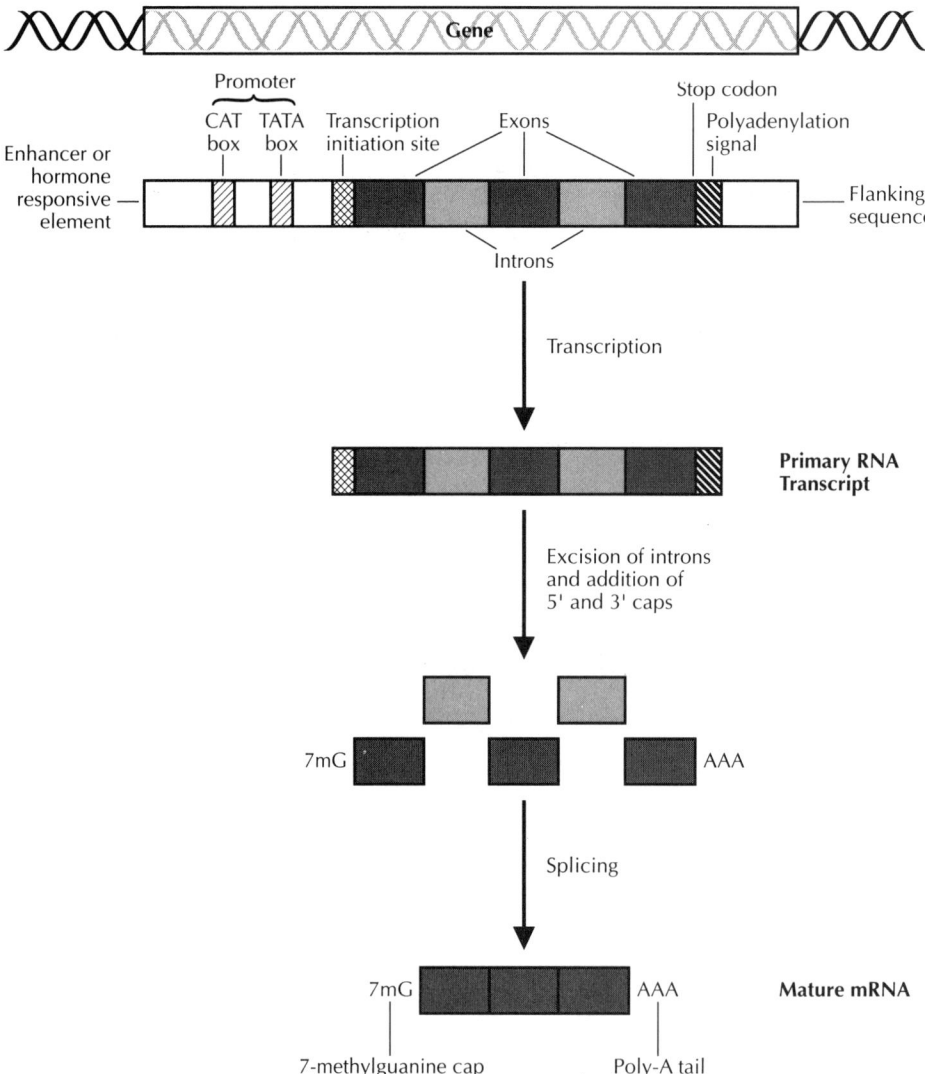

17. true   p.21

The polymerase chain reaction (PCR) is a technique to amplify (relatively quickly) small fragments or areas of DNA into quantities large enough to be analyzed with electrophoresis and blotting methods. This technique produces enormous numbers of copies of a specific DNA sequence without resorting to cloning. The sequence to be amplified must be known. Specific markers (synthesized short sequences of DNA corresponding to each end of the sequence to be studied) are selected that will delineate the region of DNA to be amplified. These flanking sequences are called primers. The DNA sample, the primers, and an excess of free single nucleotides are incubated with a DNA polymerase.

The first step involves separating DNA into its single strands by denaturation with heat (92°C), then the temperature is lowered (40°C), causing the primers to stick (anneal) to their complementary regions on the DNA. The temperature is raised to 62°C, and DNA polymerase then synthesizes a new strand beginning and ending at the primers, forming a new double-stranded DNA. Repeating the cycle many times (by alternating the reaction temperature) amplifies the amount of DNA available for study (more than 1 million-fold); the increase occurs exponentially. Thus, DNA can be analyzed from a single cell, and genes can be visualized by blotting without labeled probes.

18. false   p.22
Complementary DNA only includes the exons of a gene.

19. B p.19

Hybridization without electrophoresis by placing a drop of the cell extract directly on filter paper is called ***dot or slot blotting.***

20. E p.19

Northern blotting refers to RNA processing, Northern because RNA is the opposite image of DNA. Extracted RNA is separated by electrophoresis and transferred to a cellulose membrane as in Southern blotting for hybridization with probes (complementary DNA). Northern blotting would be used, for example, to determine whether hormone stimulation of a specific protein in a tissue is mediated by messenger RNA, i.e., gene expression.

21. C p.21

The polymerase chain reaction (PCR) is a technique to amplify (relatively quickly) small fragments or areas of DNA into quantities large enough to be analyzed with electrophoresis and blotting methods. This technique produces enormous numbers of copies of a specific DNA sequence without resorting to cloning. The sequence to be amplified must be known. Specific markers (synthesized short sequences of DNA corresponding to each end of the sequence to be studied) are selected that will delineate the region of DNA to be amplified. These flanking sequences are called primers. The DNA sample, the primers, and an excess of free single nucleotides are incubated with a DNA polymerase.

22. H p.22

A complementary DNA library is the DNA counterpart of all of the messenger RNA isolated from a particular cell or tissue. By starting with messenger RNA, the search for the gene of interest can be focused (instead of searching the entire genome). Such a library is made using reverse transcriptase. The DNA molecules then can be inserted into an appropriate vector (described below) and replicate molecules can be produced. Using probes, the complementary DNA can be selected that matches the gene of interest (keeping in mind that complementary DNA only includes the exons of a gene).

23. F p.22

Cloning means isolating a gene and making copies of it. A DNA library is a collection of DNA molecules derived from cloning methods.

24. A p.19

Electrophoresis to separate proteins is called ***Western blotting,*** and antibodies are used for the hybridization identification process. Like Northern blotting, Western blotting tests gene expression, not just the presence of a gene.

25. E p.22

Cloning the DNA simply means the production of many identical copies of a specified fragment of DNA. Cloning can also be performed using the polymerase chain reaction. Complementary DNA cloning focuses on the DNA counterpart of messenger RNA; genomic DNA cloning, using a restriction endonuclease, copies the DNA in genes. Cloning can be also used to make multiple copies of probes or unknown DNA fragments.

26. A p.25

Southern blotting reveals specific patterns of bands that reflect the varying lengths of the DNA fragments produced by restriction enzyme action. A specific site can exhibit a mutation by having a different pattern (a different length of the DNA fragment on Southern blotting). This is called a restriction fragment length polymorphism (RFLP), usually a benign variation. A polymorphism will be governed by the mendelian regulations of inheritance, and if by chance, a polymorphism is identified in a patient with a specific disease, the transmission of the disease can be studied. The RFLP, which is linked to the disease by chance, can be used to study the inheritance of a disease when the genes are unknown. This method of study requires DNA from at least one affected individual and a sufficient number of family members to trace the length polymorphism.

27. D p.26

Congenital adrenal hyperplasia is an autosomal recessive disorder with a deficiency in an enzyme necessary for adrenal steroidogenesis, most commonly the 21-hydroxylase enzyme. The 21-hydroxylase gene has been localized to the short arm of chromosome 6. Molecular analysis indicates that the genetic defect involves the structural gene for cytochrome P450c21-hydroxylase.

28. E   p.26

The commercial production of proteins from cloned genes inserted into bacteria is rapidly increasing. The production of insulin (the first) and growth hormone is a good example. Glycosylation does not occur in bacterial systems, and therefore the commercial production of recombinant glycoproteins requires a mammalian cell line for the process. This has been accomplished, and recombinant gonadotropins are now available.

29. A   p.27

Insertion of a foreign gene into an embryo results in a transgenic animal. The inserted foreign gene will be present in many tissues, and if the animal is fertile, it will be inherited. There are many applications for transgenic animals. Transgenic animals provide animal models for inherited diseases and malignant tumors and provide a means to carry out experiments in gene therapy. The transfer of new or altered genes is an important method to study gene function. Transgenic plants can even be developed to produce new pharmaceuticals, and the introduction of genes conferring resistance to insects may solve the problem of insecticide contamination.

2 Hormone Biosynthesis, Metabolism and Mechanism of Action

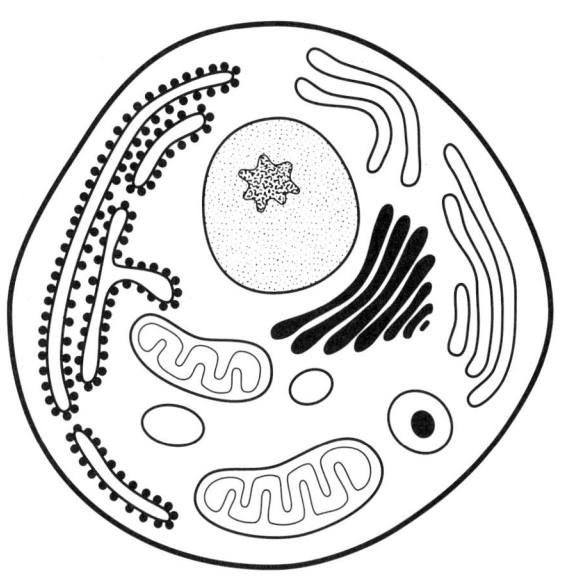

Learning Objectives

Be able to:

1. Define the differences in paracrine, autocrine, intracrine and endocrine functions.

2. Describe the synthesis, metabolism and mechanism of action of the sex steroids.

3. Understand the differences between the mechanism of action for steroids and tropic hormones.

4. Explain the regulation of tropic hormones, autocrine and paracrine factors.

5. Describe examples of hormonal agonists and antagonists, their mechanisms of action and their potential therapeutic use.

Pre-Test

A. Instructions: Fill in the blanks

1. All steroid-producing organs except the _____ can synthesize cholesterol from _____.

2. The ovary is distinguished from the adrenal gland in that it is deficient in _____ and _____ enzymes. Thus, glucocorticoids and mineralocorticoids are not produced in normal ovarian tissue.

B. Instructions: True or False

3. There are two human P450c21 genes located on chromosome 6p which include the active A gene and the inactive B gene.

4. Some of the major sex steroids in the female are secreted in a circadian cycle.

C. Instructions: For each of the following questions choose:

A. if only 1, 2 and 3 are correct
B. if only 1 and 3 are correct
C. if only 2 and 4 are correct
D. if only 4 is correct
E. if all are correct

5. The mechanism of action for steroid hormones
   1. requires the presence of intracellular receptor proteins
   2. involves c-AMP
   3. involves binding of the hormone with its protein within the nucleus
   4. is identical to the mechanism of action for glucocorticoids and mineralocorticoids

6. Cyclic AMP (c-AMP)
   1. is the intracellular messenger for FSH, LH, HCG, TSH and ACTH
   2. is produced by the action of adenylate cyclase upon ATP
   3. activates protein kinase
   4. is degraded by phosphodiesterase into 5' AMP

7. The biological activity of polypeptide or glycoprotein hormones can be altered by
   1. the heterogeneity of the molecules
   2. the up- or down-regulation of the receptors
   3. modulation of adenylate cyclase
   4. the serum concentrations of SHBG

Post-Test

A. Instructions: Match each item with the most appropriate word or phrase

A. Endocrine
B. Autocrine
C. Paracrine
D. Intracrine
E. Cyclic AMP
F. Adenylate cyclase

1. Intercellular communication involving local diffusion of regulating substances from a cell to contiguous cells.
2. Intracellular communication which occurs when unsecreted substances bind to intracellular receptors.
3. Intracellular communication where a single cell produces regulating substances that in turn act upon receptors on or within the same cell.
4. Communication by substances produced by a gland which act at distant sites.
5. Enzyme in the cell membrane.
6. A second messenger.

B. Instructions: Fill in the blanks

7. The job of the _____ is to aid in the transmission of the hormone's message to nuclear gene transcription.

8. The 21-carbon steroids include the _____ and the _____.

9. The 19-carbon steroids include the _____.

10. The 18-carbon steroids include the _____.

11. Label each carbon as numbered in the cholesterol molecule.

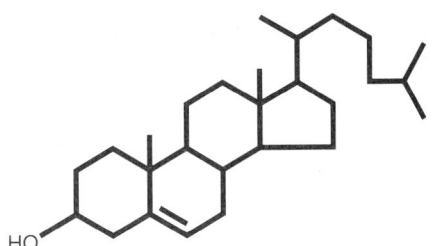

12. _____ is the basic building block in steroidogenesis.

13. The _____ are a major reason for the disparity in atherosclerosis risk between men and women. _____ and _____-cholesterol levels are lower in premenopausal women than in men, but after menopause they rise rapidly.

14. _____ can remove cholesterol by delivering cholesterol to sites for utilization (steroid-producing cells) or metabolism and excretion (liver).

15. Atherosclerotic disease is related to increased _____ and decreased _____ cholesterol concentrations. Lowering _____ levels and raising _____ levels can reduce the incidence of atherosclerotic disease.

C. Instructions: True or False

16. During steroidogenesis the number of carbon atoms in cholesterol or any other steroid molecule can be either increased or reduced.

17. Cytochrome P450 is a generic term for a family of oxidative enzymes, termed 450 because of a pigment (450) absorbance shift when reduced.

18. Cholesterol side chain cleavage enzyme (P450 scc) is a rate-limiting step in the steroid pathway.

19. The two cell system explains the sequence of events in ovarian follicular growth and adrenal steroidogenesis.

20. Insulin-like growth factor I (IGF-I) and transforming growth factors are produced by the granulosa and theca cells.

21. Sex hormone binding globulin (SHBG) concentration may be a marker for hyperinsulinemic insulin resistance.

22. The adrenal gland is the major source of circulating androgens (especially androstenedione) in the female.

23. The major androgen products of the ovary are dehydroepiandrosterone (DHA) and androstenedione which are secreted by stromal tissue derived from theca cells.

24. In the process of masculine differentiation, the development of the wolffian duct structures are dependent upon testosterone as the intracellular mediator in contrast to development of the urogenital sinus and urogenital tubercle which require DHT.

D. Instructions: For each of the following questions choose:

A. if only 1, 2 and 3 are correct
B. if only 1 and 3 are correct
C. if only 2 and 4 are correct
D. if only 4 is correct
E. if all are correct

25. Steroidogenesis
    1. c-AMP is responsible for its initiation
    2. requires cholesterol
    3. involves enzymes which are members of the cytochrome P450 group of oxidases
    4. may involve the following reactions: desmolase, dehydrogenase, hydroxylation and/or saturation

26. The cytochrome P450 group of oxidases
    1. includes a distinct number of enzymes which are essential for steroidogenesis
    2. includes aromatase, 21 hydroxylase, 11 hydroxylase, 17 hydroxylase, cholesterol side chain cleavage enzyme
    3. resides in the mitochondria or endoplasmic reticulum
    4. includes 5α-reductase

27. Aromatization
    1. is mediated by P450arom found in the mitochondria
    2. can take place in other cells in addition to granulosa and adipose cells
    3. is unaffected by the influence of growth factors, glucocorticoids and gonadotropins
    4. if blocked would result in lower levels of estrogen production

28. The two-cell, two-gonadotropin theory of the control of steroidogenesis
    1. is the current operational paradigm explaining ovarian follicular steroidogenesis
    2. states that granulosa cells must depend on theca cells to provide androgen precursors, as granulosa do not express P450c17 alpha hydroxylase
    3. states that the rate of aromatization in the granulosa layer is directly related to the androgen substrate made available by the theca cells
    4. states that LH receptors may be present on both granulosa and theca cells but FSH receptors are present only on granulosa cells.

29. Inhibin
    1. is composed of alpha and beta subunits composing a dimeric molecule
    2. is produced in the granulosa in response to FSH
    3. enhances LH stimulation of androgen synthesis in the theca cells
    4. is present in both ovarian and testicular tissues

30. Sex hormone binding globulin (SHBG)
    1. is the principal protein carrier of sex hormones
    2. is increased by hyperthyroidism, pregnancy, estrogen administration
    3. is decreased by corticoids, androgens, progestins and growth hormone
    4. concentrations are directly related to weight

31. The process of "replenishment"
    1. refers to a hormone increasing the concentration of its own receptor
    2. results in a hormone increasing target tissue responsiveness to itself
    3. is an important action of estrogen
    4. is activated by small amounts of receptor depletion

32. The steroid hormone receptor
    1. contains three domains which include the regulatory domain, the DNA-binding domain and the hormone-binding domain
    2. shares a common structure with the receptors for thyroid hormone and retinoic acid
    3. contains a hinge region
    4. is located in the cytoplasm of the target cell

33. The DNA-binding domain of the steroid receptor
    1. is not essential for activation of transcription
    2. is very similar for the thyroid receptor
    3. does not undergo a conformational change when hormone binding occurs
    4. is specific for the hormone responsive element in the gene promotor

34. The progesterone receptor
    1. is induced by estrogens at the transcriptional level
    2. is decreased by progestins at both the transcriptional and translational levels
    3. is influenced by estrogen by means of an estrogen responsive element
    4. exists as two forms

35. The androgen receptor
    1. is localized on the human X chromosome
    2. can be activated by testosterone or DHT
    3. is congenitally abnormal in the case of testicular feminization
    4. can be induced by estrogens

36. The major intracellular messenger molecules involved in the mechanism of action for tropic hormones include:
    1. c-AMP
    2. inositol 1,4,5-triphosphate (IP_3)
    3. c-GMP
    4. 1,2-diacylglycerol (1,2-DG)

37. Gonadotropin releasing hormone (GnRH)
    1. is calcium dependent in its mechanism of action
    2. utilizes IP_3 and 1,2-DG as second messengers
    3. mechanism of action involves a G protein
    4. utilizes adenylate cyclase

38. The calcium messenger system
    1. is a regulator of cyclic AMP and cyclic GMP
    2. results in a calcium flux via ionic channels
    3. is linked to hormone-receptor function by phospholipase C
    4. involves IP_3 and 1,2-DG

39. Tyrosine kinase receptors
    1. are located within the cell membrane
    2. all have a similar structure
    3. are the receptors for insulin, IGF-I, EGF
    4. are the receptors for activin and inhibin

40. Growth factors
    1. are polypeptides that act as autocrine and paracrine regulators
    2. are involved in mitogenesis, cellular differentiation and angiogenesis
    3. can operate in a cooperative or competitive fashion with other hormones
    4. such as inhibin, activin and antimullerian substance belong to the transforming growth factor-beta family.

41. Transforming growth factor-beta (TGF-ß)
    1. can either stimulate or inhibit growth and differentiation depending upon the target tissue and the company of other growth factors
    2. is a structural analog of epidermal growth factor (EGF)
    3. promotes granulosa cell differentiation by enhancing the actions of FSH and antagonizing the down-regulation of FSH receptors
    4. is not secreted by theca cells

42. Insulin-like growth factor-I (IGF-I)
    1. is a single chain polypeptide resembling insulin in structure and function
    2. is produced in greater amounts in the liver than the ovary
    3. amplifies the action of gonadotropins and coordinates the functions of theca and granulosa cells
    4. binds with circulating insulin-like growth factor binding proteins (IGFBPs)

43. Glycoproteins
    1. include interleukin-I and tumor necrosis factor
    2. consists of a family of heterogeneous forms (isoforms) of varying immunologic and biologic activity
    3. are secreted as 2–3 isoforms of both FSH and LH throughout the menstrual cycle
    4. specific biologic activity is determined by the beta-subunit and not the alpha-subunit

44. The HCG beta-subunit
    1. contains a unique carboxyl terminal tail piece of 24 amino acid groups
    2. contains a hormone response element
    3. contains 4 sites of glycosylation
    4. does not contain sialic acid

45. The half-life of
    1. whole HCG is approximately 12 hours
    2. LH is 20 mins
    3. FSH is 3–4 hours
    4. glycoproteins are heavily influenced by the presence of sialic acid

46. The isoform mixture of glycopeptides
    1. differ in their amino acid make-up
    2. can be found in the pituitary
    3. does not influence biological activity of glycopeptides
    4. is influenced both quantitatively and qualitatively by GnRH and steroid hormones

47. The heterogeneity of prolactin
    1. has little physiologic importance
    2. is due to size and structural modifications of the prolactin molecule
    3. does not explain discrepancies between prolactin bioassay and immunoassay results
    4. may explain the clinical situation of a "normal" prolactin level in a woman with galactorrhea

48. G proteins (GTP binding proteins)
    1. are critical to the functioning of adenylate cyclase
    2. are composed of alpha, beta and gama subunits, each the product of a distinct gene
    3. can be either stimulatory or inhibitory
    4. are hydrolyzed by GTPase resulting in their deactivation

49. Mutations that alter the structure and activity of G proteins
    1. are found in most adrenal and ovarian tumors
    2. can result in growth hormone-secreting pituitary tumors
    3. are of little physiologic consequence
    4. can be responsible for the McCune-Albright syndrome

50. Down-regulation
    1. is a decrease in response in the presence of continuous stimulation
    2. involves loss of unoccupied receptors by decreasing replenishment
    3. involves uncoupling of receptor binding from target cell release
    4. is an acute, rapid event

51. GnRH
    1. when altered can result in an agonist or an antagonist
    2. antagonists result from substitutions at the 6 or 10 position
    3. agonists initially stimulate then down-regulate and desensitize gonadotropin receptors
    4. agonists result from substitutions at multiple positions of the decapeptide

52. Progestins
    1. modifies estrogen action by depleting estrogen receptors
    2. convert estradiol to estrone sulfate
    3. inhibit transcription activation by the estrogen receptor
    4. bind to the androgen receptor

53. Tamoxifen
    1. has mixed agonist and antagonist bioactivity
    2. given as 20 mg daily is as potent as 2 mg of estradiol in lowering FSH levels in postmenopausal women
    3. has estrogenic actions upon the bone, vaginal mucosa and endometrium
    4. decreases antithrombin III, cholesterol, LDL cholesterol

54. RU486
    1. is a 19-nortestosterone derivative
    2. the dimethyl side chain at carbon 11 is the principal factor in its antiprogesterone action
    3. if given in large amounts can bind the glucocorticoid receptor
    4. may be useful for Cushing's syndrome and meningioma

Answers for Chapter 2 — Pre-Test Questions

1. placenta; acetate   p.37
Cholesterol is the basic building block in steroidogenesis. All steroid-producing organs except the placenta can synthesize cholesterol from acetate. Progestins, androgens, and estrogens, therefore, can be synthesized in situ in the various ovarian tissue compartments from the 2-carbon acetate molecule via cholesterol as the common steroid precursor. However, in situ synthesis cannot meet the demand, and therefore the major resource is blood cholesterol which enters the ovarian cells and can be inserted into the biosynthetic pathway or stored in esterified form for later use. The cellular entry of cholesterol is mediated via a cell membrane receptor for low-density lipoprotein (LDL), the bloodstream carrier for cholesterol.

2. 21-hydroxylase and 11β-hydroxylase   p.39
The ovary is distinguished from the adrenal gland in that it is deficient in 21-hydroxylase and 11β-hydroxylase reactions. Glucocorticoids and mineralocorticoids, therefore, are not produced in normal ovarian tissue.

3. false   p.42
Characterization of the P450c21 protein and gene cloning indicate that there is only one 21-hydroxylase enzyme, the P450c21 in the smooth endoplasmic reticulum. Two human P450c21 genes (the A and B genes) have been cloned (on chromosome 6p), and the evidence indicates that only one (the B gene) is active. The molecular genetics of 21-hydroxylase deficiency indicate that the syndrome can be due to gene conversions of material in the active B gene to resemble material in the inactive A gene, as well as deletions in the P450c21B gene. A conversion is similar to a cross-over in genetic effect. However, rather than appearing as a deletion or addition, the gene changes, but the number of gene copies does not change.

4. false   p.49
There is no circadian cycle of the major sex steroids in the female. However, short-term variations in the blood levels due to episodic secretion require multiple sampling for absolutely accurate assessment. *Although frequent sampling is necessary for a high degree of accuracy, a random sample is sufficient for clinical purposes to determine whether a level is within a normal range.*

5. B   p.52
The specificity of the reaction of tissues to sex steroid hormones is due to the presence of intracellular receptor proteins. Different types of tissues, such as liver, kidney, and uterus, respond in a similar manner. The mechanism includes: 1)

diffusion across the cell membrane, 2) transfer across the nuclear membrane to the nucleus and binding to receptor protein, 3) interaction of a hormone-receptor complex with nuclear DNA, 4) synthesis of messenger RNA (mRNA), 5) transport of the mRNA to the ribosomes, and finally, 6) protein synthesis in the cytoplasm that results in specific cellular activity. Each of the major classes of the sex steroid hormones, including estrogens, progestins, and androgens, has been demonstrated to act according to this general mechanism. Glucocorticoid and mineralocorticoid receptors, when in the unbound state, reside in the cytoplasm and move into the nucleus after hormone-receptor binding.

6. E   p.62

Cyclic AMP is the intracellular messenger for FSH, LH, human chorionic gonadotropin (HCG), thyroid-stimulating hormone (TSH), and ACTH. Union of a tropic hormone with its cell membrane receptor activates the adenylate cyclase enzyme within the membrane wall leading to the conversion of adenosine 5'-triphosphate (ATP) within the cell to cyclic AMP. Specificity of action and/or intensity of stimulation can be altered by changes in the structure or concentration of the receptor at the cell wall binding site. In addition to changes in biologic activity due to target cell alterations, changes in the molecular structure of the tropic hormone can interfere with cellular binding and physiologic activity.

The cell's mechanism for sensing the low concentrations of circulating tropic hormone is to have an extremely large number of receptors but to require only a very small percentage (as little as 1%) to be occupied by the tropic hormone. The cyclic AMP released is specifically bound to a cytoplasm receptor protein, and this cyclic AMP-receptor protein complex activates a protein kinase. The protein kinase is thought to be present in an inactive form as a tetramer containing 2 regulatory subunits and 2 catalytic subunits. Binding of cyclic AMP to the regulatory units releases the catalytic units, with the regulatory units remaining as a dimer. The catalytic units catalyze the phosphorylation of cellular proteins such as enzymes and mitochondrial, microsomal, and chromatin proteins. The physiologic event follows this cyclic AMP-mediated energy-producing event. Cyclic AMP is then degraded by the enzyme phosphodiesterase into the inactive compound, 5'-AMP.

7. A   p.79

The biologic activity of polypeptide or glycoprotein hormones (such as FSH or LH) can be altered by the heterogeneity of the molecules, up- and down-regulation of the receptors, and, finally, by modulation of the activity of the enzyme, adenylate cyclase.

Answers for Chapter 2 — Post-Test Questions

1. C   p.32

Paracrine communication:
Intercellular communication involving the local diffusion of regulating substances from a cell to nearby (contiguous) cells.

2. D   p.32

Intracrine communication:
This form of intracellular communication occurs when unsecreted substances bind to intracellular receptors.

3. B   p.32

Autocrine communication:
Intracellular communication whereby a single cell produces regulating substances that in turn act upon receptors on or within the same cell.

4. A   p.31

The classical definition of a hormone is a substance that travels from a special tissue, where it is released into the bloodstream, to distant responsive cells where the hormone exerts its characteristic effects. Hormones, therefore, are substances that provide a means of communication. The classic endocrine hormones travel through the bloodstream to distant sites.

5. F   p.32

Gonadotropin, the first messenger, activates an enzyme in the cell membrane called adenylate cyclase. This enzyme transmits the message by catalyzing the production of a second messenger within the cell, cyclic adenosine 3'5'-monophosphate (cyclic AMP). The message passes from gonadotropin to cyclic AMP, much like a baton in a relay race.

6. E   p.32

Cyclic AMP, the second messenger, initiates the process of steroidogenesis, leading to the synthesis and secretion of the hormone estradiol. This notion of message transmission has grown more and more complex with the appreciation of new physiologic concepts such as the heterogeneity of peptide hormones, the up- and down-regulation of cell membrane receptors, the regulation of adenylate cyclase activity, and the important roles for autocrine and paracrine regulating factors.

7. receptor   p.33

The biologic and metabolic effects of a hormone are determined by a cell's ability to receive and retain the hormone. The estradiol that is not bound to a protein, but floats freely in the bloodstream, readily enters cells by rapid diffusion. For estradiol to produce its effect, however, it must be grasped by a receptor within the cell. Only those cells which contain estradiol-specific receptors will respond to estradiol. The job of the receptor is to aid in the transmission of the hormone's message to nuclear gene transcription. The result is production of messenger RNA leading to protein synthesis and a cellular response characteristic of the hormone.

8. corticoids; progestins   p.34

The 21-carbon series includes the corticoids and the progestins, and the basic structure is the ***pregnane*** nucleus.

9. androgens   p.34

The 19-carbon series includes all the androgens and is based on the ***androstane*** nucleus.

10. estrogens   p.34

The estrogens are 18-carbon steroids based on the ***estrane*** nucleus. (See figure on page 21 in this Study Guide)

11.   p.40

12. Cholesterol   p.37

13. lipoproteins; Total; LDL   p.38

The protein moieties of the lipoprotein particles are strongly related to the risk of cardiovascular disease, and genetic abnormalities in their synthesis or structure can result in atherogenic conditions. The lipoproteins are a major reason for the disparity in atherosclerosis risk between men and women. Throughout adulthood, the blood HDL-cholesterol level is about 10 mg/dL higher in women, and this difference continues through the postmenopausal years. Total and LDL-cholesterol levels are lower in premenopausal women than in men, but after menopause they rise rapidly.

14. HDL   p.38

The protective nature of HDL is due to its ability to pick up free cholesterol from cells or other circulating lipoproteins. This lipid-rich HDL is known as HDL_3, which is then converted to the larger, less dense particle, HDL_2. Thus, HDL converts lipid-rich scavenger cells (macrophages residing in arterial walls) back to their low-lipid state and carries the excess cholesterol to sites (mainly liver) where it can be metabolized. Another method by which HDL removes cholesterol from the body focuses on the uptake of free cholesterol from cell membranes. The free cholesterol is esterified and moves to the core of the HDL particle. Thus HDL can remove cholesterol by delivering cholesterol to

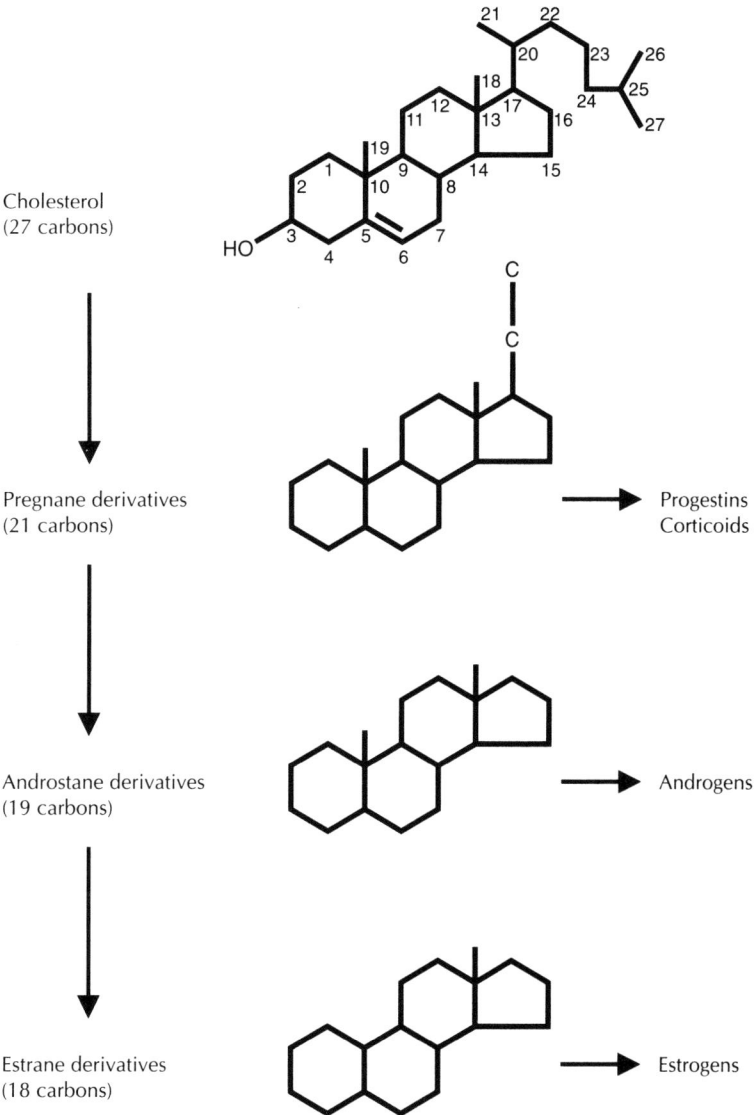

sites for utilization (steroid-producing cells) or metabolism and excretion (liver).

15. LDL; HDL; LDH; HDL   p.39
Atherosclerotic disease is related to increased LDL- and decreased HDL-cholesterol concentrations. Lowering LDL levels and raising HDL levels can reduce the incidence of atherosclerotic disease. Atherosclerosis is not a disease limited to aging people. It begins in early childhood, and its manifestation later in life can be influenced by health care behavior during younger years.

16. false   p.39
During steroidogenesis, the number of carbon atoms in cholesterol or any other steroid molecule can be reduced but never increased. The following reactions can take place.

   1. Cleavage of a side chain (desmolase reaction).
   2. Conversion of hydroxyl groups into ketones or ketones into hydroxyl groups (dehydrogenase reactions).
   3. Addition of OH group (hydroxylation reaction).
   4. Creation of double bonds (removal of hydrogen).
   5. Addition of hydrogen to reduce double bonds (saturation).

17. true   p.39

Steroidogenic enzymes are members of the cytochrome P450 group of oxidases. Cytochrome P450 is a generic term for a family of oxidative enzymes, termed 450 because of a pigment (450) absorbance shift when reduced. P450 enzymes can metabolize many substrates; e.g., in the liver, P450 enzymes metabolize toxins and environmental pollutants.

Enzyme	Cellular Location	Reactions
P450scc	Mitochondria	Cholesterol side chain cleavage
P450c11	Mitochondria	11-hydroxylase 18-hydroxylase 19-methyloxidase
P450c17	Endoplasmic reticulum	17-hydroxylase, 17,20-lyase
P450c21	Endoplasmic reticulum	21-hydroxylase
P450arom	Endoplasmic reticulum	Aromatase

18. true   p.41

Conversion of cholesterol to pregnenolone involves hydroxylation at the carbon 20 and 22 positions, with subsequent cleavage of the side chain. Conversion of cholesterol to pregnenolone by P450scc takes place within the mitochondria. It is a rate-limiting step in the steroid pathway and is one of the principal effects of tropic hormone stimulation, which also causes the uptake of the cholesterol substrate for this step.

19. false   p.43

The two cell system explains the sequence of events in ovarian follicular growth and steroidogenesis. The initial change from a primordial follicle is independent of hormones, and the stimulus governing this initial step in growth is unknown. Continued growth, however, depends upon FSH stimulation. As the granulosa responds to FSH, growth is associated with an increase in FSH receptors, a specific effect of FSH itself, but an action which is enhanced very significantly by the autocrine/paracrine peptides. The theca cells are characterized by steroidogenic activity in response to LH, specifically resulting in androgen production. Aromatization of androgens to estrogens is a distinct activity within the granulosa layer induced by FSH. Androgens produced in the theca layer, therefore, must diffuse into the granulosa layer. In the granulosa layer they are converted to estrogens, and the increasing level of estradiol in the peripheral circulation reflects release of the estrogen back toward the theca layer and into blood vessels.

20. false   p.44

The theca and granulosa cells secrete peptides that operate as both autocrine and paracrine factors. Insulin-like growth factor-I is secreted by the theca and enhances the LH stimulation of androgen production in the theca cells as well as FSH-mediated aromatization in the granulosa. Theca production of transforming growth factor can promote the growth of granulosa cells and FSH induction of LH receptors on the granulosa. The regulation of FSH receptors on granulosa cells is relatively complex. Although FSH increases the activity of its own receptor gene in a cyclic AMP-mediated mechanism, this action is influenced by inhibitory agents such as epidermal growth factor, fibroblast growth factor, and even a gonadotropin releasing hormone (GnRH)-like protein. Inhibin and activin are produced in the granulosa in response to FSH. Activin augments FSH activities, and inhibin enhances LH stimulation of androgen synthesis in the theca to serve as substrate for aromatization to estrogen in the granulosa.

21. true   p.45

The circulating level of SHBG is inversely related to weight, and thus significant weight gain can decrease SHBG and produce important changes in the unbound levels of the sex steroids. Another important mechanism for a reduction in circulating SHBG levels is insulin resistance and hyperinsulinemia (independent of age and weight). Thus, increased insulin levels in the circulation lower SHBG levels, and this may be the major mechanism that mediates the impact of increased body weight on SHBG. This relationship between the levels of insulin and SHBG is so strong that SHBG concentrations are a marker for hyperinsulinemic insulin resistance, and a low level of SHBG is a predictor for the development of type II diabetes mellitus.

Chapter 2 Hormone Biosynthesis, Metabolism and Mechanism of Action

22. true   p.46

In the female the adrenal gland remains the major source of circulating androgens, in particular androstenedione. In the male, almost all of the circulating estrogens are derived from peripheral conversion of androgens.

23. true   p.49

The major androgen products of the ovary are dehydroepiandrosterone (DHA) and androstenedione (and only a little testosterone) which are secreted mainly by stromal tissue derived from theca cells. With excessive accumulation of stromal tissue or in the presence of an androgen-producing tumor, testosterone becomes a significant secretory product. Occasionally, a nonfunctioning tumor can induce stromal proliferation and increased androgen production. The normal accumulation of stromal tissue at midcycle results in a rise in circulating levels of androstenedione and testosterone at the time of ovulation.

24. true   p.51

Not all androgen-sensitive tissues require the prior conversion of testosterone to DHT. In the process of masculine differentiation, the development of the wolffian duct structures (epididymis, the vas deferens, and the seminal vesicle) is dependent upon testosterone as the intracellular mediator, whereas development of the urogenital sinus and urogenital tubercle into the male external genitalia, urethra, and prostate requires the conversion of testosterone to DHT. Muscle development is under the direct control of testosterone.

25. E   p.37,39

Cholesterol is the basic building block in steroidogenesis. All steroid-producing organs except the placenta can synthesize cholesterol from acetate. Progestins, androgens, and estrogens, therefore, can be synthesized in situ in the various ovarian tissue compartments from the 2-carbon acetate molecule via cholesterol as the common steroid precursor. However, in situ synthesis cannot meet the demand, and therefore the major resource is blood cholesterol which enters the ovarian cells and can be inserted into the biosynthetic pathway or stored in esterified form for later use.

During steroidogenesis, the number of carbon atoms in cholesterol or any other steroid molecule can be reduced but never increased. The following reactions can take place.

1. Cleavage of a side chain (desmolase reaction).
2. Conversion of hydroxyl groups into ketones or ketones into hydroxyl groups (dehydrogenase reactions).
3. Addition of OH group (hydroxylation reaction).
4. Creation of double bonds (removal of hydrogen).
5. Addition of hydrogen to reduce double bonds (saturation).

Steroidogenic enzymes are members of the cytochrome P450 group of oxidases. Cytochrome P450 is a generic term for a family of oxidative enzymes, termed 450 because of a pigment (450) absorbance shift when reduced.

26. A   p.41

The following distinct P450 enzymes are identified with steroidogenesis: P450scc is the cholesterol side chain cleavage enzyme; P450c11 mediates 11-hydroxylase, 18-hydroxylase, and 19-methyloxidase; P450c17 mediates 17-hydroxylase and 17,20-lyase; P450c21 mediates the 21-hydroxylase; and P450arom mediates aromatization of androgens to estrogens.

27. C   p.42

Aromatization is mediated by P450arom found in the endoplasmic reticulum. The human genome has one P450arom gene, located on chromosome 15q21.1. Aromatization in different tissues with different substrates is the result of the single P450arom enzyme encoded by the single gene. Aromatase transcription is regulated by several promotor sites that respond to cytokines, cyclic nucelotides, gonadotropins, glucocorticoids, and growth factors.

28. E   p.43,44

The two cell system explains the sequence of events in ovarian follicular growth and steroidogenesis. The initial change

23

from a primordial follicle is independent of hormones, and the stimulus governing this initial step in growth is unknown. Continued growth, however, depends upon FSH stimulation. As the granulosa responds to FSH, growth is associated with an increase in FSH receptors, a specific effect of FSH itself, but an action which is enhanced very significantly by the autocrine/paracrine peptides. The theca cells are characterized by steroidogenic activity in response to LH, specifically resulting in androgen production. Aromatization of androgens to estrogens is a distinct activity within the granulosa layer induced by FSH. Androgens produced in the theca layer, therefore, must diffuse into the granulosa layer. In the granulosa layer they are converted to estrogens, and the increasing level of estradiol in the peripheral circulation reflects release of the estrogen back toward the theca layer and into blood vessels.

After ovulation the dominance of the luteinized granulosa layer is dependent upon preovulatory induction of an adequate number of LH receptors, and therefore, dependent upon adequate FSH action. Prior to ovulation the granulosa layer is characterized by aromatization activity and conversion of the theca androgens to estrogens, an FSH-mediated activity. After ovulation the granulosa layer secretes progesterone and estrogens directly into the bloodstream, an LH-mediated activity.

29. E p.44
The theca and granulosa cells secrete peptides that operate as both autocrine and paracrine factors. Insulin-like growth factor-I is secreted by the theca and enhances the LH stimulation of androgen production in the theca cells as well as FSH-mediated aromatization in the granulosa. Theca production of transforming growth factor can promote the growth of granulosa cells and FSH induction of LH receptors on the granulosa. The regulation of FSH receptors on granulosa cells is relatively complex. Although FSH increases the activity of its own receptor gene in a cyclic AMP-mediated mechanism, this action is influenced by inhibitory agents such as epidermal growth factor, fibroblast growth factor, and even a gonadotropin releasing hormone (GnRH)-like protein. Inhibin and activin are produced in the granulosa in response to FSH. Activin augments FSH activities, and inhibin enhances LH stimulation of androgen synthesis in the theca to serve as substrate for aromatization to estrogen in the granulosa.

30. A p.45
The circulating level of SHBG is inversely related to weight, and thus significant weight gain can decrease SHBG and produce important changes in the unbound levels of the sex steroids. Another important mechanism for a reduction in circulating SHBG levels is insulin resistance and hyperinsulinemia (independent of age and weight). Thus, increased insulin levels in the circulation lower SHBG levels, and this may be the major mechanism that mediates the impact of increased body weight on SHBG. This relationship between the levels of insulin and SHBG is so strong that SHBG concentrations are a marker for hyperinsulinemic insulin resistance, and a low level of SHBG is a predictor for the development of type II diabetes mellitus.

SHBG is a glycoprotein that contains a single binding site for androgens and estrogens even though it is composed of two monomers. Its gene has been localized to the short arm of chromosome 17. Transcortin, also called corticosteroid binding globulin, is a plasma glycoprotein that binds cortisol, progesterone, deoxycorticosterone, corticosterone, and some of the other minor corticoid compounds. Normally about 75% of circulating cortisol is bound to transcortin, 15% is loosely bound to albumin, and 10% is unbound or free. Binding in the circulation follows the law of mass action: the amount of the free, unbound hormone is in equilibrium with the bound hormone. Thus, the total binding capacity of SHBG will influence the amount that is free and unbound.

31. E p.54
An important action of estrogen is the modification of its own and other steroid hormone activity by affecting receptor concentration. Estrogen increases target tissue responsiveness to itself and to progestins and androgens by increasing the concentration of its own receptor and that of the intracellular progestin and androgen receptors. This process is called *replenishment*. Progesterone and clomiphene, on the other hand, limit tissue response to estrogen by blocking the replenishment mechanism, thus decreasing over time the concentration of estrogen receptors. Replenishment is very responsive to the available amount of steroid and receptors. Small amounts of receptor depletion and small amounts of steroid in the blood activate the mechanism.

32. A p.55,56
Recombinant DNA techniques have permitted the study of the gene sequences that code for the synthesis of nuclear

receptors. Steroid hormone receptors share a common structure with the receptors for thyroid hormone, 1,25-dihydroxy vitamin D_3, and retinoic acid; thus these receptors are called a superfamily. Each receptor contains characteristic domains that are similar and interchangeable. Therefore, it is not surprising that the specific hormones can interact with more than one receptor in this family. Analysis of these receptors suggests a complex evolutionary history during which gene duplication and swapping between domains of different origins occurred.

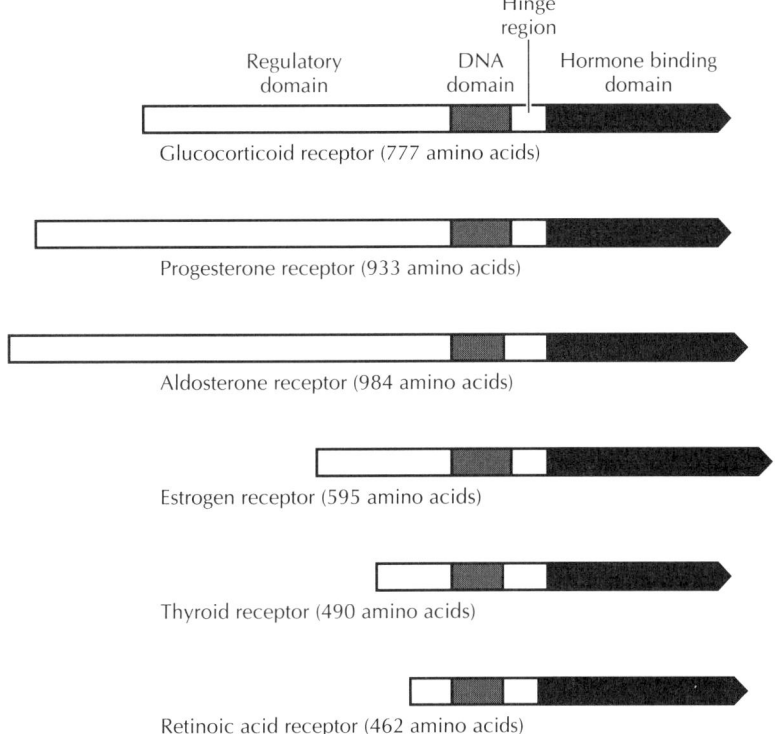

33. C p.57

The DNA-Binding Domain: The middle domain binds to DNA and consists of 66–68 amino acids with 9 cysteines in fixed positions. This domain is essential for activation of transcription. Hormone binding induces a conformational change which allows binding to the hormone responsive elements in the target gene. This domain is very similar for each member of the steroid and thyroid receptor superfamily; however, the genetic message is specific for the hormone which binds to the hormone binding domain, and this domain controls which gene will be regulated by the receptor.

34. E p.59

The progesterone receptor is induced by estrogens at the transcriptional level and decreased by progestins at both the transcriptional and translational levels (probably through receptor phosphorylation). Estrogen exerts its influence on the progesterone receptor gene by means of an estrogen responsive element in the 5' flanking region. The progesterone receptor gene encodes a collection of messenger RNAs that direct the synthesis of several structurally related receptor proteins, with two major forms, designated the A and B receptors. The two forms are each associated with a different estrogen responsive element. Each form is associated with additional proteins, which are important for folding of the polypeptide into a structure that allows hormone binding and receptor activity. Progesterone is unique in the steroid superfamily in having two forms of its receptor. Therefore, progestational agents can elicit a variety of responses determined by target tissue production and activity of the two receptor forms with dimerization as A:A and B:B (homodimers) or A:B (heterodimer).

35. A p.61

In those cells that respond only to DHT, only DHT will be found within the nucleus activating messenger RNA production. Because testosterone and DHT bind to the same high affinity androgen receptor, why is it necessary to have the DHT mechanism? One explanation is that this is a mechanism for amplifying androgen action, because the androgen receptor preferentially will bind DHT (greater affinity). The antiandrogens, including cyproterone acetate and spironolactone, bind to the androgen receptor with about 20% of the affinity of testosterone. This weak affinity is characteristic of binding without activation of the biologic response.

The amino acid sequence of the androgen receptor in the DNA-binding domain resembles that of the receptors for progesterone, mineralocorticoids, and glucocorticoids but most closely that of the progesterone receptor. Androgens and progestins can crossreact for their receptors but do so only when present in pharmacologic concentrations. Progestins not only compete for androgen receptors but also compete for the metabolic utilization of the 5α-reductase enzyme. The dihydroprogesterone which is produced in turn also competes with testosterone and DHT for the androgen receptor. A progestin, therefore, can act both as an antiandrogen and as an antiestrogen. Androgen-responsive gene expression can also be modifed by estrogen; it has been known for years that androgens and estrogens can counteract each other's biologic responses. These responses of target tissues are determined by gene interactions with the hormone-receptor complexes, androgen with its receptor and estrogen with its receptor. The ultimate biologic response reflects the balance of actions of the different hormones with their respective receptors, modified by various transcription regulators.

The syndrome of testicular feminization (androgen insensitivity) represents a congenital abnormality in the androgen intracellular receptor. The androgen receptor gene is localized on the human X chromosome, the only steroid hormone receptor to be located on the X chromosome. Thus testicular feminization is an X-linked disorder. Molecular studies of patients with testicular feminization have indicated a deletion of amino acids from the steroid binding domain due to nucleotide alterations in the gene which encodes the androgen receptor.

36. E   p.61
Tropic hormones include the releasing hormones originating in the hypothalamus and a variety of peptides and glycoproteins released by the anterior pituitary gland. The specificity of the tropic hormone depends upon the presence of a receptor in the cell membrane of the target tissue. Tropic hormones do not enter the cell to stimulate physiologic events but unite with a receptor on the surface of the cell. The receptor protein in the cell membrane can either act as the active agent and, after binding, operate as an ion channel or function as an enzyme. Alternatively, the receptor protein is coupled to an active agent, an intracellular messenger. The major intracellular messenger molecules are cyclic AMP, inositol 1,4,5-triphosphate (IP_3), 1,2-diacylglycerol (1,2,-DG), calcium ion, and cyclic GMP.

37. A   p.65
Gonadotropin releasing hormone (GnRH) is calcium dependent in its mechanism of action and utilizes IP_3 and 1,2-DG as second messengers to stimulate protein kinase activity. These responses require a G protein and are associated with cyclical release of calcium ions from intracellular stores and the opening of cell membrane channels to allow entry of extracellular calcium.

38. E   p.65
The intracellular calcium concentration is a regulator of both cyclic AMP and cyclic GMP levels. Activation of the surface receptor either opens a channel in the cell membrane that lets calcium ions into the cell, or calcium is released from internal stores (the latter is especially the case in muscle). This calcium flux is an important intracellular mediator of response to hormones, functioning itself as a second messenger in the nervous system and in muscle.

The calcium messenger system is linked to hormone-receptor function by means of a specific enzyme, phospholipase C, that catalyzes the hydrolysis of polyphosphatidylinositols, specific phospholipids in the cell membrane. Activation of this enzyme by hormone binding to its receptor leads to the generation of 2 intracellular messengers, inositol triphosphate (IP_3) and diacylglycerol (1,2-DG), which initiate the function of the 2 parts of the calcium system. The first part is a calcium activated protein kinase responsible for sustained cellular responses, and the second part involves a regulator called calmodulin responsible for acute responses. These responses are secondary to alterations in enzyme activity and in transcription factors.

39. A   p.67
The cell membrane receptors of insulin, insulin-like growth factor-I, epidermal growth factor, platelet derived growth factor, and fibroblast growth factor are tyrosine kinases. All tyrosine kinase receptors have a similar structure: an extracellular domain for ligand binding, a single transmembrane domain, and a cytoplasmic domain. The unique amino

acid sequences determine a 3-dimensional conformation that provides ligand specificity. The transmembrane domains are not highly conserved (thus differing in make-up). The cytoplasmic domains respond to ligand binding by undergoing conformational changes and autophosphorylation. The structure of the receptors for insulin and insulin-like growth factor-I is more complicated, with two alpha- and two beta-subunits, forming two transmembrane domains connected extracellularly by disulfide bridges. The receptors for the important autocrine/paracrine factors, activin and inhibin, function as serine-specific protein kinases.

40. E p.68

Growth factors are polypeptides that modulate activity either in the cells in which they are produced or in nearby cells; hence, they are autocrine and paracrine regulators. Regulation factors of this type (yet another biologic family) are produced by local gene expression and protein translation, and they operate by binding to cell membrane receptors. The receptors usually contain an intracellular component with tyrosine kinase activity which is energized by a binding-induced conformational change that induces autophosphorylation. However, some factors work through the other second messenger systems, such as cyclic AMP or IP_3. Growth factors are involved in a variety of tissue functions, including mitogenesis, tissue and cellular differentiation, chemotactic actions, and angiogenesis. TGF-β belongs to a large family of proteins that includes inhibin, activin, and antimüllerian hormone.

41. B p.68

TGF-β can either stimulate or inhibit growth and differentiation, depending on the target cell and the presence or absence of other growth factors. In the ovary, TGF-β promotes granulosa cell differentiation by enhancing the actions of FSH (especially in expression of FSH and LH receptors) and antagonizing the down-regulation of FSH receptors. TGF-β and the insulin-like growth factors are required for the maintenance of normal bone mass. EGF is a structural analog of TGF-α and is involved in mitogenesis. In the ovary, EGF, secreted by theca cells, is important for granulosa cell proliferation, an action opposed by TGF-β which is also secreted by the theca cells.

42. E p.69

The insulin-like growth factors (also called somatomedins) are single chain polypeptides that resemble insulin in structure and function. These factors are widespread and are involved in growth and differentiation in response to growth hormone, and as local regulators of cell metabolism. IGF-II is more prominent during embryogenesis, while IGF-I is more active postnatally. Only the liver produces more IGF-I than the ovary. Both IGF-I and IGF-II are secreted by granulosa cells. IGF-I amplifies the action of gonadotropins and coordinates the functions of theca and granulosa cells. IGF-I receptors on the granulosa are increased by FSH and LH and augmented by estrogen. In the theca, IGF-I increases steroidogenesis. In the granulosa, IGF-I is important for the formation and increase in numbers of FSH and LH receptors, steroidogenesis, the secretion of inhibin, and oocyte maturation. Granulosa cells also contain receptors for insulin, and insulin can bind to the IGF receptors. The IGF-I receptor is a heterotetramer with two alpha- and two beta-subunits in a structure similar to that of the insulin receptor. Insulin can bind to the alpha-subunit ligand binding domain and activate the beta-subunit which is a protein kinase. Thus, insulin can modulate ovarian cellular functions. The biologic potency and availability of the insulin-like growth factors are further modulated by a collection of IGF-binding proteins which bind circulating insulin-like growth factors and also alter cellular responsiveness. IGF-binding protein-3, for example, is secreted, bound, and processed by cells, affecting both the function of the binding protein and IGF activity.

43. C p.69

The glycoproteins, such as FSH and LH, are not single proteins but should be viewed as a family of heterogeneous forms of varying immunologic and biologic activity. The various forms (isoforms) arise in various ways, including different DNA promoter actions, alterations in RNA splicing, point mutations, and post-translational carbohydrate changes. The impact of the variations is to alter structure and metabolic clearance, thus affecting binding and activity. The isoforms have different molecular weights, circulating half-lives, and biologic activities. Throughout the menstrual cycle, the amazing number of at least 20–30 isoforms of both FSH and LH are present in the bloodstream. ***The overall activity of a glycoprotein, therefore, is due to the effects of the mixture of forms which reach and bind to the target tissue.***

The nonglycosylated subunit precursors of glycoprotein hormones are synthesized in the endoplasmic reticulum, followed by glycosylation. The glycosylated subunits combine and then are transported to the Golgi apparatus for further processing of the carbohydrate component. The units combine to form a compact heterodimer. The protein moiety binds to specific target tissue receptors, while the carbohydrate moiety plays a critical role in coupling the hormone-receptor complex to adenylate cyclase (perhaps by determining the necessary conformational structure).

The preciseness of the chemical make-up of the tropic hormones is an essential element in determining the ability of the hormone to mate with its receptor. The glycopeptides (FSH, LH, TSH, and HCG) are dimers composed of two glycosylated polypeptide subunits, the α- and β-subunits. The α- and β-subunits are tightly bound in a noncovalent association. The three-dimensional structure of the subunits is maintained by internal disulfide bonds. All of the glycopeptides of the human species (FSH, LH, TSH, and HCG) share a common α-chain, an identical structure containing 92 amino acids. The β-chains (or the β-subunits) differ in both amino acid and carbohydrate content, conferring the specificity inherent in the relationship between hormones and their receptors. Therefore, the specific biologic activity of a glycopeptide hormone is determined by the β-subunit; hypogonadism has been reported due to single amino acid substitution in the LH beta-subunit.

44. B p.70,71

β-HCG is the largest β-subunit, containing a larger carbohydrate moiety and 145 amino acid residues, including a unique carboxyl terminal tail piece of 24 amino acid groups. It is this unique part of the HCG structure which allows the production of highly specific antibodies and the utilization of highly specific immunologic assays. The extended sequence in the carboxy-terminal region of β-HCG contains 4 sites for glycosylation, the reason why HCG is glycosylated to a greater extent than LH. These differences in structure are associated with a different promoter and transcriptional site that is located upstream in the HCG beta-subunit gene compared to the site in the LH beta-subunit gene. The HCG beta-subunit site does not contain a hormone response element, allowing HCG secretion to escape feedback regulation by the sex steroids, in contrast to FSH and LH. All human tissues appear to make HCG a whole molecule, but the placenta is different in having the ability to glycosylate the protein, thus reducing its rate of metabolism and giving it biologic activity through a long half-life. The carbohydrate components of the glycoproteins are comprised of fructose, galactose, mannose, galactosamine, glucosamine, and sialic acid. Whereas the other sugars are necessary for hormonal function, sialic acid is the critical determinant of biologic half-life. Removal of sialic acid residues in HCG, FSH, and LH leads to very rapid elimination from the circulation.

45. E p.71

The half-life of α-HCG is 6–8 minutes, that of whole HCG from the placenta about 12 hours. FSH consists of the α-subunit of 92 amino acids and a β-subunit of 110 amino acids. It has four carbohydrate side chains, two on each subunit. The β-subunit of LH consists of 121 amino acids. LH has 3 carbohydrate side chains with a single glycosylation site (with less than half of the sialic acid in FSH). The initial half-life of LH is approximately 20 minutes, compared to the initial half-life of FSH of 3–4 hours.

46. C p.72

The glycopeptide hormones can be found in the pituitary existing in a variety of forms, differing in their carbohydrate make-up. Removal of carbohydrate residues from the FSH molecule produces forms of FSH with antagonistic properties. Treatment of women with a GnRH antagonist yields circulating levels of deglycosylated FSH that bind to gonadal receptors but exert no biological activity. Thus, the pituitary can secrete forms of the glycopeptide hormones which can function as naturally occurring antihormones. The isoform mixture is influenced both quantitatively and qualitatively by GnRH and the feedback of the steroid hormones.

Certain clinical conditions may be associated with alterations in the usual chemical structure of the glycopeptides, resulting in an interference with the ability to bind to receptors and stimulate biological activity. In addition to deglycosylation and the formation of antihormones, gonadotropins can be produced with an increased carbohydrate content. A low estrogen environment in the pituitary gland, for example, favors the production of so-called big gonadotropins, gonadotropins with an increased carbohydrate component and, as a result, decreased biological activity. Immunoassay in these situations may not reveal the biologic situation; an immunoassay sees only a certain set of molecules but not all. Therefore, immunologic results do not always indicate the biologic situation.

47. C p.73

In most mammalian species, prolactin consists of 197–199 amino acids, similar in structure to growth hormone and placental lactogen. All three hormones are believed to have originated in a common ancestral protein about 60–70 million years ago. Simultaneous measurements of prolactin by both bioassay and immunoassay reveal discrepancies. At first differences in prolactin were observed based on size, leading to the use of terms such as little, big, and the wonderfully sophisticated term, big big prolactin. Further chemical studies have revealed structural modifications which include glycosylation, phosphorylation, and variations in binding and charge. This heterogeneity is the result of many influences at many levels: transcription, translation, and peripheral metabolism.

Prolactin is encoded by a single gene, producing a molecule that in its major form is maintained in 3 loops by disulfide bonds. Both smaller and larger forms have been identified. Little prolactin probably represents a splicing variant resulting from the deletion of amino acids. Big prolactin can result from the failure to remove introns; it has little biologic activity and does not cross react with antibodies to the major form of prolactin. The so-called big big variants of prolactin are due to separate molecules of prolactin binding to each other, either noncovalently or by interchain disulfide bonding. Some of the apparently larger forms of prolactin are prolactin molecules complexed to binding proteins.

Other variations exist. Enzymatic cleavage of the prolactin molecule yields fragments that may be capable of biologic activity. Prolactin that has been glycosylated continues to exert activity. However, the nonglycosylated form of prolactin is the predominant form of prolactin secreted into the circulation. Posttranslational modification of prolactin also occurs and includes phosphorylation, deamidation, and sulfation.

At any one point of time, the bioactivity (e.g., galactorrhea) and the immunoactivity (circulating level by immunoassay) of prolactin represent the cumulative effect of the family of structural variants. Remember, immunoassays do not always reflect the biologic situation (e.g., a normal prolactin level in a women with galactorrhea).

48. E   p.79,81

Adenylate cyclase is composed of 3 protein units: the receptor, a guanyl nucleotide regulatory unit, and a catalytic unit. The regulatory unit is a coupling protein, regulated by guanine nucleotides (specifically GTP), and therefore it is called GTP binding protein or G protein for short. The catalytic unit is the enzyme itself which converts ATP to cyclic AMP. The receptor and the nucleotide regulatory unit are structurally linked, but inactive until the hormone binds to the receptor. Upon binding, the complex of hormone, receptor, and nucleotide regulatory unit is activated leading to an uptake of guanosine 5'-triphosphate (GTP) by the regulatory unit. The activation and uptake of GTP result in an active enzyme which can convert ATP to cyclic AMP. This result can be viewed as the outcome of the regulatory unit *coupling* with the catalytic unit, forming an intact complete enzyme. Enzyme activity is then terminated by hydrolysis of the GTP to guanosine 5'-diphosphate (GDP) returning the enzyme to its inactive state. Quick action and acute control of adenylate cyclase are assured because the G protein is a GTPase that self activates upon binding of GTP.

The G protein has been purified. From the amino acid sequence, complementary DNA clones have been produced. These studies have indicated that a family of G proteins exists that couples receptors to active proteins, playing roles in signal transduction, intracellular transport, and exocytosis. The ability of the hormone-receptor complex to work through a common messenger (cyclic AMP) and produce contrasting actions (stimulation and inhibition) is thought to be due to the presence of both stimulatory nucleotide regulatory G proteins and inhibitory nucleotide regulatory G proteins. Thus, stimulating agents bind to their receptors and interact with $G_{stimulatory}$ protein while inhibiting agents interact with $G_{inhibitory}$ protein that prohibits cyclic AMP synthesis.

The G proteins are composed of α-, β-, and γ-subunits, each the product of a distinct gene. The β- and γ-subunits are similar, but each G protein has an unique α-subunit. In the inactive state GDP is bound to the α-subunit. Hormone-receptor interaction and binding changes the α-subunit conformation. GTP replaces GDP on the α-subunit, freeing the β- and γ-subunits which allows the GTP-α-subunit to bind to the catalytic unit of adenylate cyclase, forming the active enzyme. The GTP-α-subunit can also activate other messengers, such as ion channels. Intrinsic GTPase activity quickly hydrolyzes the GTP-α to GDP-α, which leads to reassociation with the β- and γ-subunits, reforming the G protein complex for further activation. The functional specificity is due to the α-subunit which differs for each G protein, and therefore there are many different α-subunits encoded by different genes.

Another potential mechanism for influencing target tissue response is the regulation of the G protein subunits. Diversity in G protein activity is accomplished by multiple forms with different subunits encoded by different genes and by alterations due to variations in exon splicing. (See figure on page 30 in this Study Guide)

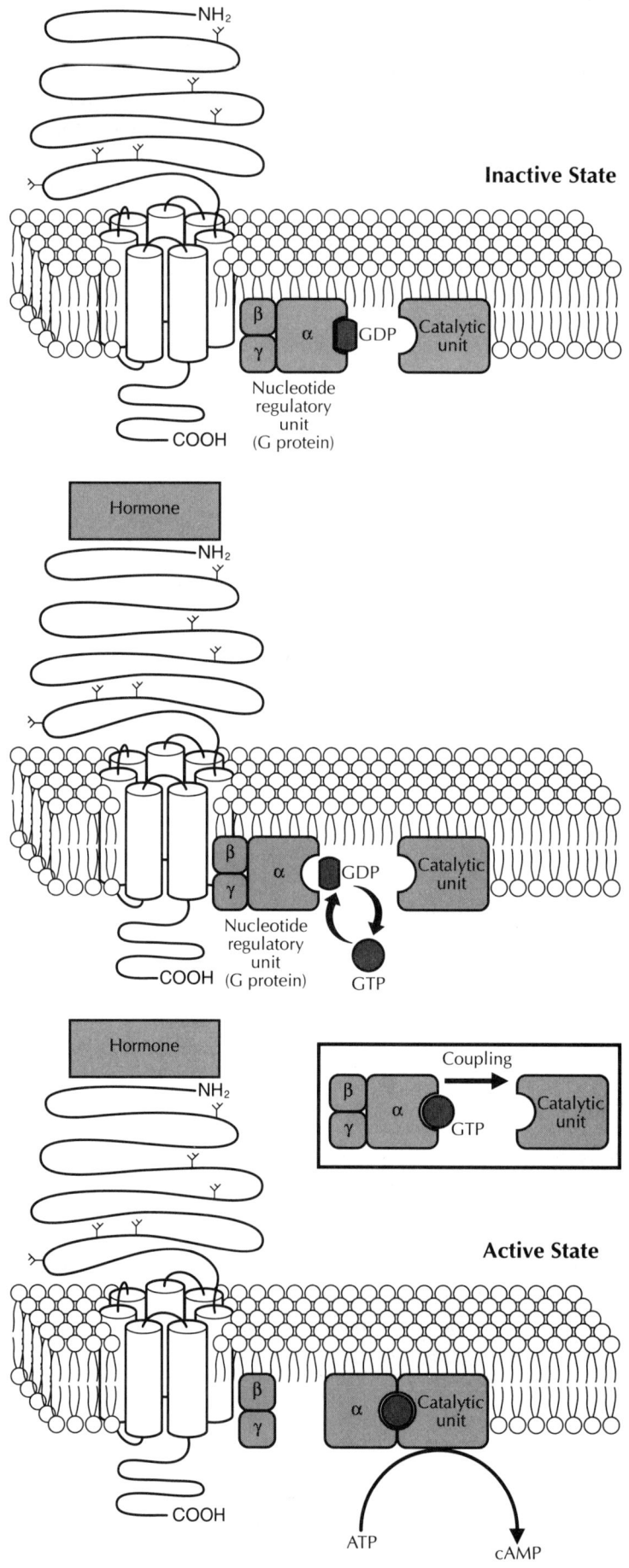

49. C p.82

Mutations that alter the structure and activity of G proteins can result in disease. A subset of growth hormone-secreting pituitary tumors has been identified with mutations (forming an oncogene) in the G protein α-subunit. The McCune-Albright syndrome (sexual precocity, polyostotic fibrous dysplasia, cafe-au-lait skin pigmentation, and autonomous functioning of various endocrine glands) can be explained by unregulated activity of the adenylate cyclase system. G protein mutations have been identified in tissues from patients with this syndrome. G protein mutations have also been found in some, but not most, adrenal and ovarian tumors. It is possible that alterations in G protein function may ultimately explain abnormalities in endocrine-metabolic functions, as well as oncogenic mutations.

50. A p.83

Down-regulation is a decrease in response in the presence of continuous stimulation. It involves the following 3 mechanisms:

1. Loss of receptors by internalization.
2. Desensitization by autophosphorylation of the cytoplasmic segment of the receptor.
3. Uncoupling of the regulatory and catalytic subunits of the adenylate cyclase enzyme.

51. B p.84

Alteration of the GnRH molecule has produced both agonists and antagonists. GnRH is a decapeptide; antagonists have substitutions at multiple positions, while agonists have substitutions at the 6 or 10 positions. The GnRH agonist molecules first stimulate the pituitary gland to secrete gonadotropins, then because of the constant stimulation, down-regulation and desensitization of the cell membrane receptors occur, and gonadotropin secretion is literally turned off. The antagonist molecules bind to the cell membrane receptor and fail to transmit a message and thus are competitive inhibitors. Various GnRH agonists are used to treat endometriosis, uterine leiomyomas, precocious puberty, cancer of the prostate gland, ovarian hyperandrogenism, and the premenstrual syndrome.

52. A p.84

Strictly speaking, a progestin is not an estrogen antagonist. It modifies estrogen action by causing a depletion of estrogen receptors. There is also evidence that a progestin can inhibit transcription activation by the estrogen receptor. In addition progestins induce enzyme activity that converts the potent estradiol to the impotent estrone sulfate which is then secreted from the cell. Androgens do block the actions of estrogen, but the mechanism is not entirely clear. Rather than a direct impact on estrogen receptor levels, the action is directed to gene activity subsequent to estrogen-receptor binding. High levels of androgen can produce estrogen and progestational effects by binding to the estrogen and progesterone receptors.

53. E p.85

Tamoxifen is very similar to clomiphene (in structure and actions), both being nonsteroidal compounds structurally related to diethylstilbestrol. Tamoxifen, in binding to the estrogen receptor, competitively inhibits estrogen binding. In vitro, the estrogen binding affinity for its receptor is 100–1,000 times greater than that of tamoxifen. Thus, tamoxifen must be present in a concentration 100–1,000 times greater than estrogen to maintain inhibition of breast cancer cells. In vitro studies demonstrate that this action is not cytocidal, but rather cytostatic (and thus its use must be long-term). The tamoxifen-estrogen receptor complex binds to DNA, but whether an agonistic, estrogenic message occurs because of gene transcription is probably determined by what promoter elements are present in specific cell types.

Serum protein changes reflect the estrogenic (agonistic) action of tamoxifen. This includes decreases in antithrombin III, cholesterol, and LDL-cholesterol, while HDL-cholesterol and sex hormone binding globulin (SHBG) levels increase (as do other binding globulins). The estrogenic activity of tamoxifen, 20 mg daily, is nearly as potent as 2 mg estradiol in lowering FSH levels in postmenopausal women, 26% vs. 34% with estradiol. The estrogenic actions of tamoxifen include the stimulation of progesterone receptor synthesis, an estrogen-like maintenance of bone, and estrogenic effects on the vaginal mucosa and the endometrium. Tamoxifen increases the frequency of hepatic carcinoma in rats at very large doses. This is consistent with its estrogenic, agonistic action, but this effect is unlikely to be a clinical problem (and it has not been observed) at doses currently used. There has been concern that tamoxifen might be associated with thrombotic events; however, the decrease in antithrombin III observed with tamoxifen is still within the normal range.

54. E p.86

RU486 (the generic name is mifepristone) is a 19 nortestosterone derivative. The dimethyl (dimethylaminophenyl) side chain at carbon 11 is the principal factor in its antiprogesterone action. There are three major characteristics of its action which are important: a long half-life, high affinity for the progesterone receptor, and active metabolites.

The affinity of RU486 for the progesterone receptor is 5 times greater than that of the natural hormone. In the absence of progesterone, it can produce an agonistic (progesterone) effect. It does not bind to the estrogen receptor, but it can act as a weak antiandrogen because of its low affinity binding to the androgen receptor. RU486 also binds to the glucocorticoid receptor, but higher doses are required to produce effects. The binding affinity of RU486 and its metabolites for the glucocorticoid receptor is very, very high. The reason why it takes such a high dose to produce an effect is because the circulating level of cortisol is so high, 1,000-fold higher than progesterone. This allows titration of clinical effects by adjustments of dose.

RU486 is most noted for its abortifacient activity and the political controversy surrounding it. However, the combination of its agonistic and antagonistic actions can be exploited for many uses, including contraception, therapy of endometriosis, induction of labor, treatment of Cushing's syndrome, and, potentially, treatment of various cancers.

3 The Ovary — Embryology and Development

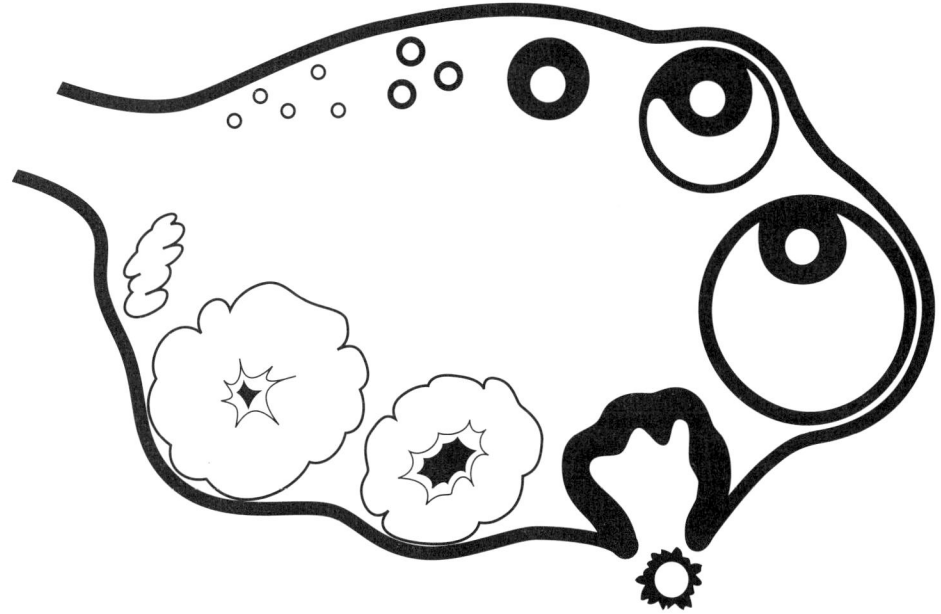

Learning Objectives

Be able to:

1. Describe the embryology of the ovary and testes.

2. Explain the stages of oogonal and oocyte maturation.

3. Describe the development of the ovary from the neonatal period to the mature adult.

Pre-Test

A. Instructions: Fill in the blanks

1. The primordial germ cells originate within the primitive _____.

2. Currently, the best candidate for the _____ gene is located within a region named _____, the sex-determining region on the Y chromosome.

B. Instructions: True or False

3. Oogonia are transformed to oocytes as they enter the first meiotic division and arrest in prophase.

4. At the time of menopause there are no remaining follicles.

C. Instructions: For the following question choose:

A. if only 1, 2 and 3 are correct
B. if only 1 and 3 are correct
C. if only 2 and 4 are correct
D. if only 4 is correct
E. if all are correct

5. Fetal gonadotropin levels
   1. are higher in female than male fetuses
   2. may cause abdominal masses in fetuses and newborns in the form of ovarian cysts
   3. are lower in males than females due to the presence of testosterone and inhibin
   4. are of similar concentrations in male and female fetuses.

Post-Test

A. Instructions: Fill in the blanks

1. The ovary consists of three major portions: the _____, the _____ and the _____.

2. Stromal tissue is composed of _____ tissue and _____ cells and has the ability to respond to LH or HCG with androgen production.

3. The earliest recognizable gonad contains somatic cells derived from at least 3 different tissues: _____ epithelium, _____ and _____ tissue.

4. The factor that determines whether the indifferent gonad will become a testis is called the _____, a product of a gene located on the Y chromosome.

5. The male phenotype is dependent upon the products of the fetal testes: _____ and _____ of the fetal testes.

6. The first and second polar bodies each contain _____ chromosomes.

7. An oocyte arrested in prophase of meiosis enveloped by a single layer of granulosa cells surrounded by a basement membrane is called a _____ follicle.

8. The development of the _____ into the fallopian tubes, uterus and upper third of the vagina is totally independent of the ovary.

B. Instructions: True or False

9. The testes begin to differentiate at weeks 6–7 of gestation.

10. Primitive germ cells are unable to survive in locations other than the gonadal ridge.

11. In the female, the loss of the wolffian system is due to the lack of locally produced testosterone.

12. The maximal oogonial content of the ovary is at 16–20 weeks in utero when there are 6–7 million oogonia resulting from meiosis.

13. Individuals with Turner syndrome experience normal migration and mitosis of germ cells, but the oogonia do not undergo meiosis.

14. The hypothalamic-pituitary portal circulation is functional by the 6th week of gestation.

15. Due to the fixed initial endowment of germ cells, the newborn female enters life having lost up to 50% of her oocytes.

16. Apoptosis (or programmed cell death) is a process probably involved in atresia of the follicle.

C. Instructions: For each of the following questions choose:

A. if only 1, 2 and 3 are correct
B. if only 1 and 3 are correct
C. if only 2 and 4 are correct
D. if only 4 is correct
E. if all are correct

17. The physical expulsion of the oocyte
    1. is dependent upon a preovulatory surge in prostaglandin synthesis within the follicle
    2. occurs regardless of gonadotropin stimulation
    3. will not occur if prostaglandin synthesis is inhibited
    4. can occur twice in one month

18. The corpus luteum
    1. is supported by LH for 14 days
    2. produces estradiol and progesterone
    3. rapidly regresses if successful implantation does not lead to hCG production
    4. is required for the first 7–9 weeks of pregnancy

19. As a premenopausal women ages
    1. there is an increase in FSH
    2. fewer follicles grow per cycle
    3. there is a decrease in inhibin
    4. her cycles often become irregular in onset

Answers for Chapter 3 — Pre-Test Questions

1. ectoderm   p.95

The primordial germ cells originate within the primitive ectoderm, but the specific cells of origin cannot be distinguished. The germ cells are first identified in the primitive endoderm at the caudal end and in the adjacent yolk sac, and soon they also appear in the splanchnic mesoderm of the hindgut. The gonadal ridge is the one and only site where the germ cells can survive. By displacement because of growth of the embryo and also by active movement, the germ cells "migrate" to their gonadal sites between weeks 4 and 6 of gestation. The factors that initiate and guide the migration of the germ cells are not known. During this "movement," the germ cells begin their proliferation.

2. TDF; SRY   p.97

Currently, the best candidate for the testicular determining factor gene is located within a region named SRY, the sex-determining region on the Y chromosome. The protein product of the TDF gene contains a DNA binding domain to activate gene transcription. The expression of the TDF gene is confined to the genital ridge during fetal life, but the gene is also active in the germ cells of the adult, perhaps playing a role in spermatogenesis. The traditional view assigns active gene control and expression for testicular differentiation and a more passive, "default" mode of development for the ovary. However, any process of differentiation requires gene expression, and therefore ovarian development, too, must involve genes and gene products.

3. true   p.98

By mitosis, the germ cells give rise to the oogonia. The oogonia are transformed to oocytes as they enter the first meiotic division and arrest in prophase. This process begins at 11–12 weeks, perhaps in response to a factor or factors produced by the rete ovarii.

4. false   p.102

At the onset of puberty, the germ cell mass has been reduced to 300,000 units. During the next 35–40 years of reproductive life, these units will be depleted further to a point at menopause where only a few hundred remain.

5. A   p.101

There is a sex difference in fetal gonadotropin levels. There are higher pituitary and circulating FSH and pituitary LH levels in female fetuses. The lower male levels are probably due to testicular testosterone and inhibin production. In infancy, the postnatal FSH rise is more marked and more sustained in females, while LH values are not as high. The FSH levels are greater than the levels reached during a normal adult menstrual cycle, decreasing to low levels usually by one year of age, sometimes later. LH levels are in the range of lower adult levels. This early activity is accompanied by inhibin levels comparable to the low range observed during the follicular phase of the menstrual cycle.

Answers for Chapter 3 — Post-Test Questions

1. outer cortex; central medulla; hilum   p.94

The ovary consists of three major portions, the outer cortex, the central medulla, and the rete ovarii (the hilum). The hilum is the point of attachment of the ovary to the mesovarium. It contains nerves and blood vessels, and hilus cells which have the potential to become active in steroidogenesis or to form tumors. These cells are very similar to the testosterone producing Leydig cells of the testes. The outermost portion of the cortex is called the tunica albuginea, topped on its surface by a single layer of cuboidal epithelium, the germinal epithelium. The oocytes, enclosed in complexes called follicles, are in the inner part of the cortex, embedded in stromal tissue.

2. connective; interstitial p.95

The stromal tissue is composed of connective tissue and interstitial cells which are derived from mesenchymal cells, and have the ability to respond to luteinizing hormone (LH) or human chorionic gonadotropin (HCG) with androgen production. The central medullary area of the ovary is derived largely from mesonephric cells.

3. coelomic; mesenchyme; mesonephric p.95

The origin of the gonadal somatic cells is still not certain. The earliest recognizable gonad contains besides the germ cells, somatic cells derived from at least 3 different tissues: coelomic epithelium, mesenchyme, and mesonephric tissue. In one model, the gonad is formed by the invasion of the "germinal epithelium" into the underlying mesenchyme. The germinal epithelium is simply that part of the coelomic epithelium which gives rise to gonadal tissue. The invading cells form the primary sex cords which contain the germ cells surrounded by somatic cells (the cells destined to form the tissue which holds the germ cells). In a newer model, the somatic cells of the gonad are believed to arise from the mesonephros and not the coelomic epithelium.

4. testes-determining factor (TDF) p.97

The factor that determines whether the indifferent gonad will become a testis is called, appropriately, the testes-determining factor (TDF), a product of a gene located on the Y chromosome.

5. testosterone; antimüllerian hormone or müllerian inhibiting substance p.97

When the Y chromosome containing the testes determining region is present, the gonads develop into testes. The male phenotype is dependent upon the products (antimüllerian hormone and testosterone) of the fetal testes, while the female phenotype is the result of an absence of these fetal gonadal products. Antimüllerian hormone (AMH), which inhibits the formation of the müllerian ducts, is secreted at the time of Sertoli cell differentiation, beginning at 7 weeks. After involution of the müllerian system, AMH continues to be secreted, but there is no known function. In the ovary, very small amounts of AMH mRNA are present early in life, and although there may be no role in female development, its production later in life by the granulosa cells raises the possibility of autocrine/paracrine actions in oocyte maturation and follicular development.

6. 23 p.99

(See figure on page 38 in this Study Guide)

7. primordial p.100

At 14–20 weeks, the highly cellular cortex is gradually perforated by vascular channels originating in the deeper medullary areas. As the finger-like vascular projections enter the cortex, it takes on the appearance of secondary sex cords. As blood vessels invade and penetrate, they divide the previously solid cortical cell mass into smaller and smaller segments. Drawn in with the blood vessels are perivascular cells that are either mesenchymal or epithelial in origin. These cells surround the oocytes that have completed the first stage of meiosis. The resulting unit is **the *primordial follicle — an oocyte arrested in prophase of meiosis enveloped by a single layer of granulosa cells, surrounded by a basement membrane.*** Eventually all oocytes are covered in this fashion. Residual mesenchyme not utilized in primordial follicle formation is noted in the interstices between follicles, forming the primitive ovarian stroma. The granulosa cells differentiate from coelomic epithelial or mesenchymal precursors (their specific origin is still disputed). This process of primordial follicular development continues until all oocytes in the diplotene stage can be found in follicles, some time shortly after birth.

8. müllerian duct p.100

Unlike the male, gonadal steroid production is not required for development of a normal phenotype. The development of the müllerian duct into the fallopian tubes, the uterus, and the upper third of the vagina is totally independent of the ovary.

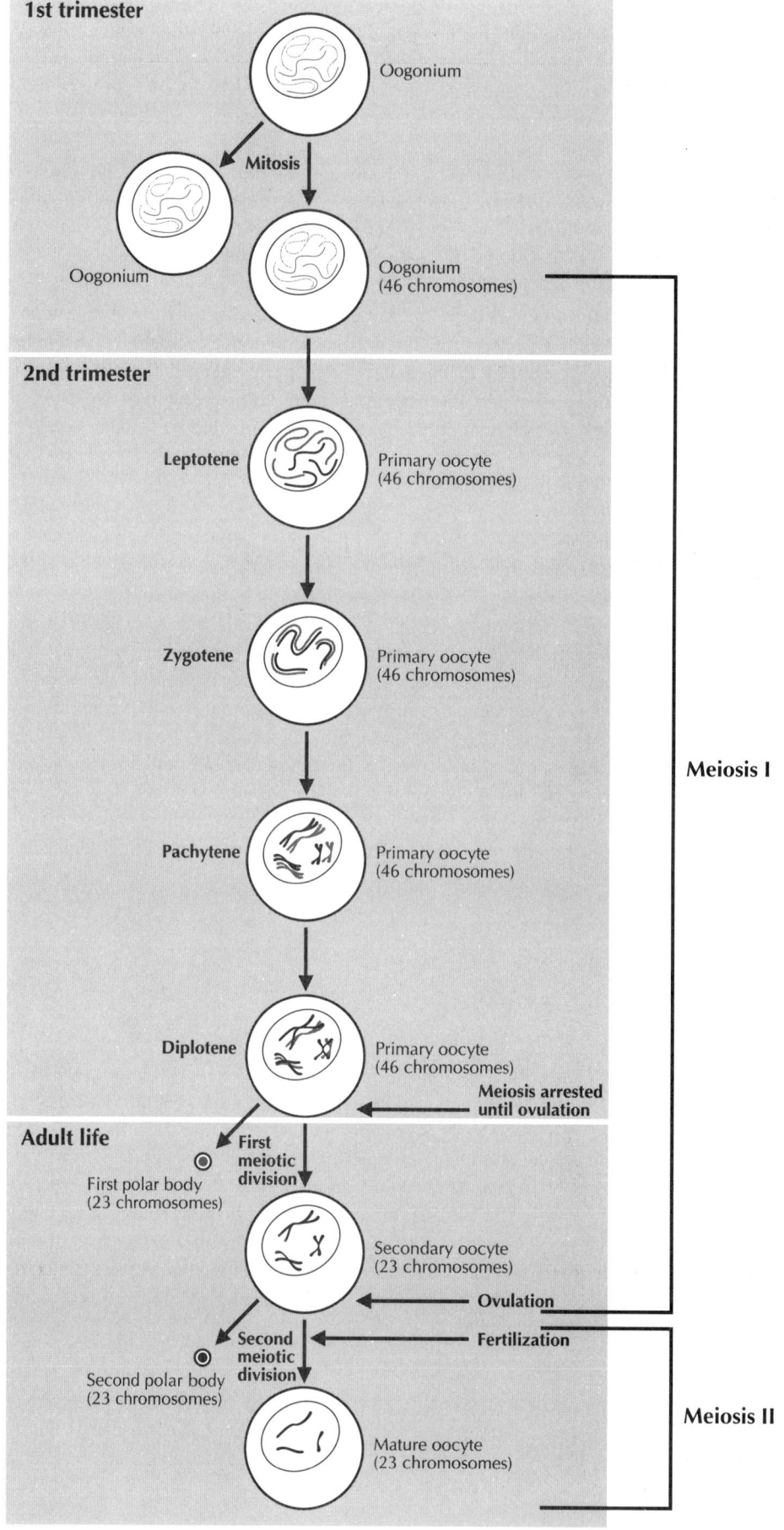

9. true   p.97

The testis begins its differentiation in week 6–7 of gestation by the appearance of Sertoli cells that aggregate to form the testicular cords. The primordial germ cells are embedded in the testicular cords that will form the Sertoli cells and spermatogonia. The mature Sertoli cells are the site of production of ABP (androgen binding protein, important in maintaining the high local androgen environment necessary for spermatogenesis) and inhibin.

10. true   p.96

If the indifferent gonad is destined to become a testis, differentiation along this line will take place at 6–9 weeks. The absence of testicular evolution (formation of medullary primary sex cords, primitive tubules, and incorporation of germ cells) gives implicit evidence of the existence of a primitive, albeit momentarily quiescent, ovary. In contrast to the male, female internal and external genitalia differentiation precedes gonadal maturation. These events are related to the genetic constitution and the territorial receptivity of the mesenchyme. If either factor is deficient or defective, improper development occurs. As has been noted, primitive germ cells are unable to survive in locations other than the gonadal ridge. If partial or imperfect gonadal tissue is formed, the resulting abnormal nonsteroidal and steroidal events have wide ranging morphologic, reproductive, and behavioral effects.

11. true   p.98

The differentiation of the wolffian system begins with the increase in testicular testosterone production. The classic experiments by Jost indicate that this effect of testosterone is due to local action, probably explaining why male internal genitalia in true hermaphrodites are only on the side of the testis. Not all androgen-sensitive tissues require the prior conversion of testosterone to dihydrotestosterone (DHT). In the process of masculine differentiation, the development of the wolffian duct structures (epididymis, the vas deferens, and the seminal vesicle) is dependent upon testosterone as the intracellular mediator, whereas development of the urogenital sinus and urogenital tubercle into the male external genitalia, urethra, and prostate requires the conversion of testosterone to DHT. In the female, the loss of the wolffian system is due to the lack of locally produced testosterone.

12. false   p.98

At 6–8 weeks, the first signs of ovarian differentiation are reflected in the rapid mitotic multiplication of germ cells, reaching 6–7 million oogonia by 16–20 weeks. This represents the maximal oogonal content of the gonad. From this point in time germ cell content will irretrievably decrease until, some 50 years later, the store of oocytes will be finally exhausted.

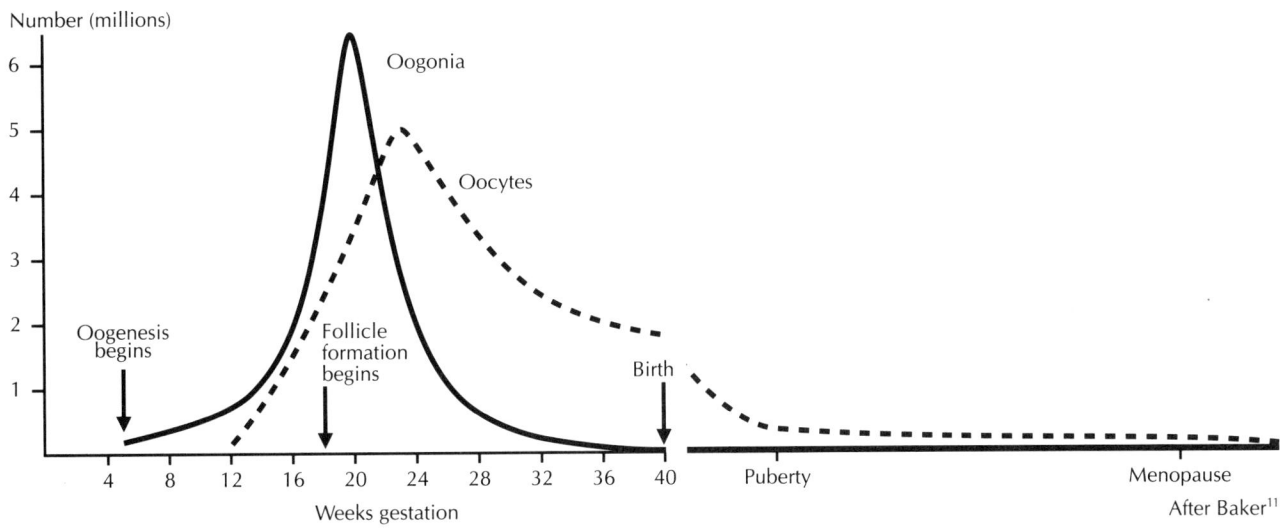

13. true   p.100

Chromosomal anomalies can accelerate germ cell loss. Individuals with Turner syndrome (45,X) experience normal migration and mitosis of germ cells, but the oogonia do not undergo meiosis, and rapid loss of oocytes leaves the gonad without follicles by birth, and it appears as a fibrous streak.

14. false   p.101

The anterior pituitary begins development between 4 and 5 weeks of fetal life. The median eminence is apparent by week 9, and the hypothalamic-pituitary portal circulation is functional by the 12th week of gestation. Pituitary levels of follicle-stimulating hormone (FSH) peak at 20–23 weeks, and circulating levels peak at 28 weeks. Levels are higher in female fetuses compared to males until the last 6 weeks of gestation. Ovaries in anencephalic fetuses (which lack gonadotropin releasing hormone [GnRH] and gonadotropin secretion) lack antral follicles and are smaller at term, but progression through meiosis and development of primordial follicles occur, apparently not dependent upon gonadotropins. The ovary develops receptors for gonadotropins only in the second half of pregnancy. Thus the loss of oocytes during fetal life cannot be solely explained by the decline in gonadotropins. The follicular growth and development observed in the second half of pregnancy, however, are gonadotropin dependent.

15. false   p.101

The total cortical content of germ cells falls to 1–2 million by birth as a result of prenatal oocyte depletion. This huge depletion of germ cell mass (close to 4–5 million) has occurred over as short a time as 20 weeks. No similar rate of depletion will be seen again. Due to the fixed initial endowment of germ cells, the newborn female enters life, still far from reproductive potential, having lost 80% of her oocytes.

16. true   p.102

The loss of oocytes (and follicles) through atresia is a response to changes in many factors. Certainly gonadotropin stimulation and withdrawal are important, but ovarian steroids and autocrine/paracrine factors are also involved. The consequence of these unfavorable changes, atresia, is a process called ***apoptosis,*** programmed cell death. This process is heralded by alterations in mRNAs required for cell proteins that maintain follicle integrity.

17. B   p.104

If gonadotropin stimulation is adequate, one of the several follicle units propelled to varying degrees of maturity will advance to ovulation. Morphologically these events include distension of the antrum by increments of antral fluid, and compression of the granulosa against the limiting membrane separating the avascular granulosa and the luteinized, vascularized theca interna. In addition, the antral fluid increment gradually pinches off the cumulus oophorous, the mound of granulosa enveloping the oocyte. The mechanisms of the thinning of the theca over the surface of the now protruding, distended follicle, the creation of an avascular area weakening the ovarian capsule, and the final acute distension of the antrum with rupture and extrusion of the oocyte in its cumulus, are multiple and complex. Repeated evaluation of intrafollicular pressures has failed to indict an explosive factor in this crucial event.

As demonstrated in a variety of animal experiments, the physical expulsion of the oocyte is dependent upon a preovulatory surge in prostaglandin synthesis within the follicle. Inhibition of this prostaglandin synthesis produces a corpus luteum with an entrapped oocyte. Both prostaglandins and the midcycle surge of gonadotropins are thought to increase the concentration and activity of local proteases, such as plasminogen conversion to plasmin. As a result of generalized tissue weakening (loss of intercellular gap junction integrity and disruption of elastic fibers), there is swift accumulation of antral fluid followed by rupture of the weakened tissue envelope surrounding the follicle.

18. E   p.104

Shortly after ovulation profound alterations in cellular organization occur in the ruptured follicle that go well beyond simple repair. After tissue integrity and continuity are retrieved, the granulosa cells hypertrophy markedly, gradually filling in the cystic, sometimes hemorrhagic, cavity of the early corpus luteum. In addition, for the first time, the granulosa becomes markedly luteinized by incorporation of lipid-rich vacuoles within its cytoplasm. Both these properties had been the exclusive features of the theca prior to ovulation. For its part, the theca of the corpus luteum becomes less prominent, vestiges being noted eventually only in the interstices of the typical scalloping of the mature corpus luteum. As a result, a new yellow body is formed, now dominated by the enlarged, lipid-rich, fully vascularized granulosa. In the 14 days of its life, dependent on the low but important quantities of LH available in the luteal phase, this unit produces estradiol and progesterone. Failing a new enlarging source of LH-like human chorionic gonadotropin (HCG) from a successful implantation, the corpus luteum rapidly ages. Its vascularity and lipid content wane, and the sequence of scarification (albicantia) ensues.

19. E p.102

In the last 10–15 years before menopause, there appears to be an acceleration of follicular loss. This loss correlates with a subtle but real increase in FSH and decrease in inhibin. The accelerated loss is probably secondary to the increase in FSH stimulation. Fewer follicles grow per cycle as a woman ages and cycles lengthen. These changes, including the increase in FSH (which is probably due to the decrease in inhibin), all reflect the reduced quality and capability of aging follicles.

4 The Uterus

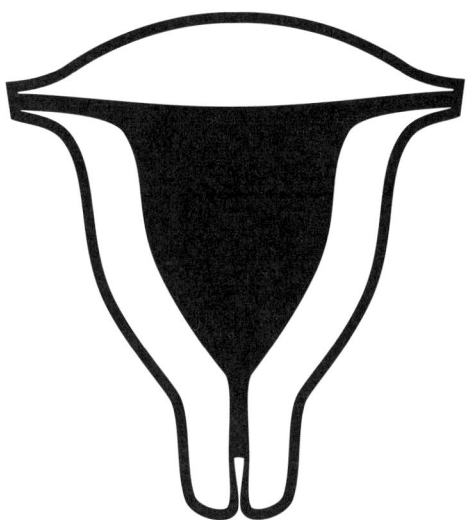

Learning Objectives

Be able to:

1. Describe the normal and abnormal development of the müllerian system.

2. Detail the histologic changes which occur in the endometrium during an ovulatory cycle.

3. Discuss the autocrine and paracrine functions within the uterus.

4. Describe what is known regarding the epidemiology, etiology, biology, medical and surgical treatment of leiomyomata.

5. Describe the mechanism of action of a GnRH-agonist, its potential side effects, its effectiveness in the treatment of leiomyomata and its limitations for long-term use.

Pre-Test

A. Instructions: Fill in the blanks

1. The critical factors secreted by the testes which direct sexual differentiation are _____ and _____.

2. The first histologic sign that ovulation has occurred is the appearance of _____ in the glandular epithelium.

B. Instructions: True or False

3. Antimüllerian hormone is synthesized by Sertoli cells and is responsible for the ipsilateral regression of the müllerian ducts by 8 weeks.

4. The purpose of the basalis layer is to provide the regenerative endometrium following menstrual loss of the functionalis.

C. Instructions: For each of the following questions, choose:

A. If only 1, 2, and 3 are correct
B. If only 1 and 3 are correct
C. If only 2 and 4 are correct
D. If only 4 is correct
E. If all are correct

5. The fertilized ovum
   1. remains unattached within the tubal lumen for at least 2 days.
   2. utilizes tubal fluids and residual cumulus cells to sustain its metabolism.
   3. enters the uterine cavity as a morula and remains unattached for another 2–3 days.
   4. 9 days following ovulation the embryo now a blastocyst is ready for implantation.

6. Leiomyomata
   1. are stimulated to grow when exposed to progestins.
   2. are infrequently associated with endometrial hyperplasia.
   3. can be reduced in size when treated with RU486.
   4. are a frequent cause of infertility.

7. GnRH agonists and steroid add-back
   1. may be a therapeutic option in selected patients.
   2. is being explored to permit long-term therapy without bone loss.
   3. has been documented to have been used up to 2 years without bone loss.
   4. may include agonist plus continuous add-back of estrogen and progestin.

Post-Test

A. Instructions: Fill in the blanks

1. The _____ and _____ ducts are discrete primordia that temporarily coexist in all embryos during the ambisexual period of development.

2. In the absence of _____, the fetus will develop fallopian tubes, uterus and upper vagina from the paramesonephric ducts.

3. In the presence of a normal ovary or the absence of any gonad, _____ duct development takes place.

4. During proliferation, the endometrium grows from approximately 0.5 mm to 3.5–5.0 mm in height. This proliferation is mainly in the _____ layer.

5. The total endometrial height is fixed after ovulation at roughly its preovulatory extent of _____ mm.

6. At the time of implantation, on days 21–22 of the cycle, the predominant morphologic feature is _____ of the _____.

7. The vasoconstriction and myometrial contractions associated with the menstrual events are mediated by _____.

8. Most women have menstrual cycles with an interval of _____ to _____ days. Only _____ % of reproductive age cycles are 28 days in length.

B. Instructions: True or False

9. Antimüllerian hormone (or müllerian inhibiting substance) is a member of the transforming growth factor-beta family of glycoprotein growth factors that include inhibin and activin.

10. The Sertoli cells secrete testosterone while the Leydig cells secrete antimüllerian hormone.

11. The fallopian tubes, uterus and the upper portion of the vagina are created by the fusion of the müllerian ducts by the 5th week of gestation.

12. The basal and spiral arteries are sensitive to hormonal changes.

13. The normal volume of menstrual blood loss is 50 mL, and greater than 100 mL is defined as abnormal.

14. Proliferation of the endometrium is marked by increased mitotic activity; increased nuclear DNA and cytoplasmic RNA synthesis with intranuclear concentrations of estrogen and progesterone receptors reaching a peak at midcycle prior to ovulation.

15. The prostaglandin content ($PGF_{2\alpha}$ and PGE_2) in the secretory endometrium reaches its highest levels at the time of menstruation.

16. Similar to postpartum bleeding, myometrial contractions are important for control of menstrual bleeding.

17. The basalis endometrium remains during menses and repair takes place from this layer.

18. The ovum must be fertilized within 12–24 hours of ovulation if a pregnancy is to take place.

C. Instructions: Match each item with the most appropriate word association:
   A. Lipid
   B. Cytokine
   C. Peptide

19. Thromboxane
20. Endorphin
21. Insulin-like growth factor
22. Interleukin-6
23. Leukotrienes

D. Instructions: For each of the following questions choose:
   A. if only 1, 2 and 3 are correct
   B. if only 1 and 3 are correct
   C. if only 2 and 4 are correct
   D. if only 4 is correct
   E. if all are correct

24. Endothelin-1
    1. is synthesized in endometrial stromal cells and glandular epithelium
    2. is a potent vasoconstrictor
    3. promotes the synthesis of endothelium-derived relaxing factor and prostacyclin
    4. is a potent stimulator of myometrial contractions and can contribute to dysmenorrhea

25. Progesterone antagonizes estrogen stimulation of proliferation by
    1. decreasing levels of estrogen receptors
    2. inducing enzymes that lead to excretion of estrogen from cells
    3. suppression of estrogen-mediated transcription of oncogenes
    4. decreasing the quality of estrogens receptors

26. Amniotic fluid prolactin
    1. is derived from the decidua
    2. reaches peak levels in the second half of gestation
    3. is unaffected by bromocriptine treatment
    4. is affected by prostaglandin and steroids

27. Congenital abnormalities of the müllerian ducts
    1. contribute to problems of infertility and recurrent pregnancy loss
    2. can produce symptoms of dysmenorrhea, dyspareunia and on occasion amenorrhea
    3. can originate in the failure of the müllerian ducts to fuse in the midline, to connect with the urogenital sinus or to resorb the septum between fused müllerian ducts
    4. has been classified into specific categories by the American Fertility Society

28. Congenital abnormality of the müllerian ducts
    1. should be treated based upon hysterosalpingography alone
    2. can often be accurately diagnosed using vaginal ultrasonography and/or magnetic resonance imaging thus avoiding the need for diagnostic laparoscopy
    3. is often associated with cardiac anomalies
    4. may involve renal agenesis on the same side as the müllerian defect

29. Leiomyomata
    1. are the indication for 10% of the hysterectomies performed in the U.S.
    2. may originate from somatic mutations in myometrial cells
    3. are thought not to be monoclonal in origin
    4. are found in over 75% of women who undergo hysterectomy

30. Leiomyomata during pregnancy
    1. usually do not grow
    2. may be accompanied by red degeneration resulting in pain
    3. are associated with a risk of premature labor depending upon their size
    4. usually regress in size following delivery

31. GnRH agonists
    1. are produced by substitution of amnio acids at the 6 position and/or replacement of the C-terminal glycine-amide in the GnRH molecule
    2. can be absorbed either intramuscularly, subcutaneously or by intranasally
    3. produce an initial increase in circulating FSH and LH within 1–3 weeks of administration
    4. cause down-regulation and desensitization of the pituitary to produce a hypogonadotropic, hypogonadal state

32. GnRH agonists in the treatment of leiomyomata
    1. can decrease uterine size by 30–64% after 3–6 months of treatment
    2. have their maximal effect upon uterine size by 3 months
    3. is associated with a return of menses 4–10 weeks following stopping their administration
    4. is associated with a return of uterine size to pretreatment levels by 4 months following discontinuation of their administration

33. Side effects associated with GnRH agonists
    1. include vaginal dryness, joint and muscle stiffness, depression, headache
    2. include hot flashes in less than 25% of patients usually 3–4 weeks after initiating treatment
    3. can include localized allergic reactions at the site of injection of depot forms in 10% of patients
    4. is never associated with bone loss if used for only 6 months

Answers for Chapter 4 — Pre-Test Questions

1. antimüllerian hormone; testosterone   p. 110
The critical factors in determining which of the duct structures stabilize or regress are the secretions from the testes: AMH (antimüllerian hormone, also known as müllerian inhibiting substance or müllerian inhibiting factor) and testosterone.

2. subnuclear intracytoplasmic glycogen vacuoles   p.116
The first histologic sign that ovulation has occurred is the appearance of subnuclear intracytoplasmic glycogen vacuoles in the glandular epithelium. Giant mitochondria and the "nucleolar channel system" appear in the gland cells. The nucleolar channel system is a unique appearance due to progesterone, presumably an infolding of the nuclear

membranes. Individual components of the tissue continue to display growth, but confinement in a fixed structure leads to progressive tortuosity of glands and intensified coiling of the spiral vessels. These structural alterations are soon followed by active secretion of glycoproteins and peptides into the endometrial cavity. Transudation of plasma also contributes to the endometrial secretions. Important immunoglobulins are obtained from the circulation and delivered to the endometrial cavity by binding proteins produced by the epithelial cells. The peak secretory level is reached 7 days after the midcycle gonadotropin surge, coinciding with the time of blastocyst implantation.

3. true   p.110

AMH is synthesized by Sertoli cells soon after testicular differentiation and is responsible for the ipsilateral regression of the müllerian ducts by 8 weeks. Despite its presence in serum up to puberty, lack of regression of the uterus and tubes is the only consistent expression of AMH gene mutations.

4. true   p.111

The endometrium can be divided morphologically into an upper two-thirds "functionalis" layer and a lower one-third "basalis" layer. The purpose of the functionalis layer is to prepare for the implantation of the blastocyst and, therefore, it is the site of proliferation, secretion, and degeneration. The purpose of the basalis layer is to provide the regenerative endometrium following menstrual loss of the functionalis.

5. A   p.121

For 2 days after fertilization, the ovum remains unattached within the tubal lumen utilizing tubal fluids and residual cumulus cells to sustain nutrition and energy for early cellular cleavage. After this stay, the solid ball of cells (morula) that is the embryo leaves the tube and enters the uterine cavity. Here the embryo undergoes another 2–3 days of unattached but active existence. Fortunately, by this time endometrial gland secretions have filled the cavity and they bathe the embryo in nutrients. This is the first of many neatly synchronized events that mark the conceptus-endometrial relationship. By 6 days after ovulation the embryo (now a blastocyst) is ready to attach and implant. At this time it finds an endometrial lining of sufficient depth, vascularity, and nutritional richness to sustain the important events of early placentation to follow. Just below the epithelial lining, a rich capillary plexus has been formed and is available for creation of the trophoblast-maternal blood interface. Later, the surrounding zona compactum, occupying more and more of the endometrium, will provide a sturdy splint to retain endometrial architecture despite the invasive inroads of the burgeoning trophoblast.

6. B   p.131

The hormone sensitivity of leiomyomas is indicated by the following clinical observations. Leiomyomas develop during the reproductive (hormonally active) years and regress after menopause. Occasionally, leiomyomas grow during pregnancy, and the hypogonadal state induced by treatment with gonadotropin releasing hormone (GnRH) agonists often causes shrinkage of myomas.

The environment within the leiomyoma is hyperestrogenic. The estradiol concentration is increased, and leiomyomas contain more estrogen receptors. Endometrial hyperplasia is frequently observed at the margins of submucous myomas. In the myometrium and in leiomyomas, peak mitotic activity occurs during the luteal phase, and mitotic activity is increased by the administration of high doses of progestational agents. These facts indicate that progesterone stimulates mitotic activity in leiomyomas, but animal studies indicate both stimulation and inhibition of myometrial growth. Similarly, clinicians have reported both regression and growth with progestational treatment. Nevertheless, most of the evidence supports a growth-promoting role for progestins (the association with estrogen can be explained by the estrogen enhancement of progesterone receptor expression). Treatment with RU486, the progesterone antagonist, is associated with a reduction in leiomyomata size.

7. E   p.134

Treatment with a GnRH agonist with steroid add-back has been explored to permit long-term therapy without bone loss. Two strategies have been employed: simultaneous agonist and steroid add-back treatment or a sequential regimen in which the agonist is used alone for 3–6 months, followed by the combination of the agonist and steroid add-back. This long-term treatment is attractive for women who are perimenopausal, perhaps avoiding surgery. In addition, long-term treatment would be useful for women with coagulopathies, and in women with medical problems who need to postpone surgery.

Simultaneous treatment with agonist and medroxyprogesterone acetate (20 mg orally daily) effectively reduced hot flushing, but was less effective in reducing uterine volume. A sequential program, adding a traditional postmenopausal hormone regimen (0.625 mg conjugated estrogens on days 1–25 and 10 mg medroxyprogesterone acetate on days 16–25) effectively reduced uterine volume and maintained the reduced volume for 2 years (and avoided any loss in bone density). Three to six months of GnRH agonist treatment is recommended followed by agonist treatment combined with a daily, continuous add-back of estrogen and progestin (0.625 mg conjugated estrogens or 1.0 mg estradiol and 2.5 mg medroxyprogesterone acetate or 0.35 mg norethindrone). In view of the sensitivity of leiomyomata tissue to progestational agents, it makes sense to keep the dose of progestin relatively low.

Answers for Chapter 4 — Post-Test Questions

1. wolffian; müllerian   p.110

The wolffian and müllerian ducts are discrete primordia that temporarily coexist in all embryos during the ambisexual period of development (up to 8 weeks). Thereafter, one type of duct system persists normally and gives rise to special ducts and glands, whereas the other disappears during the 3rd fetal month, except for nonfunctional vestiges.

2. antimüllerian hormone   p.110

In the absence of AMH, the fetus will develop fallopian tubes, uterus, and upper vagina from the paramesonephric ducts (the müllerian ducts). This development requires the prior appearance of the mesonephric ducts, and for this reason, abnormalities in development of the tubes, uterus, and upper vagina are associated with abnormalities in the renal system.

3. müllerian   p.111

The internal genitalia possess the intrinsic tendency to feminize. In the absence of a Y chromosome and a functional testis, the lack of AMH allows retention of the müllerian system and development of fallopian tubes, uterus, and upper vagina. In the absence of testosterone, the wolffian system regresses. In the presence of a normal ovary or the absence of any gonad, müllerian duct development takes place.

4. functionalis   p.115

The proliferative phase is associated with ovarian follicle growth and increased estrogen secretion. Undoubtedly as a result of this steroidal action, reconstruction and growth of the endometrium are achieved. The glands are most notable in this response. At first they are narrow and tubular, lined by low columnar epithelium cells. Mitoses become prominent and pseudostratification is observed. As a result, the glandular epithelium extends peripherally and links one gland segment with its immediate neighbor. A continuous epithelial lining is formed facing the endometrial cavity. The stromal component evolves from its dense cellular menstrual condition through a brief period of edema to a final loose syncytial-like status. Coursing through the stroma, spiral vessels extend unbranched to a point immediately below the epithelial binding membrane. Here they form a loose capillary network. All of the tissue components (glands, stromal cells, and endothelial cells) demonstrate proliferation which peaks on days 8–10 of the cycle. This proliferation is marked by increased mitotic activity and increased nuclear DNA and cytoplasmic RNA synthesis. Intranuclear concentrations of estrogen and progesterone receptors reach a peak at midcycle prior to ovulation. During proliferation, the endometrium grows from approximately 0.5 mm to 3.5–5.0 mm in height. This proliferation is mainly in the functionalis layer.

5. 5–6   p.115

After ovulation, the endometrium now demonstrates a combined reaction to estrogen and progesterone activity. Most impressive is that total endometrial height is fixed at roughly its preovulatory extent (5–6 mm) despite continued availability of estrogen. This restraint or inhibition is believed to be induced by progesterone. This limitation of growth is associated with a decline in mitosis and DNA synthesis, significantly due to progesterone interference with estrogen receptor expression and progesterone stimulation of 17β-hydroxysteroid dehydrogenase and sulfotransferase, which convert estradiol to estrone sulfate (which is rapidly excreted from the cell). In addition, estrogen stimulates many oncogenes that probably mediate estrogen-induced growth. Progesterone also antagonizes this action by suppressing the estrogen-mediated transcription of oncogene mRNA.

6. edema; endometrial stroma   p.117

At the time of implantation, on days 21–22 of the cycle, the predominant morphologic feature is edema of the endometrial stroma. This change may be secondary to the estrogen and progesterone mediated increase in prostaglandin production by the endometrium. An increase in capillary permeability is a consequence of this local increase in prostaglandins. Receptors for the sex steroids are present in the muscular walls of the endometrial blood vessels and the enzyme system for prostaglandin synthesis is present in both the muscular walls and the endothelium of the endometrial arterioles. The vascular proliferation that leads to the coiling of the spiral vessels is a response to the sex steroids, the prostaglandins, and to autocrine/paracrine factors produced in response to estrogen and progesterone.

7. prostaglandins   p.119

The withdrawal of estrogen and progesterone initiates three endometrial events: vasomotor reactions, tissue loss, and menstruation. The most prominent immediate effect of this hormone withdrawal is a modest shrinking of the tissue height and remarkable spiral arteriole vasomotor responses. The following vascular sequence has been constructed from direct observations of rhesus endometrium. With shrinkage of height, blood flow within the spiral vessels diminishes, venous drainage is decreased, and vasodilatation ensues. Thereafter, the spiral arterioles undergo rhythmic vasoconstriction and relaxation. Each successive spasm is more prolonged and profound, leading eventually to endometrial blanching. Within the 24 hours immediately preceding menstruation, these reactions lead to endometrial ischemia and stasis. White cells migrate through capillary walls, at first remaining adjacent to vessels, but then extending throughout the stroma. During arteriolar vasomotor changes, red blood cells escape into the interstitial space. Thrombin-platelet plugs also appear in superficial vessels. The prostaglandin content ($PGF_{2\alpha}$ and PGE_2) in the secretory endometrium reaches its highest levels at the time of menstruation. The vasoconstriction and myometrial contractions associated with the menstrual events are believed to be significantly mediated by the prostaglandins.

8. 21; 35; 15   p.119

Most women have menstrual cycles with an interval of 21 to 35 days. Menarche is followed by approximately 5–7 years of increasing regularity as cycles shorten to reach the usual reproductive age pattern. In the forties, cycles begin to lengthen again. The perfect 28-day cycle is the most common mode, but only 15% of reproductive age cycles are 28 days in length.

9. true   p.110

AMH is a member of the transforming growth factor-β family of glycoprotein differentiation factors that include inhibin and activin.

10. false   p.110

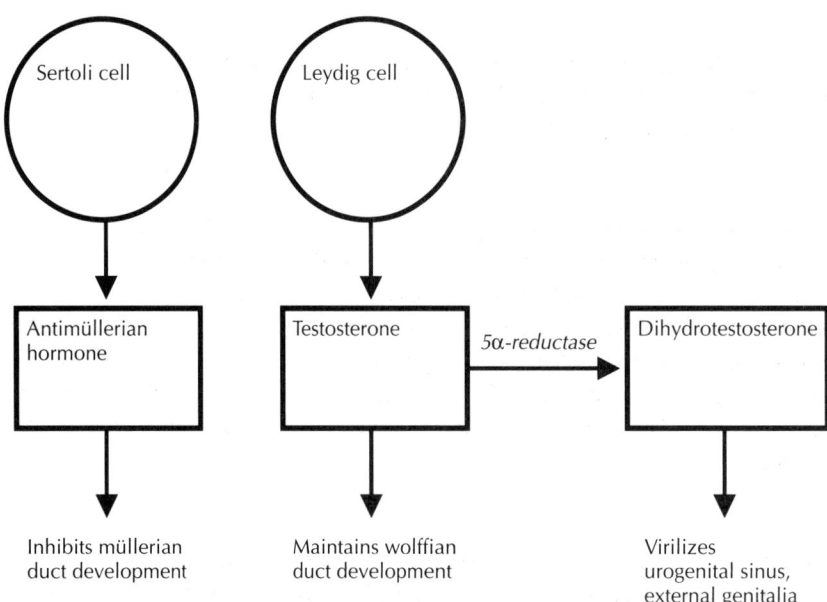

11. false   p.111
The fallopian tubes, uterus, and the upper portion of the vagina are created by the fusion of the müllerian ducts by the 10th week of gestation.

12. false   p.112
The two uterine arteries which supply the uterus are branches of the internal iliac arteries. At the lower part of the uterus, the uterine artery separates into the vaginal artery and an ascending branch that divides into the arcuate arteries. The arcuate arteries run parallel to the uterine cavity and anastomose with each other, forming a vascular ring around the cavity. Small centrifugal branches (the radial arteries) leave the arcuate vessels, perpendicular to the endometrial cavity, to supply the myometrium. When these arteries enter the endometrium, small branches (the basal arteries) extend laterally to supply the basalis layer. These basal arteries do not demonstrate a response to hormonal changes. The radial arteries continue in the direction of the endometrial surface, now assuming a corkscrew appearance (and now called the spiral arteries), to supply the functionalis layer of the endometrium. It is the spiral artery (an end artery) segment which is very sensitive to hormonal changes. One reason the functionalis layer is more vulnerable to vascular permutations is that there are no anastomoses among the spiral arteries. The endometrial glands and the stromal tissue are supplied by capillaries that emerge from the spiral arteries at all levels of the endometrium. The capillaries drain into a venous plexus and eventually into the myometrial arcuate veins and into the uterine veins. This unique vascular architecture is important in allowing a repeated sequence of endometrial growth and desquamation.

13. false   p.119
The usual duration of flow is 4–6 days, but many women flow as little as 2 days and as much as 8 days. The normal volume of menstrual blood loss is 30 mL; greater than 80 mL is abnormal.

14. true   p.113,114
The proliferative phase is associated with ovarian follicle growth and increased estrogen secretion. Undoubtedly as a result of this steroidal action, reconstruction and growth of the endometrium are achieved. The glands are most notable in this response. At first they are narrow and tubular, lined by low columnar epithelium cells. Mitoses become prominent and pseudostratification is observed. As a result, the glandular epithelium extends peripherally and links one gland segment with its immediate neighbor. A continuous epithelial lining is formed facing the endometrial cavity. The stromal component evolves from its dense cellular menstrual condition through a brief period of edema to a final loose syncytial-like status. Coursing through the stroma, spiral vessels extend unbranched to a point immediately below the epithelial binding membrane. Here they form a loose capillary network. All of the tissue components (glands, stromal cells, and endothelial cells) demonstrate proliferation which peaks on days 8–10 of the cycle. This proliferation is marked by increased mitotic activity and increased nuclear DNA and cytoplasmic RNA synthesis. Intranuclear concentrations of estrogen and progesterone receptors reach a peak at midcycle prior to ovulation.

15. true   p.119
The prostaglandin content ($PGF_{2\alpha}$ and PGE_2) in the secretory endometrium reaches its highest levels at the time of menstruation. The vasoconstriction and myometrial contractions associated with the menstrual events are believed to be significantly mediated by the prostaglandins.

16. false   p.119
Increased blood loss is a consequence of reduced platelet numbers and inadequate hemostatic plug formation. With further tissue disorganization, the endometrium shrinks further and coiled arterioles are buckled. Additional ischemic breakdown ensues with necrosis of cells and defects in vessels adding to the menstrual effluvium. A natural cleavage point exists between basalis and spongiosum, and, once breached, the loose, vascular, edematous stroma of the spongiosum desquamates and collapses. In the end, the typical deflated shallow dense menstrual endometrium results. Menstrual flow stops as a result of the combined effects of prolonged vasoconstriction, tissue collapse, vascular stasis, and estrogen-induced "healing." In contrast to postpartum bleeding, myometrial contractions are not important for control of menstrual bleeding.

17. true   p.119
The basalis endometrium remains during menses, and repair takes place from this layer. This endometrium is protected from the lytic enzymes in the menstrual fluid by a mucinous layer of carbohydrate products that are discharged from

the glandular and stromal cells. The menstrual fluid is composed of the autolysed functionalis, inflammatory exudate, red blood cells, and proteolytic enzymes (at least one of which, plasmin, lyses fibrin clots as they form). The high fibrinolytic activity advances emptying of the uterus by liquefaction of tissue and fibrin. If the rate of flow is great, clotting can and does occur.

18. true   p.121
The ovum must be fertilized within 12–24 hours of ovulation.

Failure of the appearance of human chorionic gonadotropin, despite otherwise appropriate tissue reactions, leads to the vasomotor changes associated with estrogen-progesterone withdrawal and menstrual desquamation. However, not all the tissue is lost, and, in any event, a residual basalis is always available, making resumption of growth with estrogen a relatively rapid process. Indeed, even as menses persists, early regeneration can be seen. As soon as follicle maturation occurs (in as short a time as 10 days), the endometrium is ready once again to perform its reproductive function.

19. A   p.122

20. C   p.122

21. C   p.122

22. B   p.122

23. A   p.122

Lipids	Cytokines	Peptides
Prostaglandins	Interleukin-1α	Prolactin
Thromboxanes	Interleukin-1β	Relaxin
Leukotrienes	Interleukin-6	Renin
	Interferon-γ	Endorphin
	Colony-stimulating factor-1	Epidermal growth factor
		Insulin-like growth factors
		Fibroblast growth factor
		Platelet-derived growth factor
		Transforming growth factor
		IGFBPs
		Corticotropin releasing hormone
		Fibronectin
		Tumor necrosis factor
		Parathyroid hormone-like

24. E   p.124
Endothelin-1 is a potent vasoconstrictor, but its vasoconstrictor activity is balanced by the fact that it promotes the synthesis of endothelium-derived relaxing factor and prostacyclin. Endothelin-1 is synthesized in endometrial stromal cells and the glandular epithelium, stimulated by both TGF-β and interleukin-1α. Endothelin-1 may be at least one agent that is responsible for the vasoconstriction that shuts off menstrual bleeding. It is also a potent stimulator of

myometrial contractions and can contribute to dysmenorrhea. Finally, endothelin-1 is also a mitogen and can promote the healing reepithelialization of the endometrium. Human decidual cells also synthesize and secrete endothelin-1, from where it may be transported into the amniotic fluid.

25. A p.125

Progesterone antagonizes estrogen stimulation of proliferation and metabolism. This antagonism can be explained by the effects of progestins on the estrogen receptor (a decrease in levels) and on the enzymes that lead to excretion of estrogen from cells and by progesterone suppression of estrogen-mediated transcription of oncogenes.

26. B p.126

There is good reason to believe that the amniotic fluid prolactin is derived from the decidua. In vitro experiments indicate that the passage of prolactin across the fetal membranes is in the direction of the amniotic cavity. The amniotic fluid concentration correlates with the decidual content, not maternal circulating levels. Amniotic fluid prolactin reaches peak levels in the first half of gestation (about 4,000 ng/mL [180 nmol/L]) when maternal plasma levels are approximately 50 ng/mL (2,220 pmol/L) and fetal levels about 10 ng/mL (440 pmol/L). Maternal circulating prolactin reaches maximal levels near term. Finally, amniotic fluid prolactin is unaffected by bromocriptine treatment (which reduces both fetal and maternal circulating levels to baseline levels).

27. E p.127,130

Congenital abnormalities of the müllerian ducts are relatively common and contribute to the problems of infertility, recurrent pregnancy loss, and poor outcome in pregnancy (encountered in approximately 25% of women with uterine anomalies). The problems encountered in pregnancy include preterm labor, breech presentations, and complications that lead to interventions and greater perinatal mortality. Cervical cerclage is often indicated for prevention of preterm labor due to these anomalies. In addition, these abnormalities can produce the symptoms of dysmenorrhea and dyspareunia, and even amenorrhea. Because the embryologic origin of the ovaries is separate and distinct from that of the müllerian structures, patients with müllerian anomalies have normal ovaries and ovarian function.

Anomalies can originate in the failure of the müllerian ducts to fuse in the midline, to connect with the urogenital sinus, or to create the appropriate lumen in the upper vagina and uterus by resorption of the central vaginal cells and the septum between the fused müllerian ducts. Because fusion begins in the midline and extends caudally and cephalad, abnormal results can exist at either end. Formation of the uterine cavity begins at the lower pole and extends cephalad with dissolution of midline tissue; hence, incomplete resorption of tissue commonly yields persistence of midline uterine wall intruding into the cavity. The molecular pathophysiology of these abnormalities has been insufficiently studied; however, the association with other somatic anomalies and occasional reports of familial transmission suggest genetic linkages.

Vaginal outflow tract obstruction can be minimal with a transverse septum or complete due to agenesis. A septum is the result of a defect in the connection of the fused müllerian ducts to the urogenital sinus or a failure of canalization of the vagina. Vaginal agenesis is the result of a complete failure in canalization. These patients present with amenorrhea or pain due to accumulated menstrual effluvium. Surgical correction is frequently necessary to relieve the relative constriction (and obstruction) of the vaginal canal. An absent vagina is usually accompanied by an absent uterus and tubes, the classic müllerian agenesis of the Mayer-Rokitansky-Kuster-Hauser syndrome

28. C p.130

Hysterosalpingography is relatively inaccurate, and decisions should not be based upon hysterosalpingography alone. Congenital anomalies of the müllerian ducts are frequently accompanied by abnormalities in the urinary tract. Renal agenesis is often present on the same side as a müllerian defect. In the past full diagnosis has required surgical intervention, first laparotomy and then, more recently, laparoscopy. Today, vaginal ultrasonography and magnetic resonance imaging are highly accurate, and surgical intervention is usually not necessary.

29. C p.130,131

Uterine leiomyomas are benign neoplasms that arise from uterine smooth muscle. It is hypothesized that leiomyomas originate from somatic mutations in myometrial cells, resulting in progressive loss of growth regulation. The tumor grows as genetically abnormal clones of cells derived from a single progenitor cell (in which the original mutation took place). Studies indicate that leiomyomas are monoclonal. Different rates of growth can reflect the different cytogenetic abnormalities present in individual tumors. Multiple myomas within the same uterus are not clonally related; each myoma arises independently. The presence of multiple myomas (which have a higher recurrence rate than single myomas) argues in favor of a genetic predisposition for myoma formation; however, the familial inheritance of uterine myomas has not been well studied. It is not certain whether leiomyosarcomas arise independently or from leiomyomas.

If surgical specimens are serially sectioned, about 77% of women who come to hysterectomy will have myomas, many of which are occult. Overall, about 17% of hysterectomies are performed for myomas in the U.S. (44% in women 45–54 years old). The peak incidence for myomas requiring surgery occurs around age 45, approximately 8 cases per 1,000 women each year. In the U.S., approximately 10–15% of women require hysterectomy for myomas.

Myomas will be encountered in about 1% of pregnant women. The risk of myoma is decreased with increasing parity and with increasing age at last term birth. Women with at least two full term pregnancies have half the risk for myomas. Smoking decreases the risk (presumably by decreasing estrogen levels), and obesity increases the risk (presumably by increasing estrogen levels). Indeed, a lower risk for myomas is associated with factors that decrease estrogen levels, including leanness, smoking, and exercise. The use of oral contraceptives is not associated with an increased risk of uterine myomas.

30. E   p.132

Most myomas do not grow during pregnancy. When they do, most of the growth is in the first trimester, and most myomas regress in size after the pregnancy. The size of a myoma will not predict its course; large myomas will not necessarily grow more than a small one. So-called red degeneration of myomas is occasionally observed during pregnancy, a condition due to central hemorrhagic infarction of the myoma. Pain is the hallmark of this condition, occasionally associated with rebound tenderness, mild fever, leukocytosis, nausea, and vomiting. Usually pain is the only symptom and resolution follows rest and analgesic treatment. Surgery should be a last resort. The larger the myoma, the greater the risk of premature labor.

31. E   p.132

The short half-life of GnRH is due to rapid cleavage of the bonds between amino acids 5–6, 6–7, and 9–10. By altering amino acids at these positions, analogues of GnRH can be synthesized with different properties. Substitution of amino acids at the 6 position or replacement of the C-terminal glycine-amide (inhibiting degradation) produces agonists. The GnRH agonists are administered either intramuscularly, subcutaneously, or by intranasal absorption. An initial agonistic action (the so-called flare effect) is associated with an increase in the circulating levels of follicle-stimulating hormone (FSH) and luteinizing hormone (LH). This response is greatest in the early follicular phase when GnRH and estradiol have combined to create a large reserve pool of gonadotropins. After 1–3 weeks, down-regulation and desensitization of the pituitary produce a hypogonadotropic, hypogonad state. The initial response is due to a loss of receptors, while the sustained response is due to desensitization, the uncoupling of the receptor from its effector system. Furthermore, postreceptor mechanisms lead to secretion of biologically inactive gonadotropins, which, however, can still be detected by immunoassay.

The GnRH analogues cannot escape destruction if administered orally. Higher doses administered subcutaneously can achieve nearly equal effects as observed with intravenous treatment; however, the smaller blood peaks are slower to develop and take longer to return to baseline. Other forms of administration include nasal spray, sustained release implants, and injections of biodegradable microspheres.

32. E   p.133

Summarizing the experience with GnRH agonist treatment of leiomyomata, the mean uterine size decreases 30–64% after 3–6 months of treatment. Maximal response is usually achieved by 3 months. The reduction in size correlates with the estradiol level and with body weight. Menorrhagia, anemia, pelvic pressure, and urinary frequency all respond favorably to GnRH agonist treatment. A decrease in operative blood loss is significant when the uterus is the size of a 16 week pregnancy. Why is there a variation in response? When one considers the many factors involved in myoma growth (estrogen, progesterone, growth factors, receptors), it makes sense that not every myoma is the same. After cessation of GnRH agonist therapy, menses return in 4–10 weeks, and myoma and uterine size return to pretreatment levels in 3–4 months.

Preoperative GnRH agonist therapy offers several advantages for hysteroscopic removal of submucous tumors. In addition to a decrease in myoma size, endometrial atrophy will improve visualization, and decreased vascularity will reduce blood loss.

33. B p.133

Hot flushes are experienced by more than 75% of patients, usually in 3–4 weeks after beginning treatment. Approximately 5–15% of patients will complain of headache, vaginal dryness, joint and muscle stiffness, and depression. About 30% of patients will continue to have irregular (although light) vaginal bleeding. It is useful to measure the circulating estradiol level. If the level is greater than 30 pg/mL (110 pmol/L), suppression is inadequate. On the other hand, Friedman and colleagues have suggested that maintaining the estradiol level in the early follicular phase range (30–50 pg/mL [110–180 pmol/L]) can protect against osteoporosis and reduce hot flushes, but not allow the growth of myomas. The efficacy of this titration of response requires validation by clinical studies.

A small number (10%) of patients will experience a localized allergic reaction at the site of injection of depot forms of GnRH analogues. More serious reaction is rare, but immediate and delayed anaphylaxis can occur, requiring intense support and management.

Bone loss occurs with GnRH therapy, but not in everyone, and it is reversible (although it is not certain if it is totally reversible in all patients). A significant vaginal hemorrhage 5–10 weeks after beginning treatment is encountered in about 2% of treated women, due to degeneration and necrosis of submucous myomas. A disadvantage of agonist treatment is a delay in diagnosis of a leiomyosarcoma. Keep in mind that almost all leiomyosarcomas present as the largest or only uterine mass. Close monitoring is necessary and surgery is indicated when either enlargement or no shrinkage of myomas occurs during GnRH agonist treatment. The use of Doppler ultrasonography or magnetic resonance imaging offer greater accuracy of evaluation.

Escape of suppression can result in an unexpected pregnancy. No adverse effects of fetal exposure to GnRH agonists have been reported, even when exposure has persisted throughout the early weeks of pregnancy.

5 Neuroendocrinology

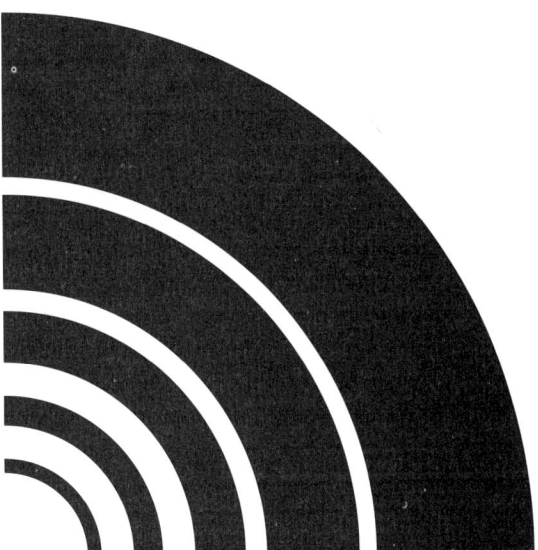

Learning Objectives

1. Describe the components, their anatomical relationship and function composing the hypothalamic-hypophyseal portal circulation.

2. Describe the structure, mechanism of action, and regulation of gonadotropin releasing hormone (GnRH) and its analogues.

3. Detail the role of dopamine as it affects the action of GnRH and prolactin.

4. Discuss the following and their role in regulating timing of GnRH pulses: arcuate nucleus, tuberoinfundibular tract, norepinephrine tract, estrogen, progesterone.

5. Detail the role endogenous opiates may play in the regulation of the menstrual cycle.

6. Describe the anatomy and function of the posterior pituitary pathway.

7. Discuss the possible function and physiology of the pineal gland.

8. Describe the pattern of gonadotropin secretion in fetal life, prepuberty and puberty.

Pre-Test

A. Instructions: Fill in the blanks

1. The cells which produce GnRH originate from the _____ area.

2. There are 3 classes of opiates: _____, _____ and _____.

B. Instructions: True or False

3. Prolactin gene expression occurs in lactotrophs of the anterior pituitary gland, in decidualized endometrium and the myometrium.

4. Dopamine does not exert a direct effect on gonadotropin secretion by the anterior pituitary but directly supressess GnRH release in the hypothalamus.

C. Instructions: For each of the following questions choose:

A. if only 1, 2 and 3 are correct
B. if only 1 and 3 are correct
C. if only 2 and 4 are correct
D. if only 4 is correct
E. if all are correct

5. Inhibin
   1. contains two identical beta-subunits
   2. is peptide member of the transforming growth factor beta family
   3. inhibits both FSH and LH
   4. is secreted by granulosa cells

6. Tanycytes
   1. are part of the tuberoinfundibular tract
   2. are specialized ependymal cells lining the third ventricle area the median eminence
   3. do not change morphologically in response to steroids
   4. terminate on portal vessels and transport materials from ventricular CSF to the portal system

7. The onset of female puberty
   1. is associated with a rise in serum DHA, DHAS beginning at 6–8 years of age
   2. is dependent upon the onset of secretion of melatonin
   3. is preceded by an increase in pulse frequency, amplitude and regularity of gonadotropins
   4. is marked by an equal rise in biologically and immunoreactive LH

Chapter 5 Neuroendocrinology

Post-Test

A. Instructions: Fill in the blanks

1. The superior _____ arteries form a dense network of capillaries within the median eminence, which then drains into the _____ vessels that descend along the pituitary stalk to the _____ pituitary.

2. The neurohormone that controls prolactin is called _____ _____ hormone and is probably _____.

3. The _____ is the part of the _____ at the base of the brain that forms the floor of the _____ ventricle and part of its lateral walls.

4. The _____ _____ together with the _____ _____ can be viewed as a unit where GnRH secretion into the portal circulation is initiated.

5. Like GnRH, gonadotropins are also secreted in a _____ fashion.

6. Normal menstrual cycle require the maintenance of the pulsatile release of _____ within a critical range of _____ and _____.

7. The dopamine _____ tract arises within the _____ _____ hypothalamus and projects into the _____ _____.

8. The current concept is that the biogenic catecholamines modulate GnRH pulsatile release. _____ is thought to exert stimulatory effects on GnRH, while _____ and _____ exert inhibitory effects.

B. Instructions: True or False

9. Human corticotropin releasing hormone (CRH) suppresses gonadotropin secretion, an action mediated by endorphin inhibition of GnRH.

10. Purified or synthesized GnRH stimulates both FSH and LH secretion.

11. Pituitary secretion prolactin is chiefly under the stimulatory control of hypothalamic dopamine released into the portal circulation.

12. Other factors besides dopamine that are involved in regulation of prolactin secretion include TRH and vasoactive intestinal peptide (VIP).

13. Kallman's syndrome is due to a mutation of a single gene on the short arm of the X chromosome in the Xp 22.3 region, which encodes for a protein necessary for neuronal migration.

14. The arcuate nucleus is the central site of action, releasing GnRH in a pulsatile fashion into the portal circulation.

15. Pulsatile secretion of LH and/or GnRH is less frequent but greater amplitude during the follicular phase compared to the luteal phase.

16. For an understanding of clinical problems, it is best to view dopamine as an inhibitor of prolactin and GnRH.

17. GnRH is calcium dependent in its mechanism of action and utilizes inositol 1,4,5-triphosphate (IP_3) and cyclic AMP as second messengers to stimulate a protein kinase.

18. Opioid tone plays a minor role in regulation of menstrual function and cyclicity.

19. The principal endogenous opiates affecting GnRH release are beta-endorphin and enkephalins.

C. Instructions: *Match each brain peptide with the appropriate phrase*

A. Somatostatin
B. Activin
C. Inhibin
D. Neuropeptide Y
E. Follistatin
F. Endothelins

20. Exists as three forms.
21. Produced by granulosa cells and selectively inhibits FSH.
22. Inhibits release of prolactin, TSH and growth hormone from the pituitary.
23. Elevated in the cerebrospinal fluid of women with anorexia and bulimia nervosa.

D. Instructions: *For each of the following questions choose:*

A. if only 1, 2 and 3 are correct
B. if only 1 and 3 are correct
C. if only 2 and 4 are correct
D. if only 4 is correct
E. if all are correct

24. GnRH
    1. requires a G protein receptor as part of its mechanism of action
    2. involves cyclic AMP as a second messenger
    3. involves protein kinase and calmodulin as mediators of its action
    4. promotes the synthesis of gonadotropins to take place in the golgi

25. The endogenous opiates
    1. stimulate gonadotropin secretion
    2. are derived from one of 3 precursor peptides
    3. act exclusively through mu receptors
    4. play a role in regulating the menstrual cycle

26. Proopiomelanocortin (POMC)
    1. is the source of endorphins
    2. is found in highest concentration in the pituitary
    3. is split into 2 fragments: ACTH and beta-lipoprotein
    4. gene expression is regulated by sex steroids

27. GnRH secretion can be inhibited by
    1. corticotropin-releasing hormone (CRH)
    2. the administration of naltrexone
    3. an increase in endogenous opioid tone
    4. norepinephrine

28. Beta-endorphin
    1. can cause release of prolactin
    2. reaches highest levels just before ovulation
    3. is a principal endogenous opiate which affects GnRH release
    4. is derived from beta-lipoprotein

29. Pulses of GnRH
    1. are required at a critical range of frequency and amplitude for normal menstrual function
    2. is under the influence of a dual catecholaminergic system
    3. are influenced by endogenous opioid activity
    4. are influenced by steroids possibly mediated through catecholsteroid messengers or various neurotransmitters

30. GnRH agonists
    1. are produced by substituting amnio acids which result in inhibiting degradation of the analogue molecule
    2. undergoes cleavage of the bonds between amnio acids 9–10 by endopeptidase and between 5–6 and 6–7 by carboxyamide peptidase
    3. initially cause down-regulation followed by desensitization
    4. post receptor mechanisms lead to secretion of biologically active gonadotropins

31. GnRH antagonists
    1. do not cause an initial increase in FSH or LH
    2. bind to the GnRH receptor and provide competitive inhibition to the endogenous GnRH
    3. produce an immediate therapeutic effect
    4. in combination with testosterone hold promise as a potential male contraceptive

32. The posterior pituitary
    1. is limited to the transport of vasopressin and oxytocin to the posterior pituitary
    2. connects to tanycytes
    3. receives direct transmission of signals from the pineal gland
    4. is a direct prolongation of the hypothalamus via the pituitary stalk

33. Oxytocin and vasopressin
    1. consists of 9 amnio acid residues
    2. have genes which are closely linked on the same chromosome
    3. circulate as the free peptides with rapid half-lives of less than 4 minutes
    4. have similar physiological functions

34. Estrogen
    1. at low levels enhance FSH and LH synthesis and storage while having little effect on LH secretion and inhibiting FSH secretion
    2. at low levels act at the level of the pituitary gland to enhance the LH response to GnRH
    3. at high levels induces the LH surge at midcycle
    4. at high levels are responsible for the FSH surge at midcycle

35. The pineal gland
    1. may be the source of gonadal inhibiting substances
    2. contains an enzyme essential for melatonin synthesis
    3. tends to become calcified with age
    4. responses to photic and hormonal stimuli and exhibits circadian rhythms

36. Melatonin
    1. synthesis requires the presence of hydroxyindole-o-methyltransferase (HIOMT)
    2. synthesis is controlled by norepinephrine stimulation of adenylate cyclase
    3. is synthesized mainly in pineal parenchymal cells
    4. secretion increases in daylight

37. Fetal gonadotropins
    1. are peaked at 28 weeks in utero
    2. peak after maximum numbers of oogonia and oocytes are produced in utero
    3. are lower in males than females probably due to testosterone and inhibin
    4. begin to be produced in the pituitary by 12 weeks of intrauterine life

38. Female puberty
    1. has the following typical sequence of events: thelarche, pubarche, menarche, growth spirit
    2. begins between 8 and 14 years of age
    3. is associated with a rise in LH and little change in FSH
    4. usually takes 2 to 4 years from its onset to completion

39. Women with gonadal dysgenesis
    1. demonstrate augmented gonadotropin secretion during sleep
    2. have normal serum FSH levels between ages 2 and 6
    3. have elevated serum FSH levels consistent with normal menopausal values as teenagers
    4. have rises and declines in their gonadotropins at different points of their development which support the concept of a central nervous system inhibitory force suppressing GnRH pulsatile secretion

Answers for Chapter 5 — Pre-Test Questions

1. olfactory $\hfill$ p.145
The cells which produce GnRH originate from the olfactory area. By migration during embryogenesis, the cells move along cranial nerves connecting the nose and the forebrain to their primary location, the arcuate nucleus of the hypothalamus.

2. enkephalins; endorphin; dynorphin $\hfill$ p.155
There are 3 classes of opiates: enkephalins, endorphin, and dynorphin. Proopiomelanocortin is split into 2 fragments, an ACTH intermediate fragment and β-lipotropin. β-Lipotropin has no opioid activity but is broken down in a series of steps to β-melanocyte-stimulating hormone (β-MSH), enkephalin, and α-, γ-, and β-endorphins. Melanocyte-stimulating hormone acts in lower animals to stimulate melanin granules within cells, causing darkening of the skin. In humans, there is no known function.

Enkephalin and the α- and γ-endorphins are as active as morphine on a molar basis, while β-endorphin is 5–10 times more potent. In the adult pituitary gland, the major products are ACTH and β-lipotropin, with only small amounts of endorphin. Thus, ACTH and β-lipotropin blood levels show similar courses, and they are major secretion products of the anterior pituitary in response to stress. In the intermediate lobe of the pituitary (which is prominent only during fetal life), ACTH is cleaved to CLIP (corticotropin-like intermediate lobe peptide) and β-MSH. In the placenta and adrenal medulla, POMC processing yields α-MSH-like and β-endorphin peptides. β-Endorphin has also been detected in the ovaries and in the testes.

In the brain, the major products are the opiates, with little ACTH. In the hypothalamus the major products are β-endorphin and α-MSH in the region of the arcuate nucleus and the ventromedial nucleus. The pituitary system is a system for secretion into the circulation while the hypothalamic system allows for distribution via axons to regulate other brain regions and the pituitary gland.

β-Endorphin is appropriately considered a neurotransmitter, a neurohormone, and a neuromodulator. β-Endorphin influences a variety of hypothalamic functions, including regulation of reproduction, temperature, cardiovascular and respiratory function, as well as extrahypothalamic functions such as pain perception and mood. POMC gene expression in the anterior pituitary is controlled mainly by adrenal hormones, stimulated by CRH (corticotropin releasing hormone) and influenced by the feedback effects of glucocorticoids. In the hypothalamus, regulation of POMC gene expression is via the sex steroids. In the absence of sex steroids, little, if any, secretion occurs.

Proenkephalin A is produced in the adrenal medulla, the brain, the posterior pituitary, the spinal cord, and the gastrointestinal tract. It yields several enkephalins: methionine-enkephalin, leucine-enkephalin, and other variants. The enkephalins are the most widely distributed endogenous opioid peptides in the brain and are probably mainly involved as inhibitory neurotransmitters in the modulation of the autonomic nervous system. Prodynorphin, found in the brain (concentrated in the hypothalamus) and the gastrointestinal tract, yields dynorphin, an opioid peptide with high analgesic potency and behavioral effects, as well as α-neoendorphin, β-neoendorphin, and leumorphin. The last 13 amino acids of leumorphin constitute another opioid peptide, rimorphin. The prodynorphin products probably function in a fashion similar to endorphin.

3. true   p.144
Prolactin gene expression occurs in the lactotrophs of the anterior pituitary gland, in decidualized endometrium, and the myometrium. The prolactin secreted in these various sites is identical, but there are differences in mRNA indicating differences in prolactin gene regulation.

Transcription of the prolactin gene is regulated by a transcription factor (named Pit-1) which binds to the 5' promoter region and which is specific for the pituitary and also necessary for growth hormone. In addition, prolactin gene transcription is regulated by the interaction of estrogen and glucocorticoid receptors with 5' flanking sequences. Mutations in the sequences of these flanking regions or in the gene for the Pit-1 protein can result in the failure to secrete prolactin. The Pit-1 gene is also involved in differentiation and growth of anterior pituitary cells, and therefore mutations in this gene can lead not only to absent secretion of growth hormone and prolactin but to an absence of their trophic cells in the pituitary.

4. true   p.148,149
Dopamine does not exert a direct effect on gonadotropin secretion by the anterior pituitary; thus, this effect is mediated through GnRH release in the hypothalamus. Athough the exact chemical nature of the endogenous prolactin inhibiting hormone is still not known, evidence is rather overwhelming that dopamine is the hypothalamic inhibitor of prolactin secretion. It is directly secreted into the portal blood, thus behaving like a neurohormone. Therefore, dopamine may directly suppress arcuate GnRH activity, and also be transported via the portal system to directly and specifically suppress pituitary prolactin secretion. The hypothalamic tuberoinfundibular dopamine pathway is not the only dopamine pathway in the CNS, and it is only one of two major dopamine pathways in the hypothalamus. But it is this pathway that directly participates in the regulation of prolactin secretion. Ergot derivatives, such as bromocriptine, used clinically to treat high prolactin levels, activate dopaminergic receptors and directly inhibit the secretion of prolactin in a fashion identical to dopamine. Whether the peptide associated with GnRH (GAP) plays a role in physiologic prolactin regulation is not known.

5. C   p.153
Inhibin consists of two dissimilar peptides (known as alpha- and beta-subunits) linked by disulfide bonds. Two forms of inhibin (inhibin A and inhibin B) have been purified, each containing an identical alpha-subunit and distinct but related beta-subunits. Thus, there are three subunits for inhibins: alpha, beta-A, and beta-B. Each subunit is a product of different messenger RNA; therefore, each is derived from its own large precursor molecule. Inhibin is secreted by granulosa cells, but messenger RNA for the alpha and beta chains has also been found in pituitary gonadotropes.

6. C   p.161
Tanycytes are specialized ependymal cells whose ciliated cell bodies line the third ventricle over the median eminence. The cells terminate on portal vessels, and they can transport materials from ventricular CSF to the portal system, e.g., substances from the pineal gland, or vasopressin, or oxytocin. Tanycytes change morphologically in response to steroids and exhibit morphological changes during the ovarian cycle.

7. B   p.173,174

The precise signal that initiates the events of puberty is unknown. In girls, the first steroids to rise in the blood are dehydroepiandrosterone (DHA) and its sulfate (DHAS) beginning at 6–8 years of age, at the same time that FSH begins to increase. Estrogen levels, as well as LH, do not begin to rise until 10–12 years of age. If the onset of puberty is triggered by the first hormone to increase in the circulation, then a role for adrenal steroids must be considered. However, there is no evidence to suggest that the adrenal steroids are necessary for the proper timing of puberty, and adrenarche appears to be independent, not controlled by the same mechanism which turns on the gonads. Neither is there a definite relationship demonstrated between melatonin secretion and puberty. Because the studies have focused on the amount of melatonin secreted rather than the rhythm of secretion, this question remains open.

Prior to puberty, gonadotropin levels are low but still associated with pulses (although quite irregular). The clinical onset of puberty is preceded by an increase in pulse frequency, amplitude, and regularity, especially during the night. At the time of appearance of secondary sex characteristics, the mean LH levels are 2 to 4 times higher during sleep than during wakefulness. This pattern is not present before or after puberty and is an early sign of changes taking place in the hypothalamus, where there is increasing coordination of GnRH neurons with increasing GnRH pulsatile secretion. This pattern can be detected in individuals who develop increasing and decreasing degrees of hypothalamic suppression (such as in individuals with worsening and improving anorexia nervosa). FSH levels plateau by midpuberty, while LH and estradiol levels continue to rise until late puberty. Biologically active LH has been found to rise proportionately more than immunoactive LH with the onset of puberty.

Answers for Chapter 5 — Post-Test Questions

1. hypophyseal; portal; anterior   p.142

The hypothalamus is at the base of the brain just above the junction of the optic nerves. In order to influence the anterior pituitary gland, the brain requires a means of transmission or connection. A direct nervous connection does not exist. The blood supply of the anterior pituitary, however, originates in the capillaries that richly lace the median eminence area of the hypothalamus. The superior hypophyseal arteries form a dense network of capillaries within the median eminence, which then drain into the portal vessels that descend along the pituitary stalk to the anterior pituitary. The direction of the blood flow in this hypophyseal portal circulation is from the brain to the pituitary. Section of the neural stalk which interrupts this portal circulation leads to inactivity and atrophy of the gonads, along with a decrease in adrenal and thyroid activity to basal levels. With regeneration of the portal vessels, anterior pituitary function is restored. Thus, the anterior pituitary gland is under the influence of the hypothalamus by means of neurohormones released into this portal circulation. There also exists retrograde flow so that pituitary hormones can be delivered directly to the hypothalamus, creating the opportunity for pituitary feedback upon the hypothalamus. An additional blood supply is provided by short vessels which originate in the posterior pituitary that in turn receives its arterial supply from the inferior hypophyseal arteries.

A considerable body of evidence indicates that influence of the pituitary by the hypothalamus is achieved by materials secreted in the cells of the hypothalamus and transported to the pituitary by the portal vessel system. In addition to the stalk section experiments cited above, transplantation of the pituitary to ectopic sites (e.g., under the kidney capsule) results in failure of gonadal function. With retransplantation to an anatomic site under the median eminence, followed by regeneration of the portal system, normal pituitary function is regained. This retrieval of gonadotropic function is not accomplished if the pituitary is transplanted to other sites in the brain. Hence, there is something very special about the blood draining the basal hypothalamus. An exception to this overall pattern of positive influence is the control of prolactin secretion. Stalk secretion and transplantation cause release of prolactin from the anterior pituitary, implying a negative hypothalamic control. Furthermore, cultures of anterior pituitary tissue release prolactin in the absence of hypothalamic tissue or extracts.

2. prolactin inhibiting; dopamine   p.142

Neuroendocrine agents originating in the hypothalamus have positive stimulatory effects on growth hormone, thyroid-stimulating hormone (TSH), adrenocorticotropin hormone (ACTH), as well as the gonadotropins, and represent the individual neurohormones of the hypothalamus. The neurohormone that controls gonadotropins is called gonadotropin releasing hormone (GnRH). The neurohormone that controls prolactin is called prolactin inhibiting hormone and is probably dopamine.

3. hypothalamus; diencephalon; third p.145

The hypothalamus is the part of the diencephalon at the base of the brain that forms the floor of the third ventricle and part of its lateral walls. Within the hypothalamus are peptidergic neural cells that secrete the releasing and inhibiting hormones. These cells share the characteristics of both neurons and endocrine gland cells. They respond to signals in the bloodstream, as well as to neurotransmitters within the brain, in a process known as neurosecretion. In neurosecretion, a neurohormone or neurotransmitter is synthesized on the ribosomes in the cytoplasm of the neuron, packaged into a granule in the Golgi apparatus, and then transported by active axonal flow to the neuronal terminal for secretion into a blood vessel or across a synapse.

4. arcuate nucleus; median eminence p.146

In primates, the primary network of GnRH cell bodies is located within the medial basal hypothalamus. Most of these cell bodies can be seen within the arcuate nucleus where GnRH is synthesized in GnRH neurons. The delivery of GnRH to the portal circulation is via an axonal pathway, the GnRH tuberoinfundibular tract. *A most useful concept is to view the arcuate nucleus as the central site of action, releasing GnRH into the portal circulation in pulsatile fashion.*

5. pulsatile p.148

Like GnRH, gonadotropins are also secreted in pulsatile fashion, and indeed, the pulsatile pattern of gonadotropin release is believed to reflect the pulsatile GnRH pattern. Initiation of the pulsatile pattern of gonadotropin secretion occurs just before puberty with nighttime increases in LH. After puberty, pulsatile secretion is maintained throughout the 24-hour period, but it varies in both amplitude and frequency. In puberty, arcuate activity begins with a low frequency of GnRH release and proceeds through a cycle of acceleration of frequency, characterized by passage from total inactivity, to nocturnal activation, to the full adult pattern. The progressive changes in FSH and LH reflect this activation of GnRH pulsatile secretion.

6. GnRH; frequency; amplitude p.148

Normal menstrual cycles require the maintenance of the pulsatile release of GnRH within a critical range of frequency and amplitude. This pulsatile release is mediated by a catecholaminergic mechanism and can be modified by gonadal steroids and a variety of brain peptides. Pulsatile secretion is more frequent but smaller in amplitude during the follicular phase compared to the luteal phase. It should be emphasized that these numbers are not inviolate. There is considerable variability between and within individuals and a large normal range exists. Despite the handicap of the long half-life, it has been ascertained that FSH secretion is correlated with LH secretion.

7. tuberoinfundibular; medial basal; median eminence p.148

Cell bodies for dopamine synthesis can be found in the arcuate and periventricular nuclei. The dopamine tuberoinfundibular tract arises within the medial basal hypothalamus and projects to the median eminence.

8. Norepinephrine; dopamine; serotonin p.150

The current concept is that the biogenic catecholamines modulate GnRH pulsatile release. Norepinephrine is thought to exert stimulatory effects on GnRH, while dopamine and serotonin exert inhibitory effects. Little is known, however, about the role of serotonin. The probable mode of action of catecholamines is to influence the frequency (and perhaps the amplitude) of GnRH discharge. Thus, pharmacologic or psychologic factors that affect pituitary function probably do so by altering catecholamine synthesis or metabolism, and thus the pulsatile release of GnRH.

9. true p.143

Human corticotropin releasing hormone (CRH) is a 41 amino acid peptide which, besides being the principal regulator of ACTH secretion, also activates the sympathetic nervous system. CRH suppresses gonadotropin secretion, an action mediated by endorphin inhibition of GnRH. CRH is found in many tissues outside the central nervous system, including pancreas, gastrointestinal tract, liver, placenta, and adrenal gland.

10. true   p.143

Initially, it was believed that there were two separate releasing hormones for follicle-stimulating hormone (FSH) and luteinizing hormone (LH). It is now apparent that there is a single neurohormone (GnRH) for both gonadotropins. GnRH is a small peptide with 10 amino acids with some variation in the amino acid sequence among various mammals. Purified or synthesized GnRH stimulates both FSH and LH secretion. The divergent patterns of FSH and LH in response to a single GnRH are due to the modulating influences of the endocrine environment, specifically the feedback effects of steroids on the anterior pituitary gland.

11. false   p.145

Pituitary secretion of prolactin is chiefly under the inhibitory control of hypothalamic dopamine released into the portal circulation. The action of dopamine in the pituitary is mediated by receptors that are coupled to the inhibition of adenylate cyclase activity. Dopamine-regulated prolactin gene transcription, therefore, involves modulation of the promoter activity by cyclic AMP, intracellular calcium, and phosphatidyl inositol. Pit-1 binding sites are involved in this dopamine response. Molecular studies indicate that Pit-1 participates in mediating both stimulatory and inhibitory hormone signals for prolactin gene transcription.

12. true   p.145

The secretion of prolactin is inhibited and stimulated by the association and dissociation of dopamine from its receptors. Other factors are also involved in the regulation of prolactin secretion, especially TRH, vasoactive intestinal peptide (VIP), and perhaps GnRH. These factors interact with each other, affecting the overall lactotroph responsiveness.

13. true   p.146

The GnRH neurons appear in the medial olfactory placode (a thickened plate of ectoderm from which a sense organ develops) and enter the brain with the nervus terminalis, a cranial nerve that projects from the nose to the septal-preoptic nuclei in the brain. This amazing journey accounts for Kallmann's syndrome, an association between an absence of GnRH and a defect in smell (a failure of both olfactory axonal and GnRH neuronal migration from the olfactory placode). The mutations responsible for this syndrome involve a single gene on the short arm of the X chromosome in the Xp22.3 region, which encodes a protein (homologous to members of the fibronectin family) responsible for cell adhesion and protease inhibition, functions necessary for neuronal migration. Location on the X chromosome explains why the syndrome occurs 5 to 7 times more frequently in males than in females.

14. true   p.147

(See figure on page 67 in this Study Guide)

15. false   p.148

The measurement of LH pulses is utilized as an indication of GnRH pulsatile secretion (the long half-life of FSH precludes its use for this purpose). The characteristics of LH pulses (and presumably of GnRH pulses) during the menstrual cycle are as follows:

LH pulse mean amplitude:
        Early follicular phase: 6.5 IU/L.
        Mid follicular phase: 5.1 IU/L.
        Late follicular phase: 7.2 IU/L.
        Early luteal phase: 14.9 IU/L.
        Mid luteal phase: 12.2 IU/L.
        Late luteal phase: 7.6 IU/L.

LH pulse mean frequency:
        Early follicular phase: 94 minutes.
        Late follicular phase: 71 minutes.
        Early luteal phase: 103 minutes.
        Late luteal phase: 216 minutes.

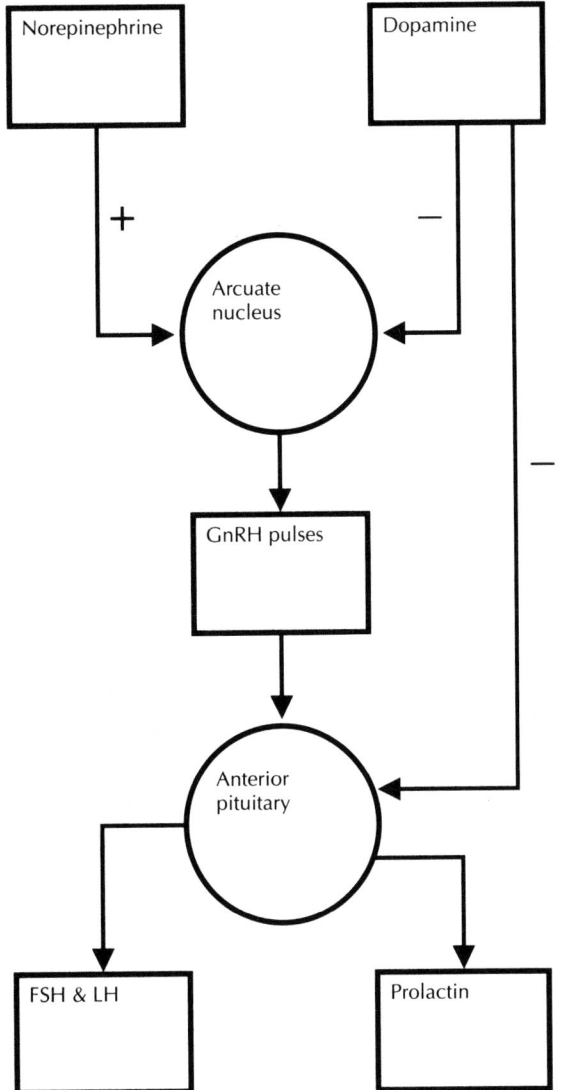

16. true p.149

Many studies, including specific *in vitro* systems, have indicated that dopamine stimulates the release of GnRH from the hypothalamus. This appears to be a paradox, but it simply indicates that the ultimate GnRH response reflects the complex interactions of steroids and neurotransmitters. For an understanding of clinical problems, it is best to view dopamine as an inhibitor of both GnRH and prolactin.

17. false p.150

Both LH and FSH are secreted by the same cell, the gonadotrope, localized primarily in the lateral portions of the pituitary gland and responsive to the pulsatile stimulation by GnRH. GnRH is calcium dependent in its mechanism of action and utilizes inosistol 1,4,5-triphosphate (IP_3) and 1,2-diacylglycerol (1,2-DG) as second messengers to stimulate protein kinase activity. These responses require a G protein receptor, and are associated with cyclical release of calcium ions from intracellular stores and the opening of cell membrane channels to allow entry of extracellular calcium. Thus both protein kinase and calmodulin are mediators of GnRH action. GnRH receptors are regulated by many agents, including GnRH itself, inhibin, activin, and the sex steroids. A decreased gonadotropin response to continued excessive GnRH stimulation is not due to a loss of GnRH receptors alone but includes desensitization and uncoupling of the receptors.

18. false p.156

The opioid tone is an important part of menstrual function and cyclicity. Endogenous endorphin levels, therefore, increase throughout the cycle from nadir levels during menses to highest levels during the luteal phase. Normal cyclicity thus requires sequential periods of high (luteal phase) and low (during menses) hypothalamic opioid activity.

19. false   p.156

The principal endogenous opiates affecting GnRH release are β-endorphin and dynorphin, and it is probable that the major effect is modulation of the catecholamine pathway, principally norepinephrine. The action does not involve dopamine receptors, acetylcholine receptors, or alpha-adrenergic receptors. On the other hand, endorphin may affect GnRH release directly, without the involvement of any intermediary neuroamine.

20. B   p.153

The Two Forms of Inhibin
    Inhibin-A: Alpha-Beta$_A$
    Inhibin-B: Alpha-Beta$_B$

The Three Forms of Activin
    Activin-A: Beta$_A$-Beta$_A$
    Activin-AB: Beta$_A$-Beta$_B$
    Activin-B: Beta$_B$-Beta$_B$

21. C   p.153

Inhibin selectively inhibits FSH, but not LH, secretion.

22. A   p.152

Somatostatin inhibits the release of growth hormone, prolactin, and TSH from the pituitary. It is also a typical gut-brain peptide, being found in neurons throughout the brain, stomach, intestine, and pancreas. It inhibits secretion of glucagon, insulin, and gastrin. It is also located in sensory neurons and may be a transmitter of pain sensation.

23. D   p.153

The secretion and gene expression of neuropeptide Y in hypothalamic neurons is regulated by gonadal steroids. Neuropeptide Y stimulates pulsatile release of GnRH and in the pituitary potentiates gonadotropin response to GnRH. It thus may facilitate pulsatile secretion of GnRH and gonadotropins. In the absence of estrogen, neuropeptide Y inhibits gonadotropin secretion. Because undernutrition is associated with an increase in neuropeptide Y and increased amounts have been measured in cerebrospinal fluid of women with anorexia and bulimia nervosa, it has been proposed that neuropeptide Y is at least one link between nutrition and reproductive function.

24. B   p.151

GnRH is calcium dependent in its mechanism of action and utilizes inosistol 1,4,5-triphosphate (IP$_3$) and 1,2-diacylglycerol (1,2-DG) as second messengers to stimulate protein kinase activity. These responses require a G protein receptor, and are associated with cyclical release of calcium ions from intracellular stores and the opening of cell membrane channels to allow entry of extracellular calcium. Thus both protein kinase and calmodulin are mediators of GnRH action. GnRH receptors are regulated by many agents, including GnRH itself, inhibin, activin, and the sex steroids. A decreased gonadotropin response to continued excessive GnRH stimulation is not due to a loss of GnRH receptors alone but includes desensitization and uncoupling of the receptors.

Synthesis of gonadotropins takes place on the rough endoplasmic reticulum. The hormones are packaged into secretory granules by the Golgi cisternae of the Golgi apparatus and then stored as secretory granules. Secretion requires migration (activation) of the mature secretory granules to the cell membrane where an alteration in membrane permeability results in extrusion of the secretory granules in response to GnRH. The rate limiting step in gonadotropin synthesis is the GnRH-dependent availability of the beta-subunits.

Binding of GnRH to its receptor in the pituitary activates multiple messengers and responses. The immediate event is a secretory release of gonadotropins, while delayed responses prepare for the next secretory release. One of these delayed responses is the self-priming action of GnRH that leads to even greater responses to subsequent GnRH pulses due to a complex series of biochemical and biophysical intracellular events. This self-priming action is important to achieve the large surge in secretion at midcyle; it requires estrogen exposure, and it can be augmented by progesterone.

This important action of progesterone depends upon estrogen exposure (for an increase in progesterone receptors) and activation of the progesterone receptor by GnRH stimulated phosphorylation. This latter action is an example of crosstalk between peptide and steroid hormone receptors.

25. C p.154

Opiate production is regulated by gene transcription and the synthesis of precursor peptides and at a posttranslational level where the precursors are processed into the various bioactive smaller peptides. All opiates derive from one of 3 precursor peptides.

Proopiomelanocortin (POMC) — the source of endorphins.

Proenkephalin A and B — the source of several enkephalins.

Prodynorphin — yields dynorphins.

Opioid peptides are able to act through different receptors, although specific opiates bind predominantly to one of the various receptor types. Naloxone, used in most human studies, does not bind exclusively to any one receptor type, and thus results with this antagonist are not totally specific. Localization of opioid receptors explains many of the pharmacological actions of the opiates. Opioid receptors are found in the nerve endings of sensory neurons, in the limbic system (site of euphoric emotions), in brainstem centers for reflexes such as respiration, and widely distributed in the brain and the spinal cord.

A reduction in LH pulse frequency is linked to increased endorphin release. Naloxone increases both the frequency and the amplitude of LH pulses. *Thus, the endogenous opiates inhibit gonadotropin secretion by suppressing the hypothalamic release of GnRH.* Opiates have no effect on the pituitary response to GnRH. The gonadal steroids modify endogenous opioid activity, and the negative feedback of steroids on gonadotropins appears to be mediated by endogenous opiates. Because the fluctuating levels of endogenous opiates in the menstrual cycle are related to the changing levels of estradiol and progesterone, it is attractive to speculate that the sex steroids directly stimulate endogenous opioid receptor activity. There is an absence of opioid effect on postmenopausal and oophorectomized levels of gonadotropins, and the response to opiates is restored with the administration of estrogen, progesterone, or both. Both estrogen and progesterone alone increase endogenous opiates, but estrogen enhances the action of progesterone, which explains the maximal suppression of GnRH and gonadotropin pulse frequency during the luteal phase. Experiments with naloxone administration suggest that the suppression of gonadotropins during pregnancy and the recovery during the postpartum period reflect steroid-induced opioid inhibition, followed by a release from central opioid suppression.

26. E p.154

POMC was the first precursor peptide to be identified. It is made in the anterior and intermediate lobes of the pituitary, in the hypothalamus and other areas of the brain, in the sympathetic nervous system, and in other tissues including the gonads, the placenta, the gastrointestinal tract, and the lungs. The highest concentration is in the pituitary gland. In the hypothalamus, regulation of POMC gene expression is via the sex steroids. In the absence of sex steroids, little, if any, secretion occurs.

Proopiomelanocortin is split into 2 fragments, an ACTH intermediate fragment and β-lipotropin. β-Lipotropin has no opioid activity but is broken down in a series of steps to β-melanocyte-stimulating hormone (β-MSH), enkephalin, and α-, γ-, and β-endorphins. Melanocyte-stimulating hormone acts in lower animals to stimulate melanin granules within cells, causing darkening of the skin. In humans, there is no known function.

27. B p.157

A change in opioid inhibitory tone is not important in the changes of puberty because the responsiveness to naloxone does not develop until after puberty. A change in opioid tone does seem to mediate the hypogonadotropic state seen with elevated prolactin levels, exercise, and other conditions of hypothalamic amenorrhea, while endogenous opioid inhibition does not seem to play a causal role in delayed puberty or hereditary problems such as Kallmann's syndrome. Treatment of patients with hypothalamic amenorrhea (suppressed GnRH pulsatile secretion) with a drug (naltrexone) which blocks opioid receptors restores normal function (ovulation and pregnancy). Thus, the reduced GnRH secretion associated with hypothalamic amenorrhea is mediated by an increase in endogenous opioid inhibitory tone. Experimental evidence indicates that corticotropin-releasing hormone (CRH) directly inhibits hypothalamic GnRH secretion, probably by augmenting endogenous opioid secretion. Women with hypothalamic amenorrhea demonstrate hypercortisolism, suggesting that this could be the pathway by which stress interrupts reproductive function.

28. E p.154–157

β-Endorphin is appropriately considered a neurotransmitter, a neurohormone, and a neuromodulator. β-Endorphin influences a variety of hypothalamic functions, including regulation of reproduction, temperature, cardiovascular and respiratory function, as well as extrahypothalamic functions such as pain perception and mood. POMC gene expression in the anterior pituitary is controlled mainly by adrenal hormones, stimulated by CRH (corticotropin releasing hormone) and influenced by the feedback effects of glucocorticoids. In the hypothalamus, regulation of POMC gene expression is via the sex steroids. In the absence of sex steroids, little, if any, secretion occurs.

A reduction in LH pulse frequency is linked to increased endorphin release. Naloxone increases both the frequency and the amplitude of LH pulses. ***Thus, the endogenous opiates inhibit gonadotropin secretion by suppressing the hypothalamic release of GnRH.*** Opiates have no effect on the pituitary response to GnRH. The gonadal steroids modify endogenous opioid activity, and the negative feedback of steroids on gonadotropins appears to be mediated by endogenous opiates. Because the fluctuating levels of endogenous opiates in the menstrual cycle are related to the changing levels of estradiol and progesterone, it is attractive to speculate that the sex steroids directly stimulate endogenous opioid receptor activity. A change in opioid inhibitory tone is not important in the changes of puberty because the responsiveness to naloxone does not develop until after puberty. A change in opioid tone does seem to mediate the hypogonadotropic state seen with elevated prolactin levels, exercise, and other conditions of hypothalamic amenorrhea, while endogenous opioid inhibition does not seem to play a causal role in delayed puberty or hereditary problems such as Kallmann's syndrome.

29. E p.158

The key concept is that normal menstrual function requires GnRH pulsatile secretion in a critical range of frequency and amplitude. The normal physiology and pathophysiology of the menstrual cycle, at least in terms of central control, can be explained by mechanisms which affect the pulsatile secretion of GnRH. The pulses of GnRH appear to be directly under the influence of a dual catecholaminergic system: norepinephrine facilatory and dopamine inhibitory. In turn, the catecholamine system can be influenced by endogenous opioid activity. The feedback effects of steroids may be mediated through this system via catecholsteroid messengers or directly by influencing the various neurotransmitters. (See figure on page 71 in this Study Guide)

30. B p.160

The short half-life of GnRH is due to rapid cleavage of the bonds between amino acids 5–6, 6–7, and 9–10. By altering amino acids at these positions, analogues of GnRH can be synthesized with different properties. Thousands of GnRH analogues have been produced. Substitution of amino acids at the 6 position or replacement of the C-terminal glycine-amide (inhibiting degradation) produces agonists. The GnRH agonists are administered either intramuscularly or subcutaneously or by intranasal absorption. An initial agonistic action (the so-called flare effect) is associated with an increase in the circulating levels of FSH and LH. This response is greatest in the early follicular phase when GnRH and estradiol have combined to create a large reserve pool of gonadotropins. After 1–3 weeks, down-regulation and desensitization of the pituitary produce a hypogonadotropic, hypogonad state. The initial response is due to a loss of receptors, while the sustained response is due to desensitization and the uncoupling of the receptor from its effector system. Furthermore, postreceptor mechanisms lead to secretion of biologically inactive gonadotropins, which, however, can still be detected by immunoassay. (See figure on page 72 in this Study Guide)

31. E p.161

GnRH antagonists are synthesized by multiple amino acid substitutions. GnRH antagonists bind to the GnRH receptor and provide competitive inhibition of the naturally occurring GnRH. Thus GnRH antagonists produce an immediate decline in gonadotropin levels with an immediate therapeutic effect. The early products either lacked potency or were associated with undesirable side effects due to histamine release. New analogues continue to be developed and tested, aimed toward the control of fertility.

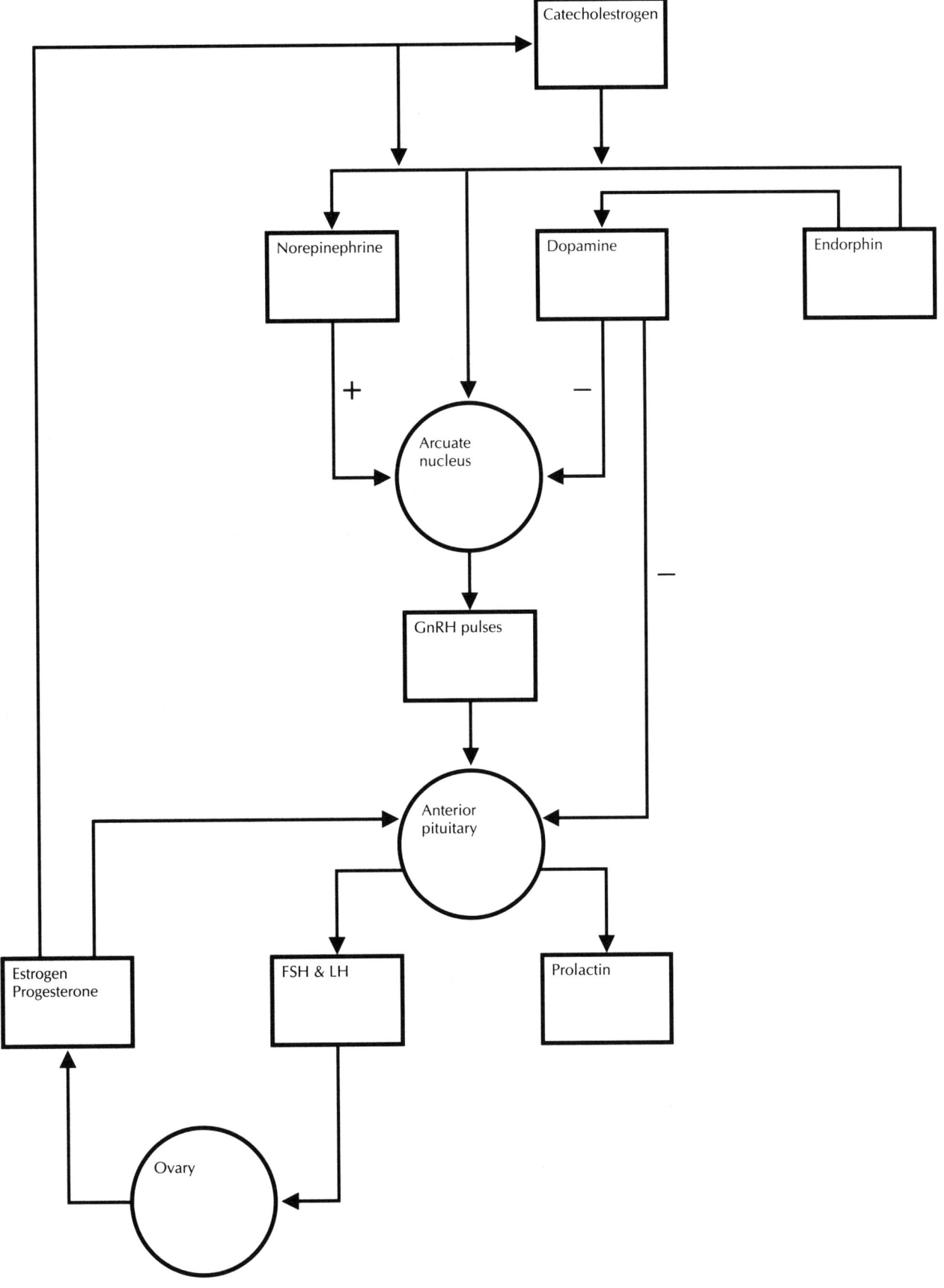

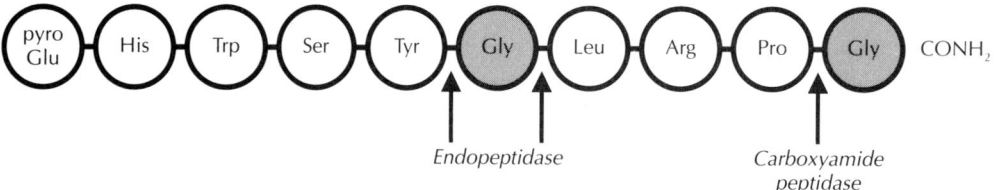

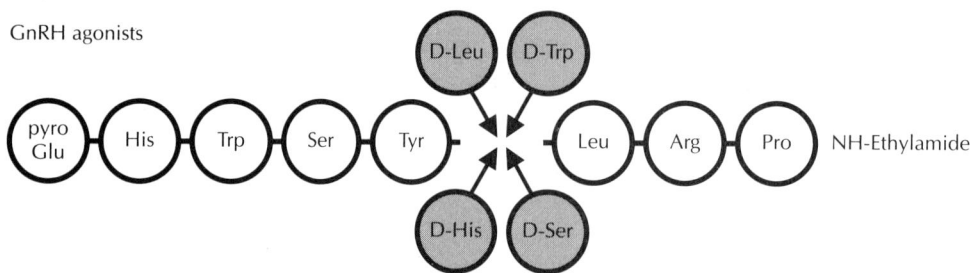

32. D p.162

The posterior pituitary is a direct prolongation of the hypothalamus via the pituitary stalk, whereas the anterior pituitary arises from pharyngeal epithelium that migrates into position with the posterior pituitary. Separate neurosecretory cells in both the supraoptic and paraventricular nuclei make vasopressin and oxytocin as parts of large precursor molecules that also contain the transport peptide, neurophysin. The neurophysins are polypeptides with a molecular weight of about 10,000. There are two distinct neurophysins, estrogen-stimulated neurophysin known as neurophysin I, and nicotine-stimulated neurophysin, known as neurophysin II.

The genes for oxytocin and vasopressin are closely linked on the same chromosome. The transcriptional activity of these genes is regulated by endocrine factors, such as the sex steroids and thyroid hormone, through hormone-response elements located upstream. The neurons secrete two large protein molecules, a precursor called pro-pressophysin, which contains vasopressin and its neurophysin, and a precursor called pro-oxyphysin, which contains oxytocin and its neurophysin. Neurophysin I is specifically related to oxytocin, and neurophysin II accompanies vasopressin. Because of this unique packaging, the hormones and their neurophysins are stored together and released at the same time into the circulation. The neurophysins are cleaved from their associated neurohormones during axonal transport from the neuronal cell bodies in the supraoptic and paraventricular nuclei to the posterior pituitary. The only known function for the neurophysins is axonal transport for oxytocin and vasopressin.

The posterior pathway is complex and not limited to the transmission of vasopressin and oxytocin to the posterior pituitary. The transportation of vasopressin and oxytocin to the posterior pituitary occurs via nerve tracts which emanate from the supraoptic and paraventricular nuclei and descend through the median eminence to terminate in the posterior pituitary. However, these hormones are also secreted into the cerebrospinal fluid and directly into the portal system. Therefore, vasopressin and oxytocin can reach the anterior pituitary and influence, in the case of vasopressin, ACTH secretion, and in the case of oxytocin, gonadotropin secretion. Vasopressin cooperates with corticotropin releasing hormone to cause an increased yield of ACTH. Vasopressin and oxytocin-like materials are also found in the ovary, the oviduct, the testis, and the adrenal gland, suggesting that these neurohypophyseal peptides have roles as paracrine or autocrine hormones. The concentrations of these substances in the cerebrospinal fluid exhibit a circadian rhythm (with peak levels occurring during the day), suggesting a different mechanism for CSF secretion compared to posterior pituitary release.

33. A p.164

Both oxytocin and vasopressin consist of 9 amino acid residues. In the human, vasopressin contains arginine, unlike animals that have lysine vasopressin. Both oxytocin and vasopressin circulate as the free peptides with a rapid half-life (initial component less than 1 minute, second component of 2–3 minutes). Three major stimuli for vasopressin secretion are changes in osmolality of the blood, alterations in blood volume, and psychogenic stimuli such as pain and fear. The osmoreceptors are located in the hypothalamus; the volume receptors are in the left atrium, aortic arch, and carotid sinus. Angiotensin II also produces a release of vasopressin, suggesting another mechanism for the link between fluid balance and vasopressin. Cortisol may modify the osmotic threshold for the release of vasopressin.

The major functions of vasopressin involve the regulation of osmolality and blood volume. Vasopressin is a powerful vasoconstrictor and antidiuretic hormone. Vasopressin release increases when plasma osmolality rises and is inhibited by water loading (resulting in diuresis). Diabetes insipidus is a condition marked by loss of water because of a lack of vasopressin action in the tubules of the kidney, secondary to a defect in synthesis or secretion of vasopressin. The opposite condition is the continuous and autonomous secretion of vasopressin, the syndrome of inappropriate ADH (antidiuretic hormone) secretion. This syndrome, with its resultant retention of water, is associated with a variety of brain disorders as well as the production of vasopressin and its precursor by malignant tumors.

Oxytocin stimulates muscular contractions in the uterus and myoepithelial contractions in the breast. Thus it is involved in parturition and the letdown of milk. The release of oxytocin is so episodic that it is described as spurts. Ordinarily, there are about 3 spurts every 10 minutes. Oxytocin is released during coitus, probably by the Ferguson reflex (vaginal and cervical stimulation) but also by olfactory, visual, and auditory pathways. Perhaps oxytocin has some role in muscle contractions during orgasm. In the male, release of oxytocin during coitus may contribute to sperm transport during ejaculation.

34. B p.170

Summary of key neuroendocrine events:
1. Pulsatile GnRH secretion must be within a critical range for frequency and concentration (amplitude).
2. GnRH has only positive actions on the anterior pituitary: synthesis and storage, activation, and secretion of gonadotropins. The gonadotropins are secreted in a pulsatile fashion in response to the similar pulsatile release of GnRH.
3. Low levels of estrogen enhance FSH and LH synthesis and storage, have little effect on LH secretion, and inhibit FSH secretion.
4. High levels of estrogen induce the LH surge at midcycle, and high steady levels of estrogen lead to sustained elevated LH secretion.
5. Low levels of progesterone acting at the level of the pituitary gland enhance the LH response to GnRH and are responsible for the FSH surge at midcycle.
6. High levels of progesterone inhibit pituitary secretion of gonadotropins by inhibiting GnRH pulses at the level of the hypothalamus. In addition, high levels of progesterone antagonize pituitary response to GnRH by interfering with estrogen action. (See figure on page 74 in this Study Guide)

35. E p.170

Although no physiologic role has been firmly established in the human, the reproductive functions of the hypothalamus may also be under inhibitory control of the brain via the pineal gland. The pineal arises as an outgrowth of the roof of the third ventricle, but soon after birth it loses all afferent and efferent neural connections with the brain. Instead the parenchymal cells receive a new and unusual sympathetic innervation which allows the pineal gland to be an active neuroendocrine organ that responds to photic and hormonal stimuli and exhibits circadian rhythms. Hydroxyindole-o-methyltransferase (HIOMT), an enzyme essential for melatonin synthesis, is found mainly in pineal parenchymal cells, and its products are essentially unique to the pineal. Calcification of the pineal gland is common. It is frequently present in young children, and almost all elderly people have pineal calcification. Possible roles in humans may be to give circadian rhythmicity to other functions such as temperature and sleep. In all vertebrates tested so far, there is a daily and seasonal rhythm in melatonin secretion: high values during the dark and low during light, greater secretion in the winter compared to the summer. Desynchronization with travel across time zones may contribute to the symptom complex known as jet lag.

36. A p.171

Norepinephrine stimulates tryptophan entry into the pineal cell and also adenylate cyclase activity in the membrane.

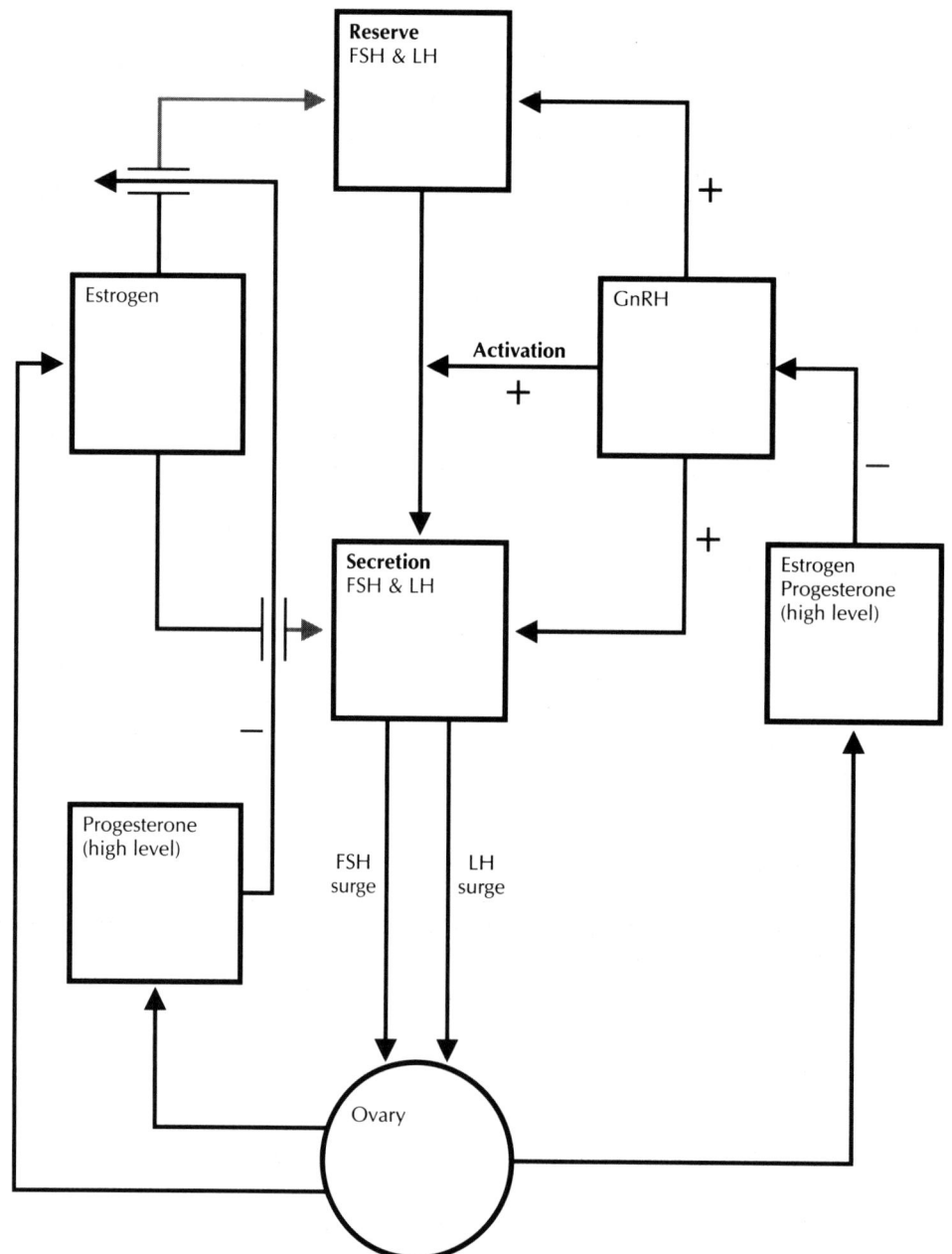

The resulting increase in cyclic AMP leads to *N*-acetyltransferase activity, the rate-limiting step in melatonin synthesis. Thus, melatonin synthesis is controlled by norepinephrine stimulation of adenylate cyclase, and the norepinephrine is liberated by sympathetic stimulation due to the absence of light. HIOMT is also found in the retina where melatonin may serve to regulate the pigment in retinal cells, and in the intestine. However, pinealectomy completely eliminates detectable levels of melatonin in the circulation. A rat in constant light develops a small pineal with decreased HIOMT and melatonin, while the ovarian weight increases. A rat in constant dark has the opposite result, increased pineal size, HIOMT, and melatonin, with decreased ovarian weight and pituitary function. A rhythm is established in pineal HIOMT activity by the presence or absence of light. Short days and long nights result in gonadal atrophy, and this is the major mechanism governing seasonal breeding.

37. E   p.172

Remarkable levels of FSH and LH, similar to postmenopausal levels, can be measured in the fetus. GnRH is detectable in the hypothalamus by 10 weeks of gestation, and by 10–13 weeks when the vascular connection is complete, FSH and LH are being produced in the pituitary. The peak pituitary concentrations of FSH and LH occur at about 20–23 weeks of intrauterine life, and peak circulating levels occur at 28 weeks.

The increasing production rate of gonadotropins until midgestation reflects the growing ability of the hypothalamic-pituitary axis to perform at full capacity. Beginning at midgestation, there is an increasing sensitivity to inhibition by steroids and a resultant decrease in gonadotropin secretion. Full sensitivity to steroids is not reached until late in infancy. The rise in gonadotropins after birth reflects loss of the high levels of placental steroids. Thus, in the first year of life there is considerable follicular activity in the ovaries in contrast to later in childhood when gonadotropin secretion is suppressed. Furthermore, the postnatal rise in gonadotropins is even greater in infants born prematurely.

Testicular function in the fetus can be correlated with the fetal hormone patterns. Initial testosterone production and sexual differentiation are in response to the fetal levels of HCG, whereas further testosterone production and masculine differentiation appear to be maintained by the fetal pituitary gonadotropins. Decreased testosterone levels in late gestation probably reflect the decrease in gonadotropin levels. The fetal generation of Leydig cells somehow avoids down-regulation and responds to high levels of HCG and LH by increased steroidogenesis and cell multiplication. This generation of cells is replaced by the adult generation which becomes functional at puberty and responds to high levels of HCG and LH with down-regulation and decreased steroidogenesis.

There is a sex difference in fetal gonadotropin levels. There are higher pituitary and circulating FSH and pituitary LH levels in female fetuses. The lower male levels are probably due to testicular testosterone and inhibin production. In infancy, the postnatal FSH rise is more marked and more sustained in females, while LH values are not as high. This early activity is accompanied by inhibin levels comparable to the low range observed during the follicular phase of the menstrual cycle. After the postnatal rise, gonadotropin levels reach a nadir during early childhood (by about 6 months of age in males and 1–2 years in females) and then rise slightly between 4 and 10 years. This childhood period is characterized by low levels of gonadotropins in the pituitary and in the blood, little response of the pituitary to GnRH, and maximal hypothalamic suppression.

38. C   p.174

The trend toward lowering of the menarcheal age and the period of acceleration of growth has halted. In a 10-year prospective study of middle class contemporary American girls, the mean age of menarche was 12.8 with a range of 9.1–17.7 years. The age of onset of puberty is variable and influenced by genetic factors, socioeconomic conditions, and general health. The earlier menarche today compared to the past is undoubtedly due to improved nutrition and better health. It has been suggested that initiation of growth and menarche occur at a particular body weight (48 kg) and percent of body fat (17%). It is thought that this relationship reflects a required stage of metabolism. Although this hypothesis of a critical weight is a helpful concept, the extreme variability in onset of menarche indicates that there is no particular age or size at which an individual girl should be expected to experience menarche.

In the female, the typical sequence of events is growth initiation, thelarche, pubarche, and finally menarche. This generally begins sometime between 8 and 14 years of age. The length of time involved in this evolution is usually 2–4 years. During this time span, puberty is said to occur. Individual variation in the order of appearance of this sequence is great. For example, growth of pubic hair and breast development are not always correlated.

39. E   p.173,175

The rise of gonadotropins at puberty appears to be independent of the gonads in that the same response can be observed in patients with gonadal dysgenesis (who lack functional steroid-producing gonadal tissue). Adolescent girls with Turner syndrome (45,X) also demonstrate augmented gonadotropin secretion during sleep. Thus, maturation at puberty must involve changes in the hypothalamus that are independent of ovarian steroids. Because agonadal children show a rise in gonadotropins at pubertal age following suppression to a nadir during childhood, the dominant mechanism must be a CNS inhibitory force. The initial maturational change in the hypothalamus would then be a decrease in this inhibitory influence. A search for this mechanism continues. Some have argued that, rather than a chronic state of inhibition prior to puberty, the GnRH neurons exist in an unrestrained but uncoordinated pattern of activity that prevents adequate secretion.

6 Regulation of the Menstrual Cycle

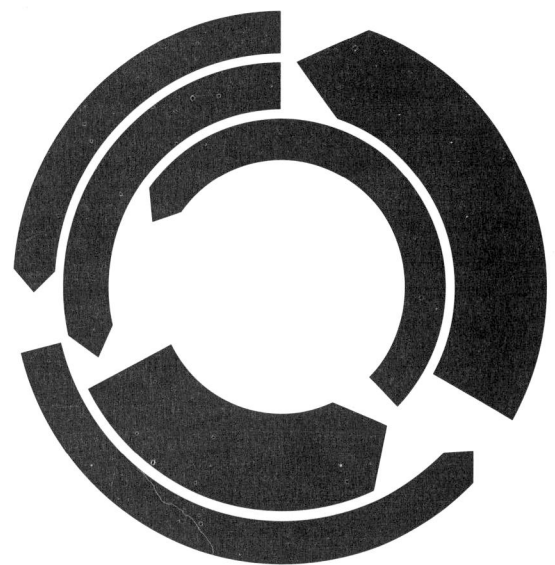

Learning Objectives

Be able to:

1. Describe the development and natural history of the primordial follicle.

2. Explain the two-cell, two-gonadotropin system and its relevance to ovarian physiology.

3. Discuss the potential roles for inhibin, activin, follistatin, and insulin-like growth factors in the regulation of the menstrual cycle.

4. Describe the process of selection of the dominant follicle.

5. Detail the hormonal events involved in the ovulatory process.

Pre-Test

A. Instructions: Fill in the blanks

1. The _____ _____ serve as the pathway for nutritional and metabolite interchange between the granulosa cells and the oocyte.

2. _____ synergizes with LH to increase _____ production by the theca.

B. Instructions: True or False

3. The most rapid decrease in the germ cell pool occurs after birth, resulting in a decline from 2 million at birth to 300,000 at puberty.

4. Androgens serve not only as substrate for FSH-induced aromatization but, in low concentrations can enhance aromatase activity.

C. Instructions: For each of the following questions choose:

A. if only 1, 2 and 3 are correct
B. if only 1 and 3 are correct
C. if only 2 and 4 are correct
D. if only 4 is correct
E. if all are correct

5. P450c17
    1. is expressed by granulosa and theca cells
    2. is the enzyme capable of converting a 21-carbon substrate to androgens
    3. is not required for normal granulosa-theca cell function
    4. is found in the endoplasmic reticulum not the mitochondria

6. Insulin-like growth factor binding proteins
    1. are 6 nonglycosylated peptides
    2. serve to carry insulin-like growth factors in serum, prolong half-lives, and regulate their tissue effects
    3. do not bind insulin
    4. change with age and pregnancy

7. Human granulosa cells retrieved from women undergoing in vitro fertilization
    1. contain large amounts of P450c17 mRNA
    2. are luteinized
    3. produce a minimum amount of progesterone
    4. express P450scc, 3β-hydroxysteroid and aromatase

Chapter 6 Regulation of the Menstrual Cycle

Post-Test

A. Instructions: Fill in the blanks

1. The primordial germ cells originate in the _____ of the yolk sac, allantois and hindgut of the embryo.

2. The primordial follicle consists of an oocyte, arrested in the _____ stage of meiotic _____, surrounded by a single layers of spindle-shaped granulosa cells.

3. In the presence of _____, estrogen becomes the dominant substance in the follicular fluid.

4. In the absence of FSH, _____ predominate in the follicular fluid.

5. In response to _____, theca tissue is stimulated to produce _____ that can be converted through _____ -induced aromatization to _____ in the granulosa cells.

6. _____ is defined as programmed cell death and believed to be the process responsible for atresia.

7. In women, the estradiol concentration necessary, to achieve a LH surge is greater than _____ sustained for approximately _____ hours.

8. There is a well-established relationship between the activity and half-life of glycoprotein hormones and their _____ _____ content.

9. _____ suppresses FSH activity, probably by binding activin.

10. The inhibin-activin family of peptides _____ cell growth.

11. _____ _____ are polypeptides that modulate cell _____ and _____, operating through binding to specific cell membrane receptors. They are not classic endocrine substances, but function as _____ and _____ substances.

12. Laron-type dwarfism is characterized by a deficiency in _____ due to an abnormality in the _____ _____ receptor.

13. The inability to suppress gonadotropins to a normal range during estrogen treatment of postmenopausal women reflects a loss of _____.

B. Instructions: True or False

14. Follicular growth and atresia are interrupted by pregnancy, ovulation and periods of anovulation.

15. The initiation of follicular growth is dependent upon gonadotropin stimulation.

16. Aromatization is induced or activated through the action of FSH.

17. FSH initiates steroidogenesis in granulosa cells and stimulates granulosa cell growth.

18. FSH operates through the G protein, adenylate cyclase system, that is subject to down-regulation by a calcium-calmodulin intermediary.

19. The steroids present in follicular fluid are found in concentrations several orders of magnitude higher than those in the plasma.

20. Ovarian steroidogenesis is always LH dependent.

21. The successful conversion to an androgen dominant follicle marks the selection of a follicle destined to ovulate.

22. Gonadotropins are secreted in a pulsatile fashion with a frequency and magnitude that vary with the phase of the cycle.

23. Pulsatile secretion of LH is less frequent but greater in amplitude during the follicular phase compared to the luteal phase.

24. The inhibitory action of luteal phase steroids appears to be mediated by an increase in hypothalamic endogenous opioid peptides.

25. There is a disparity between the patterns of FSH and LH secretion as determined by immunoassay and bioassay, indicating that more biologically active gonadotropins are secreted during the late luteal phase than at other times in the cycle.

26. There is a diurnal rhythm in FSH and LH secretion.

C. Instructions: Match each growth factor with the most appropriate word association.

A. Insulin-like growth factor I (IGF-I)
B. Antimüllerian hormone
C. Activin
D. Inhibin
E. Transforming growth factor-beta
F. Transforming growth factor-alpha

27. Augments FSH actions in granulosa cells.
28. Augments LH stimulation of thecal androgen production.
29. May inhibit oocyte meiosis.
30. Describes the name of the gene family to which inhibin, activin and antimüllerian hormone belong.
31. The structural analogue of epidermal growth factor.

D. Instructions: For each of the following questions choose:

A. if only 1, 2 and 3 are correct
B. if only 1 and 3 are correct
C. if only 2 and 4 are correct
D. if only 4 is correct
E. if all are correct

32. Androgens
   1. at low concentrations enhance their own aromatization and contribute to estrogen production
   2. increase the FSH receptor content of the follicle
   3. at higher levels cause follicular atresia
   4. may serve as substrate for progesterone

33. The dominant follicle
    1. has a greater content of FSH receptors
    2. contains granulosa cells with a rate of proliferation greater than its cohorts
    3. contains high concentrations of local autocrine paracrine peptides
    4. is selected prior to recruitment of a cohort of follicles

34. Inhibin
    1. is produced by FSH stimulated granulosa cells
    2. secretion is inhibited by GnRH and epidermal growth factor
    3. exists as two isoforms (inhibin A and inhibin B)
    4. rises throughout the follicular phase to reach a midcycle peak followed by a greater midluteal peak

35. Activin
    1. represses the release of FSH and GnRH receptor number
    2. contains 2 subunits different from the beta-subunits of inhibin
    3. regulates growth but not differentiation
    4. augments FSH stimulation of aromatization and inhibin production within the ovarian follicle

36. Follistatin
    1. is expressed by granulosa cells in response to FSH
    2. is a single chain, glycosylated polypeptide produced in the pituitary
    3. has a structure distinct from inhibin and activin
    4. modifies FSH activity by binding activin

37. Insulin-like growth factors (somatomedins)
    1. have structural and functional similarity to insulin and mediate growth hormone action
    2. are double chain polypeptides
    3. are composed of insulin-like growth factor I which mediates the action of growth hormone and insulin-like growth factor II which has little growth hormone dependence
    4. are not influenced by the presence or absence of insulin-like growth factor binding proteins.

38. IGF receptors
    1. consists of an IGF-I receptor and an IGF-II receptor
    2. are both similar in structure and resemble the insulin receptor
    3. are critical to the functioning of insulin-like growth factors
    4. are both present in the corpus luteum

39. Insulin-like growth factor-I
    1. is of thecal origin
    2. can move from theca to granulosa thus functioning in a paracrine fashion
    3. augments LH stimulation of androgen production
    4. is involved in both estradiol and progesterone synthesis

40. Insulin-like growth factor-II
    1. circulating levels vary according to phase of the menstrual cycle
    2. is the most abundant IGF in human follicles
    3. mediates the growth promoting actions of growth hormone
    4. is synthesized by luteinized granulosa cells

41. Human follicular fluid has been shown to contain
    1. beta-endorphin
    2. prorenin
    3. antimüllerian hormone
    4. pregnancy-associated plasma protein A

42. The preovulatory follicle
    1. as it approaches maturity produces decreasing amounts of estrogen
    2. contains granulosa cells which enlarge and acquire lipid inclusions and theca which becomes vacuolated and vascular
    3. does not produce progesterone prior to ovulation
    4. contains an oocyte which resumes meiosis

43. Ovulation
    1. is most reliably predicted by the onset of the LH surge which occurs 34–36 hours prior to rupture
    2. occurs approximately 10–12 hours after the LH peak
    3. requires a threshold of LH concentration to be maintained for 14–27 hours in order for full maturation of the oocyte to occur
    4. involves considerable variation in timing from cycle to cycle within the same woman.

44. Events in the luteal-follicular transition
    1. involve removal of inhibin and estradiol and increasing GnRH pulses to allow a greater secretion of FSH compared to LH
    2. involve a demise of the corpus luteum resulting in peak of activin
    3. involve an increase in FSH which is instrumental in rescuing a group of follicles from atresia and allowing a dominant follicle to occur
    4. do not involve demise of the corpus luteum

45. Menstrual cycle length
    1. of less than 21 days long or greater than 35 days in less than 2% of cycling women
    2. is determined primarily by duration of the luteal phase
    3. is irregular in at least 20% of women
    4. is 28 days in approximately 50% of reproductive age cycles

46. Women with "incipient" ovarian failure have
    1. elevated FSH levels
    2. decreased inhibin levels
    3. normal estradiol levels
    4. elevated LH levels

Answers for Chapter 6 — Pre-Test

1. gap junctions   p.184

The first visible signs of follicular recruitment are when the oocyte increases in size and when the granulosa cells become cuboidal rather than squamous in shape. At this same time, in response to FSH, small gap junctions develop between the granulosa cells and the oocyte. The gap junctions serve as the pathway for nutritional and metabolite interchange between the granulosa cells and the oocyte. With multiplication of the cuboidal granulosa cells, the primordial follicle becomes a primary follicle. The granulosa layer is separated from the stromal cells by a basement membrane called the basal lamina. The surrounding stromal cells differentiate into concentric layers designated the theca interna (closest to the basal lamina) and the theca externa (the outer portion).

2. IGF-I; androgen   p.188

As the follicle develops, theca cells begin to express the genes for LH receptors, P450scc, and 3β-hydroxysteroid dehydrogenase. Insulin-like growth factor-I (IGF-I) synergizes with LH to increase enzyme gene transcription; however IGF-I does not stimulate steroidogenesis. The separately regulated (by LH) entry of cholesterol into mitochondria, utilizing internalization of LDL-cholesterol, is essential for steroidogenesis. Therefore, ovarian steroidogenesis is always LH-dependent.

3. false   p.184
Until their numbers are exhausted, follicles begin to grow and undergo atresia under all physiologic circumstances. From the maximal number at 16–20 weeks of pregnancy, the number of oocytes will irretrievably decrease. The rate of decrease is proportional to the total number present; thus, the most rapid decrease occurs before birth, resulting in a decline from 6–7 million to 2 million at birth and to 300,000 at puberty. From this large reservoir, fewer than 500 follicles will ovulate during a woman's reproductive years.

4. true   p.186
At low concentrations, androgens enhance their own aromatization and contribute to estrogen production. At higher levels, the limited capacity of aromatization is overwhelmed, and the follicle becomes androgenic and ultimately atretic. Follicles will progress in development only if emerging when FSH is elevated and LH is low. Those follicles arising at the end of the luteal phase or early in the subsequent cycle would be favored by an environment in which aromatization in the granulosa cell can prevail. The success of a follicle depends upon its ability to convert an androgen microenvironment to an estrogen microenvironment.

5. C   p.189 and p.41 in Chapter 2
As the follicle emerges, the theca cells are characterized by their expression of P450c17, the enzyme step which is rate-limiting for the conversion of 21-carbon substrate to androgens. Granulosa cells do not express this enzyme and thus are dependent upon androgens from the theca in order to make estrogen. Increasing expression of the aromatization system (P450arom) is a marker of increasing maturity of granulosa cells.

Enzyme	Cellular Location	Reactions
P450scc	Mitochondria	Cholesterol side chain cleavage
P450c11	Mitochondria	11-hydroxylase 18-hydroxylase 19-methyloxidase
P450c17	Endoplasmic reticulum	17-hydroxylase, 17,20-lyase
P450c21	Endoplasmic reticulum	21-hydroxylase
P450arom	Endoplasmic reticulum	Aromatase

6. E   p.196
There are 6 known nonglycosylated peptides which function as IGF binding proteins: IGFBP-1 to IGFBP-6. These binding proteins serve to carry the IGFs in serum, prolong half-lives, and regulate tissue effects of the IGFs. The regulating action appears to be due to binding and sequestering of the IGFs, preventing their access to the cell membrane surface receptors, and thus not permitting the synergistic actions that result when gonadotropins and growth factors are combined. The IGFBPs may also exert direct actions on cellular functions, independently of growth factor functions. IGFBP-1 is the principal BP in amniotic fluid; IGFBP-3 is the main BP in serum and its synthesis, primarily in the liver, is dependent on growth hormone. Circulating levels of IGFBP-3 reflect the total IGF concentration (IGF-I plus IGF-II) and carry at least 90% of the circulating IGFs. These BPs do not bind insulin. The BPs change with age (decreasing levels of BP-3) and during pregnancy (decreasing BP-3 due to a circulating protease unique to pregnancy).

7. C   p.214
Human granulosa cells (already luteinizing when recovered from in vitro fertilization patients) contain minimal amounts of P450c17 mRNA. This is consistent with the two cell explanation which assigns androgen production (and P450c17) to the cells derived from thecal cells. With luteinization, expression of P450scc and 3β-hydroxysteroid dehydrogenase markedly increases as expected, to account for the increasing production of progesterone, and the continued expression of mRNAs for these enzymes requires LH. The aromatase system (P450arom), of course, continues to be active in luteinized granulosa cells.

Answers for Chapter 6 — Post-Test

1. endoderm　　　p.184
The primordial germ cells originate in the endoderm of the yolk sac, allantois, and hindgut of the embryo, and by 5–6 weeks of gestation, they have migrated to the genital ridge. A rapid mitotic multiplication of germ cells occurs at 6–8 weeks of pregnancy, and by 16–20 weeks, the maximal number of oocytes is reached: a total of 6–7 million in both ovaries.

2. diplotene; prophase　　　　　　　　　　　　　　　　　　　　　　　　　　　　　　　　　　　　　　p.184
The primordial follicle consists of an oocyte, arrested in the diplotene stage of meiotic prophase, surrounded by a single layer of spindle-shaped granulosa cells.

3. FSH　　　p.187
In the presence of FSH, estrogen becomes the dominant substance in the follicular fluid. Antral follicles with the greatest rates of granulosa proliferation contain the highest estrogen concentrations and the lowest androgen:estrogen ratios, and are the most likely to house a healthy oocyte. An androgenic milieu antagonizes estrogen-induced granulosa proliferation and, if sustained, promotes degenerative changes in the oocyte.

4. androgens　　p.187
In the absence of FSH, androgens predominate. LH is not normally present in follicular fluid until the midcycle. If LH is prematurely elevated in plasma and antral fluid, mitotic activity in the granulosa decreases, degenerative changes ensue, and intrafollicular androgen levels rise. Therefore, the dominance of estrogen and FSH is essential for sustained accumulation of granulosa cells and continued follicular growth.

5. LH; androgens; FSH; estrogens　　　　　　　　　　　　　　　　　　　　　　　　　　　　　　　　　p.187
Although each compartment (theca and granulosa) retains the ability to produce progestins, androgens, and estrogens, the aromatase activity of the granulosa far exceeds that observed in the theca. In human preantral and antral follicles, LH receptors are present only on the theca cells and FSH receptors only on the granulosa cells. Thecal interstitial cells, located in the theca interna, have approximately 20,000 LH receptors in their cell membranes. In response to LH, thecal tissue is stimulated to produce androgens that can then be converted, through FSH-induced aromatization, to estrogens in the granulosa cells.

The interaction between the granulosa and theca compartments, with resulting accelerated estrogen production, is not fully functional until later in antral development. Like preantral granulosa cells, the granulosa of small antral follicles exhibits an in vitro tendency to convert significant amounts of androgen to the more potent 5α-reduced form. In contrast, granulosa cells isolated from large antral follicles readily and preferentially metabolize androgens to estrogens. The conversion from an androgen microenvironment to an estrogen microenvironment (a conversion essential for further growth and development) is dependent upon a growing sensitivity to FSH brought about by the action of FSH and the enhancing influence of estrogen. (See figure on page 85 in this Study Guide)

6. Apoptosis　　　p.189
The loss of oocytes (and follicles) through atresia is a response to changes in many factors. Certainly gonadotropin stimulation and withdrawal are important, but ovarian steroids and autocrine/paracrine factors are also involved. The consequence of these unfavorable changes, atresia, is a process called apoptosis, programmed cell death. This process is heralded by alterations in mRNAs required for cell proteins which maintain follicle integrity. This type of "natural death" is a physiologic process, in contrast to the pathologic cell death of necrosis.

7. 200 pg/ml; 50 hours　　　　　　　　　　　　　　　　　　　　　　　　　　　　　　　　　　　　　　p.191
The transition from suppression to stimulation of LH release occurs as estradiol rises during the midfollicular phase. There are two critical features in this mechanism: 1) the concentration of estradiol and 2) the length of time during which the estradiol elevation is sustained. In women, the estradiol concentration necessary to achieve a positive feedback is more than 200 pg/mL (730 pmol/L), and this concentration must be sustained for approximately 50 hours.

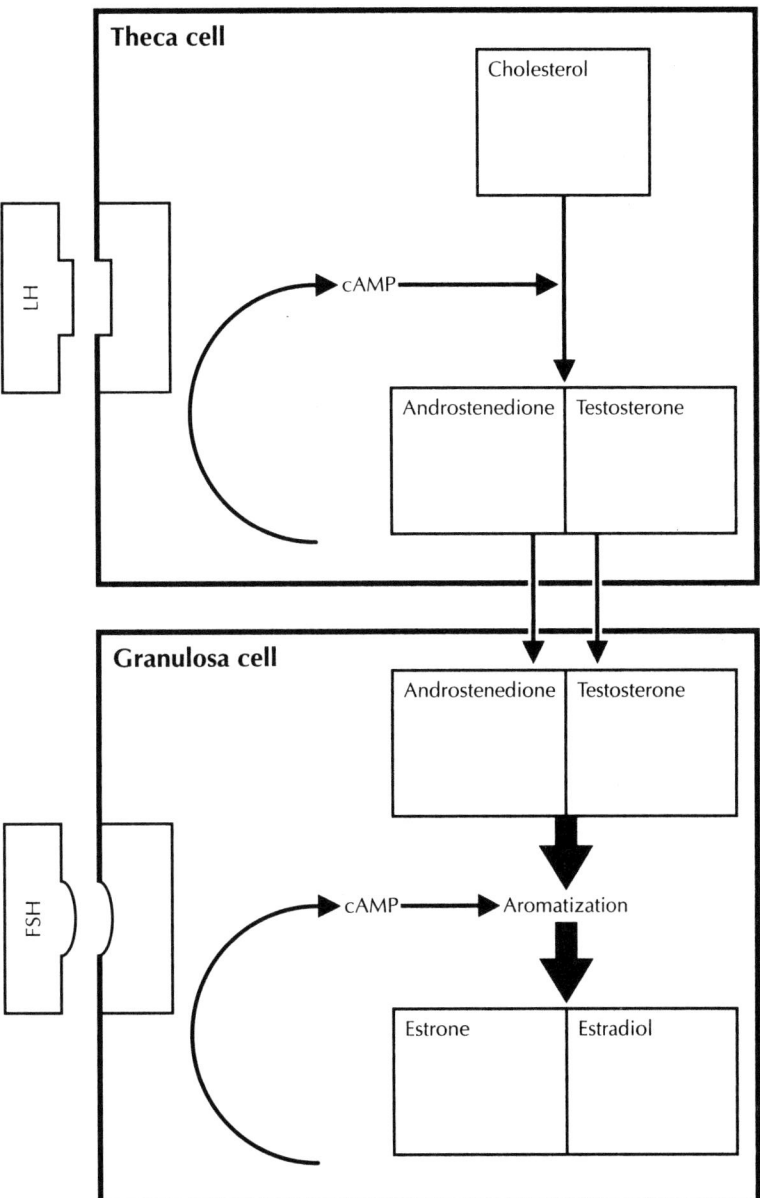

The estrogen stimulus must be applied until after the surge actually begins. Otherwise, the LH surge is abbreviated or fails to occur at all.

8. sialic acid   p.192
There is an important action of estrogen. A disparity exists between the patterns of FSH and LH secretion as determined by immunoassay and bioassay, indicating that more biologically active gonadotropins are secreted at midcycle than at other times in the cycle. This quality, bioactivity vs immunoactivity, is determined by the molecular structure of the gonadotropin molecule, a concept referred to as heterogeneity of the tropic hormones. There is a well-established relationship between the activity and half-life of glycoprotein hormones and their sialic acid content. The feedback effects of estrogen include modulation of sialylation and the size and activity of the gonadotropins subsequently released, as well as an augmentation of GnRH-stimulated secretory release of biologically active gonadotropin. It certainly makes sense to intensify the gonadotropin effect at midcycle. The positive feedback action of estrogen, therefore, both increases the quantity and the quality (the bioactivity) of FSH and LH.

9. Follistatin   p.193,195
A family of peptides is synthesized by granulosa cells in response to FSH and secreted into the follicular fluid and

ovarian venous effluent. The expression of these peptides is not limited to the ovary; they are present in many tissues throughout the body serving as autocrine/paracrine regulators. Inhibin is an important inhibitor of FSH secretion. Activin stimulates FSH release in the pituitary and augments FSH action in the ovary. Follistatin suppresses FSH activity, probably by binding activin.

Follistatin is a single chain, glycosylated polypeptide produced in the pituitary but found primarily in preovulatory follicles. It is expressed by granulosa cells in response to FSH. Its structure is distinct from that of inhibin and activin, and shows homology to epidermal growth factor. It modifies FSH activity by binding activin thus removing this enhancing agent from cellular activity. It also possesses weak activity similar to inhibin. Thus, follistatin, like inhibin and activin, functions locally in the follicle and in the pituitary. Its circulating blood levels parallel estrogen and inhibin.

10. inhibits   p.195
The inhibin-activin family of peptides (also including antimüllerian hormone and transforming growth factor-β) inhibits cell growth and can be considered as a class of tumor-suppressor proteins. Mice have been generated that are deficient in the inhibin alpha-subunit gene. The mice that are homozygous and lack inhibin are susceptible to the development of gonadal stromal tumors which appear after normal sexual differentiation and development. Thus, the alpha-inhibin gene is a specific tumor-suppressor gene for the gonads. A contributing factor to this tumor development could be the high FSH levels associated with the deficiency in inhibin.

11. Growth factors; proliferation; differentiation; paracrine; autocrine   p.196
Growth factors are polypeptides that modulate cell proliferation and differentiation, operating through binding to specific cell membrane receptors. They are not classic endocrine substances; they act locally and function in paracrine and autocrine modes. There are multiple growth factors, and most cells contain multiple receptors for the various growth factors.

12. IGF-I; growth hormone   p.200
The insulin-like growth factor story is fascinating and compelling. However, its contribution may be facilitory and not essential. Laron-type dwarfism is characterized by a deficiency in IGF-I due to an abnormality in the growth hormone receptor. Despite low levels of IGF-I and high levels of IGFBP, a woman with Laron-type dwarfism responded to exogenous gonadotropin stimulation with the production of multiple, mature follicles with good estrogen production and fertilizable oocytes. Another explanation for this observation is that IGF-II, rather than IGF-I, is the important factor in the human dominant follicle. This possibility is supported by evidence indicating that IGF-II is the most abundant IGF in human ovarian follicles. Another possibility is that the Laron-type dwarf is deficient only in growth hormone-dependent IGF-I, and ovarian IGFs may not be totally dependent on growth hormone.

13. inhibin   p.220
The rise in FSH during the later years is believed to represent declining inhibin production by the less competent ovarian follicles. Inhibin levels are lower in the follicular phase in women 45–49 years old compared to younger women. This decline begins early but accelerates after 40 years of age. The rise in FSH is not apparent until age 40, and there is no change in LH levels until menopause. The inability to suppress gonadotropins to a normal range during estrogen treatment of postmenopausal women reflects this loss of inhibin.

14. false   p.184
Growth and atresia are not interrupted by pregnancy, ovulation, or periods of anovulation. This dynamic process continues at all ages, including infancy and around the menopause.

15. false   p.184
The mechanism for determining which follicles and how many will start growing during any one cycle is unknown. The number of follicles that starts growing each cycle appears to be dependent upon the size of the residual pool of inactive primordial follicles. Reducing the size of the pool (e.g., unilateral oophorectomy) causes the remaining follicles to redistribute their availability over time. It is possible that the follicle which is singled out to play the leading role in a particular cycle is the beneficiary of a timely match of follicle "readiness" and appropriate tropic hormone stimulation. The first follicle able to respond to stimulation may achieve an early lead that it never relinquishes.

16. true   p.185

The granulosa cells of the preantral follicle have the ability to synthesize all 3 classes of steroids; however, significantly more estrogens than either androgens or progestins are produced. An aromatase enzyme system acts to convert androgens to estrogens and appears to be a factor limiting ovarian estrogen production. Aromatization is induced or activated through the action of FSH.

17. true   p.185

The binding of FSH to its receptor and activation of the adenylate cyclase mediated signal is followed by expression of multiple mRNAs which encode proteins responsible for cell proliferation, differentiation, and function. Thus FSH both initiates steroidogenesis (estrogen production) in granulosa cells and stimulates granulosa cell growth.

18. true   p.186

FSH operates through the G protein, adenylate cyclase system, that is subject to down-regulation and modulation by many factors, including a calcium-calmodulin intermediary. Although steroidogenesis in the ovarian follicle is mainly regulated by the gonadotropins, multiple signaling pathways are involved which respond to many factors besides the gonadotropins. Besides the adenylate cyclase enzyme system, these pathways include ion gate channels, tyrosine kinase receptors, and the phospholipase system of second messengers. These pathways are utilized by a multitude of regulating factors, including the growth factors, prostaglandins, and peptides such as gonadotropin releasing hormone (GnRH), angiotensin II, tissue necrosis factor-α, and vasoactive intestinal peptide. The binding of luteinizing hormone (LH) to its receptor in the ovary is also followed by activation of the adenylate cyclase-cyclic AMP pathway in the G protein mechanism. Continuous exposure of receptors to gonadotropins results in down-regulation, involving loss of receptors by internalization, desensitization of the receptor by autophosphorylation of the cytoplasmic segment of the receptor, and uncoupling of the regulatory and catalytic subunits of the adenylate cyclase enzyme.

19. true   p.187

The steroids present in follicular fluid can be found in concentrations several orders of magnitude higher than those in plasma and reflect the functional capacity of the surrounding granulosa and theca cells. The synthesis of steroid hormones is functionally compartmentalized within the follicle — the two cell system.

20. true   p.188

As the follicle develops, theca cells begin to express the genes for LH receptors, P450scc, and 3β-hydroxysteroid dehydrogenase. Insulin-like growth factor-I (IGF-I) synergizes with LH to increase enzyme gene transcription; however IGF-I does not stimulate steroidogenesis. The separately regulated (by LH) entry of cholesterol into mitochondria, utilizing internalization of LDL-cholesterol, is essential for steroidogenesis. Therefore, ovarian steroidogenesis is always LH-dependent.

21. false   p.189

The successful conversion to an estrogen dominant follicle marks the "selection" of a follicle destined to ovulate, the process whereby, with rare exception, only a single follicle succeeds. An asymmetry in ovarian estrogen production, an expression of the emerging dominant follicle, can be detected in ovarian venous effluent on day 5 of the cycle, corresponding with the gradual fall of FSH levels observed at the midfollicular phase and preceding the increase in diameter that marks the physical emergence of the dominant follicle. This is a crucial time in the cycle

The negative feedback of estrogen on FSH serves to inhibit the development of all but the dominant follicle. The selected follicle remains dependent upon FSH and must complete its preovulatory development in the face of declining plasma levels of FSH. The dominant follicle, therefore, must escape the consequences of FSH suppression induced by its own accelerating estrogen production. The dominant follicle has two significant advantages, a greater content of FSH receptors acquired because of a rate of granulosa proliferation that surpasses that of its cohorts and enhancement of FSH action because of its high intrafollicular estrogen concentration (the nonprimate model) or because of local autocrine/paracrine peptides (the primate model). As a result, the stimulus for aromatization, FSH, can be maintained, while at the same time it is being withdrawn from among the less developed follicles. A wave of atresia among the lesser follicles, therefore, is seen to parallel the rise in estrogen.

22. **true** p.191

Within the well-established monthly pattern, the gonadotropins are secreted in a pulsatile fashion with a frequency and magnitude that vary with the phase of the cycle. The pulsatile pattern is directly due to a similar pulsatile secretion of GnRH, but amplitude and frequency modulation is probably the consequence of steroid feedback on both hypothalamus and anterior pituitary.

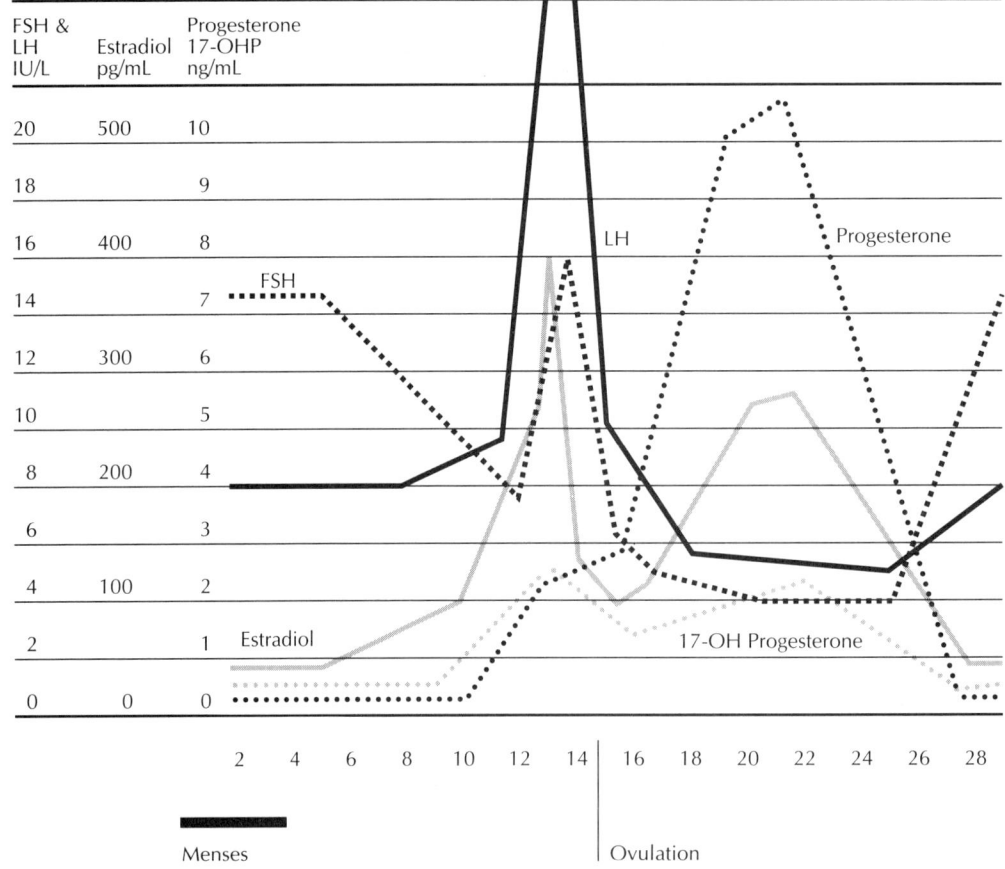

23. **false** p.191

Pulsatile secretion is more frequent but smaller in amplitude during the follicular phase compared to the luteal phase, with a slight increase in frequency observed as the follicular phase progresses to ovulation.

24. **true** p.192

The GnRH pulse frequency changes in the luteal phase correlate with duration of exposure to progesterone, while pulse amplitude changes appear to be influenced by changes in progesterone levels. Both estradiol and progesterone are required to achieve the low, suppressed secretory pattern of GnRH during the luteal phase. The studies suggest that steroids influence the hypothalamic release of GnRH for frequency changes and the pituitary for action on amplitude of the gonadotropin pulses. The inhibitory action of luteal phase steroids appears to be mediated by an increase in hypothalamic endogenous opioid peptides. Both estrogen and progesterone can increase endogenous opiates, and administration of clomiphene (an estrogen antagonist) during the luteal phase increases the LH pulse frequency with no effect on amplitude. Thus, estrogen appears to enhance the stimulatory action of progesterone in the luteal phase on endogenous opioid peptides, creating relatively high levels of endogenous opiates during the luteal phase.

Plasma endorphin begins to rise in the 2 days before the LH peak, coinciding with the midcycle gonadotropin surge. The maximal level is reached just after the LH peak, coinciding with ovulation. Levels then gradually decline until the nadir is reached during menses and the early follicular phase. Monkeys have their highest beta-endorphin levels in the hypophyseal portal blood at midcycle. Normal cyclicity requires sequential periods of high (midcycle and luteal phase) and low (during menses) hypothalamic opioid activity.

25. false   p.192

A disparity exists between the patterns of FSH and LH secretion as determined by immunoassay and bioassay, indicating that more biologically active gonadotropins are secreted at midcycle than at other times in the cycle. This quality, bioactivity vs immunoactivity, is determined by the molecular structure of the gonadotropin molecule, a concept referred to as heterogeneity of the tropic hormones. There is a well-established relationship between the activity and half-life of glycoprotein hormones and their sialic acid content. The feedback effects of estrogen include modulation of sialylation and the size and activity of the gonadotropins subsequently released, as well as an augmentation of GnRH-stimulated secretory release of biologically active gonadotropin. It certainly makes sense to intensify the gonadotropin effect at midcycle. The positive feedback action of estrogen, therefore, both increases the quantity and the quality (the bioactivity) of FSH and LH.

26. true   p.193

There is a diurnal rhythm in FSH and LH secretion. In contrast to the nocturnal rise seen with ACTH, thyroid-stimulating hormone (TSH), growth hormone, and prolactin, FSH and LH exhibit nocturnal decline, probably mediated by endogenous opiates. This diurnal rhythm for LH is present only in the early follicular phase, while FSH maintains a circadian rhythm throughout the menstrual cycle (and thus it is not influenced by steroid hormone feedback) and even in the postmenopausal period of life.

27. C   p.195

In the ovarian follicle, activin increases FSH binding in granulosa cells (by regulating receptor numbers) and augments FSH stimulation of aromatization and inhibin production. Considerable evidence derived from human cells exists to indicate that inhibin and activin act directly on thecal cells to regulate androgen synthesis. Inhibin enhances the stimulatory action of LH and/or IGF-I, while activin suppresses this action. Inhibin in increasing doses can overcome the inhibitory action of activin. Prior to ovulation, activin suppresses granulosa progesterone production, perhaps preventing premature luteinization. There is a repertoire of cell transmembrane kinase receptors for activin, with differing binding affinities and domain structures. This receptor heterogeneity allows the many different responses elicited by a single peptide. (See figure on page 90 in this Study Guide)

28. A   p.198

In whole human ovary studies, IGF-I is of thecal origin in the preovulatory phase, which together with its known biochemical actions suggests that IGF-I moves from the theca to the granulosa to function in a paracrine fashion. IGF-II, on the other hand, is synthesized by luteinized granulosa and appears to function locally in an autocrine fashion. Human thecal cells express mRNA transcripts which encode receptors for both IGF-I and insulin. Thus IGF-I exerts a paracrine influence on granulosa cells and autocrine activity in the theca (augmenting LH stimulation of androgen production). These actions are augmented by growth hormone, which increases IGF production and thus indirectly enhances gonadotropin stimulation of ovarian follicles. (See figure on page 91 in this Study Guide)

29. B   p.202

Antimüllerian hormone is produced by granulosa cells and may play a role in oocyte maturation (it inhibits oocyte meiosis) and follicular development. Antimüllerian hormone directly inhibits proliferation of granulosa and luteal cells, as well as epidermal growth factor-stimulated proliferation.

30. E   p. 194,201

The structure of the inhibin-activin genes is homologous to that of transforming growth factor-β, indicating that these products all come from the same gene family. Another important member of this family is the antimüllerian hormone, as well as a protein active during insect embryogenesis, and a protein active in frog embryos.

TGF-β utilizes a receptor distinct from the epidermal growth factor receptor. These factors are thought to be autocrine growth regulators. Inhibin and activin are derived from the same gene family. TGF-β, secreted by theca cells, enhances FSH induction of LH receptors on granulosa cells, an action which is opposite that of epidermal growth factor. While this action can be viewed as a positive impact on granulosa cells, in the theca, TGF-β has a negative action, inhibiting androgen production.

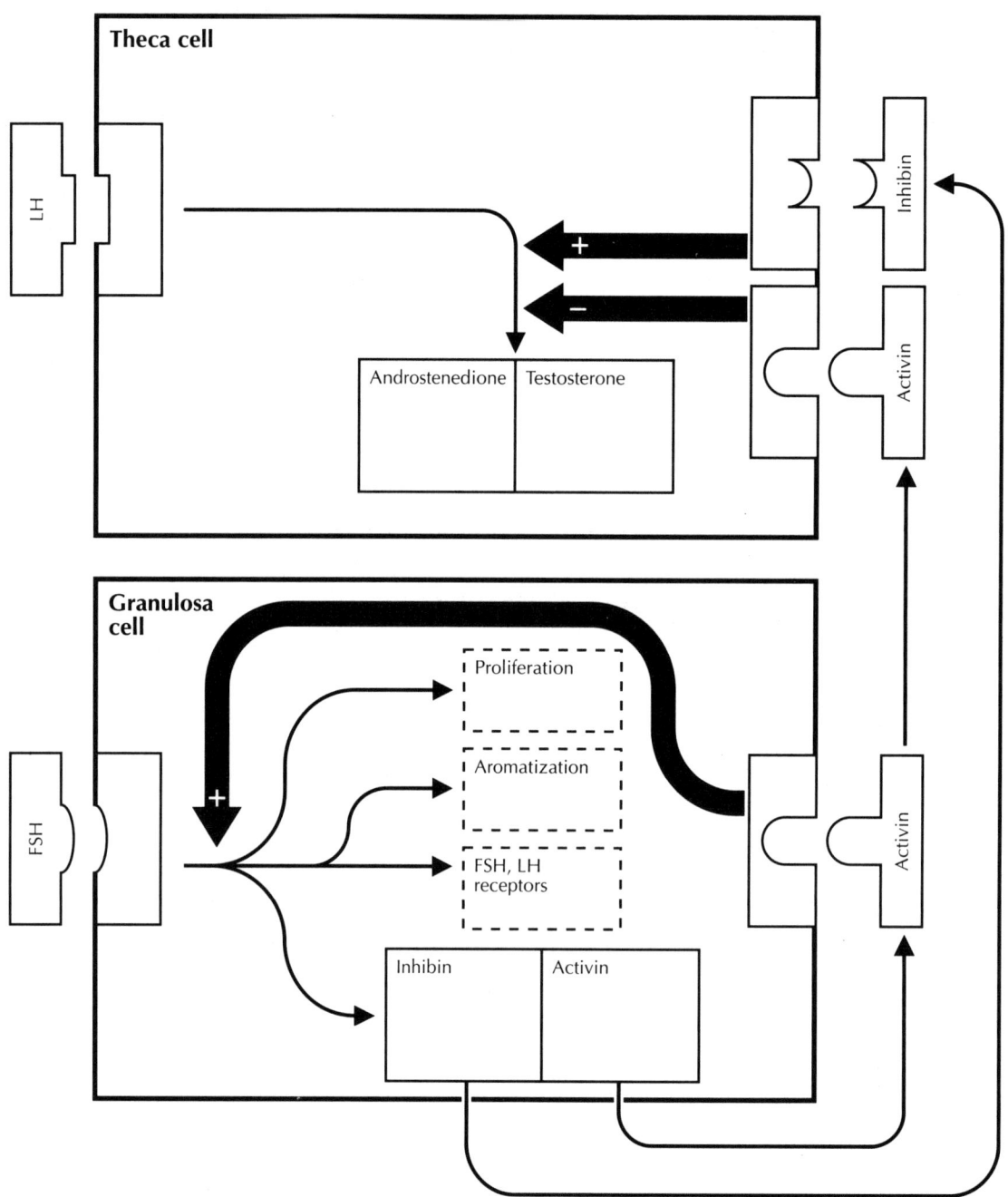

Early Follicular Phase

31. F p.201
TGF-α is a structural analogue of epidermal growth factor and can bind to the epidermal growth factor receptor.

32. B p.186
The role of androgens in early follicular development is complex. Specific androgen receptors are present in the granulosa cells. The androgens serve not only as substrate for FSH-induced aromatization but, in low concentrations, can further enhance aromatase activity. When exposed to an androgen-rich environment, preantral granulosa cells favor the conversion of androgens to more potent 5α-reduced androgens rather than to estrogens. These androgens cannot be converted to estrogen and, in fact, inhibit aromatase activity. They also inhibit FSH induction of LH receptor formation, another essential step in follicular development.

Early Follicular Phase

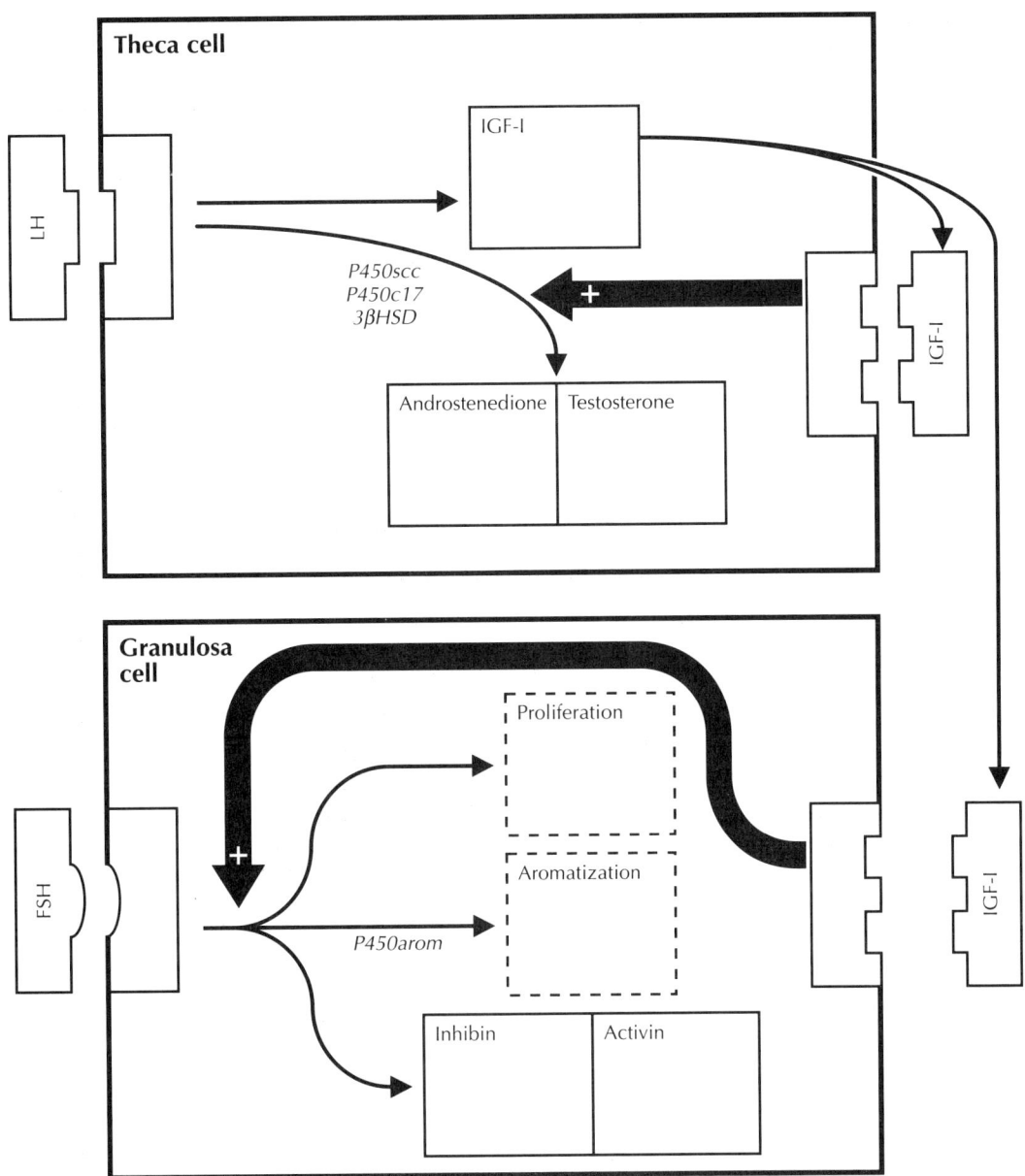

33. A   p.189,190

The negative feedback of estrogen on FSH serves to inhibit the development of all but the dominant follicle. The selected follicle remains dependent upon FSH and must complete its preovulatory development in the face of declining plasma levels of FSH. The dominant follicle, therefore, must escape the consequences of FSH suppression induced by its own accelerating estrogen production. The dominant follicle has two significant advantages, a greater content of FSH receptors acquired because of a rate of granulosa proliferation that surpasses that of its cohorts and enhancement of FSH action because of its high intrafollicular estrogen concentration (the nonprimate model) or because of local autocrine/paracrine peptides (the primate model). As a result, the stimulus for aromatization, FSH, can be maintained, while at the same time it is being withdrawn from among the less developed follicles. A wave of atresia among the lesser follicles, therefore, is seen to parallel the rise in estrogen.

34. E   p.193,194

Inhibin consists of two dissimilar peptides (known as alpha- and beta-subunits) linked by disulfide bonds. Two forms of inhibin (inhibin-A and inhibin-B) have been purified, each containing an identical alpha-subunit and distinct but related beta-subunits. Thus, there are three subunits for inhibins: alpha, beta-A, and beta-B. Each subunit is a product of different messenger RNA, each derived from its own precursor molecule.

The 2 Forms of Inhibin:
    Inhibin-A: Alpha-Beta$_A$
    Inhibin-B: Alpha-Beta$_B$

FSH stimulates the secretion of inhibin from granulosa cells and, in turn, is suppressed by inhibin — a reciprocal relationship. The secretion of inhibin is further regulated by local autocrine/paracrine control. GnRH and epidermal growth factor diminish FSH stimulation of inhibin secretion, while insulin-like growth factor-I enhances inhibin production. The inhibitory effects of GnRH and epidermal growth factor are consistent with their known ability to decrease FSH-stimulated estrogen production and LH receptor formation. The action of GnRH lends some support for an endogenous ovarian GnRH-like substance (which is found in follicular fluid) and which is involved in inhibin production.

The secretion of inhibin into the circulation further amplifies the withdrawal of FSH from other follicles, another mechanism by which an emerging follicle secures dominance. Inhibin rises slowly but steadily throughout the follicular phase to reach a midcycle peak that coincides with the gonadotropin surge. With development of the follicle into a corpus luteum, inhibin expression comes under the control of LH. The circulating levels of inhibin drop slightly from the midcycle peak, then rise to reach a level at the midluteal phase that is at least two times greater than the midcycle peak. After conception, even higher circulating levels of inhibin are achieved. There is some question whether the luteal levels of immunoactive inhibin represent true inhibin bioactivity or whether inactive subunits of inhibin are being measured.

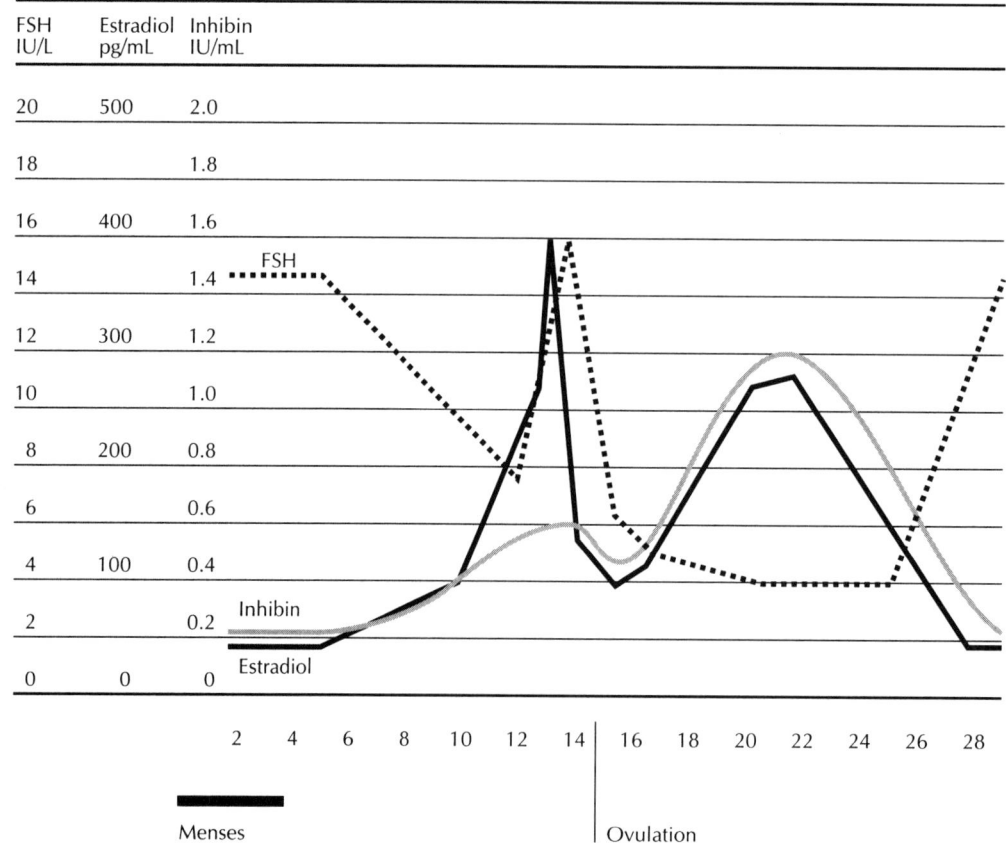

35. D   p.194,195
Activin is a peptide that is related to inhibin but has an opposite action (the stimulation of FSH release and GnRH receptor number). This peptide contains two subunits that are identical to the beta-subunits of inhibins A and B. Thus,

when each of the beta-subunits of the inhibins is combined with an alpha-subunit, the resulting molecule, inhibin A or B, inhibits the release of FSH. If the beta-subunits are paired together, the molecule stimulates the release of FSH. Each inhibin and activin subunit is encoded by a distinct gene.

The 3 Forms of Activin:

Activin-A: $Beta_A$-$Beta_A$
Activin-AB: $Beta_A$-$Beta_B$
Activin-B: $Beta_B$-$Beta_B$

Activin is present in many cell types, regulating growth and differentiation. In the ovarian follicle, activin increases FSH binding in granulosa cells (by regulating receptor numbers) and augments FSH stimulation of aromatization and inhibin production.

36. E   p.195

Follistatin is a single chain, glycosylated polypeptide produced in the pituitary but found primarily in preovulatory follicles. It is expressed by granulosa cells in response to FSH. Its structure is distinct from that of inhibin and activin, and shows homology to epidermal growth factor. It modifies FSH activity by binding activin thus removing this enhancing agent from cellular activity. It also possesses weak activity similar to inhibin. Thus, follistatin, like inhibin and activin, functions locally in the follicle and in the pituitary. Its circulating blood levels parallel estrogen and inhibin.

The pituitary secretion of FSH can be significantly regulated by the balance of activin and inhibin, with follistatin playing a role by inhibiting activin and enhancing inhibin activity. Within the ovarian follicle, activin and inhibin influence growth and development by modulating thecal and granulosal responses to the gonadotropins.

37. B   p.196

The insulin-like growth factors (also called somatomedins) are peptides that have structural and functional similarity to insulin and mediate growth hormone action. Insulin-like growth factor-I (IGF-I) and insulin-like growth factor-II (IGF-II) are single chain polypeptides containing 3 disulfide bonds. IGF-I is encoded on the long arm of chromosome 12 and IGF-II on the short arm of chromosome 11 (which also contains the insulin gene). The genes are subject to a variety of promoters, and thus differential regulation can govern ultimate actions.

IGF-I mediates the growth promoting actions of growth hormone. The majority of circulating IGF-I is derived from the growth hormone dependent synthesis in the liver. However, IGF-I is synthesized in many tissues where production can be regulated in conjunction with growth hormone or independently by other factors.

IGF-II has little growth hormone dependence. It is believed to be more important in fetal growth and development. Both IGFs induce the expression of cellular genes responsible for cellular proliferation and differentiation.

There are 6 known nonglycosylated peptides which function as IGF binding proteins: IGFBP-1 to IGFBP-6. These binding proteins serve to carry the IGFs in serum, prolong half-lives, and regulate tissue effects of the IGFs. The regulating action appears to be due to binding and sequestering of the IGFs, preventing their access to the cell membrane surface receptors, and thus not permitting the synergistic actions that result when gonadotropins and growth factors are combined. The IGFBPs may also exert direct actions on cellular functions, independently of growth factor functions. IGFBP-1 is the principal BP in amniotic fluid; IGFBP-3 is the main BP in serum and its synthesis, primarily in the liver, is dependent on growth hormone. Circulating levels of IGFBP-3 reflect the total IGF concentration (IGF-I plus IGF-II) and carry at least 90% of the circulating IGFs. These BPs do not bind insulin. The BPs change with age (decreasing levels of BP-3) and during pregnancy (decreasing BP-3 due to a circulating protease unique to pregnancy).

38. B   p.196

The Type I receptor preferentially binds IGF-1 and can be called the IGF-I receptor. The Type II receptor in a similar fashion can be called the IGF-II receptor. IGF-I also binds to the insulin receptor but with low affinity. Insulin binds to the IGF-I receptor with moderate affinity. The IGF-I receptor and the insulin receptor are similar in structure: tetramers composed of two α-subunits and two β-subunits linked by disulfide bonds. The intracellular component of the β-subunit is a tyrosine kinase that is activated by autophosphorylation. The IGF-II receptor does not bind insulin.

It is a single chain glycoprotein, with 90% of its structure extending extracellularly. This receptor functions as a receptor coupled to a G protein. The physiologic effects of IGF-I are mediated by its own receptor, but IGF-II can exert its actions via both receptors. In human cells, the IGF-I receptor is present in theca and granulosa cells and in luteinized granulosa cells. IGF-II receptor expression is marked in luteinized granulosa cells, and only IGF-II is found in the corpus luteum. Ovarian stromal tissue contains IGF-I receptors.

39. E   p.197–200

IGF-I has been demonstrated to stimulate the following events in ovarian theca and granulosa cells: DNA synthesis, steroidogenesis, aromatase activity, LH receptor synthesis, and inhibin secretion. IGF-II stimulates granulosa mitosis. In human ovarian cells, IGF-I, in synergy with FSH, stimulates protein synthesis and steroidogenesis. After LH receptors appear, IGF-I enhances LH-induced progesterone synthesis and stimulates proliferation of granulosa-luteal cells. IGF-I, in synergy with FSH, is very active in stimulating aromatase activity in preovulatory follicles. Thus, IGF-I is involved in both estradiol and progesterone synthesis.

Summary of Insulin-Like Growth Factor Action in the Ovary
1. IGF-I stimulates granulosa cell proliferation, aromatase activity, and progesterone synthesis.
2. IGF-I is produced in theca cells; luteinized granulosa cells produce IGF-II. In the pig and rat, the sites are reversed; granulosa produces IGF-I and theca produces IGF-II.
3. Gonadotropins stimulate IGF production, and in animal experiments, this stimulation is enhanced by estradiol and growth hormone.
4. IGF-I receptors are present in theca and granulosa cells, and only IGF-II receptors are present in luteinized granulosa.
5. The most abundant IGF in human follicles is IGF-II.
6. FSH inhibits binding protein synthesis, and thus maximizes growth factor availability.

40. C   p.198–200

IGF-II is synthesized by luteinized granulosa and appears to function locally in an autocrine fashion. There are no menstrual cycle changes in the circulating levels of IGF-I and IGF-II; high levels in the dominant follicle are not associated with an increase in circulating levels. IGF-II, rather than IGF-I may be the important factor in the human dominant follicle. This possibility is supported by evidence indicating that IGF-II is the most abundant IGF in human ovarian follicles.

41. E   p.201–202

Follicular fluid contains prorenin, the inactive precursor of renin, in a concentration that is about 12 times higher than plasma levels. It appears that LH stimulates its synthesis in the follicle, and there is a midcycle peak in prorenin plasma levels. The circulating levels of prorenin also increase (10-fold) during the early stages of pregnancy, the result of ovarian stimulation by the rise in human chorionic gonadotropin (HCG). These increases in prorenin from the ovary are not responsible for any significant changes in the plasma levels of the active form, renin. Possible roles for this ovarian prorenin-renin-angiotensin system include stimulation of steroidogenesis to provide androgen substrate for estrogen production, regulation of calcium and prostaglandin metabolism, and stimulation of angiogenesis. This system may affect vascular and tissue functions both within and outside the ovary.

Members of the proopiomelanocortin family are found in human follicular fluid. Follicular levels of ACTH and β-lipotropin remain constant throughout the cycle, but β-endorphin levels peak just before ovulation. In addition, enkephalin is present in relatively unchanging concentrations.

Antimüllerian hormone is produced by granulosa cells and may play a role in oocyte maturation (it inhibits oocyte meiosis) and follicular development. Antimüllerian hormone directly inhibits proliferation of granulosa and luteal cells, as well as epidermal growth factor-stimulated proliferation.

Follicular fluid prevents resumption of meiosis until the preovulatory LH surge either overcomes or removes this inhibition. This action is attributed to oocyte maturation inhibitor (OMI). Pregnancy-associated plasma protein A, found in the placenta, is also present in follicular fluid. It may inhibit proteolytic activity within the follicle before ovulation. Endothelin-1 is a peptide, originally isolated from vascular endothelial cells, which may be the substance previously known as luteinization inhibitor; endothelin gene expression is induced by the hypoxia associated with the avascular granulosa, and it inhibits LH-induced progesterone production. It is uncertain whether GnRH-like peptides have a follicular role or represent sequestered GnRH. Oxytocin is found in preovulatory follicles and the corpus luteum, but its function is unknown. Growth hormone-binding protein is present in follicular fluid and similar in characteristics to the same binding protein in serum.

42. C   p.207

Granulosa cells in the preovulatory follicle enlarge and acquire lipid inclusions while the theca becomes vacuolated and richly vascular, giving the preovulatory follicle a hyperemic appearance. The oocyte resumes meiosis, approaching completion of its reduction division.

Approaching maturity, the preovulatory follicle produces increasing amounts of estrogen. During the late follicular phase, estrogens rise slowly at first, then rapidly, reaching a peak approximately 24–36 hours prior to ovulation. The onset of the LH surge occurs when the peak levels of estradiol are achieved. In providing the ovulatory stimulus to the selected follicle, the LH surge seals the fate of the remaining follicles, with their lower estrogen and FSH content, by further increasing androgen superiority.

43. E   p.209

The preovulatory follicle, through the elaboration of estradiol, provides its own ovulatory stimulus. Considerable variation in timing exists from cycle to cycle, even in the same woman. A reasonable and accurate estimate places ovulation approximately 10–12 hours after the LH peak and 24–36 hours after peak estradiol levels are attained. The onset of the LH surge appears to be the most reliable indicator of impending ovulation, occurring 34–36 hours prior to follicle rupture. A threshold of LH concentration must be maintained for 14–27 hours in order for full maturation of the oocyte to occur. Usually the LH surge lasts 48–50 hours.

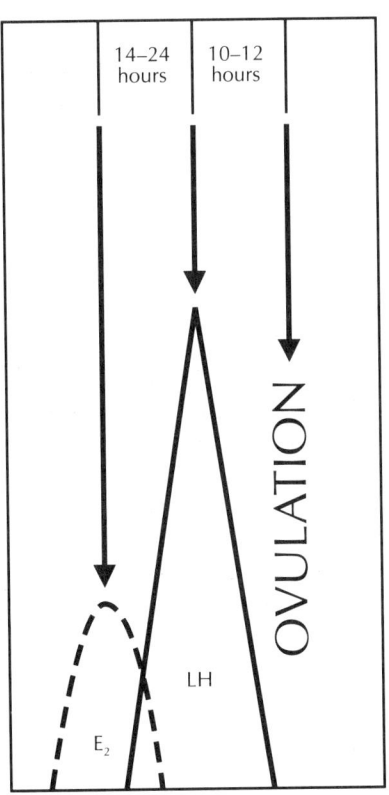

44. B   p.219

Summary of Events in the Luteal-Follicular Transition
1. The demise of the corpus luteum results in a nadir in the circulating levels of estradiol, progesterone, and inhibin.
2. The decrease in inhibin removes a suppressing influence on FSH secretion in the pituitary.
3. The decrease in estradiol and progesterone allows a progressive and rapid increase in the frequency of GnRH pulsatile secretion and a removal of the pituitary from negative feedback suppression.
4. The removal of inhibin and estradiol and increasing GnRH pulses combine to allow greater secretion of FSH compared to LH, with an increase in the frequency of the episodic secretion.
5. The increase in FSH is instrumental in rescuing a group of follicles from atresia, allowing a dominant follicle to begin its emergence.

45. B   p.219

Menstrual cycle length is determined by the rate and quality of follicular growth and development, and it is normal for the cycle to vary in individual women. Menarche is followed by approximately 5–7 years of increasing regularity as cycles shorten to reach the usual reproductive age pattern. In the 40s, cycles begin to lengthen again. The highest incidence of anovulatory cycles is under age 20 and over age 40. At age 25, over 40% of cycles are between 25 and 28 days in length; from 25 to 35, over 60% are between 25 and 28 days. The perfect 28-day cycle is indeed the most common mode, but it totals only 12.4%. Overall, approximately 15% of reproductive age cycles are 28 days in length. Only 0.5% of women experience a cycle less than 21 days long, and only 0.9% a cycle greater than 35 days. Most women have cycles that last from 24 to 35 days, but at least 20% of women experience irregular cycles.

The duration of the follicular phase is the major determinant of cycle length. Cycle lengths are the shortest (with the least variability) in the late 30s, a time when subtle but real increases in FSH and decreases in inhibin are occurring. This can be pictured as accelerated follicular growth (because of the changes in FSH and inhibin). At the same time, fewer follicles grow per cycle as a woman ages. Approximately 2–4 years (6–8 years according to Trelolar) prior to menopause, the cycles lengthen again. Eventually menopause occurs because the supply of follicles is depleted.

46. A   p.220

The rise in FSH during the later years is believed to represent declining inhibin production by the less competent ovarian follicles. Inhibin levels are lower in the follicular phase in women 45–49 years old compared to younger women. This decline begins early but accelerates after 40 years of age. The rise in FSH is not apparent until age 40, and there is no change in LH levels until menopause. The inability to suppress gonadotropins to a normal range during estrogen treatment of postmenopausal women reflects this loss of inhibin.

7 Sperm and Egg Transport, Fertilization and Implantation

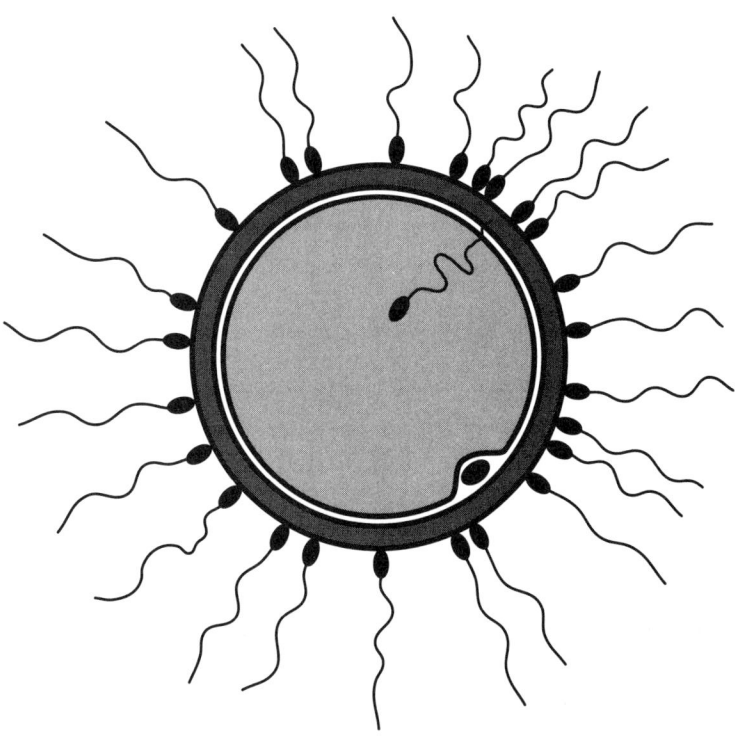

Learning Objectives

Be able to:

1. Detail the anatomy of the sperm and oocyte prior to fertilization.

2. Describe the significance of capacitation and the acrosome reaction as they relate to sperm physiology.

3. Describe the time course of oocyte transport throughout the fallopian tube following ovulation.

4. Detail the processes of the zona reaction and cortical reaction and their relevance to normal fertilization of the oocyte.

5. Discuss the role of the blastocyst as it relates to timing of implantation within the uterus.

6. Describe the incidence and etiology of post-implantation pregnancy loss.

Pre-Test

A. Instructions: Fill in the blanks

1. Motility and the ability to fertilize are acquired gradually as the sperm pass into the _____.

2. The initiation of the block to penetration of the zona by additional sperm is mediated by the _____ reaction.

B. Instructions: True or False

3. During the act of coitus, of the 200–300 million sperm deposited in the vagina, fewer than 200 achieve proximity to the egg.

4. The fertilizable life of the mature human ovum is unknown, but most estimates range between 24 and 48 hours.

D. Instructions: For each of the following questions choose:

A. if only 1, 2 and 3 are correct
B. if only 1 and 3 are correct
C. if only 2 and 4 are correct
D. if only 4 is correct
E. if all are correct

5. Capacitation
    1. allows sperm to undergo the acrosome reaction
    2. allows sperm to acquire hypermotility
    3. allows sperm to be able to bind to the zona pellucida
    4. requires breakdown and merging of the plasma membrane and the outer acrosomal membrane

6. Implantation
    1. occurs in the uterus in the upper, anterior wall in the midsagittal phase
    2. is associated with an endometrium that is 10–14mm thick in the midluteal phase
    3. is a well understood process
    4. has a "window" of endometrial receptivity restricted to days 16–19 of a 28-day cycle

Chapter 7 Sperm and Egg Transport, Fertilization and Implantation

Post-Test

A. Instructions: Fill in the blanks

1. The sperm reach the caudal epididymis approximately _____ days after the initiation of spermatogenesis.

2. The _____ is a large vesicle of proteolytic enzymes located within the _____ of the sperm.

3. Preservation of optimal sperm function during storage requires adequate _____ levels in the circulation and maintenance of the normal _____ _____.

4. Semen is liquefied following ejaculation due to enzymes derived from the _____.

5. _____ is the process by which sperm becomes capable of penetrating an ovum.

6. The _____ reaction is a process which allows enzymes to egress from a cap-like structure that covers a portion of sperm nucleus.

7. _____ syndrome is a congenital absence of dynein arms in the _____.

8. Sperm receptors in the zona pellucida are glycoproteins known as _____, _____, and _____.

B. Instructions: True or False

9. The caudal epididymis stores sperm available for ejaculation.

10. The epididymis is limited to a storage role because sperm which has bypassed the epididymis by epididymal aspiration can fertilize the human oocyte in vitro.

11. Following insemination sperm take at least 30 minutes before they are in the tube.

12. Enzymes stored in the acrosome include hyaluronidase and acrosin which play a role in sperm penetration of the zona pellucida.

13. Ectopic pregnancies occur with similar frequency in humans as compared to other animals.

14. Fusion of the sperm and oocyte membrane triggers the cortical reaction and completion of meiosis.

15. Implantation occurs 10 days after fertilization.

C. Instructions: Match each phrase with the most appropriate word association

A. perivitelline
B. zona pellucida
C. corona radiata
D. ZP3
E. polyspermy

16. its gene is expressed only in growing oocytes
17. is a space located between the zona pellucida and the plasma membrane of the oocyte

D. Instructions: For each of the following questions choose:
- A. if only 1, 2 and 3 are correct
- B. if only 1 and 3 are correct
- C. if only 2 and 4 are correct
- D. if only 4 is correct
- E. if all are correct

18. Semen
    1. has an alkaline PH
    2. contains sperm and seminal plasma
    3. liquefies within 20–30 minutes
    4. is a product of the testicles and seminal vesicles

19. The oocyte
    1. is surrounded by specialized granulosa cells called the mural oophorus
    2. communicates metabolically with granulosa cells by gap junctions
    3. following ovulation the cumulus cells retract their cellular contacts from the oocyte
    4. disruption of gap junctions induces maturation and migration of the cortical granules to the outer cortex of the oocyte

20. The zona pellucida
    1. contains receptors for sperm which are species-specific
    2. undergoes the zona reaction which blocks polyspermia from occurring
    3. is penetrated by sperm having undergone capacitation and the acrosome reaction
    4. is a noncellular porous layer of glycoproteins

21. The acrosome
    1. reaction requires an influx of calcium ions, an efflux of hydrogen ions
    2. completely surrounds the nucleus of the sperm
    3. reaction requires a change in pH
    4. reaction occurs prior to sperm-egg binding

22. The cortical reaction
    1. involves hardening of the extracellular layer by cross-linking proteins
    2. prevents polyspermy
    3. is associated with a rapid depolarization of the oocyte membrane
    4. is mediated by the release of hydrolytic enzymes from the cortical granules

23. True statements regarding the reproductive process are:
    1. the total rate of pregnancy loss after implantation is approximately 30%
    2. the generally accepted figure for spontaneous abortion in the first trimester is 15%
    3. 50–60% of first trimester abortions have chromosome abnormalities
    4. in each ovulatory cycle, 33% of normally fertile couples can achieve a live birth

24. The human blastocyst
    1. initially develops within the ampullary portion of the fallopian tube
    2. remains in the uterine secretions for approximately 72 hours prior to implantation
    3. develops prior to the morula stage
    4. must hatch from its zona pellucida in preparation for attachment

Answers for Chapter 7 — Pre-Test

1. epididymis p.231–232

The sperm reach the caudal epididymis approximately 72 days after the initiation of spermatogenesis. At this time, the head of the sperm contains a membrane bound nucleus capped by the acrosome, a large vesicle of proteolytic enzymes. The inner acrosomal membrane is closely opposed to the nuclear membrane, and the outer acrosomal membrane is next to the surface plasma membrane. The flagellum is a complex structure of microtubules and fibers, surrounded at the proximal end by mitochondria. Motility and the ability to fertilize are acquired gradually as the sperm pass into the epididymis.

2. cortical p.239

The initiation of the block to penetration of the zona (and the vitellus) by other sperm is mediated by the cortical reaction, a release of materials from the cortical granules, lysosome-like organelles which are found just below the egg surface. As with other lysosome-like organelles, these materials include various hydrolytic enzymes. Changes brought about by these enzymes lead to the zona reaction, the hardening of the extracellular layer by cross-linking of proteins, and inactivation of sperm receptors. Thus the zona block to polyspermy is accomplished. The initial change in this zona block is a rapid depolarization of the oocyte membrane associated with a release of calcium ions from calmodulin. The increase in intracellular calcium acts as a signal or trigger to activate protein synthesis in the oocyte. The depolarization of the membrane initiates only a transient block to sperm entry. The permanent block is a consequence of the cortical reaction and release of enzymes, also apparently triggered by the increase in calcium.

3. true p.233

The attrition in sperm numbers from vagina to tube is substantial. Of an average of 200 million to 300 million sperm deposited in the vagina, fewer than 200 achieve proximity to the egg. The major loss occurs in the vagina, with expulsion of semen from the introitus playing an important role. Other causes for loss are digestion of sperm by vaginal enzymes and phagocytosis of sperm along the reproductive tract. There are also reports of sperm burrowing into or being engulfed by endometrial cells. Sperm are not stored in the fallopian tube, and indeed many sperm continue past the oocyte to be lost into the peritoneal cavity. However, the cervix does serve as a reservoir providing a supply of sperm for up to 72 hours.

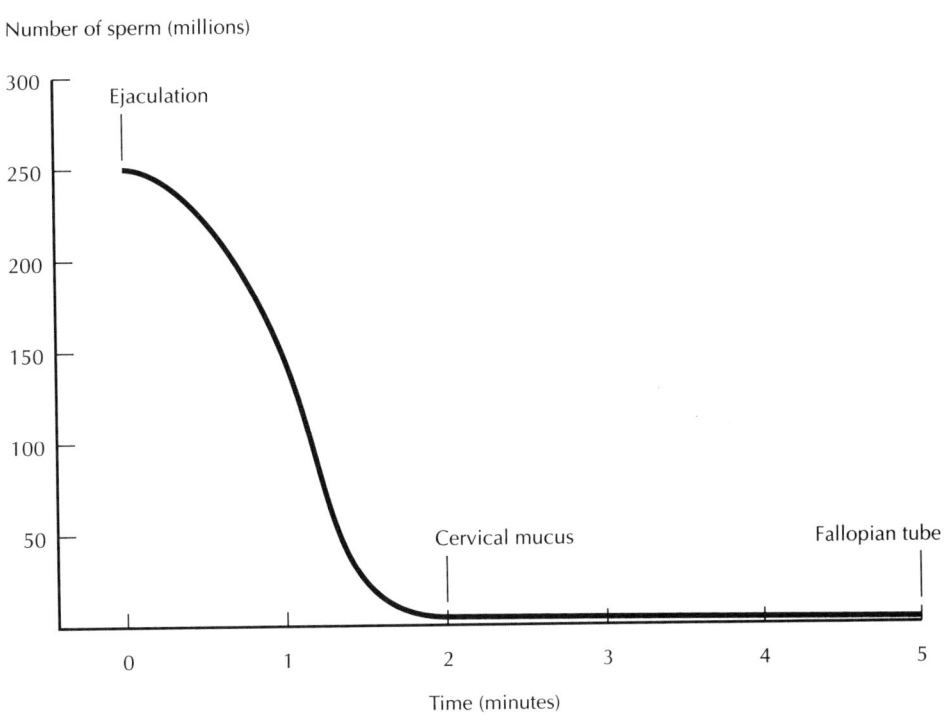

4. false p.238

Following ovulation, the fertilizable lifespan of the rabbit egg is between 6 and 8 hours. The fertilizable life of the human ovum is unknown, but most estimates range between 12 and 24 hours. However, immature human eggs recovered for in vitro fertilization can be fertilized even after 36 hours of incubation. Equally uncertain is knowledge of the fertilizable lifespan of human sperm. The most common estimate is 48–72 hours, although motility can be maintained after the sperm have lost the ability to fertilize.

5. A p.234

Capacitation is characterized by 3 accomplishments:
1. The ability to undergo the acrosome reaction.
2. The ability to bind to the zona pellucida.
3. The acquisition of hypermotility.

Capacitation changes the surface characteristics of sperm, as exemplified by removal of seminal plasma factors that coat the surface of the sperm, modification of their surface charge, and restriction of receptor mobility. This is associated with decreased stability of the plasma membrane and the membrane lying immediately under it, the outer acrosomal membrane. The membranes undergo further, more striking, modifications when capacitated sperm reach the vicinity of an ovum or when they are incubated in follicular fluid. There is a breakdown and merging of the plasma membrane and the outer acrosomal membrane, the acrosome reaction. This allows egress of the enzyme contents of the acrosome, the cap-like structure that covers the sperm nucleus. These enzymes, which include hyaluronidase, a neuraminidase-like factor, corona-dispersing enzyme, and a protease called acrosin, are all thought to play roles in sperm penetration of the egg investments. The changes in the sperm head membranes also prepare the sperm for fusion with the egg membrane. It is the inner acrosomal membrane that fuses with the oocyte plasma membrane. In addition, capacitation endows the sperm with hypermotility, and the increased velocity of the sperm may be the most critical factor in mediating zona penetration. The acrosome reaction can be induced by zona pellucida proteins of the oocyte and by human follicular fluid in vitro.

6. C p.241

The endometrium is 10–14 mm thick at the time of implantation in the midluteal phase. By this time, secretory activity has reached a peak, and the endometrial cells are rich in glycogen and lipids. Understanding the dynamic endocrine behavior of the endometrium increases the appreciation for its active participation in the implantation process. The window of endometrial receptivity is restricted to days 16–19 (of a 28-day cycle).

Answers for Chapter 7 — Post-Test

1. 72 p.231

The sperm reach the caudal epididymis approximately 72 days after the initiation of spermatogenesis.

2. acrosome; head p.231

The head of the sperm contains a membrane bound nucleus capped by the acrosome, a large vesicle of proteolytic enzymes. The inner acrosomal membrane is closely opposed to the nuclear membrane, and the outer acrosomal membrane is next to the surface plasma membrane. The flagellum is a complex structure of microtubules and fibers, surrounded at the proximal end by mitochondria. (See figure on page 103 in this Study Guide)

3. testosterone; scrotal temperature p.232

The caudal epididymis stores sperm available for ejaculation. The ability to store functional sperm provides a capacity for repetitive fertile ejaculations. Preservation of optimal sperm function during this period of storage requires adequate testosterone levels in the circulation and maintenance of the normal scrotal temperature. The importance of temperature is emphasized by the correlation of reduced numbers of sperm associated with episodes of body fever.

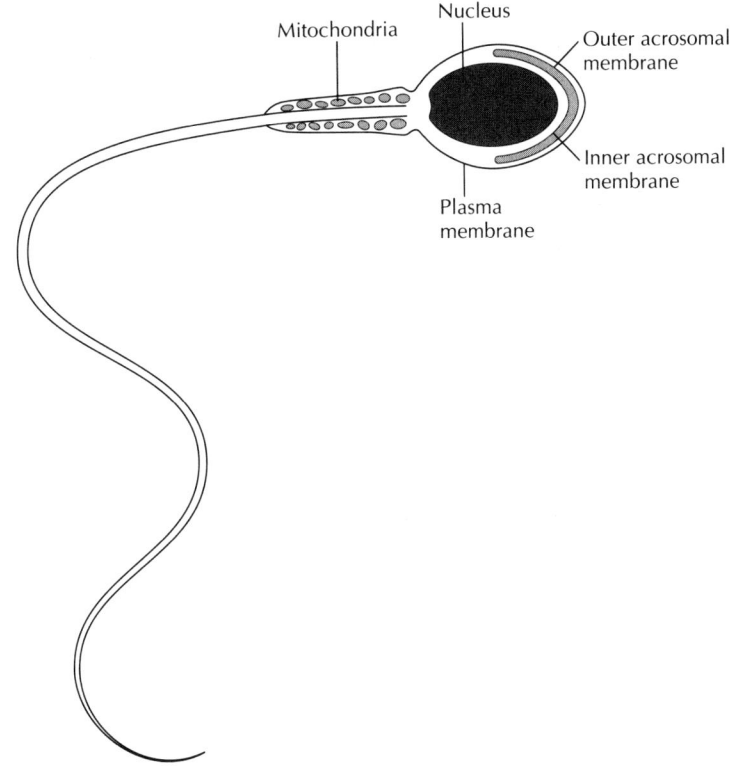

4. prostate p.232

Semen forms a gel almost immediately following ejaculation but then is liquefied in 20–30 minutes by enzymes derived from the prostate gland. The alkaline pH of semen provides protection for the sperm from the acid environment of the vagina. This protection is transient, and most sperm left in the vagina are immobilized within 2 hours. The more fortunate sperm, by their own motility, gain entrance into the tongues of cervical mucus that layer over the ectocervix. These are the sperm that enter the uterus; the seminal plasma is left behind in the vagina.

5. Capacitation p.233

The discovery in 1951 that rabbit and rat spermatozoa must spend some hours in the female tract before acquiring the capacity to penetrate ova stimulated intensive research efforts to delineate the environmental conditions required for this change in the sperm to occur. The process by which the sperm were transformed was called capacitation.

6. acrosome p.234

Capacitation is associated with decreased stability of the plasma membrane and the membrane lying immediately under it, the outer acrosomal membrane. The membranes undergo further, more striking, modifications when capacitated sperm reach the vicinity of an ovum or when they are incubated in follicular fluid. There is a breakdown and merging of the plasma membrane and the outer acrosomal membrane, the acrosome reaction. This allows egress of the enzyme contents of the acrosome, the cap-like structure that covers the sperm nucleus.

7. Kartagener's; cilia p.236

Ciliary beat is crucial for egg transport in the rabbit. Cilia play, in all likelihood, a less important role in the human. There are *fertile* women who have Kartagener's syndrome in which there is a congenital absence of dynein arms in cilia, and thus the cilia do not beat. This deficiency in the cilia is found in the fallopian tubes as well as in the respiratory tract.

8. ZP1; ZP2; ZP3 p.238

The initial contact between the sperm and the oocyte is a receptor-mediated process. The sperm receptors in the zona pellucida are glycoproteins, known as ZP1, ZP2, and ZP3, with ZP3 being the most abundant. Structural alteration of these glycoproteins leads to a loss of receptor activity; inactivation of these receptors after fertilization is probably accomplished by one or more cortical granule enzymes. The zona pellucida is a porous structure, due to the many receptor glycoproteins assembled into long, interconnecting filaments.

9. true   p.232

The caudal epididymis stores sperm available for ejaculation. The ability to store functional sperm provides a capacity for repetitive fertile ejaculations.

10. true   p.232

The epididymis is limited to a storage role because sperm that have never passed through the epididymis and that have been obtained from the vasa efferentia in men with a congenital absence of the vas deferens can fertilize the human oocyte in vitro and result in pregnancy with live birth.

11. false   p.232

The more fortunate sperm, by their own motility, gain entrance into the tongues of cervical mucus that layer over the ectocervix. These are the sperm that enter the uterus; the seminal plasma is left behind in the vagina. This entry is rapid, and sperm have been found in mucus within 90 seconds of ejaculation. The destruction of all sperm in the vagina 5 minutes after ejaculation does not interfere with fertilization in the rabbit, further attesting to the rapidity of transport.

12. true   p.234

The acrosomal enzymes, which include hyaluronidase, a neuraminidase-like factor, corona-dispersing enzyme, and a protease called acrosin, are all thought to play roles in sperm penetration of the egg investments. The changes in the sperm head membranes also prepare the sperm for fusion with the egg membrane. It is the inner acrosomal membrane that fuses with the oocyte plasma membrane. In addition, capacitation endows the sperm with hypermotility, and the increased velocity of the sperm may be the most critical factor in mediating zona penetration. The acrosome reaction can be induced by zona pellucida proteins of the oocyte and by human follicular fluid in vitro.

13. false   p.238

Animal and human reproduction differ in the occurrence of ectopic pregnancy. Ectopic pregnancies are rare in animals, and in rodents they are not induced even if the uterotubal junction is occluded immediately following fertilization. The embryos reach the blastocyst stage and then degenerate.

14. true   p.240

Fusion of the sperm and oocyte membrane triggers the cortical reaction, metabolic activation of the oocyte, and completion of meiosis. The second polar body is released at the time of fertilization and leaves the egg with a haploid complement of chromosomes. The addition of chromosomes from the sperm restores the diploid number to the now fertilized egg.

15. false   p.242

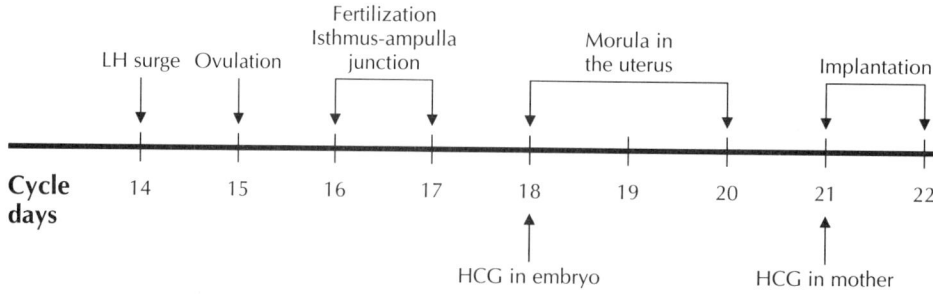

16. D   p.239

The ZP3 gene is expressed only in growing oocytes. DNA sequence similarities of the ZP3 gene in various mammals indicates that this gene has been evolutionarily conserved and that the sperm-receptor interaction is a common mechanism among mammals.

17. A   p.239

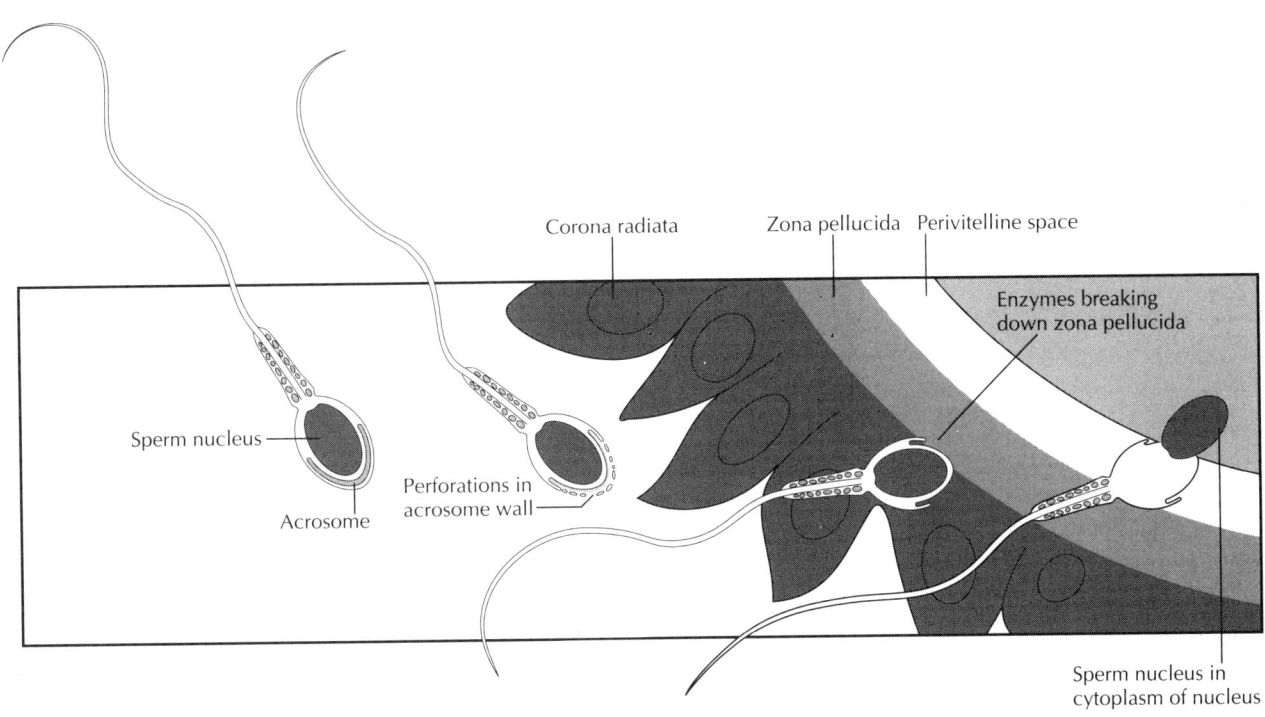

18. E   p.232
Semen forms a gel almost immediately following ejaculation but then is liquefied in 20–30 minutes by enzymes derived from the prostate gland. The alkaline pH of semen provides protection for the sperm from the acid environment of the vagina. This protection is transient, and most sperm left in the vagina are immobilized within 2 hours.

19. C   p.235
The oocyte, at the time of ovulation, is surrounded by granulosa cells (the cumulus oophorus) that attach the oocyte to the wall of the follicle. The granulosa cells communicate metabolically with the oocyte by means of gap junctions between the oocyte plasma membrane and the cumulus cells. In response to the midcycle surge in luteinizing hormone (LH), maturation of the oocyte proceeds with the resumption of meiosis as the oocyte enters into the second meiotic division and arrests in the second metaphase. Just before ovulation, the cumulus cells retract their cellular contacts from the oocyte. The disruption of the gap junctions induces maturation and migration of the cortical granules to the outer cortex of the oocyte. Prior to ovulation, the oocyte and its cumulus mass of cells prepare to leave their long residence in the ovary by becoming detached from the follicular wall.

20. E   p.235,238
The zona pellucida, a noncellular porous layer of glycoproteins, separates the oocyte from the granulosa cells. The acellular zona pellucida that surrounds the egg at ovulation and remains in place until implantation has two major functions in the fertilization process:

   1. The zona pellucida contains receptors for sperm which are, with some exceptions, relatively species-specific.
   2. The zona pellucida undergoes the **zona reaction** in which the zona becomes impervious to other sperm once the fertilizing sperm penetrates, and thus it provides a bar to polyploidy.

Penetration through the zona is rapid and possibly is mediated by acrosin, a trypsin-like proteinase that is bound to the inner acrosomal membrane of the sperm.

21. B   p.238,239

The acrosome is a lysosome-like organelle in the anterior region of the sperm head, lying just beneath the plasma membrane. The acrosome contains many enzymes that are exposed by the acrosome reaction, the loss of the acrosome immediately before fertilization. This reaction requires an influx of calcium ions, the efflux of hydrogen ion, an increase in pH, and fusion of the plasma membrane with the outer acrosomal membrane, leading to the exposure and escape of the enzymes contained on the inner acrosomal membrane. Binding to the zona pellucida is required to permit a component of the zona to induce the acrosomal reaction. This component is believed to be a glycoprotein sperm receptor, which thus serves a dual function.

22. E   p.239

The initiation of the block to penetration of the zona (and the vitellus) by other sperm is mediated by the cortical reaction, a release of materials from the cortical granules, lysosome-like organelles which are found just below the egg surface. As with other lysosome-like organelles, these materials include various hydrolytic enzymes. Changes brought about by these enzymes lead to the zona reaction, the hardening of the extracellular layer by cross-linking of proteins, and inactivation of sperm receptors. Thus the zona block to polyspermy is accomplished. The initial change in this zona block is a rapid depolarization of the oocyte membrane associated with a release of calcium ions from calmodulin. The increase in intracellular calcium acts as a signal or trigger to activate protein synthesis in the oocyte. The depolarization of the membrane initiates only a transient block to sperm entry. The permanent block is a consequence of the cortical reaction and release of enzymes, also apparently triggered by the increase in calcium.

23. A   p.240

By using sensitive pregnancy tests, it has been suggested that the total rate of pregnancy loss after implantation is approximately 30%. When the loss of fertilized oocytes before implantation is included, approximately 46% of all pregnancies end before the pregnancy is clinically perceived.

In the postimplantation period, if only clinically diagnosed pregnancies are considered, the generally accepted figure for spontaneous abortion in the first trimester is 15%. Approximately 50–60% of these abortions have chromosome abnormalities. This suggests that a minimum of 7.5% of all human conceptions are chromosomally abnormal. The fact that only 1 in 200 newborns has a chromosome abnormality attests to the powerful selection mechanisms operating in early human gestation. In each ovulatory cycle, only 25% of normally fertile couples can achieve a live birth.

24. C   p.242

The human blastocyst remains in the uterine secretions for approximately 72 hours and then hatches from its zona pellucida in preparation for attachment. Implantation is marked initially by apposition of the blastocyst to the uterine epithelium. A prerequisite for this contact is a loss of the zona pellucida, which, in vitro, can be ruptured by contractions and expansions of the blastocyst. In vivo this activity is less critical, because the zona can be lysed by components of the uterine fluid. The exact nature and function of these components and related proteins that are thought to mediate the implantation process (implantation-initiating factor, fibronectin, uteroglobin and blastokinin) are uncertain. Their production is, however, known to be dependent upon the secretion of ovarian steroid hormones. Even if the hormonal milieu and protein composition of the uterine fluid are hospitable to the implantation, it may not occur if the embryo is not at the proper stage of development. It has been inferred from this information that there must be developmental maturation of the surface of the embryo before it is able to achieve attachment and implantation.

8 The Endocrinology of Pregnancy

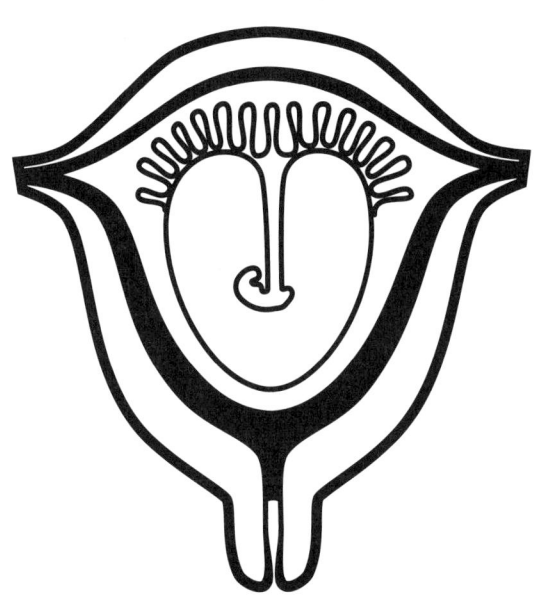

Learning Objectives

Be able to:

1. Describe the origin and clinically relevant metabolic steps of estrogen and progesterone within the fetal-placental-maternal unit.

2. Detail the development and physiology of the fetal adrenal cortex.

3. Understand the potential benefits and limitations of estriol testing during pregnancy.

4. Explain the etiology, incidence and clinical presentation of placental sulfatase deficiency.

5. Give examples of specific proteins associated with pregnancy produced by the fetal placental and maternal compartments.

6. Describe the structural configuration of HCG and its secretion throughout normal and abnormal pregnancies.

7. Discuss the clinical importance of alpha-fetoprotein.

8. Understand the possible role growth factors and cytokines may play in supporting a pregnancy.

Pre-Test

A. Instructions: Fill in the blanks

1. Normal range of maternal plasma progesterone is _____–_____ mg during the first trimester, _____–_____ mg during the second and _____–_____ mg during the last trimester of pregnancy.

2. There is a virtual absence of the cytochrome P450 enzyme _____ in the placenta.

B. Instructions: True or False

3. The fetus borrows progesterone from the placenta while the placenta borrows 19-carbon compounds from the fetus to serve as precursors for estrogens.

4. HCG levels close to term are lower in women bearing female fetuses.

C. Instructions: For each of the following questions choose:

A. if only 1, 2 and 3 are correct
B. if only 1 and 3 are correct
C. if only 2 and 4 are correct
D. if only 4 is correct
E. if all are correct

5. Maternal plasma unconjugated estrogens concentrations
   1. are highest for estriol
   2. consist of estriol, estrone and estradiol
   3. appear earliest for estriol
   4. are excreted at 100 to 1000-fold during pregnancy compared to the nonpregnant state

6. The placenta contains
   1. corticotropin releasing hormone
   2. somatostatin
   3. gonadotropin releasing hormone
   4. relaxin

Post-Test

A. Instruction: Fill in the blanks

1. _____ is obtained from the maternal bloodstream for progesterone synthesis by the placenta.

2. Exogenous support for an early pregnancy up till 10 weeks requires _____ mg progesterone daily.

3. _____ serves as the substrate for fetal adrenal gland production of gluco- and mineralocorticoids.

4. The vast majority of estrogen exerted in maternal urine is derived from _____ androgens.

5. The principal mission of the fetal adrenal may be to provide _____ as the basic precursor for placental estrogen production.

6. The _____ is the functional cell of the placenta and major site of hormone and protein production.

7. Alterations in the _____ component change the half-life of HCG.

8. The maternal circulation HCG concentration is approximately _____ IU/L at the time of the expected but missed period.

9. Relaxin is a peptide hormone produced by the _____ _____ of pregnancy and not detected in men or nonpregnant women.

10. _____ is the principal growth factor binding protein in pregnancy in contrast to _____ which is the main circulating growth factor binding protein in the nonpregnant state.

11. _____ is now recognized to be the same as placental protein-12, a decidual protein.

12. Fetal _____ is the principal requisite for surfactant biosynthesis.

B. Instructions: True or False

13. Progesterone production by the placenta is largely independent on the quantity of precursor available, the uteroplacental perfusion, fetal well-being or the presence of a healthy fetus.

14. The cholesterol utilized for progesterone synthesis enters the trophoblast from the maternal bloodstream as high-density lipoprotein cholesterol.

15. In the first 5–6 weeks of pregnancy, hCG stimulation of the corpus luteum results in the daily secretion of about 25 mg progesterone and 0.5 mg estradiol.

16. Cortisol, corticosterone and aldosterone are secreted by the fetal adrenal gland independently of the mother.

17. Amniotic fluid estriol is correlated with maternal estrogen pattern rather than the fetus.

18. Placental sulfatase deficiency is an autosomal recessive metabolic disease.

19. The syncytiotrophoblast is the basic placental stem cell from which the cytotrophoblasts arise by differentiation.

20. Only primates and horses have genes for beta chorionic gonadotropin.

21. Levels of maternal circulating HCG concentration reach a level of 200,000 IU/L by 20 weeks of pregnancy.

22. Human placental lactogen is secreted by the syncytiotrophoblast and responsible in part for carbohydrate metabolism of the mother.

23. Screening for fetal aneuploidy using a combination of three markers: AFP, HCG and unconjugated estriol will also detect 85% of open neural tube defects.

24. Prolactin is synthesized by decidualized endometrium.

C. Instructions: Match the compartment of origin with each hormone, enzyme description or protein associated with pregnancy.

A. fetal
B. placental
C. maternal

25. progesterone
26. absence of 17-hydroxylase
27. estriol
28. DHAS
29. maternal blood prolactin
30. unable to perform 16α-hydroxylation
31. cholesterol
32. alpha-fetoprotein

D. Instructions: For each of the following questions choose:

A. if only 1, 2 and 3 are correct
B. if only 1 and 3 are correct
C. if only 2 and 4 are correct
D. if only 4 is correct
E. if all are correct

33. Progesterone concentrations
    1. in the amniotic fluid are maximal between 10 and 20 weeks then decrease gradually
    2. are about 3 times higher in the myometrium than in the maternal plasma
    3. in the serum increase with advancing gestation
    4. depends upon the availability of maternal LDL cholesterol

34. The fetal adrenal cortex
    1. during development undergoes specific morphologic changes which are associated with specific steroidogenic characteristics
    2. requires the presence of ACTH after 20 weeks for normal development
    3. near term is capable of de novo synthesis of cholesterol
    4. is differentiated by 4 weeks in utero

35. ACTH
    1. is essential for the morphologic development and function of the fetal adrenal gland
    2. growth promoting effects upon the fetal adrenal are mediated in part by insulin-like growth factors
    3. action results in an increase in LDL receptors leading to an uptake of LDL-cholesterol by the fetal adrenal
    4. levels in the fetus increase throughout pregnancy

36. Clinical uses of estriol assays
    1. are limited to specific clinical situations
    2. provide greater predictive value than biophysical fetal profile for fetal distress
    3. are limited because specific steroids and antibiotics interfere with normal metabolism of estriol
    4. may provide useful information from a single sample

37. Women with placental sulfatase deficiency
    1. are unable to hydrolyze DHAS
    2. fail to go into labor at term and usually require cesarean sections
    3. deliver males much more often than females
    4. have low plasma estriol with high amniotic fluid DHAS and normal amniotic DHA and androstenedione

38. HCG
    1. has a half-life of approximately 48 hours compared to a half-life of 2 hours for LH
    2. has a half-life which is determined in part by its sialic acid content
    3. is coded by genes for the alpha and beta subunits which are located on the same chromosome
    4. has unique biological activity attributed to molecular differences in the beta subunits

39. Cytokines
    1. are believed to have little if any role in the establishment or maintenance of pregnancy
    2. include colony-stimulating factor-I and tumor necrosis factor-alpha
    3. are known to be produced by the placenta in response to circulating levels of prorenin
    4. may be important for embryonic growth and in the maternal immune response essential for survival of the pregnancy

---

Answers for Chapter 8 — Pre-Test

1. 25–30 mg; 30–75 mg; 75–150 mg figure on p.252

2. P450c17 p.255
The basic precursors of estrogens are 19-carbon androgens. However, there is a virtual absence of 17-hydroxylation and 17–20 desmolase activity (P450c17) in the human placenta. As a result, 21 carbon products (progesterone and pregnenolone) cannot be converted to 19 carbon steroids (androstenedione and dehydroepiandrosterone). Like progesterone, estrogen produced by the placenta P450arom enzyme system must derive precursors from outside the placenta.

3. true p.254
The fetal zone in the adrenal gland is extremely active, but produces steroids with a 3β-hydroxy-Δ^5 configuration like pregnenolone and dehydroepiandrosterone, rather than 3-keto-Δ^4 products such as progesterone. The fetus therefore lacks significant activity of the 3β-hydroxysteroid-dehydrogenase, Δ^{4-5} isomerase system. Thus, the fetus must borrow progesterone from the placenta to circumvent this lack in order to synthesize the biologically important corticosteroids. In return the fetus supplies what the placenta lacks: 19-carbon compounds to serve as precursors for estrogens.

4. false p.270
HCG levels close to term are higher in women bearing female fetuses. This is true of serum levels, placental content, urinary levels, and amniotic fluid concentrations. The mechanism and purpose of this difference are not known.

5. C p.258
The profiles of the unconjugated compounds in the maternal compartment for the three major estrogens in pregnancy are:

   1. A rise in estrone begins at 6–10 weeks, and individual values range from 2 to 30 ng/mL at term. This wide range in normal values precludes the use of estrone measurements in clinical applications.
   2. A rise in estradiol begins in weeks 6–8 when placental function becomes apparent. Individual estradiol values vary between 6 and 40 ng/mL (22–147 nmol/L) at 36 weeks of gestation and then undergo an accelerated rate of increase. At term, an equal amount of estradiol arises from maternal DHAS and fetal

DHAS, and its importance in fetal monitoring is negligible.
3. Estriol is first detectable at 9 weeks when the fetal adrenal gland secretion of precursor begins. Estriol concentrations plateau at 31–35 weeks, and then increase again at 35–36 weeks.

During pregnancy, estrone and estradiol excretion is increased about 100 times over nonpregnant levels. However, the increase in maternal estriol excretion is about a thousand-fold. The traditional view that estriol is a weak estrogen metabolite is not accurate. A weak estrogen provided in high concentrations can produce a biologic response equivalent to that of estradiol. Because of its high production and concentration, estriol is an important hormone in pregnancy. The maternal level of estradiol is higher than the level in the fetus; in contrast, the estriol level in the fetus is greater than in the mother.

6. A   p.266

Proteins Associated with Pregnancy

Fetal Compartment	Placental Compartment	Maternal Compartment

Alpha-fetoprotein	Hypothalamic-like hormones
	  GnRH
	  CRH
	  TRH
	  Somatostatin
	
	Pituitary-like hormones
	  HCG
	  HPL
	  HGH
	  HCT
	  ACTH
	
	Growth factors
	  IGF-I
	  Epidermal growth factor
	  Platelet-derived growth factor
	  Fibroblast growth factor
	  Transforming growth factor-β
	  Inhibin
	  Activin
	
	Cytokines
	  Interleukin-1
	  Interleukin-6
	  Colony stimulating factor-1
	
	Other
	  Opiates
	  Prorenin
	  Pregnancy-specific β_1-glycoprotein
	  Pregnancy-associated plasma protein A
		Decidual proteins
		  Prolactin
		  Relaxin
		  IGFBP-1
		  Interleukin-1
		  Colony stimulating factor-1
		  Progesterone-associated endometrial protein
		
		Corpus luteum proteins
		  Relaxin
		  Prorenin

Answers for Chapter 8 — Post-Test

1. Cholesterol p.252

In its key location as a way station between mother and fetus, the placenta can utilize precursors from either mother or fetus to circumvent its own deficiencies in enzyme activity. The placenta converts little, if any, acetate to cholesterol or its precursors. Cholesterol as well as pregnenolone are obtained from the maternal bloodstream for progesterone synthesis. The fetal contribution is negligible since progesterone levels remain high after fetal demise. Thus, the massive amount of progesterone produced in pregnancy depends upon placental-maternal cooperation.

2. 100 p.252

Progesterone is largely produced by the corpus luteum until about 10 weeks of gestation. Indeed, until approximately the 7th week, the pregnancy is dependent upon the presence of the corpus luteum. Exogenous support for an early pregnancy (until 10 weeks) requires 100 mg progesterone daily, associated with a maternal circulating level of approximately 10 ng/mL (32 nmol/L). Despite this requirement, patients pregnant after ovarian stimulation with one of the techniques of assisted reproductive technology have concluded a successful pregnancy after experiencing extremely low progesterone levels. Thus, individual variation is great, and very low circulating levels of progesterone can be encountered occasionally in women who experience normal pregnancies. The predictive value, therefore, of progesterone measurements is limited.

3. Progesterone p.254

Progesterone serves as the substrate for fetal adrenal gland production of gluco- and mineralocorticoids; however, most of the cortisol synthesis is derived from low-density lipoprotein cholesterol (LDL-cholesterol) obtained from the fetal circulation and synthesized in the fetal liver.

4. fetal p.255

The fetal adrenal provides DHAS as precursor for placental production of estrone and estradiol. However, the placenta lacks a 16α-hydroxylation ability, and estriol with its 16α-hydroxyl group must be derived from an immediate fetal precursor. The fetal adrenal, with the aid of 16α-hydroxylation in the fetal liver, provides the 16α-hydroxy-dehydroepiandrosterone sulfate for placental estriol formation. After birth, neonatal 16-hydroxylation activity rapidly disappears. The maternal contribution of DHAS to total estrogen synthesis must be negligible because in the absence of normal fetal adrenal glands (as in an anencephalic infant) maternal estrogen levels and excretion are extremely low. The fetal adrenals secrete more than 200 mg of DHAS daily, about 10 times more than the mother.

5. DHAS p.261

The principal mission of the fetal adrenal may be to provide DHAS as the basic precursor for placental estrogen production. Estrogen, in turn, feeds back to the adrenal to direct steroidogenesis along the Δ^5 pathway to provide even more of its precursor, DHAS. Thus far this is the only known function for DHAS. With birth and loss of exposure to estrogen, the fetal adrenal gland quickly changes to the adult type of gland.

6. syncytiotrophoblast p.265

The two main trophoblastic layers consist of the cytotrophoblast, separate mononuclear cells prominent early in pregnancy and sparse late in pregnancy, and the syncytiotrophoblast, a continuous multinuclear layer on the surface of the villi. Control of this important cellular differentiation is still not understood; however, the process is influenced by HCG and, undoubtedly, a variety of growth factors. The releasing hormones, neurohormones, inhibin, and activin are produced in the cytotrophoblast. The surface of the syncytiotrophoblast is in direct contact with the maternal blood in the intervillous space. This may be a reason why placental proteins are secreted preferentially into the mother.

7. carbohydrate or sialic acid p.267

Human chorionic gonadotropin is a glycoprotein, a peptide framework to which carbohydrate side chains are attached. Alterations in the carbohydrate components (about one-third of the molecular weight) change the biologic properties.

8. 100 p.269

HCG is secreted by the syncytiotrophoblast. The maternal circulating HCG concentration is approximately 100 IU/L at the time of the expected but missed menses. A maximal level of about 100,000 IU/L in the maternal circulation is reached at 8–10 weeks of gestation. Why does the corpus luteum involute at the time that HCG is reaching its highest levels? One possibility is that a specific inhibitory agent becomes active at this time. Another is down-regulation of receptors by the high levels of HCG. In early pregnancy, down-regulation may be avoided because HCG is secreted in an episodic fashion. For unknown reasons, the fetal testes escape desensitization; no receptor down regulation takes place.

9. corpus luteum p.276

Relaxin is a peptide hormone produced by the corpus luteum of pregnancy, and not detected in men or nonpregnant women. It is composed of two short peptide chains (24 and 29 amino acids, respectively) linked by disulfide bridges. While it has been argued that the human corpus luteum is the sole source of relaxin in pregnancy, it has also been identified in human placenta, decidua, and chorion. The maternal serum concentration rises during the first trimester when the corpus luteum is dominant and declines in the second trimester. This suggests a role in maintaining early pregnancy, but its function is not really known. In animals, relaxin softens the cervix, inhibits uterine contractions, and relaxes the pubic symphysis. The cervical changes are comparable to those seen with human labor. To examine the contribution of the corpus luteum, normally pregnant women were compared to women pregnant with donated oocytes (and therefore without corpora lutea). Relaxin was undetectable in the women without functioning ovaries, confirming that its major source is the corpus luteum. No effect on prolactin secretion was observed, but it did appear that relaxin enhanced growth hormone secretion by the pituitary. Obviously relaxin is not necessary for the maintenance of pregnancy and labor because the rest of pregnancy and the outcomes did not differ between those women with circulating levels of relaxin and those with undetectable levels. However, recombinant relaxin is being tested for ripening of the cervix.

10. IGFBP-1; IGFBP-3 p.278

The IGF binding proteins transport IGFs in the circulation, protect IGFs against metabolism and clearance, and importantly, affect the biologic activity of IGFs by modulating IGF availability at the cellular level. Pregnancy is marked by a rise in maternal levels of insulin-like growth factor binding protein-1 (IGFBP-1), beginning at the end of the first trimester and reaching a peak at term. The prominence of IGFBP-1 in the pregnant state is in contrast to the nonpregnant state when IGFBP-3 is the main circulating IGFBP. During pregnancy, the levels of IGFBP-3 and IGFBP-2 decrease, apparently due to the activity of a pregnancy-associated serum protease.

11. IGFBP-1 p.278

IGFBP-1 is now recognized to be the same as placental protein-12, a decidual protein. Thus IGFBP-1 originates in the decidua, regulated by progesterone, as well as in the liver.

12. cortisol p.281

It has become recognized that fetal cortisol is the principal requisite for surfactant biosynthesis. This is true despite the fact that no increase in fetal cortisol can be demonstrated to correlate with the increases in fetal lung maturation. For that reason, fetal lung maturation can be best viewed as the result of not only cortisol, but the synergistic action of cortisol, prolactin, thyroxine, estrogens, prostaglandins, growth factors, and perhaps other yet unidentified agents. Insulin directly inhibits surfactant protein expression in fetal lung tissue, which explains the increase in respiratory distress syndrome associated with hyperglycemia in pregnancy (although this effect can be overcome by the stress associated with advanced diabetes).

13. true p.252

In contrast to estrogen, progesterone production by the placenta is largely independent of the quantity of precursor available, the uteroplacental perfusion, fetal well-being, or even the presence of a live fetus. This is because the fetus contributes essentially no precursor. The majority of placental progesterone is derived from maternal cholesterol that is readily available. At term a small portion (3%) is derived from maternal pregnenolone.

14. false p.253

The cholesterol utilized for progesterone synthesis enters the trophoblast from the maternal bloodstream as low-density lipoprotein (LDL)-cholesterol, by means of the process of endocytosis (internalization) involving the LDL cell membrane receptors, a process enhanced in pregnancy by estrogen. Hydrolysis of the protein component of LDL may yield amino acids for the fetus, and essential fatty acids may be derived from hydrolysis of the cholesterol esters. Unlike steroidogenesis elsewhere, it is not clear whether placental progesterone production requires the control of tropic hormones. While some evidence suggests tropic hormone support is not necessary, other evidence indicates that a small amount of human chorionic gonadoatropin (HCG) must be present.

15. true   p.254

Since implantation normally occurs about 6–7 days after ovulation, and human chorionic gonadotropin (HCG) must appear by the 10th day after ovulation to rescue the corpus luteum, the blastocyst must successfully implant and secrete HCG within a narrow window of time. In the first 5–6 weeks of pregnancy, HCG stimulation of the corpus luteum results in the daily secretion of about 25 mg progesterone and 0.5 mg estradiol. Whereas estrogen levels begin to increase at 4–5 weeks due to placental secretion, progesterone production by the placenta does not significantly increase until about 10–11 weeks after ovulation.

16. true   p.255

Steroid levels have been compared in maternal blood, fetal blood, and amniotic fluid obtained at fetoscopy in women undergoing termination of pregnancy at 16–20 weeks gestation. Cortisol, corticosterone, and aldosterone are definitely secreted by the fetal adrenal gland independently of the mother. The fetal arterial-venous differences confirm that placental progesterone is a source for fetal adrenal cortisol and aldosterone.

17. false   p.263

Amniotic fluid estriol is correlated with the fetal estrogen pattern rather than the maternal. Most of the estriol in the amniotic fluid is present as 16-glucosiduronate or as 3-sulfate-16-glucosiduronate. A small amount exists as 3-sulfate. Very little unconjugated estriol is present in the amniotic fluid because free estriol is rapidly transferred across the placenta and membranes. Estriol sulfate is low in concentration because the placenta and fetal membranes hydrolyze the sulfated conjugates, and the free estriol is then passed out of the fluid. Because the membranes and the placenta have no glucuronidase activity, the glucosiduronate conjugates are removed slowly from the fetus. The glucosiduronates therefore predominate in the fetal urine and the amniotic fluid. Because of the slow changes in glucosiduronates, measurements of amniotic fluid estriol have wide variations in both normal and abnormal pregnancies. An important clinical use for amniotic fluid estrogen measurements has not emerged.

18. false   p.264

There is an X-linked metabolic disease expressed by a placental sulfatase deficiency, and postnatally, ichthyosis, occurring in about 1 in 2,000–6,000 newborns.

19. false   p.265

The cytotrophoblast is the basic placental stem cell from which the syncytiotrophoblasts arise by differentiation. The syncytiotrophoblast is, therefore, the functional cell of the placenta, the major site of hormone and protein production.

20. true   p.267

A single gene on chromosome 6 encodes the α-subunit for the four glycoprotein tropic hormones. The genes that encode for the beta-subunits of HCG, LH, and TSH are located in a cluster on chromosome 19. There is one gene for β-LH, but there are 6 genes for the β-subunit of HCG, each with different promotor activity. Only two of the genes are actively transcribed, and it is not certain why there are two active genes for β-HCG. It may be necessary for the high output of HCG during pregnancy, and it may reflect the relatively recent and rapid evolution of the β-HCG cluster. Only primates and horses have genes for β-CG. In contrast to the primate, the equine β-CG gene is identical to the equine β-LH gene, i.e., a single gene produces the β-subunits for both LH and CG. The primate β-CG gene is thus believed to have evolved from an ancestral β-LH gene. The most logical reason for this evolvement is development of new control mechanisms for gene expression in the placenta producing a glycosylated gonadotropin with a longer half life. In this process, a single base deletion caused a read-through mutation of a stop signal in the β-LH gene, leading to the extended carboxy terminal sequence of β-HCG.

21. false   p.270

HCG levels decrease to about 10,000–20,000 IU/L by 18–20 weeks and remain at that level to term. It is not certain why HCG levels are decreased in the second half of pregnancy. Advancing gestation is associated with increasing amounts of "nicked" HCG molecules in the maternal circulation. These molecules are missing a peptide linkage on the beta-subunit, and therefore, they dissociate into free α- and β-subunits. At any one point in time the maternal circulation contains HCG, nicked HCG, free subunits, and fragments of HCG. The production of normal molecules is maximal in early gestation when the biologic actions of HCG are so important.

22. true   p.271–272

Human placental lactogen (sometimes called human chorionic somatomammotropin), also secreted by the syncytiotrophoblast, is a single chain polypeptide of 191 amino acids held together by two disulfide bonds. In the mother, HPL stimulates IGF-I production and induces insulin resistance and carbohydrate intolerance. Experimentally, the maternal level of HPL can be altered by changing the circulating level (chronically, not acutely) of glucose. HPL is elevated with hypoglycemia and depressed with hyperglycemia.

23. true   p.276

Down syndrome is a very common genetic cause of abnormal development. The majority of cases are due to trisomy 21, an extra chromosome usually due to nondisjunction in maternal meiosis. A low maternal level of AFP is associated with trisomy 21. However, there is extensive overlap between normal and affected pregnancies responsible for a significant false positive rate. Several placental products are secreted in increased amounts in pregnancies with trisomy 21, including HCG and HPL, whereas the maternal circulating level of unconjugated estriol is lower in affected pregnancies. With trisomy 18, all markers are decreased. Modern screening for fetal aneuploidy combines three markers: AFP, HCG, and unconjugated estriol. This protocol will also detect 85% of open neural tube defects.

24. true   p.277

Following ovulation, the endometrium becomes a secretory organ and remains so throughout pregnancy. Decidualized endometrium secretes renin which may be involved in the regulation of water and electrolytes in the amniotic fluid, and relaxin, which may influence prostaglandin production in the membranes. One of the best studied special endocrine functions of the decidual endometrium is the secretion of prolactin. Prolactin is synthesized by endometrium during a normal menstrual cycle, but this synthesis is not initiated until histologic decidualization begins about day 23. The control of prolactin secretion by decidual tissue has not been definitively established. Some argue that once decidualization is established, prolactin secretion continues in the absence of either progesterone or estradiol, although there is evidence for an inhibitory feedback by decidual proteins (perhaps prolactin itself). Others indicate that endometrial prolactin production requires the combined effects of progestin and estrogen hormones plus the presence of other placental and decidual factors including relaxin, IGF-I, and specific stimulatory and inhibitory proteins.

25. B   p.252

Progesterone is largely produced by the corpus luteum until about 10 weeks of gestation. Indeed, until approximately the 7th week, the pregnancy is dependent upon the presence of the corpus luteum. After a transition period of shared function between the 7th week and 10th week during which there is a slight decline in circulating maternal progesterone levels, the placenta emerges as the major source of progesterone and levels progressively increase.

26. A   p.257

27. B   p.257

(See figure on page 117 in this Study Guide)

28. B   p.255

There is a virtual absence of 17-hydroxylation and 17–20 desmolase activity (P450c17) in the human placenta. As a result, 21 carbon products (progesterone and pregnenolone) cannot be converted to 19 carbon steroids (androstenedione and dehydroepiandrosterone). Like progesterone, estrogen produced by the placenta P450arom enzyme system must derive precursors from outside the placenta.

29. C   p.277

During pregnancy, prolactin secretion is limited to the fetal pituitary, the maternal pituitary, and the uterus. Neither trophoblast nor fetal membranes synthesize prolactin, but both the myometrium and endometrium can produce prolactin. The endometrium requires the presence of progesterone to initiate prolactin, while progesterone suppresses

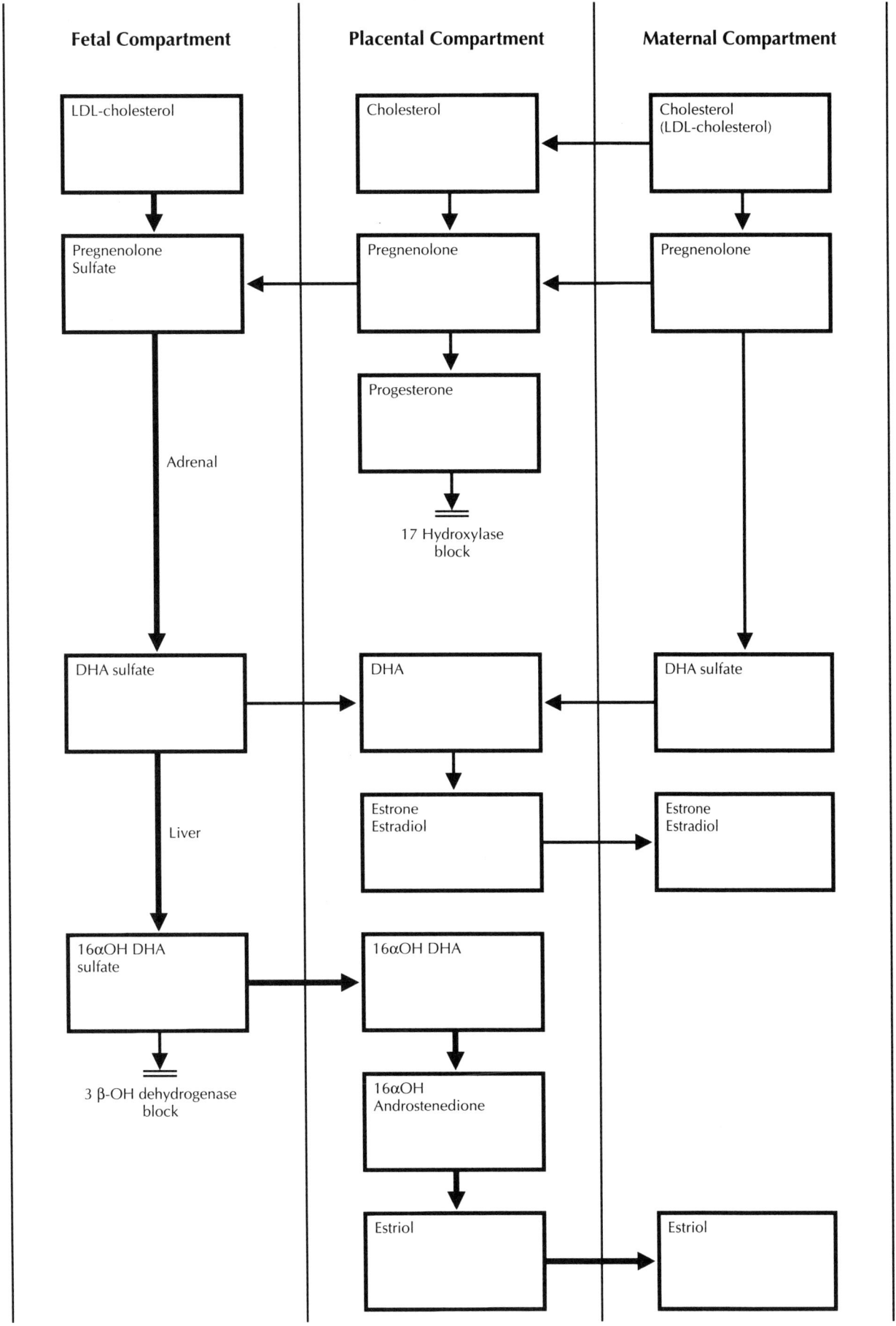

prolactin synthesis in the myometrium. Prolactin derived from the decidua is the source of prolactin found in the amniotic fluid. The prolactin in the fetal circulation is derived from the fetal pituitary.

Amniotic fluid concentrations of prolactin parallel maternal serum concentration until the 10th week of pregnancy, rise markedly until the 20th week, and then decrease. The maternal and fetal blood levels of prolactin are derived from the respective pituitary glands. Bromocriptine suppression of pituitary secretion of prolactin throughout pregnancy produces minimal maternal and fetal blood levels, yet there are normal fetal growth and development, and amniotic fluid levels are unchanged. Fortunately decidual secretion of prolactin is unaffected by dopamine agonist treatment because decidual prolactin may be important for fluid and electrolyte regulation of the amniotic fluid. This decidual prolactin is transported across the membranes in a process which requires the intact state of amnion and chorion with adherent decidua.

30. B p.255

The fetal adrenal provides DHAS as precursor for placental production of estrone and estradiol. However, the placenta lacks a 16α-hydroxylation ability, and estriol with its 16α-hydroxyl group must be derived from an immediate fetal precursor. The fetal adrenal, with the aid of 16α-hydroxylation in the fetal liver, provides the 16α-hydroxy-dehydroepiandrosterone sulfate for placental estriol formation. After birth, neonatal 16-hydroxylation activity rapidly disappears. The maternal contribution of DHAS to total estrogen synthesis must be negligible because in the absence of normal fetal adrenal glands (as in an anencephalic infant) maternal estrogen levels and excretion are extremely low. The fetal adrenals secrete more than 200 mg of DHAS daily, about 10 times more than the mother.

31. C p.252

The placenta converts little, if any, acetate to cholesterol or its precursors. Cholesterol as well as pregnenolone is obtained from the maternal bloodstream for progesterone synthesis. The fetal contribution is negligible since progesterone levels remain high after fetal demise.

32. A p.275

Alpha-fetoprotein (AFP) is a relatively unique glycoprotein (590 amino acids and 4% carbohydrate) derived largely from fetal liver and partially from the yolk sac until it degenerates at about 12 weeks. In early pregnancy (5–12 weeks), amniotic fluid AFP is mainly from yolk sac origin, whereas maternal circulating AFP is mainly from the fetal liver. Its function is unknown, but it is comparable in size to albumin and contains 39% sequence homology; it may serve as a protein carrier of steroid hormones in fetal blood. AFP may also be a modulator of cell proliferation, synergizing with various growth factors.

33. E p.253,254

The cholesterol utilized for progesterone synthesis enters the trophoblast from the maternal bloodstream as low-density lipoprotein (LDL)-cholesterol, by means of the process of endocytosis (internalization) involving the LDL cell membrane receptors, a process enhanced in pregnancy by estrogen. After a transition period of shared function between the 7th week and 10th week during which there is a slight decline in circulating maternal progesterone levels, the placenta emerges as the major source of progesterone and levels progressively increase. Amniotic fluid progesterone concentration is maximal between 10 and 20 weeks, then decreases gradually. Myometrial levels are about 3 times higher than maternal plasma levels in early pregnancy, remain high, and are about equal to the maternal plasma concentration at term.

34. A p.259

The fetal adrenal cortex is differentiated by 7 weeks into a thick inner fetal zone and a thin outer definitive zone, the source of cortisol and the forerunner of the adult cortex. Early in pregnancy, adrenal growth and development are remarkable, and the gland achieves a size equal to or larger than that of the kidney by the end of the first trimester. After the first trimester the adrenal glands slowly decrease in size until a second spurt in growth begins at about 34–35 weeks. The gland remains proportionately larger than the adult adrenal glands. After delivery, the fetal zone (about 80% of the bulk of the gland) rapidly involutes to be replaced by the adult definitive zone of the adrenal cortex. Thus, the specific steroidogenic characteristics of the fetus are associated with a specific morphologic change of the adrenal gland.

Early in pregnancy, the adrenal gland can function without ACTH, perhaps in response to HCG. After 20 weeks, fetal

ACTH is required. However, during the last 12–14 weeks of pregnancy when fetal ACTH levels are declining, the adrenal quadruples in size. Because pituitary prolactin is the only fetal pituitary hormone to increase throughout pregnancy, paralleling fetal adrenal gland size changes, it has been proposed that fetal prolactin is the critical tropic substance. In experimental preparations, however, only ACTH exerts a steroidogenic effect. There is no fetal adrenal response to prolactin, HCG, growth hormone, melanocyte-stimulating hormone (MSH), or thyrotropin releasing hormone (TRH). Furthermore, in patients treated with bromocriptine, fetal blood prolactin levels are suppressed, but DHAS levels are unchanged. Nevertheless, interest in prolactin persists because both ACTH and prolactin can stimulate steroidogenesis in vivo in the fetal baboon.

35. A   p.259,260

There is no question that ACTH is essential for the morphologic development and the steroidogenic mechanism of the fetal adrenal gland. ACTH activates adenylate cyclase, leading to steroidogenesis. Soon the supply of cholesterol becomes rate limiting. Further ACTH action results in an increase in LDL receptors leading to an increased uptake of circulating LDL-cholesterol. With internalization of LDL-cholesterol, hydrolysis by lysosomal enzymes of the cholesterol ester makes cholesterol available for steroidogenesis. For this reason, fetal plasma levels of LDL are low, and after birth newborn levels of LDL rise as the fetal adrenal involutes. In the presence of low levels of LDL-cholesterol, the fetal adrenal is capable of synthesizing cholesterol de novo. Thus near term, both de novo synthesis and utilization of LDL-cholesterol are necessary to sustain the high rates of DHAS and estrogen formation. The tropic support of the fetal adrenal gland by ACTH from the fetal pituitary is protected by placental estrogen. The placenta prevents maternal cortisol from reaching the fetus by converting cortisol to cortisone. This 11β-hydroxysteroid dehydrogenase activity is stimulated by placental estrogen. Adrenal gland steroidogenesis involves autocrine and paracrine regulation. Fetal adrenal cells produce inhibin, and the α-subunit is preferentially increased by ACTH.

36. B   p.262,263

There are two essential aspects to the clinical use of estriol assays. First, a single specimen is meaningless. Daily assays must be performed to provide a serial assessment of sequential changes. Second, to be significant, there must be a decrease of approximately 40% from the mean of the three highest consecutive values. While estrogen levels in the mother are related to the size of the fetal adrenal gland and its production of precursor, there is a poor correlation between birth weight and plasma estriol levels. Macrosomia is not always associated with high estriol levels. However, excessive adrenal activity as in congenital adrenal hyperplasia can be associated with unusually high levels.

Drugs that affect the maternal estrogen level include corticosteroids and antibiotics. Corticosteroids administered to the mother cross the placenta poorly, and large amounts (the equivalent of 75 mg cortisol daily) are required to suppress fetal adrenal production of estriol precursor. The synthetic steroids, dexamethasone and betamethasone, however, cross the placenta more easily, and maternal estriol assessment is not reliable for at least 1 week, and sometimes 2 weeks, after the last dose. Antibiotics which affect the flora of the maternal gastrointestinal tract depress maternal total estriol levels by interfering with the enterohepatic circulation. Such antibiotics inhibit hydrolysis of the biliary estriol conjugates in the gut, preventing their reabsorption and reconjugation, leading to loss of estriol in the feces. Total blood and urinary estriol decline, but unconjugated estriol is unaffected. Falsely elevated blood total estriols will be encountered in the presence of renal disease or when a patient is receiving oxytocin for the induction of labor because of the antidiuretic action of oxytocin, but the levels of unconjugated estriol will not be affected.

Assessment of maternal estriol levels has been superseded by various biophysical fetal monitoring techniques such as nonstress testing, stress testing, and measurement of fetal breathing and activity. Nevertheless, in certain clinical situations the addition of estriol assays is useful. The combination of a low estriol and a positive stress test is ominous. Certainly patients should not be managed by estriols alone. While a low estriol and a positive stress test indicate a fetus in jeopardy, a low estriol with a negative stress test allows postponement of intervention. Modern screening for fetal aneuploidy utilizes 3 markers in the maternal circulation: alpha fetoprotein, human chorionic gonadotropin, and unconjugated estriol.

37. E   p.264

Patients with the placental sulfatase disorder are unable to hydrolyze DHAS or 16α-hydroxy-DHAS, and, therefore, the placenta cannot form normal amounts of estrogen. A deficiency in placental sulfatase is usually discovered when patients go beyond term and are found to have extremely low estriol levels and no evidence of fetal distress. The patients usually fail to go into labor and require delivery by cesarean section. Most striking is the failure of cervical softening and dilatation; thus a cervical dystocia occurs that is resistant to oxytocin stimulation. There are many case reports of this deficiency, almost all detected by finding low estriol levels. All newborn children, with a few exceptions, have been male. The steroid sulfatase X-linked recessive ichthyosis locus has been mapped on the distal short arm portion of the X chromosome. There are no known geographic or racial factors which affect the gene frequency.

38. C   p.267

For example, the long half-life of HCG is approximately 24 hours as compared to 2 hours for luteinizing hormone (LH), a 10-fold difference which is due mainly to the greater sialic acid content of HCG. As with the other glycoproteins, follicle-stimulating hormone (FSH), LH, and thyroid-stimulating hormone (TSH), HCG consists of two noncovalently linked subunits, called alpha (α) and beta (β). The α-subunits in these glycoprotein hormones are identical, consisting of 92 amino acids. Unique biological activity as well as specificity in radioimmunoassays is attributed to the molecular and carbohydrate differences in the β-subunits. A single gene on chromosome 6 encodes the α-subunit for the four glycoprotein tropic hormones. The genes that encode for the beta-subunits of HCG, LH, and TSH are located in a cluster on chromosome 19.

39. C   p.278

Local placental cytokine production is believed to be important for embryonic growth and in the maternal immune response essential for survival of the pregnancy. Interleukin-1β is produced in the decidualized endometrium during pregnancy, and colony-stimulating factor-1 (CSF-1) is produced by both decidua and placenta. CSF-1 gene expression in response to interleukin-1β has been localized to mesenchymal fibroblasts from the core of placental villi. Thus, a system of communication is present between maternal decidual and fetal tissue to provide growth factor support for the placenta which would include fetal hematopoiesis, a known response to CSF-1. The placenta also produces interleukin-6, and both interleukins stimulate HCG release by activation of the interleukin-6 receptor. Thus, the interleukin-1 influence on HCG secretion is mediated by the interleukin-6 system. Both trophoblast derived interleukin-1 and tumor necrosis factor-α (TNFα) synergistically release interleukin-6 and activate the interleukin-6 system to secrete HCG.

9 Prostaglandins

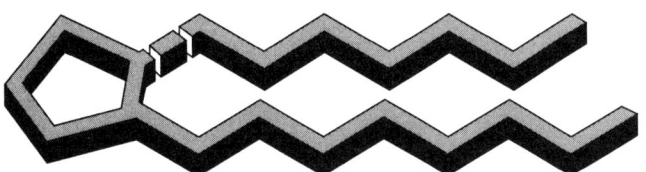

Learning Objectives

Be able to:

1. Discuss the clinical relevance of the role of prostaglandins in reproductive medicine with regard to luteal regression, parturition, and preeclampsia.

2. Describe the roles thromboxane and prostacyclin play in prostaglandin physiology.

3. Explain the mechanisms of action of steroids, aspirin and nonsteroidal anti-inflammatory agents in prostaglandin inhibition and their potential therapeutic roles.

4. Discuss the therapeutic roles prostaglandin analogues may offer in obstetrics and gynecology with respect to cervical ripening, therapeutic abortion and postpartum hemorrhage.

Clinical Gynecologic Endocrinology and Infertility: Self Assessment and Study Guide

Pre-Test

A. Instructions: Fill in the blanks

1. The predominant effect of prostaglandins on the fetal and maternal cardiovascular system is maintenance of arteries in a _____ state.

2. E prostaglandins and prostacyclin are potent _____, _____ the peripheral resistance and systemic blood pressure by directly _____ the smooth muscle of the arterial walls.

B. Instructions: True of False

3. Platelets produce prostacyclin (PGI_2) while endothelium produces thromboxane (TXA_2).

4. Prostaglandins have two direct actions associated with labor: ripening of the cervix and a direct oxytocic action.

C. Instructions: For the following question choose:

A. if only 1, 2 and 3 are correct
B. if only 1 and 3 are correct
C. if only 2 and 4 are correct
D. if only 4 is correct
E. if all are correct

5. An imbalance of thromoboxane-prostacyclin may be involved in the pathogenesis of:
   1. cardiovascular disease
   2. diabetes
   3. preeclampsia
   4. incompetent cervix

Post-Test

A. Instructions: Fill in the blanks

1. The immediate precursor of prostaglandins is _____ _____.

2. The rate-limiting step in the formation of the prostaglandin family is the release of free _____ _____.

3. The prostaglandin family includes _____, _____, _____, and the _____.

4. The _____ pathway leads to the prostaglandins.

5. Thromboxane A_2 (TXA_2) is the most powerful _____ known.

6. Ripening of the cervix is the result of a change which includes an _____ in hyaluronic acid and water and a _____ in dermatan sulfate and chondroitin sulfate.

7. Altered _____ cell function and _____ cell injury are responsible for the characteristic pathologic lesions of preeclampsia.

B. Instructions: True or False

8. Prostaglandins are secretory products of only the prostate gland.

9. All leukotrienes increase microvascular permeability.

10. The first true prostaglandin compounds formed in the cyclooxygenase pathway are PGG_2 and PGH_2.

11. Thromboxane and prostacyclin can be viewed as agonists.

12. The metabolism of prostaglandins occurs primarily in the lungs, kidney and liver.

13. Corticosteroids block the action of cyclooxygenase, thus blocking prostaglandin synthesis.

14. Prostaglandin $F_{2\alpha}$ causes luteal regression in many species.

15. The concentration of oxytocin receptors in the myometrium is low in the nonpregnant state and increases steadily throughout gestation.

16. Low dose aspirin may offer effective prophylaxis against preeclampsia because it inhibits prostacyclin production.

C. Instructions: For each of the following questions choose:

A. if only 1, 2 and 3 are correct
B. if only 1 and 3 are correct
C. if only 2 and 4 are correct
D. if only 4 is correct
E. if all are correct

17. The following clinical situations may be better understood within the context of the prostacyclin-thromboxane mechanism
    1. smokers who use oral contraceptives have increased platelet aggregation
    2. the well-known association between LDL- and HDL-cholesterol and cardiovascular disease
    3. the potential benefits of garlic upon cardiovascular disease
    4. the beneficial effects of antioxidants upon cardiovascular disease

18. Prostaglandin inhibition can be achieved with
    1. steroids by blocking phospholipase A_2
    2. aspirin which irreversibly blocks the action of cyclooxygenase
    3. indomethacin which reversibly blocks the action of cyclooxygenase
    4. antihistamines which reversibly block phospholipase A_2

19. The use of postcoital estrogen for contraception
    1. may work through a mechanism of increasing prostaglandin $F_{2\alpha}$ which antagonizes LH action
    2. may be effective within the 7 days prior to implantation
    3. is not effective if the corpus luteum is subject to rescue by HCG
    4. represents an example supporting the role prostaglandins play in promoting luteal regression

20. Evidence for a role of prostaglandin in parturition includes the following:
    1. prostaglandin levels in maternal blood and amniotic fluid increase in association with labor
    2. women taking high doses of aspirin have increased length of gestation and incidence of postmaturity
    3. arachidonate injected into the amniotic sac of animals initiates parturition
    4. indomethacin stops premature labor in women

21. Intravaginal PGE_2
    1. is useful in evacuating fetal demise and anencephalic fetuses
    2. can cause marked vasodilatation
    3. should not be used in conjunction with oxytocin unless 6 hours pass from the last prostaglandin
    4. can be given safely by intravenous administration

22. Prostin 15M
    1. is useful in the management of postpartum hemorrhage due to uterine atony
    2. can be used in patients with symptomatic asthma
    3. is administered either intramuscularly or directly into the myometrium
    4. may result in constipation

Answers for Chapter 9 — Pre-Test

1. relaxed or dilated p.298
The predominant effect of prostaglandins on the fetal and maternal cardiovascular system is to maintain the ductus arteriosus, renal, mesenteric, uterine, placental, and probably the cerebral and coronary arteries in a relaxed or dilated state.

2. vasodilators; decreasing; relaxing p.308
Two properties of certain classes of prostaglandins are noteworthy in searching for the mechanism of vasodilatation and regulation of blood flow in pregnancy. First, E prostaglandins and prostacyclin are potent vasodilators, decreasing the peripheral resistance and systemic blood pressure by directly relaxing the smooth muscle of the arterial walls. Second, the majority of the activity of these prostaglandins appears to be limited to the immediate vicinity of the synthesizing tissue itself.

3. false p.295
Because platelets synthesize TXA_2, a potent stimulator of platelet aggregation, the natural tendency of platelets is to clump and plug defects and damaged spots. The endothelium, on the other hand, produces PGI_2 and its constant presence inhibits platelet aggregation and adherence, keeping blood vessels free of platelets and ultimately clots. Thus, prostacyclin has a defensive role in the body. It is 4 to 8 times more potent a vasodilator than the E prostaglandins, and it prevents the adherence of platelets to healthy vascular endothelium. However, when the endothelium is damaged, platelets gather, beginning the process of thrombus formation. Even in this abnormal situation, prostacyclin strives to fulfill its protective role because increased PGI_2 can be measured in injured endothelium, thrombosed vessels, and in the vascular tissues of hypertensive animals.

4. true p.306
Pharmacologically and physiologically, prostaglandins have two direct actions associated with labor: ripening of the cervix and a direct oxytocic action. Successful parturition requires organized changes in both the upper uterus and in

the cervix. The cervical changes are in response to the estrogen/progesterone ratio and the local release of prostaglandins.

5. A p.295, 309

Conditions associated with vascular disease can be understood through the prostacyclin-thromboxane mechanism. For example, atheromatous plaques and nicotine inhibit prostacyclin synthesis. Increasing the cholesterol content of human platelets increases the sensitivity to stimuli which cause platelet aggregation due to increased thromboxane production. The well-known association between low-density and high-density lipoproteins (LDL-cholesterol and HDL-cholesterol) and cardiovascular disease may also be partly explained in terms of PGI_2. LDL from men and postmenopausal women inhibits and HDL stimulates prostacyclin production. Platelets from diabetics and from Class A diabetic pregnant women make more TXA_2 than platelets from normal pregnant women. Smokers who use oral contraceptives have increased platelet aggregation and an inhibition of prostacyclin formation. It is proposed that a fundamental disturbance in preeclampsia is an imbalance between the vasodilator and vasoconstrictor members of the prostaglandin family, prostacyclin (PGI_2) and thromboxane A_2 (TXA_2). Many investigators have reported a general decrease in prostacyclin associated with preeclampsia. Lower levels of this potent vasodilator and inhibitor of platelet activity could explain three of the most significant clinical consequences of preeclampsia: hypertension, platelet consumption, and reduced uteroplacental blood flow.

Answers for Chapter 9 — Post-Test

1. arachidonic acid p.292
(See figure on page 126 in this Study Guide)

2. arachidonic acid p.292

The rate-limiting step in the formation of the prostaglandin family is the release of free arachidonic acid. A variety of hydrolases may be involved in arachidonic acid release, but phospholipase A_2 activation is an important initiator of prostaglandin synthesis because of the abundance of arachidonate in the 2 position of phospholipids. Types of stimuli that activate such lipases include burns, infusions of hypertonic and hypotonic solutions, thrombi and small particles, endotoxin, snake venom, mechanical stretching, catecholamines, bradykinin, angiotensin, and the sex steroids.

3. prostaglandins, leukotrienes, thromboxane, and prostacyclin p.292, 294, 295

"Eicosanoids" refer to all the 20-carbon derivatives, while "prostanoids" indicate only those containing a structural ring. After the release of arachidonic acid the synthetic path can go in two different directions: the lipoxygenase pathway or the cyclooxygenase (prostaglandin endoperoxide H synthetase) pathway. The leukotrienes are formed by 5-lipoxygenase oxygenation of arachidonic acid at C-5, forming an unstable intermediate, LTA_4. LTB_4 is formed by hydration and LTC_4 by the addition of gluathione. The remaining leukotrienes are metabolites of LTC_4. Thromboxanes are not true prostaglandins due to the absence of the pentane ring, but prostacyclin (PGI_2) is a legitimate prostaglandin.

4. cyclooxygenase p.294

The cyclooxygenase pathway leads to the prostaglandins. The first true prostaglandin (PG) compounds formed are PGG_2 and PGH_2 (half-life of about 5 minutes), the mothers of all other prostaglandins. The numerical subscript refers to the number of double bonds. This number depends on which of the three precursor fatty acids has been utilized. Besides arachidonic acid, the other two precursor fatty acids are linoleic acid, which gives rise to the PG_1 series, and pentanoic acid, the PG_3 series. The latter two series are of less importance in physiology, hence the significance of the arachidonic acid family. The prostaglandins of original and continuing relevance to reproduction are PGE_2 and $PGF_{2\alpha}$ and possibly PGD_2. The α in $PGF_{2\alpha}$ indicates the α steric configuration of the hydroxyl group at the C-9 position. The A, B, and C prostaglandins either have little biologic activity or do not exist in significant concentrations in biologic tissues. In the original work, the prostaglandin more soluble in ether was named PGE, and the one more soluble in phosphate (spelled with an F in Swedish) buffer was named PGF. Later, naming became alphabetical.

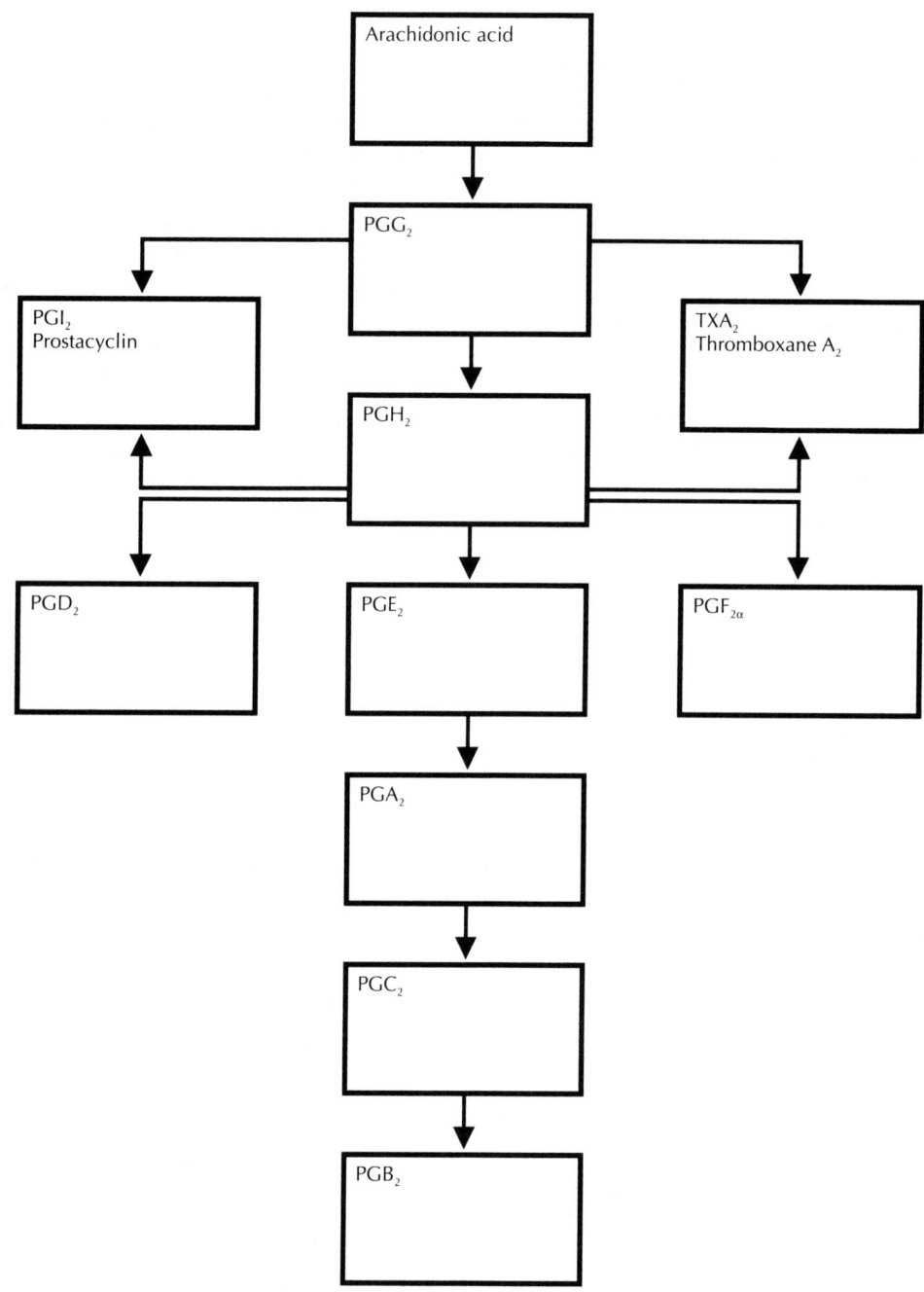

5. vasoconstrictor p.295
TXA_2 is the most powerful vasoconstrictor known, while PGI_2 is a potent vasodilator.

6. increase; decrease p.306
Ripening of the cervix is the result of a change which includes an increase in hyaluronic acid and water and a decrease in dermatan sulfate and chondroitin sulfate (these compounds hold the collagen fibers in a rigid structure). How prostaglandins operate in this change is unknown, but enzyme activation must be involved. For ripening of the cervix, PGE_2 is very effective, while $PGF_{2\alpha}$ has little effect. The purpose of achieving ripening of the cervix is to increase the success rate with induction of labor and lower the proportion of cesarean sections. Intravaginal prostaglandin E_2 administered as tablets, suppositories, and mixed in gels has been very effective for cervical ripening. The commercial formulation currently available in the U.S. consists of 0.5 mg PGE_2 dissolved in a triacetin viscous gel base, also containing a colloid silicone dioxide, provided in a prefilled syringe for application (Prepidil Gel, The Upjohn Company).

7. endothelial; endothelial p.308
Besides the vasospasm and hypertension, preeclampsia is associated with increased activation of platelets and the coagulation system in the microvasculature. The endothelium is a target of the alterations in preeclampsia and is important role in the pathogenesis of preeclampsia. Altered endothelial cell function and endothelial cell injury are responsible for the characteristic pathologic lesions of preeclampsia.

8. false p.291
Prostaglandins play fundamental roles in the regulation of reproductive events. Given the name prostaglandins because of the erroneous belief they were the secretory products of only the prostate gland, these substances have widespread actions in keeping with their ubiquitous presence.

9. true p.292
All leukotrienes increase microvascular permeability. Thus, the leukotrienes are major agonists, synthesized in response to antigens and provoking asthma and airway obstruction. Leukotrienes are 100–1000 times more potent than histamine in the pulmonary airway.

10. true p.294
The cyclooxygenase pathway leads to the prostaglandins. The first true prostaglandin (PG) compounds formed are PGG_2 and PGH_2 (half-life of about 5 minutes), the mothers of all other prostaglandins.

11. false p.295
Thromboxane (TX) (half-life about 30 seconds) and PGI_2 (half-life about 2–3 minutes) can be viewed as opponents, each having powerful biologic activity that counters or balances the other.

12. true p.296
The metabolism of prostaglandins occurs primarily in the lungs, kidney, and liver. The lungs are important in the metabolism of E and F prostaglandins. Indeed, there is an active transport mechanism which specifically carries E and F prostaglandins from the circulation into the lungs. Any active prostaglandins in the circulation are metabolized during one passage through the lungs. Therefore, members of the prostaglandin family have a short half-life, and in most instances, exert autocrine/paracrine actions at the site of their synthesis. Because of the rapid half-lives, studies are often performed by measuring the inactive end products, for example 6-keto-$PGF_{1\alpha}$, the metabolite of prostacyclin, and TXB_2, the metabolite of thromboxane A_2.

13. false p.296
Corticosteroids were previously thought to inhibit the prostaglandin family by stabilizing membranes and preventing the release of phospholipase. It is now recognized that corticosteroids induce the synthesis of proteins called lipocortins (or annexins) which block the action of phospholipase. Thus far, steroids and some local anesthetic agents are the only substances known to work at this step.

Aspirin is an irreversible inhibitor, selectively acetylating the cyclooxygenase involved in prostaglandin synthesis. The other inhibiting agents, nonsteroidal anti-inflammatory agents such as indomethacin and naproxen, are reversible agents, forming a reversible bond with the active site of the enzyme. Acetaminophen inhibits cyclooxygenase in the central nervous system, accounting for its analgesic and antipyretic properties, but has no anti-inflammatory properties nor does it affect platelets. However, acetaminophen does reduce prostacyclin synthesis; the reason for this preferential effect is unknown.

14. true p.297
Prostaglandin $F_{2\alpha}$ causes luteal regression in many species. It is the agent responsible for terminating the life span of the corpus luteum if fertilization fails to take place, so that a subsequent repeat ovulation can follow rapidly. The $PGF_{2\alpha}$ originates in the endometrium, and its synthesis is stimulated by the estrogen produced in growing follicles. It is transported directly to the corpus luteum through the vasculature connecting the ovary and the uterus, thus achieving an effective concentration at the corpus luteum and avoiding rapid clearance in the systemic circulation.

15. true   p.304

It is likely that oxytocin action during the inital stages of labor may depend on myometrial sensitivity to oxytocin in addition to the levels of oxytocin in the blood. The concentration of oxytocin receptors in the myometrium is low in the nonpregnant state and increases steadily throughout gestation (an 80-fold increase), and during labor the concentration doubles. This receptor concentration correlates with the uterine sensitivity to oxytocin. The mechanism for the increase is unknown, but it likely is due to a change in the prostaglandin and hormonal milieu of the uterus. In addition, oxytocin is synthesized in the amnion, chorion, and significantly, in the decidua. The local production and effects of oxytocin, estrogen, and progesterone combine in a complicated process of autocrine, paracrine, and endocrine actions to result in parturition.

16. false   p.310

A low dose of aspirin (40–80 mg daily) that selectively inhibits platelet cyclooxygenase results in a marked reduction in thromboxane levels in maternal blood (but not in fetal blood), with minimal but transient impact on prostacyclin metabolites and no impairment of prostacyclin synthesis in the umbilical artery. Low doses of aspirin that inhibit thromboxane production (in platelets and perhaps in trophoblastic tissue), unbalancing the ratio in favor of prostacyclin, offer prophylaxis against preeclampsia. The measurement of the pressor response to angiotensin II indicates that pregnant women with preeclampsia can have an underlying imbalance of thromboxane and prostacyclin corrected by low dose aspirin. This dose of aspirin appears to be safe for the fetus because it takes 100 mg daily to decrease levels of thromboxane in cord bloods (leaving prostacyclin unaffected) and 500 mg to inhibit both thromboxane and prostacyclin in the fetus. Low dose aspirin (60 mg per day) has been demonstrated to be effective in some clinical trials, but not all, in preventing preeclampsia and intrauterine growth retardation. This treatment is especially indicated for women with a previous history of significant preeclampsia. Large scale clinical trials are underway to determine efficacy and adverse effects.

17. A   p.295

Conditions associated with vascular disease can be understood through the prostacyclin-thromboxane mechanism. For example, atheromatous plaques and nicotine inhibit prostacyclin synthesis. Increasing the cholesterol content of human platelets increases the sensitivity to stimuli which cause platelet aggregation due to increased thromboxane production. The well-known association between low-density and high-density lipoproteins (LDL-cholesterol and HDL-cholesterol) and cardiovascular disease may also be partly explained in terms of PGI_2. LDL from men and postmenopausal women inhibits and HDL stimulates prostacyclin production. Platelets from diabetics and from Class A diabetic pregnant women make more TXA_2 than platelets from normal pregnant women. Smokers who use oral contraceptives have increased platelet aggregation and an inhibition of prostacyclin formation. Onion and garlic inhibit platelet aggregation and TXA_2 synthesis.

18. E   p.296,297

(See figure on page 129 in this Study Guide)

19. E   p.297,298

Luteolysis has not been demonstrated in the primate, and it is well-known that removal of the uterus does not interfere with normal ovulatory cycles. However, high doses of estrogen can induce luteolysis in the monkey and perhaps in the human. In the monkey, estrogen induces a drop in progesterone during the luteal phase, mirrored by a rise in F prostaglandin. Furthermore, indomethacin can block this effect of estrogen. There is considerable evidence to support a role for estrogen in the decline of the human corpus luteum. The premature elevation of circulating estradiol levels in the early luteal phase results in a prompt fall in progesterone concentrations. Direct injections of estradiol into the ovary bearing the corpus luteum induces luteolysis, while similar treatment of the contralateral ovary produces no effect. Prostaglandin $F_{2\alpha}$ produced within the ovary bearing the corpus luteum or within the corpus luteum may serve as the luteolytic agent, and the production of the prostaglandin is initiated by the luteal estrogen. However, the absence of estrogen receptors in luteal tissue argues against a luteolytic role in the primate for physiologic concentrations of estrogen.

The human application of these findings can be found in the use of postcoital estrogen for contraception. High doses of estrogen can decrease progesterone levels in human cycles. It is important to remember that the mechanism of estrogen is through $PGF_{2\alpha}$, and since the mechanism of $PGF_{2\alpha}$ is antagonism of LH action, human chorionic

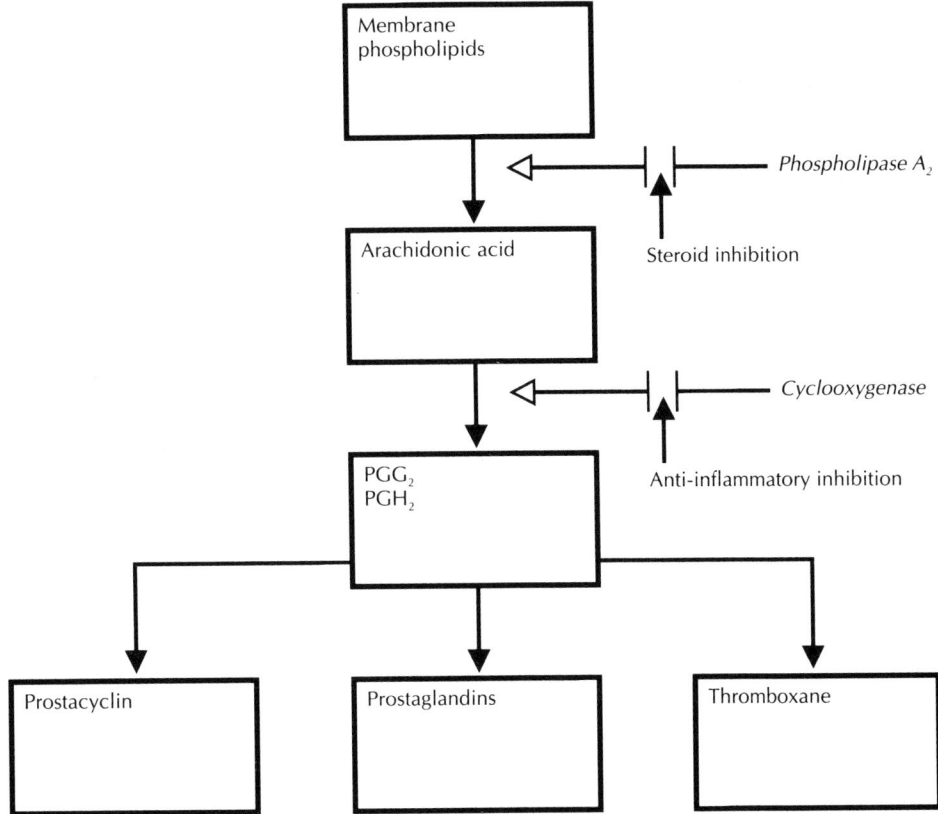

gonadotropin (HCG) can overcome this effect of estrogen. Hence, the effective action of estrogen when used for postcoital contraception is limited to the 7 days prior to implantation, before the corpus luteum is subject to rescue by HCG.

20. E   p.301

Evidence for a role of prostaglandin in parturition includes the following:

1. Prostaglandin levels in maternal blood and amniotic fluid increase in association with labor.
2. Arachidonic acid levels in the amniotic fluid also rise in labor, and arachidonate injected into the amniotic sac initiates parturition.
3. Patients taking high doses of aspirin have a highly significant increase in the average length of gestation, incidence of postmaturity, and duration of labor.
4. Indomethacin prevents the normal onset of labor in monkeys and stops premature labor in human pregnancies.
5. Stimuli known to cause the release of prostaglandins (cervical manipulation, stripping of membranes, and rupture of membranes) augment or induce uterine contractions.
6. Prostaglandins induce labor.

21. A   p.306

A major clinical application for the induction of labor in the United States is the use of intravaginal PGE_2 in cases of fetal demise and anencephalic fetuses. Based on our own experience, certain precautions have been developed. The patient should be well hydrated with an electrolyte solution to counteract the induced vasodilatation and decreased peripheral resistance. If satisfactory uterine activity is established, the next application should be withheld. And, finally, because there is a synergistic effect when oxytocin is used shortly after prostaglandin administration, there should be a minimum of 6 hours between the last prostaglandin dose and beginning oxytocin augmentation.

Prostaglandins are used to induce term labor. Intravenous prostaglandins are not an acceptable method due to the side effects achieved by the high dosage necessary to reach the uterus. The intravaginal and oral administration of PGE_2 is as effective as intravenous oxytocin, even including patients with previous cesarean sections. These methods, plus intracervical administration, are in routine use in many parts of the world.

22. B p.307

When routine methods of management for postpartum hemorrhage caused by uterine atony have failed, an analogue of prostaglandin $F_{2\alpha}$ has been used with excellent results (80–90% successful). Prostin 15 M is (15-S)-15-methyl prostaglandin $F_{2\alpha}$-tromethamine. The dose is 0.25–0.5 mg, repeated up to 4 times and given with equal efficacy either intramuscularly or directly into the myometrium. It can also be used after the replacement of an inverted uterus. Failures are usually associated with infections or magnesium sulfate therapy. It should not be used in patients with severe hypertension or symptomatic asthma. Diarrhea is a frequent side effect.

10 Normal and Abnormal Sexual Development

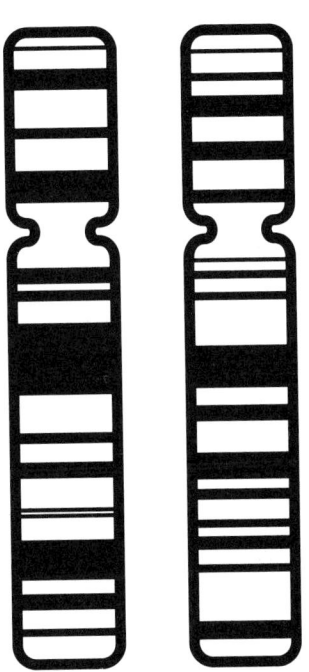

Learning Objectives

Be able to:

1. Understand the processes of normal sexual differentiation.

2. Detail the board categories of abnormal sexual differentiation.

3. Describe the types and clinical significance of enzymatic abnormalities within the adrenal which result in female pseudohermaphrodism.

4. Describe the workup, diagnosis and management plan of both nonpregnant and pregnant women with congenital adrenal hyperplasia.

5. Explain the differences in clinical presentations of individuals with complete versus incomplete androgen insensitivity.

6. Detail what is known regarding the anatomy and genetics of true hermaphrodites.

7. Discuss the clinical challenges involved in diagnosing and treating individuals with gonadal dysgenesis.

8. Describe the clinical challenges involved in diagnosing and treating individuals with ambiguous genitalia.

Clinical Gynecologic Endocrinology and Infertility: Self Assessment and Study Guide

Pre-Test

A. Instructions: Fill in the blanks

1. The critical factors in determining which of the duct structures stabilize or regress are secretions from the testis: _____ and _____.

2. An absent uterus in a normal appearing female is encountered in only two conditions: _____ and _____.

B. Instructions: True or False

3. A variety of mutations affecting CYP21A lead to 21-hydroxylase deficiency.

4. Androgen insensitivity accounts for 25% of all cases of primary amenorrhea, third most common after gonadal dysgenesis and congenital absence of the vagina.

C. Instructions: For each of the following questions choose:

A. if only 1, 2 and 3 are correct
B. if only 1 and 3 are correct
C. if only 2 and 4 are correct
D. if only 4 is correct
E. if all are correct

5. Late-onset 21-hydroxylase deficiency
   1. becomes apparent prior to adolescence
   2. causes hirsutism, menstrual irregularities and infertility
   3. can be a life threatening condition
   4. is the same as attenuated, acquired or nonclassical 21-hydroxylase deficiency

6. Medical treatment of congenital adrenal hyperplasia (CAH)
   1. may be complicated by Cushing's syndrome and poor growth
   2. requires pharmacologic dosages of steroids
   3. may be complicated by short stature, hirsutism and infertility
   4. does not involve mineralocorticoid supplementation

Post-Test

A. Instructions: Fill in the blanks

1. At _____ weeks of fetal life the gonads are bipotential, capable of differentiation into either testes or ovaries. After _____ weeks of fetal life they are no longer bipotential.

2. A single gene determinant on the _____ chromosome called _____ is necessary for testicular differentiation.

3. In an XX individual, without the influence of a Y chromosome, the bipotential gonad develops into an ovary about _____ weeks _____ than testicular development.

4. Testosterone secretion stimulates development of the wolffian duct system into _____, _____ and _____.

5. In the absence of a Y chromosome and a functional testis, the lack of _____ allows retention of the _____ system and development of _____, _____ and _____ vagina.

6. Of all infants with ambiguous genitalia _____% have adrenal hyperplasia.

7. There are two 21-hydroxylase genes called _____ and _____ which are both located on chromosome _____ between HLA-B and DR.

8. In adults, 17-OHP must be measured in early morning to avoid later elevations due to the _____ pattern of ACTH secretion.

9. Treatment of adrenal hyperplasia is to supply _____. This decreases _____ secretion and lowers production of _____ precursors.

10. In the newborn, the clinical signs of adrenal failure being due to some form of adrenal enzyme defect are _____ and hyponatremia or hypertension and _____.

B. Instructions: True or False

11. Prenatally, sexual differentiation follows the following order: genetic sex, gonadal differentiation, differentiation of the internal duct system and finally formation of the external genitalia.

12. The embryonic brain is not sexually differentiated.

13. The testes-determining gene is located on the distal long arm of the Y chromosome.

14. Testes formation is an active event whereas female sex differentiation is a passive event if SRY is absent or deficient.

15. A complete 46, XX chromosomal complement is necessary for normal development.

16. Abnormalities in the renal system are associated with abnormalities in development of the tubes, uterus, and upper vagina.

17. Serum measurement of antimüllerian hormone is a sensitive marker for the presence of testicular tissue and thus helpful in gender assignment of an infant with ambiguous genitalia.

18. In the absence of testosterone, the wolffian system regresses while in the presence of a normal ovary or absence of any gonad, müllerian duct development takes place.

19. Deficiency of 17α-hydroxylase may result in the following syndrome: hypertension, hypokalemia, infantile female external genitalia; elevated FSH and primary amenorrhea.

20. Deficiency of 20–22 desmolase is incompatible with life.

21. The immunoassay of blood 17-hydroxyprogesterone has become the primary assessment for the diagnosis and management of congenital adrenal hyperplasia.

22. Fertility in women with late onset adrenal hyperplasia is significantly reduced.

23. Masculinization of the female fetus may be produced by an androgen-secreting maternal tumor or by an intake of exogenous progestins or danazol.

24. Treatment for female infants who suffer from congenital adrenal hyperplasia does not involve surgery.

25. Congenital insensitivity to androgens is transmitted by a maternal X-linked dominant gene responsible for the androgen intracellular receptor.

C. Instructions: Match each classification with each disorder.

A. female pseudohermaphroditism
B. male pseudohermaphroditism
C. gonadal dysgenesis

26. androgen insensitivity
27. P450c17 deficiency
28. placental aromatase deficiency
29. 21-hydroxylase deficiency
30. mosaicism
31. 5α-reductase

D. Instructions: For each of the following questions choose:

A. if only 1, 2 and 3 are correct
B. if only 1 and 3 are correct
C. if only 2 and 4 are correct
D. if only 4 is correct
E. if all are correct

32. Gender identity is the result of
    1. gonadal sex
    2. genetic sex
    3. internal and external genitalia
    4. secondary sex characteristics

33. Testes-determining factor (TDF) gene
    1. is located on the distal long arm of the Y
    2. if lost results in gonadal dysgenesis
    3. must be present in Swyer's syndrome
    4. if transferred to the X chromosome results in an XX male

34. Antimüllerian hormone has several extra müllerian functions which include:
    1. inhibitory effect on oocyte meiosis
    2. a role in the descent of the testes
    3. inhibits surfactant accumulation in the lungs
    4. sexual differentiation of the brain

35. Congenital adrenal hyperplasia
    1. may appear in utero or develop postnatally
    2. is not associated with abnormal secretion of antimüllerian hormone
    3. may be characterized by fusion of the labioscrotal folds and hypospadias
    4. if untreated, will result in early epiphysial closure and shortened stature in adulthood

36. Deficiency of 21-hydroxylase
    1. is responsible for 90% of congenital adrenal hyperplasia
    2. is not the most frequent cause of sexual ambiguity
    3. is the most frequent endocrine cause of neonatal death
    4. is recognized as two different clinical forms

37. Deficiency of 11β-hydroxylase
    1. is associated with hypertension and hypokalemic acidosis
    2. is associated with virilization similar to that seen in 21-hydroxylase deficiency
    3. has a gene close to the HLA complex on chromosome 6
    4. is associated with a mild nonclassic form characterized by mild biochemical abnormalities

38. Prenatal diagnosis of 21-hydroxylase deficiency
    1. can be demonstrated by elevated levels of 17 OHP and androstenedione in the amniotic fluid
    2. can be made through chorion villus biopsy utilizing DNA probes
    3. may allow therapy to be instituted before the critical period of fetal genital differentiation
    4. may allow prenatal treatment with dexamethasone thus precluding genital ambiguity in the affected fetus

39. The use of dexamethasone in the prenatal treatment of 21-hydroxylase deficiency
    1. may be associated with significant maternal side effects
    2. usually requires greater than 1.5 mg/day
    3. is appropriate for only 1 of 8 fetuses who will ultimately require treatment
    4. is usually kept at a constant dosage throughout pregnancy

40. Serum 17-hydroxyprogesterone
    1. is drawn in early AM for most accurate assessment
    2. baseline level should be less than 400 ng/dl (12nmol/L)
    3. levels over 800 ng/dl (24nmol/L) are virtually diagnostic of 21-hydroxylase deficiency
    4. is elevated in patients with 17-hydroxylase or 3β-hydroxysteroid dehydrogenase deficiencies

41. Medical treatment of congenital adrenal hyperplasia (CAH)
    1. may involve hydrocortisone or 9-fluorohydrocortisone
    2. needs to maintain 17-OHP level in range of 500–4,000 ng/dL
    3. should be supplemented with additional steroids during major stress
    4. is directed toward decreasing ACTH secretion

42. Patients with complete androgen insensitivity
    1. have normal antimüllerian hormone activity
    2. vagina is short and ends blindly
    3. is a cause of primary amenorrhea
    4. the testes are normally developed

43. Incomplete androgen insensitivity
    1. represent a spectrum of disorders, all due to x-linked recessive tract
    2. is only one-tenth as common as the complete syndrome
    3. has a clinical presentation which involves an endocrine profile similar to complete androgen insensitivity
    4. does not often result in a newborn with ambiguous genitalia

44. 5α-reductase deficiency
    1. is characterized by severe perineal hypospadias and underdevelopment of the vagina
    2. results in masculinization at puberty
    3. can be diagnosed by an increased testosterone to dihydrotestosterone ratio
    4. if present in homozygous 46 XX females results in infertility

45. Swyer Syndrome
    1. have normal female external but abnormal internal genitalia
    2. present with primary amenorrhea but have age appropriate Tanner breasts and pubic hair
    3. have male levels of serum testosterone
    4. require gonadectomy as soon as the diagnosis is made

46. True hermaphrodites
    1. have internal structures corresponding to the adjacent gonad
    2. in the majority of cases have external genitalia which are not ambiguous
    3. are genetic females (XX) in the majority of cases
    4. can not contain both ovarian and testicular tissue in one gonad

47. Turner syndrome
    1. results from total loss on one X chromosome in 40% of patients with this syndrome
    2. patients have normal intelligence
    3. is not commonly associated with autoimmune disorders
    4. patients should have a diagnostic workup which includes: thyroid antibodies, intravenous pyelogram or renal ultrasound and echocardiography

48. Mosaicism
    1. may explain the presence of menstrual function and reproduction in a patient with a Turner phenotype
    2. may be seen in a large variety of patterns with gonadal dysgenesis
    3. within the gonad can be missed in a karyotype derived from leukocyte culture
    4. involving a Y chromosome requires gonadectomy to avoid the 25% incidence of later development of a gonadal tumor

49. Gonadectomy
    1. should be performed for intra-abdominal testes
    2. is performed to avoid the development of a gonadoblastoma or dysgerminoma in a mosaic individual with a Y cell line
    3. in selected cases may be performed laparoscopically with an effort to preserve the uterus and tubes
    4. is usually recommended immediately except in a prepubertal individual with testicular feminization

50. Hormone treatment of young patients without ovaries
    1. is directed to promoting the development of secondary sexual characteristics while avoiding closure of the epiphyses
    2. initially requires small amounts of unopposed estrogen (0.3 mg conjugated estrogens or 0.5 mg estradiol daily).
    3. after 6 months to 1 year of small amounts of unopposed estrogen should be progressed to a sequential program similar to replacement in a postmenopausal woman
    4. may be supplemented by recombinant growth hormone in selected cases

51. Diagnosis of ambiguous genitalia in the newborn
    1. requires palpation of the inguinal regions or scrotal folds
    2. results in the patient being assigned to one of four categories: female or male pseudohermaphroditism, true hermaphroditism or gonadal dysgenesis
    3. must consider foremost the possibility of congenital adrenal hyperplasia
    4. is accompanied by the difficult problem of correct sex assignment

52. Assignment of sex rearing
    1. should be male in cases of masculinized females
    2. should be delayed rather than reversed when presented with a difficult case
    3. can probably be reversed up to age 3
    4. should depend on future fertility, projected appearance of genitalia after puberty and penile adequacy for coitus

Answers for Chapter 10 — Pre-Test

1. antimüllerian hormone; testosterone　　　　　　　　　　　　　　　　　　　　　　　　　　　　p.325,326

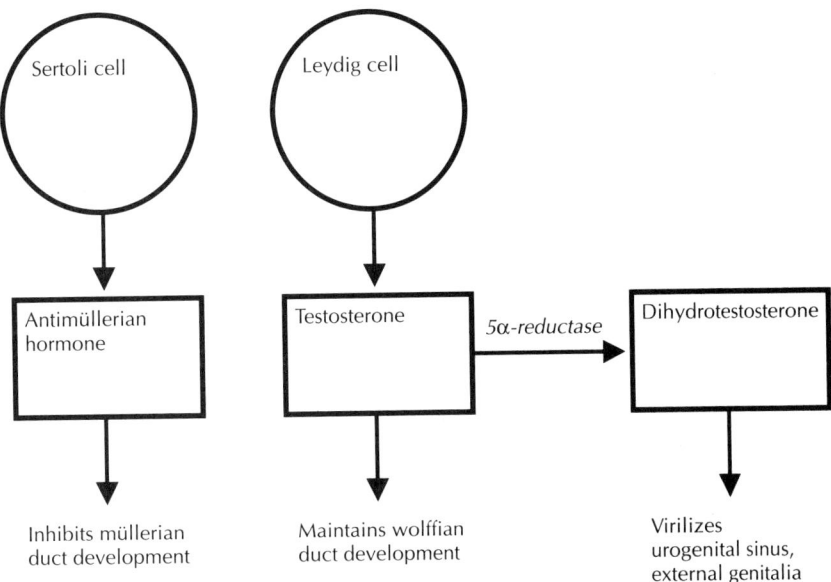

2. androgen insensitivity; müllerian agenesis　　　　　　　　　　　　　　　　　　　　　　　　　　p.340
An absent uterus in a normal appearing female is encountered in only two conditions: androgen insensitivity and müllerian agenesis (the Mayer-Rokitansky-Kuster-Hauser syndrome). The latter is easily diagnosed because of the presence of pubic and axillary hair and a normal 46,XX karyotype.

3. false　　p.331
As a result of the close genetic linkage between 21-hydroxylase deficiency and the human leukocyte antigen (HLA) complex located on the short arm of chromosome 6, we have learned the following:

   1. The disorder is inherited as a monogenic autosomal recessive trait.
   2. HLA typing can be used to determine the carrier status of family members and for early prenatal diagnosis prior to virilization.
   3. Two 21-hydroxylase genes exist, designated CYP21A and CYP21B, located on chromosome 6 between HLA-B and DR, and are in tandem duplication with the genes encoding the fourth component of

complement. Only CYP21B is active in adrenal steroidogenesis; CYP21A is not involved (a pseudogene because its product is enzymatically inactive).

4. A variety of mutations affecting CYP21B (deletions, gene conversion [material from CYP21A to CYP21B], point mutations) lead to 21-hydroxylase deficiency.

4. false   p.340

Androgen insensitivity accounts for about 10% of all cases of primary amenorrhea, third most common after gonadal dysgenesis and congenital absence of the vagina. The hormone profile in these individuals is typical: high LH, normal to slightly elevated male testosterone levels, high estradiol (for men), and normal to elevated FSH.

5. C   p.331

Three different clinical forms are recognized: the salt-wasting, the simple virilizing, and the late-onset (also known as nonclassic, attenuated, or acquired adrenal hyperplasia). The first and second are associated with female pseudohermaphroditism at birth, while the third usually becomes apparent at adolescence or beyond and causes hirsutism, menstrual irregularities, and infertility.

6. B   p.338

Overtreatment causes Cushing's syndrome and poor growth; undertreatment is associated with short stature, hirsutism, and infertility. In some cases, undertreatment and increased androgen secretion lead to premature pubertal maturation that may require treatment with a gonadotropin-releasing hormone (GnRH) agonist. The adult height achieved by most patients is less than normal, testimony to overtreatment and undertreatment (which both compromise growth). Mineralocorticoid therapy should be maximized (maintaining the plasma renin activity at its lower limit of normal) to eliminate hypovolemia as a stimulus for ACTH secretion. A treatment approach is being investigated that adds an antiandrogen and an aromatase inhibitor in an effort to avoid hypercortisolism and block excess sex steroid action on growth.

Answers for Chapter 10 — Post-Test

1. 6; 8   p.322, 325

In human embryos, the gonads begin development during the 5th week of gestation as protuberances overlying the mesonephric ducts. The migration of primordial germ cells into these gonadal ridges occurs between weeks 4 and 6 of gestation. Although germ cells do not induce gonadal development, if the germ cells fail to arrive, gonads do not develop and only the fibrous streak of gonadal agenesis will exist. At 6 weeks of fetal life the gonads are indifferent but bipotential, possessing both cortical and medullary areas, and are capable of differentiation into either testes or ovaries. They are composed of germ cells, special epithelia (potential granulosa/Sertoli cells), mesenchyme (potential theca/Leydig cells), and the mesonephric duct system. Wolffian and müllerian ducts exist side by side; external genitalia are undifferentiated.

The wolffian and müllerian ducts are discrete primordia which temporarily coexist in all embryos during the ambisexual period of development (up to 8 weeks). Thereafter, one type of duct system persists normally and gives rise to special ducts and glands, whereas the other disappears during the 3rd fetal month, except for nonfunctional vestiges.

2. Y; TDF   p.323

Sexual differentiation requires direction by various genes, with a single gene determinant on the Y chromosome (testes determining factor — TDF) necessary for testicular differentiation.

3. 2; later   p.324

In an XX individual, without the active influence of a Y chromosome, the bipotential gonad develops into an ovary about 2 weeks later than testicular development. The cortical zone develops and contains the germ cells, while the medullary portion regresses with its remnant being the rete ovarii, a compressed nest of tubules and Leydig cells in the hilus of the ovary. The germ cells proliferate by mitosis, reaching a peak of 5–7 million by 20 weeks. By 20 weeks, the fetal ovary achieves mature compartmentalization with primordial follicles containing oocytes, initial evidence of follicle maturation and atresia, and an incipient stroma. Degeneration (atresia) begins even earlier, and by birth, approximately 1–2 million germ cells remain. These have become surrounded by a layer of follicular cells, forming primordial follicles with oocytes which have entered the first meiotic division. Meiosis is arrested in the prophase of the first meiotic division until reactivation of follicular growth that may not occur until years later. Excessively rapid atresia (germ cell attrition) in gonadal dysgenesis (45,X) accounts for the streak gonad seen in these cases. A complete 46,XX chromosomal complement is necessary for normal ovarian development. The second X chromosome, therefore, contains elements essential for ovarian maintenance.

4. epididymis, vas deferens, seminal vesicles   p.326

Testosterone is secreted by the fetal testes soon after Leydig cell formation (at 8 weeks) and rapidly rises to peak concentrations at 15–18 weeks. This testosterone secretion stimulates development of the wolffian duct system into epididymis, vas deferens, and seminal vesicles. Testosterone levels in the male fetus correlate with Leydig cell development, overall gonadal weight, 3β-hydroxysteroid dehydrogenase activity, and chorionic gonadotropin (HCG) concentrations. As HCG declines (approximately 20 weeks) the fetal pituitary lutinizing hormone (LH) assumes control of Leydig cell testosterone secretion; anencephalics and other forms of congenital hypopituitarism display diminished androgen effects on internal and external genitalia.

The wolffian ducts receive testosterone signals directly from nearby Leydig cells as well as the general fetal circulation. This local paracrine effect is essential to the stimulation of ipsilateral differentiation into the epididymis, vas deferens, and seminal vesicles. Duct system differentiation will proceed, therefore, according to the nature of the adjacent gonad. The wolffian ducts do not form dihydrotestosterone, so the direct high concentration is crucial for normal development. Because of this local paracrine action, wolffian development cannot be stimulated in females exposed to adrenal or exogenous androgens.

5. antimüllerian hormone, müllerian, uterus, tubes, upper   p.326

The internal genitalia possess the intrinsic tendency to feminize. In the absence of a Y chromosome and a functional testis, the lack of AMH allows retention of the müllerian system and development of fallopian tubes, uterus, and upper vagina. In the absence of testosterone, the wolffian system regresses. In the presence of a normal ovary or the absence of any gonad, müllerian duct development takes place.

6. 40–45%   p.329

Masculinized females possess ovaries and are female by genetic sex (XX), but the external genitalia are not those of a normal female. Of all infants with ambiguous genitalia, 40–45% have adrenal hyperplasia. Rarer causes of female pseudohermaphroditism are excess maternal androgen caused by drug ingestion, tumor secretion, or possibly placental aromatase deficiency.

7. CYP2IA; CYP21B; 6   p.331

Two 21-hydroxylase genes exist, designated CYP21A and CYP21B, located on chromosome 6 between HLA-B and DR, and are in tandem duplication with the genes encoding the fourth component of complement. Only CYP21B is active in adrenal steroidogenesis; CYP21A is not involved (a pseudogene because its product is enzymatically inactive).

8. diurnal   p.336

In adults, 17-OHP must be measured first thing in the morning to avoid later elevations due to the diurnal pattern of ACTH secretion. The baseline 17-OHP level should be less than 200 ng/dL (6 nmol/L). Levels greater than 200 ng/dL, but less than 800 ng/dL (24 nmol/L), require ACTH testing. Levels over 800 ng/dL (24 nmol/L) are virtually diagnostic of the 21-hydroxylase deficiency. The DHAS level is usually normal. The hallmarks of late-onset adrenal hyperplasia are elevated levels of 17-OHP and a dramatic increase after ACTH stimulation. The elevated levels of 17-OHP are often not impressive (e.g., overlapping with those found in women with polycystic ovaries due to anovulation), and a simple ACTH stimulation test must be utilized.

9. cortisol; ACTH; androgenic   p.337

Treatment of adrenal hyperplasia is to supply the deficient hormone, cortisol. This decreases ACTH secretion and lowers production of androgenic precursors. The addition of salt-retaining hormone to glucocorticoid therapy has improved the control of the disease. When the plasma renin activity is normalized, ACTH and androgen levels are further decreased, and a decrease in the glucocorticoid dose is also possible. Therefore, the modern management of hormonal control requires the measurement of the blood levels of 17-OHP, androstenedione, testosterone, and plasma renin activity. The drugs of choice are hydrocortisone (approximately 10 mg per day) and 9-fluorohydrocortisone (approximately 100 mg/day). This method of treatment and monitoring applies to all forms of adrenal hyperplasia. The standard dose of cortisol is 12–18 mg/m^2 or 3.5–5 mg/m^2 of prednisone, but larger doses given on alternate days (14 mg/m^2 of prednisone, about 20 mg) can maintain adrenal androgen suppression and perhaps achieve better growth and pubertal development, despite higher levels of 17-hydroxyprogesterone. The 17-OHP level should be maintained in the range of 500 to 4,000 ng/dL, thereby avoiding both overtreatment and undertreatment. Minor stresses will cause brief elevations of adrenal androgens but usually do not require readjustment of dosage. With major stress, such as surgery, additional hormonal support is necessary.

10. hyperkalemia; hypokalemia p.352

Clinical signs of adrenal failure indicate that the newborn has some form of adrenal enzyme defect regardless of the steroid pattern. The diagnosis is certain if such an infant is hyperkalemic and hyponatremic (due to aldosterone deficiency) or hypertensive and hypokalemic (secondary to elevated deoxycorticosterone).

11. true p.322

Prenatally, sexual differentiation follows a specific sequence of events. First is the establishment of the genetic sex. Second, under the control of the genetic sex the gonads differentiate, determining the hormonal environment of the embryo, the differentiation of internal duct systems, and the formation of the external genitalia.

12. false p.322

It has become apparent that the embryonic brain is also sexually differentiated, perhaps via a control mechanism very similar to that which determines the sexual development of the external genitalia. The inductive influences of hormones on the central nervous system may have an effect on the patterns of hormone secretion and sexual behavior in the adult.

13. false p.323,324

The distal end of the short arm of the Y chromosome is called the pseudoautosomal region because during meiosis the homologous distal short arms of the X and Y chromosomes pair, and interchange of genetic material occurs. The genes in the pseudoautosomal regions are doubly present in both sexes, and therefore escape X inactivation. Gene deletions in this area of the X chromosome (Xp22.3) are associated with various conditions, known as contiguous gene syndromes: short stature, mental retardation, X-linked ichthyosis, Kallmann's syndrome. The testis-determining gene is located on the distal short arm of the Y, immediately adjacent to the pseudoautosomal region. Loss of the TDF gene causes gonadal dysgenesis. Transfer of the TDF gene to the X results in an XX male.

14. true p.324

SRY participation in morphogenesis and pattern formation leading to a testis from the bipotential genital ridge is a model "genetic switch" between alternative inherent programs. Whereas testes formation is an active event, female sex determination is the default pathway occurring if SRY is absent or deficient. The formation of the testicle precedes any other sexual development in time, and a functionally active testis controls subsequent sexual development. Testicular hormones activate or repress genes to direct development away from an otherwise predetermined course of female differentiation.

15. true p.325

Proteins other than SRY are required for proper gonadogenesis. In the human, autosomal genes are essential for gonadal development. These autosomal genes regulate migration of the germ cells and coding of the steroidogenic enzymes.

16. true p.325

AMH is a member of the transforming growth factor-β family of glycoprotein differentiation factors that include inhibin and activin. The gene for AMH has been mapped to the short arm of chromosome 19. AMH is synthesized by Sertoli cells soon after testicular differentiation and is responsible for the ipsilateral regression of the müllerian ducts by 8 weeks, before the emergence of testosterone and stimulation of the wolffian ducts. Despite its presence in serum up to puberty, lack of regression of the uterus and tubes is the only consistent expression of AMH gene mutations. In the absence of AMH, the fetus will develop fallopian tubes, uterus, and upper vagina from the paramesonephric ducts (the müllerian ducts). This development requires the prior appearance of the mesonephric ducts, and for this reason, abnormalities in the renal system are associated with abnormalities in development of the tubes, uterus, and upper vagina.

17. true p.325

AMH is detectable in the serum of males during infancy, childhood, adolescence, and adulthood. In contrast, AMH is not measureable until the second decade of life in females. This difference allows serum measurement to be a sensitive marker for the presence of testicular tissue in intersex anomalies.

18. true p.326

The internal genitalia possess the intrinsic tendency to feminize. In the absence of a Y chromosome and a functional testis, the lack of AMH allows retention of the müllerian system and development of fallopian tubes, uterus, and upper vagina. In the absence of testosterone, the wolffian system regresses. In the presence of a normal ovary or the absence of any gonad, müllerian duct development takes place.

19. true p.334

With block of the 17α-hydroxylase enzyme (P450c17), synthesis of cortisol, androgens, and estrogens is curtailed. Only the non-17-hydroxylated corticoids, DOC and corticosterone, are formed. The molecular basis for this enzyme deficiency is due to a variety of mutations which result in multiple base deletions and duplications in the gene on chromosome 10. The resulting syndrome is composed of hypertension (due to hypernatremia and hypervolemia), hypokalemia, infantile female external genitalia, which do not mature at puberty, and primary amenorrhea with elevated follicle-stimulating hormone (FSH) and luteinizing hormone (LH). Genital ambiguity is a problem only in male infants.

20. true p.334

A block in this step prevents conversion of cholesterol to pregnenolone, the necessary precursor to all biologically active steroids. The adrenals are enlarged and filled with cholesterol esters. Predictably, the internal and external genitalia are female, and death occurs.

21. true p.336

For years the demonstration of a metabolic defect and its location depended upon the study of urinary steroid excretion. Today, the immunoassay of blood 17-hydroxyprogesterone (17-OHP) has become the primary assessment for the diagnosis and management of congenital adrenal hyperplasia. With the 21-hydroxylase and 11β-hydroxylase deficiencies, the 17-OHP level will be 50–400-fold above normal.

22. false p.337

Normal reproduction is possible with replacement therapy of the cortisol deficiency. Unfortunately poor compliance with therapy and less than satisfactory surgical reconstruction of the vagina result in decreased fertility and sexuality. Greater attention to these factors is needed to improve the sexual experience and fertility of these women. Many cases come to cesarean section because normal anatomy of the perineum may be obscured by scar tissue from earlier plastic surgery; therefore, greater blood loss and the risk of a hematoma with a vaginal delivery are significant factors. A masculine pelvis is not expected since the adult form and size of the inlet of the pelvis are assumed largely during the growth spurt in puberty. However, a small pelvis might be anticipated if the bone age is up to age 13–14 when treatment is initiated. Fertility in women with late onset adrenal hyperplasia is only slightly reduced, dependent upon the degree of hormonal dysfunction (which is promptly corrected with glucocorticoid therapy).

23. true p.338

Masculinization of the female fetus, although in most cases due to fetal virilizing adrenal hyperplasia, may be produced by an androgen-secreting maternal tumor or may be due to the intake of exogenous androgenic substances, such as progestins and danazol. When not caused by an error in the metabolism of the fetal adrenal gland, virilization is not progressive, blood steroids are not elevated, and no hormonal therapy is needed. Subsequent development will be normal. Therefore, surgical correction of abnormalities in the external genitalia is the only indicated treatment.

The occurrence of an androgen-secreting tumor in a mother during pregnancy is rarely seen. On the other hand, the iatrogenic cause of masculinization is a well-known story. The majority of these cases resulted from antenatal maternal treatment of threatened or recurrent abortion with various progestin compounds. In view of the lack of evidence for positive results with such therapy, the use of progestin compounds in pregnancy is contraindicated.

24. false p.337

The surgical treatment of the anatomical abnormalities should be carried out in the first few years of life, when the patient is still too young to remember the procedure and too young to have developed psychological problems centered about the abnormal external genitalia. If clitoridectomy is necessary, the clitoral recession procedure, conserving the glans and its innervation, should be employed. It is important to know that women who undergo total clitoral amputations have no subsequent impairment of erotic responsiveness or capacity for orgasm. Significant vaginal reconstruction, if necessary, is best accomplished after puberty when mature compliance is possible.

25. false p.340

The phenotype of this condition is female, despite the normal male karyotype 46,XY. There is a congenital insensitivity to androgens, transmitted by means of a maternal X-linked recessive gene responsible for the androgen intracellular receptor. Therefore, androgen induction of wolffian duct development does not occur. However, antimüllerian hormone activity is present, and the individual does not have müllerian development (a natural experiment that indicates the presence of an antimüllerian hormone). Frequently the testes have descended to the inguinal ring because AMH mediates the transabdominal descent of the testes. The vagina is short (derived from the urogenital sinus only) and ends blindly. The uterus and tubes are absent. The testes are normally developed but abnormally positioned. Testosterone production is normal or slightly increased. There is no problem of sex assignment because there is no trace of androgen activity. The diagnosis is likely when an individual presents following breast development at puberty, with primary amenorrhea, scanty or absent pubic and axillary hair, a short vagina, and an absent cervix and uterus.

26. B p.329

27. B p.329

28. A p.329

29. A p.329

30. C p.329

31. B p.329

Disorders of Fetal Endocrinology

Female pseudohermaphroditism (partial virilization)
Congenital adrenal hyperplasia
    21-Hydroxylase deficiency (P450c21)
    11β-Hydroxylase deficiency (P450c11β)
    3β-Hydroxysteroid dehydrogenase deficiency
Drug intake
Maternal disease
Placental aromatase deficiency

Male pseudohermaphroditism (inadequate virilization)
Antimüllerian hormone defect
Impaired androgenization
Androgen insensitivity syndromes
5α-Reductase deficiency
Testosterone biosynthesis defects
P450scc deficiency
3β-Hydroxysteroid dehydrogenase deficiency
17α-Hydroxylase deficiency (P450c17)
17β-Hydroxysteroid dehydrogenase deficiency

Disorders of Gonadal Development

Male pseudohermaphroditism
Primary gonadal defect
Y Chromosome defect

True hermaphroditism

Gonadal dysgenesis
Turner syndrome
Mosaicism
Structural abnormality — X chromosome
Normal karyotype

---

32. E   p.322
The gender identity of a person (whether an individual identifies as a male or a female) is the end result of genetic, hormonal, and morphologic sex as influenced by the environment of the individual. It includes all behavior with any sexual connotation, such as body gestures and mannerisms, habits of speech, recreational preferences, and content of dreams. Sexual expression, both homosexual and heterosexual, can be regarded as the result of all influences on the individual, both prenatal and postnatal. Specifically, gender identity is the result of the following determinants: genetic sex, gonadal sex, the internal genitalia, the external genitalia, the secondary sexual characteristics that appear at puberty, and the role assigned by society in response to all of these developmental manifestations of sex.

33. C   p.324
The testis-determining gene is located on the distal short arm of the Y, immediately adjacent to the pseudoautosomal region. Loss of the TDF gene causes gonadal dysgenesis. Transfer of the TDF gene to the X results in an XX male.

34. A   p.325
AMH may have extra müllerian functions. AMH exerts an inhibitory effect on oocyte meiosis, plays a role in the descent

of the testes, and inhibits surfactant accumulation in the lungs. Proteolytic cleavage of AMH produces fragments which have the ability to inhbit growth of various tumors (a potential therapeutic application). Testicular descent occurs in stages. Transabdominal movement of the testes is the result of rapid gubernacular growth, apparently under AMH control. Movement through the inguinal canal is mediated by androgens.

35. E p.330

Congenital adrenal hyperplasia in females is characterized by masculinized external genitalia, and is diagnosed by demonstrating excessive androgen production by the adrenal cortex, caused by either tumor or hyperplasia. The syndrome may appear in utero or develop postnatally.

Depending on the time of onset, quantity available, and duration of exposure, the presence of excessive androgens is manifested by varying degrees of fusion of the labioscrotal folds, clitoral enlargement, and anatomical changes of the urethra and vagina. Generally, the urethra and vagina share a urogenital sinus formed by the fusion of labial folds. This sinus opens at the base of the clitoris, which is usually enlarged. The degree of urogenital sinus deformity is related to the timing in prenatal development of the onset of masculinizing androgen effect. Because there is no anomalous secretion of antimüllerian hormone in females with congenital adrenal hyperplasia, the fallopian tubes, uterus, and upper vagina develop normally. Since wolffian duct development and maintenance depend on high local androgen levels provided by the male gonad, the excessive androgens of adrenal hyperplasia origin cannot stimulate this process, and no wolffian development is retained. The external genitalia on the other hand can be substantially altered by adrenal hyperplasia. After the 10th week, when the vagina and urethra have separated, the emerging excess androgen effect may be limited to clitoral hypertrophy. High androgen levels earlier than the 12th week of fetal age, however, can cause progressive fusion of the labia (anteriorly-posteriorly), formation of a urogenital sinus, and even variable closure of the urethra along the phallus (hypospadias). The absence of palpable testes may be the only clinical marker suggesting female pseudohermaphroditism.

Only the external genitalia are affected because internal genitalia differentiation is completed by the 10th week of gestation, while the adrenal cortex begins function by the 12th week. Since the female external genitalia phenotype is not completed until 140 days of fetal age, early androgen excess (7–12 weeks) may fully masculinize, whereas late (18–20 weeks) androgen may create limited ambiguity of the basically female appearance of the urogenital sinus and genital folds. The size of the clitoris depends on the quantity rather than timing of androgen excess. Cases of incorrect sex assignment in the female are due to the similarity between these external genitalia and hypospadias and bilateral cryptorchidism in a male infant.

If untreated, the female with adrenal hyperplasia will develop signs of progressive virilization postnatally. Pubic hair will appear by age 2–4, followed by axillary hair, then body hair and beard. Bone age is advanced by age 2, and because of early epiphyseal closure, height in childhood is achieved at the expense of shortened stature in adulthood. Progressive masculinization continues with the development of the male habitus, acne, deepened voice, and primary amenorrhea and infertility.

36. B p.331

The 21-hydroxylase block is the most common form of congenital adrenal hyperplasia (90% of cases), the most frequent cause of sexual ambiguity, and the most frequent endocrine cause of neonatal death. With severe uncompensated blocks of this type, salt-wasting and shock accompany significant virilization. In less severe variations, when sufficient cortisol can be produced, virilization due to excess androgen is still present in utero, at birth, or later in life. Three different clinical forms are recognized: the salt-wasting, the simple virilizing, and the late-onset (also known as nonclassic, attenuated, or acquired adrenal hyperplasia). The first and second are associated with female pseudo-hermaphroditism at birth, while the third usually becomes apparent at adolescence or beyond and causes hirsutism, menstrual irregularities, and infertility.

37. C p.332

The final step in cortisol synthesis is blocked in this condition. In classic 11β-hydroxylase deficiency, 11-deoxycortisol is not converted to cortisol. Accumulated precursors are shunted into androgen biosynthesis with virilization similar to that seen with 21-hydroxylase deficiency. However, a parallel defect also exists so that deoxycorticosterone (DOC) is not converted to corticosterone. This pathway is used in the zona glomerulosa to synthesize aldosterone, and the degree to which aldosterone levels are affected lends clinical heterogeneity to the classic presentation of 11β-hydroxylase deficiency (virilization, hypertension, volume overload).

Usually as a result of 11β-hydroxylase deficiency, metabolically active precursors of corticosterone and cortisol add to excess androgen synthesis as further liabilities of ACTH-induced hyperplasia. Hypertension and hypokalemic alkalosis are induced by elevated DOC with reduced renin and aldosterone. Virilization is caused by androgens of the "deoxy" type (dehydroepiandrosterone [DHA], dehydroepiandrosterone sulfate [DHAS], and androstenedione). The diagnosis is confirmed by high plasma DOC and compound S (11-deoxycortisol) levels.

About two-thirds of untreated patients with 11β-hydroxylase deficiency become hypertensive, usually of mild to moderate degree (150/90 mm Hg) and only after several years of life. A mild nonclassic form of 11β-hydroxylase deficiency, as in 21-hydroxylase defects, has also been documented; it is characterized by mild biochemical abnormalities, and the patients are only mildly virilized and rarely hypertensive.

Contrary to 21-hydroxylase deficiency, the 11β-hydroxylase deficiency locus is remote from the HLA complex. The gene for the enzyme is on the long arm of chromosome 8, and the deficiency is inherited in autosomal recessive fashion.

38. E p.336
The diagnosis of congenital adrenal hyperplasia due to 21-hydroxylase deficiency can be obtained prenatally by demonstrating elevated levels of 17-OHP, 21-deoxycortisol, and androstenedione in the amniotic fluid. 17-OHP may be elevated only in the salt-losing form of adrenal hyperplasia, but androstenedione is increased with all forms. HLA genotyping of amniotic cells can yield confirmation by showing that the fetus is HLA identical to an affected sibling. Prenatal diagnosis of the 21-hydroxylase deficiency by chorion villus biopsy utilizing DNA probes offers the timely options of termination or in utero therapy. With chorion villus biopsy, diagnosis can be made and therapy instituted before the critical period of fetal genital differentiation with avoidance of genital ambiguity in affected female fetuses. In addition, masculinization of the fetal brain can be avoided which might have an impact on gender identity and adult sexual behavior.

39. B p.336
Despite the very real limitations of HLA-specific and cDNA probes, prenatal treatment has been administered with dexamethasone in fetuses at risk for 21-hydroxylase deficiency. Using multiple daily doses of dexamethasone (total no greater than 1.5 mg/day), complete prevention has been achieved in some newborns and diminished virilization in others. No congenital malformations, fetal death, or low birth weight or height have resulted from pregnancy-long cortisol derivative therapy. However, this treatment is associated with significant maternal side effects, such as severe striae with permanent scarring, hyperglycemia, hypertension, gastrointestinal symptoms, and emotional lability. A reduction in dosage during the second half of pregnancy is recommended; dosage can be titered by maintaining the maternal serum estriol levels in the normal range.

40. B p.337
During delivery of affected infants, the concentration of 17-OHP is elevated in cord blood (1,000–3,000 ng/dL [30–90 nmol/L]), but it rapidly decreases to 100–200 ng/dL (3–6 nmol/L) after 24 hours. A delay in measurement gains accuracy. In contrast to 17-ketosteroids in the urine where the delay must be several days, with 17-OHP the delay need be only a day or two. In affected infants, 17-OHP ranges from 3,000 to 40,000 ng/dL (90–1,200 nmol/L). Measurement of 17-OHP is the basis for the newborn screening programs currently in place in many countries and some states in the U.S.

In adults, 17-OHP must be measured first thing in the morning to avoid later elevations due to the diurnal pattern of ACTH secretion. The baseline 17-OHP level should be less than 200 ng/dL (6 nmol/L). Levels greater than 200 ng/dL, but less than 800 ng/dL (24 nmol/L), require ACTH testing (discussed in Chapter 14). Levels over 800 ng/dL (24 nmol/L) are virtually diagnostic of the 21-hydroxylase deficiency. The DHAS level is usually normal. The hallmarks of late-onset adrenal hyperplasia are elevated levels of 17-OHP and a dramatic increase after ACTH stimulation. The elevated levels of 17-OHP are often not impressive (e.g., overlapping with those found in women with polycystic ovaries due to anovulation), and a simple ACTH stimulation test must be utilized.

Of course, in patients with 3β-hydroxysteroid dehydrogenase or 17-hydroxylase blocks, the 17-OHP level will not be elevated. With the 3β-hydroxysteroid dehydrogenase block, the blood levels of DHA and DHA sulfate (DHAS) will be markedly increased. In the 11β-hydroxylase deficiency, in addition to elevated 17-OHP, elevation of 11-deoxycortisol is diagnostic. In this deficiency, plasma renin activity will be low, whereas in 21-hydroxylase and 3β-hydroxysteroid dehydrogenase deficiencies plasma renin activity is elevated in the salt-losing forms.

41. E   p.337

The modern management of hormonal control requires the measurement of the blood levels of 17-OHP, androstenedione, testosterone, and plasma renin activity. The drugs of choice are hydrocortisone (approximately 10 mg per day) and 9-fluorohydrocortisone (approximately 100 mg/day). This method of treatment and monitoring applies to all forms of adrenal hyperplasia. The standard dose of cortisol is 12–18 mg/m^2 or 3.5–5 mg/m^2 of prednisone, but larger doses given on alternate days (14 mg/m^2 of prednisone, about 20 mg) can maintain adrenal androgen suppression and perhaps achieve better growth and pubertal development, despite higher levels of 17-hydroxyprogesterone. The 17-OHP level should be maintained in the range of 500 to 4,000 ng/dL, thereby avoiding both overtreatment and undertreatment. Minor stresses will cause brief elevations of adrenal androgens but usually do not require readjustment of dosage. With major stress, such as surgery, additional hormonal support is necessary.

42. A   p.340

Frequently the testes have descended to the inguinal ring because AMH mediates the transabdominal descent of the testes. The vagina is short (derived from the urogenital sinus only) and ends blindly. The uterus and tubes are absent. The testes are normally developed but abnormally positioned. Testosterone production is normal or slightly increased. There is no problem of sex assignment because there is no trace of androgen activity. The diagnosis is likely when an individual presents following breast development at puberty, with primary amenorrhea, scanty or absent pubic and axillary hair, a short vagina, and an absent cervix and uterus. Androgen insensitivity accounts for about 10% of all cases of primary amenorrhea, third most common after gonadal dysgenesis and congenital absence of the vagina. The hormone profile in these individuals is typical: high LH, normal to slightly elevated male testosterone levels, high estradiol (for men), and normal to elevated FSH.

The "complete" form indicates that there is no androgen response; therefore, normal external female development occurs, and these infants should be reared as females. The testes (azoospermic with hyperplastic Leydig cells) may be present in the inguinal canals. Children with inguinal hernias and/or inguinal masses should be suspected of testicular feminization. There is no virilization at puberty because of the lack of androgen response. In contrast to dysgenetic gonads with a Y chromosome, the occurrence of gonadal tumors is relatively late, rarely before age 25, and the overall incidence is less, about 5%. Therefore, gonadectomy should be performed at approximately age 16–18, to allow endogenous hormonal changes and a smooth transition through puberty. Individuals with complete androgen insensitivity perform less well in tests of visual-spatial ability, suggesting that androgens exert an organizing effect in the brain during development.

43. A   p.341

A spectrum of disorders, all due to an X-linked recessive trait, are known as incomplete forms of testicular feminization. It is one-tenth as common as the complete syndrome. The clinical presentation ranges from almost complete failure of virilization to essentially complete phenotypic masculinization. Between these poles exist examples of mild clitoromegaly and slight labial fusion to significant genital ambiguity. Reifenstein's syndrome is now applied to all the intermediate forms that were initially given individual names (such as Lubs syndrome). Recently, males have been described whose only indication of androgen insensitivity was azoospermic or severe oligospermic infertility. Indeed the incidence may approach 40% or more of men with infertility due to azoospermia or severe oligospermia. However, the defect in androgen receptor function may be so subtle that some affected men are fertile. The undervirilized fertile male syndrome is another manifestation of this androgen receptor disorder. The diversity of presentation represents variable manifestations of the same mutant gene. The biochemical abnormality lies in the degree of function of the androgen receptor or postreceptor events.

Molecular analysis of the androgen receptor gene in individuals with androgen insensitivity has demonstrated a spectrum of disorders in which both the complete and partial forms result from androgen receptor gene mutations. The gene encoding the androgen receptor is localized to the q11–12 region (the long arm) of the X chromosome and encodes a receptor protein comprised of discrete functional domains which mediate steroid binding, DNA binding, and transcriptional activation of target genes.

Two types of defective androgen receptor function are recognized: abnormalities of androgen binding and abnormalities of DNA binding. The molecular defects responsible for these deficiencies have been identified and characterized. These include major structural abnormalities of the androgen receptor gene in which complete deletion of the gene or deletions of the exons encoding the androgen binding domain or the DNA binding domain each result in the clinical picture of complete androgen insensitivity. In addition, point mutations that result in a defective receptor or alter receptor mRNA and cause reduced receptor protein production also result in complete androgen insensitivity. On the other hand, single base mutations that change a single amino acid yield subjects displaying either complete or partial androgen insensitivity. Alterations in receptor function, therefore, range from complete loss to subtle qualitative changes in the stimulation and transcription of androgen dependent target genes. Less understandable, however, is the poor correlation between receptor levels (and androgen binding affinity) with the degree of masculinization seen in partial androgen insensitivity. Nevertheless, the same mode of inheritance, despite differences in androgen receptor functioning, indicates that all forms originate in changes in the structural gene responsible for the androgen receptor.

Sex assignment may be a problem when ambiguous genitalia exist because of a partial response of the receptor. If sex assignment is female, early gonadectomy is performed to avoid neoplasia. In Reifenstein syndrome, the phallus may be large enough to allow a male sex assignment at birth, despite the perineal hypospadias. After puberty, however, the inadequate androgen receptor resource becomes evident and feminization with gynecomastia occurs. The receptor function is inadequate to respond to the surge of androgen at puberty; without androgen effect, estrogen activity prevails. These individuals are infertile and cannot react to exogenous androgen. The karyotype is male XY, distinguishing it from other feminizing syndromes of puberty in phenotypic males (e.g., Klinefelter's syndrome).

The endocrine profiles of both the complete and incomplete forms are similar: high blood levels of testosterone, normal to elevated FSH levels, mildly elevated LH (due to absence of negative androgen feedback), and high levels of estradiol (increased testicular response to LH and increased peripheral conversion).

44. A p.342

This form of familial incomplete male (46,XY) pseudohermaphroditism is due to an autosomal recessive trait that leads to a deficiency of the 5α-reductase enzyme (and, in some individuals, enzyme that is present but unstable) and is characterized by severe perineal hypospadias and underdevelopment of the vagina. In the past it was known as pseudovaginal perineoscrotal hypospadias (PPH). It differs from the incomplete forms of testicular feminization because, at puberty, masculinization occurs (the breasts remain male). Normal testicular function occurs, and there is no lack of response to endogenous or exogenous androgen. At birth, however, the external genitalia are similar to that of incomplete testicular feminization; i.e., hypospadias, varying failure of fusion of labioscrotal folds and a urogenital opening, or separate urethral and vaginal openings. The cleft in the scrotum appears to be a vagina (there are no müllerian ducts), and these patients have been reared as girls with an enlarged clitoris. At birth, steroid levels are normal, ruling out adrenal disorders.

Diagnosis can be established by demonstrating an elevated T:DHT ratio based upon the blood levels of testosterone and dihydrotestosterone, especially after HCG stimulation. The karyotype is XY, and, as with other incompletely masculinized males, the sex assignment is female if the phallus is inadequate. Gonadectomy is necessary to avoid not only neoplasia but the virilization that is certain to appear at puberty. The deficiency is believed to be due to the homozygous state, manifest clinically only in males. Homozygous 46,XX females have normal fertility.

45. D p.344, 348

Affected individuals have an XY karyotype but normal (infantile) female external and internal genitalia. There are fibrous bands in place of the gonads yielding primary amenorrhea and lack of secondary sexual development at puberty. It is a matter of prudent practice to avoid the possibility of virilization or neoplasm; therefore, removal of these band areas is advocated as soon as the diagnosis is made. Presumably, testes failed to develop or were eliminated (testicular regression) before internal or external genital differentiation. Estrogen and progestin sequential therapy supports female secondary sex development.

46. B p.345,346

Abnormal sexual differentiation can occur as a result of a mixture of gonadal sex (true hermaphroditism) or complete uncertainty of gonadal sex (gonadal dysgenesis with some virilization). A true hermaphrodite possesses both ovarian and testicular tissue. Both types may be contained in one gonad (ovotestis) or less often, one side may be an ovary, the other a testis. The internal structures correspond to the adjacent gonad. In the majority, external genitalia are ambiguous with sufficient male character to allow male sex assignment. However, three-fourths develop gynecomastia and half menstruate after puberty. Sixty percent are genetic females (XX), few are XY, the rest are mosaics with at least one cell line XX. 46,XX individuals without SRY may have a mutation of an autosomal gene that permits testicular determination in the absence of the testis determining factor.

47. C p.346, 347

Gonadal dysgenesis with bilateral rudimentary streak gonads due to an abnormality in or absence of one of the X chromosomes in all cell lines is called Turner syndrome. Approximately 60% of Turner patients have the total loss of one X chromosome; the remainder have either a structural abnormality in one of the X chromosomes or mosaicism with an abnormal X. In the absence of gonadal development, these individuals are phenotypic females. The well-known characteristics are short stature (142–147 cm, 56–58 inches), sexual infantilism, and streak gonads. The streak gonad is composed of white fibrous stromal tissue, 2–3 cm long and about 0.5 cm wide, containing no ova or follicular derivatives. Other congenital problems in this syndrome are a webbed neck, a high arched palate, cubitus valgus, a broad shield-like chest with widely spaced nipples, a low hairline on the neck, short fourth metacarpal bones, disproportionately short legs, and renal abnormalities (horseshoe kidney, unilateral pelvic kidney, rotational abnormalities, and partial or complete duplication of the collecting system). Autoimmune disorders are common, such as Hashimoto's thyroiditis, Addison's disease, alopecia, and vitiligo. Hypothyroidism is present in about 10% of patients. Mild insulin resistance and hearing loss are also common. One-third of patients with Turner syndrome have cardiovascular abnormalities, including bicuspid aortic valves, coarctation of the aorta, mitral valve prolapse, and aortic aneurysms. Usually the diagnosis is not made until puberty when amenorrhea and lack of sexual development become apparent. At birth, however, lymphedema (due to hypoplasia of superficial vessels) of the extremities may indicate the condition. It is important to assess the aorta, aortic root, and aortic valve with ultrasonography at least in infancy and again during the teens. Patients with Turner syndrome have normal intelligence; however, there may be difficulty with mathematical ability, visual-motor coordination, and spatial-temporal processing.

Because of the high incidence of assorted abnormalites in patients with Turner syndrome, the following evaluations should be performed, some only once at the time of diagnosis, and others annually as part of on-going surveillance: thyroid function testing (annually) and antibodies (at least once), intravenous pyelogram or renal ultrasonography (once if normal), echocardiography, audiometry, and annual evaluation of the lipid profile and glucose metabolism.

48. E p.346, 347

The presence of menstrual function and reproduction in a patient with Turner phenotype must be due to a mosaic complement, such as a 46,XX line in addition to 45,X. When pregnancy does occur in an X deficient subject, the incidence of aneuploidy in the conceptus is almost 50%.

A large variety of mosaic patterns is seen with gonadal dysgenesis. From analysis of the various combinations, it is apparent that short stature is related to loss of regions on the short arm of one X chromosome. Distal long arm deletions of one of the X chromosomes are associated with amenorrhea (usually secondary after some ovarian function) and streak gonads, but the patients are not always growth compromised nor do they display other Turner somatic malformations. Long arm deletions near the centromere are associated with primary amenorrhea. Thus, loss of material from the short arms of the X chromosome leads to short stature and the other stigmata of Turner syndrome. This suggests that normal ovarian development requires two loci, one on the long arm and one on the short arm; loss of either results in gonadal failure. Thyroid autoimmunity is common in Turner syndrome, but Hashimoto's thyroiditis may be specific to 46,XXqi cases.

Just as X chromosome monosomy, with deletion of the second X chromosome, results in Turner's phenotype, the same will apply to loss of the Y chromosome. The 45,X karyotype derived from leukocyte culture does not guarantee that a mosaic does not exist with a gonadal line containing XY. For this reason, annual pelvic examinations and appropriate screening are required to detect incipient signs of gonadal neoplasia as an adnexal mass. If a presumed 45,X patient develops breasts or sexual hair without exogenous therapy, a gonadoblastoma or dysgerminoma should be considered and ruled out. Heterosexual signs require scrutiny in all 45,X individuals. Expert consultation should be obtained to pursue further analysis with X- and Y-specific DNA probes.

49. E   p.348, 349

Patients with mosaic patterns in the karyotype have a reduced risk of tumor, but it still amounts to 15–20%. The most common tumor is the often bilateral gonadoblastoma, but dysgerminomas and even the more threatening embryonal carcinoma are also seen. Intra-abdominal testes should be removed as early in life as possible because of the known risk of tumor development. There is no debate that gonadal tissue having any Y chromosome component in phenotypic females requires removal as soon as the diagnosis is made to avoid the risk of malignant gonadal tumors. There is one exception to this rule. Because gonadal tumors occur relatively late in patients with complete androgen insensitivity, surgery is delayed until after puberty. An accomplished laparoscopist can attempt this procedure, with the option of laparotomy if the gonads prove to be inaccessible. Streak gonads have been removed in this fashion, as well as the testes in androgen insensitivity. With androgen insensitivity, the gonads can be close to the external iliac artery and herniated into the inguinal canals. The procedure is more difficult, and care must be taken to extract the gonad from the inguinal canal to secure complete excision. It may also be necessary to make a small abdominal incision or a culdotomy to extract the gonad in order to avoid morcellation. The uterus and tubes should be retained for the possibility of pregnancy with donor oocytes.

50. E   p.349, 350

When ovaries are absent in individuals being reared as females, either because of surgery or streak gonads, hormonal treatment will be necessary at puberty and thereafter. Estrogen will initiate and sustain maturation and function of secondary sexual characteristics, and promote the achievement of the full height potential. The adolescent increase in bone density is a very important determinant of an indivdual's later risk for osteoporosis. This alone is sufficient reason for treatment. Very small amounts of estrogen will promote growth and development. Start at about age 10 with unopposed estrogen (0.3 mg conjugated estrogens or 0.5 mg estradiol daily). After 6 months to 1 year, move to a sequential program with 0.625 mg conjugated estrogens or 1.0 mg estradiol daily and 10 mg medroxyprogesterone acetate for the first 12 days each month (if a uterus is present). Adequacy of treatment can be assessed by following bone age changes, although this is unnecessary in most cases. In patients with genetic shortness in stature (e.g., Turner syndrome), estrogen treatment is not started until bone age is 11–12 to avoid epiphysial closure and to allow a longer period of time for long bone growth.

Short stature occurs in virtually all patients with a 45,X karyotype and nearly all patients with Turner syndrome who have other karyotypes. This growth impairment begins in utero, is apparent throughout childhood, and results in a short adult height (a mean of 143 cm). This attenuation of growth is partly due to insufficient growth hormone secretion due to the deficiency in sex steroids and also to an end organ resistance to insulin-like growth factor-I. Anabolic steroids have been used to stimulate growth, especially in patients with Turner syndrome. Short-term growth can be stimulated by anabolic steroids; however, the effect on final adult height is equivocal because epiphyseal maturation is also enhanced. Furthermore, virilizing side effects are a drawback. The combination of low doses of estrogen and recombinant growth hormone offer the best prospect. Treatment with growth hormone (50 mg/kg/day) yields significant growth acceleration that can be sustained for at least 6 years, achieving an adult height of over 150 cm (59 inches), which is a low normal range for women. The future may see effective use of growth hormone-releasing hormone for this purpose. It is worth noting that adolescents with Turner syndrome being treated with growth hormone do not lose bone mineral density prior to estrogen treatment; hence, it is unnecessary to begin estrogen treatment at an early age (when it might counteract the goal of growth hormone therapy, achieving maximal height).

51. E   p.350–354

The most important point to remember when confronted with a newborn infant with ambiguous genitalia, or an apparently male infant with bilateral cryptorchidism, is that the prime diagnosis until ruled out is congenital adrenal hyperplasia. The reason is clear: adrenal hyperplasia is the only condition which is life-threatening. Although the appearance of the external genitalia in intersex infants may be similar regardless of etiology, and a definitive diagnosis unachievable by physical examination alone, certain useful clues can be discerned.

Palpation of the genital and inguinal regions is the most important part of the physical examination. Gonads in the inguinal regions or in scrotal folds are almost certainly testes. Ovaries are not found in scrotal folds or in the inguinal regions. The testicles, however, may be intra-abdominal. If testicles are not palpable, the infant should be considered to have congenital adrenal hyperplasia until demonstrated otherwise. (See figure on page 151 in this Study Guide)

52. C p.354, 355

In a newborn who presents a problem of correct sex assignment, it is better to delay than to reverse the sex assignment at a later date. Generally, the decision can be made within a few days, at most a few weeks. In dealing with the parents, terms with unfortunate connotations, such as hermaphrodite, should be avoided. An easy way to explain ambiguous genital development to parents is to indicate that the genitals are unfinished, rather than abnormal from a sexual point of view. Chromosome discrepancies are probably best left unmentioned.

When all the information is in place, gender assignment will rest on:

1. Future fertility,
2. The projected appearance of genitalia after puberty,
3. Penile adequacy for coital function.

The future fertility in all masculinized females is unaffected. With proper treatment, reproduction is possible, since the internal genitalia and gonads are those of a normal female. Therefore, all masculinized females should be reared as females.

All decisions regarding sex of rearing and the overall treatment program should be made early in life. If a case has been neglected, sex reassignments must be made according to the gender identity in which a child has developed. Reassignment of sex can probably be made safely up to age 18 months.

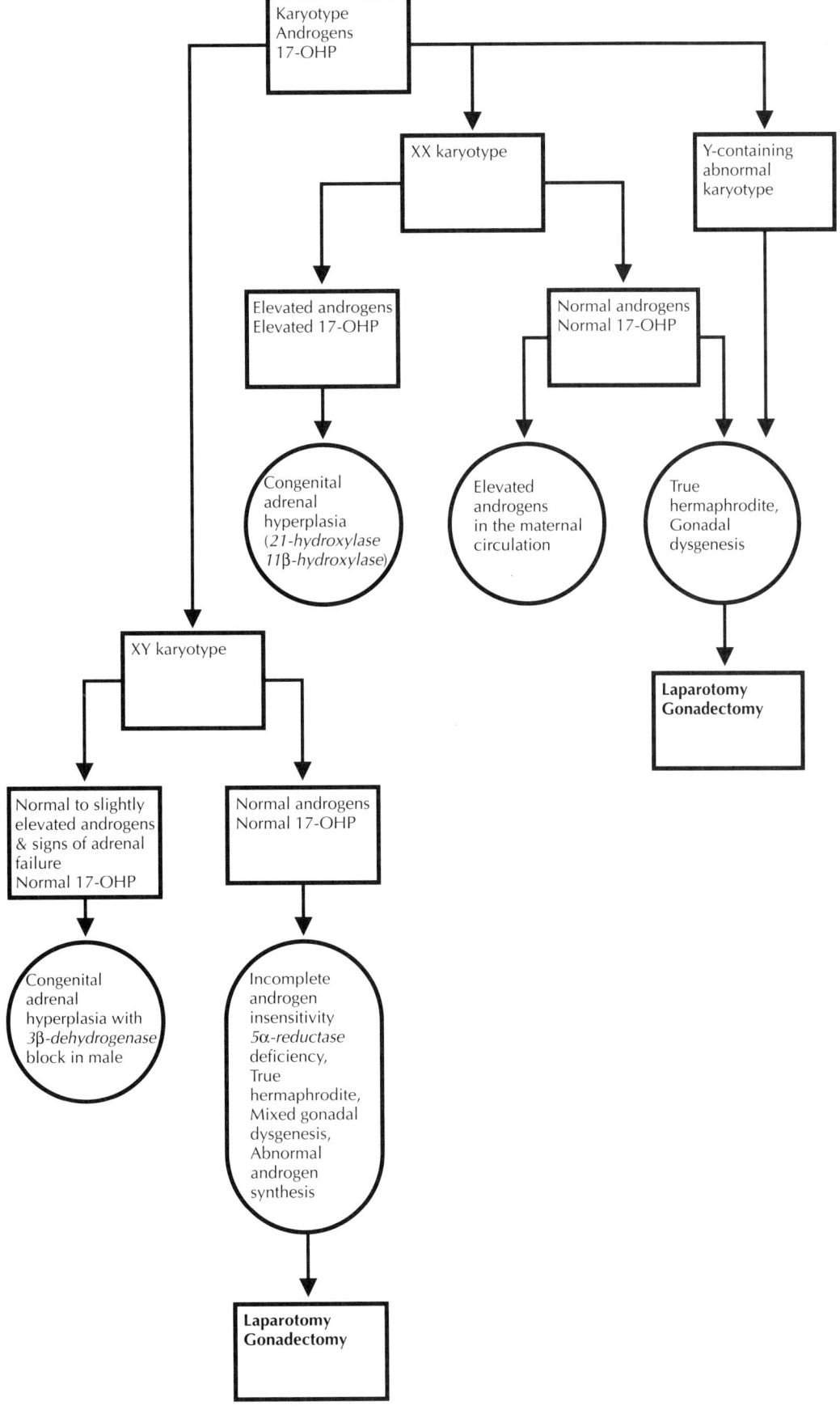

11 Abnormal Puberty and Growth Problems

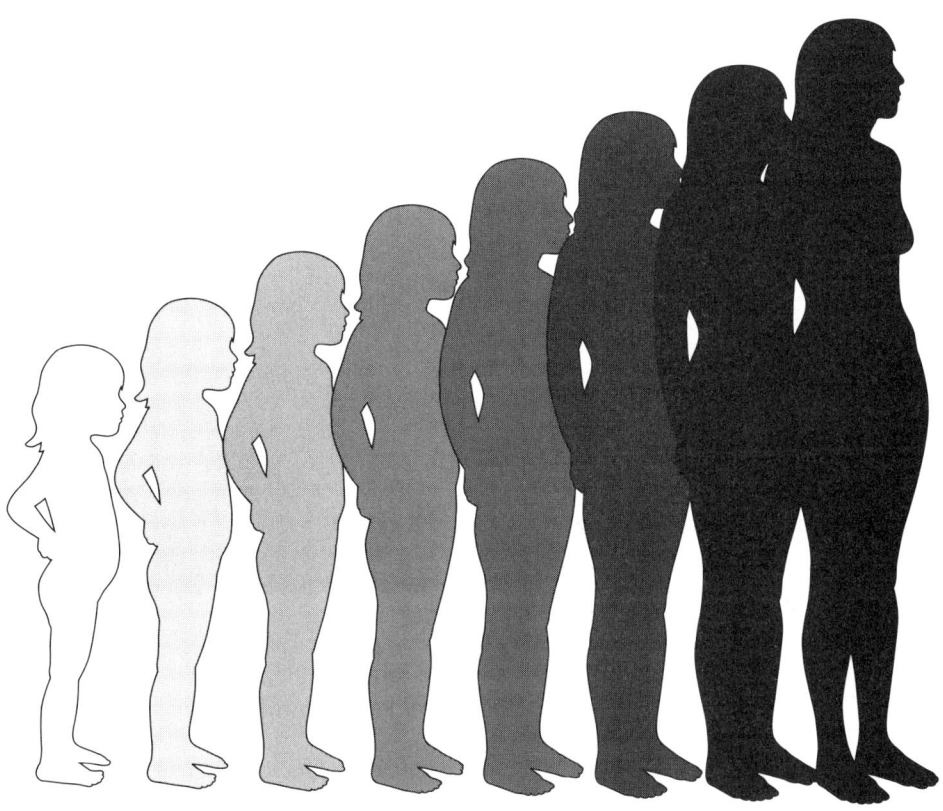

Learning Objectives

1. Describe the hormonal changes relative to the reproductive cycle beginning with the fetal period progressing to infancy, childhood and the onset and completion of puberty.

2. Define the concepts of the gonadostat, adrenarche, premature adrenarche, premature thelarche.

3. Describe the normal sequence and age of onset of female pubertal milestones.

4. Detail the differential diagnosis, workup and treatment of disorders producing precocious puberty.

5. Detail the differential diagnosis, workup and treatment of disorders producing delayed puberty.

Pre-Test

A. Instructions: Fill in the blanks

1. On the average, the pubertal sequence of accelerated growth, breast development, adrenarche and menarche requires a period of _____ years.

2. _____% of girls with precocious puberty have an ovarian tumor.

B. Instructions: True or False

3. As the pubertal transition advances there is a disproportionate rise of immunologic LH to bioactive LH.

4. Because delayed puberty is a rare condition in girls, a genetic problem or hypothalamic-pituitary disorder must be suspected.

C. Instructions: For each of the following questions choose:

A. if only 1, 2 and 3 are correct
B. if only 1 and 3 are correct
C. if only 2 and 4 are correct
D. if only 4 is correct
E. if all are correct

5. Effective pharmacologic agent(s) which are available for the treatment of precocious puberty include
   1. medroxyprogesterone acetate
   2. cyproterone acetate
   3. danazol
   4. GnRH analogues

6. Craniopharyngioma
   1. is a common neoplasm associated with precocious puberty
   2. has a peak incidence between ages 15–25
   3. has an abnormal appearance on imaging in less than 50% of cases
   4. is treated by a combination of surgery and irradiation

Post-Test

A. Instructions: Fill in the blanks

1. Low levels of FSH and LH are present in hypogonadal children with gonadal dysgenesis between the ages of _____ and _____ years and are similar to the low levels in normal infants of this age.

2. Premature adrenarche is defined as pubic and axillary hair _____ any other sign of sexual development.

3. The normal pubertal timing of gonadarche results from the combined reduction in intrinsic _____ of _____ and decreased sensitivity to the negative feedback of _____.

4. Like the gonadotropins, growth hormone is secreted in a _____ fashion.

5. Pubertal changes in a female before age _____ are regarded as precocious. Increased _____ is often the first change in precocious puberty.

6. Various tumors can induce precocity including _____ in the hypothalamus which is the most common lesion in very young girls. _____ is the most sensitive method for detection of these small tumors.

7. Neoplasms of the _____, _____ and adrenal must be ruled out as potential causes of precocious puberty.

8. _____ hypogonadism is the most frequent etiology of delayed puberty.

9. Hormone treatment may be discontinued in the treatment of short stature when the _____ age matches the _____ age.

B. Instructions: True or False

10. During fetal life, serum concentrations of FSH and LH reach adult levels at midgestation.

11. In gonadal dysgenesis or Kallmann's syndrome adrenarche occurs despite the absence of gonadarche.

12. There is evidence that melatonin is important in the physiologic onset of normal puberty.

13. By mid to late puberty, maturation of the positive feedback relationship between estradiol and FSH is established.

14. Growth hormone is the most abundant hormone produced by the pituitary gland.

15. Precocity occurs in boys more frequently than in girls and delayed puberty occurs in girls more frequently than in boys.

16. The most common form of sexual precocity in females is idiopathic or constitutional precocity.

17. Sexual precocity is associated with premature menopause and adult short stature.

18. When signs of sexual precocity are accompanied by virilization adrenal hyperplasia or an adrenal or ovarian tumor must be considered.

19. If breast and genital development, pubic hair growth and vaginal bleeding are seen in a short child with a delayed bone age, primary hypothyroidism is the most likely diagnosis.

20. GnRH agonist treatment is effective for McCune-Albright syndrome or noncentral forms of precocious puberty.

21. The prognosis for young girls with precocious puberty is uniformly poor.

22. The Bayley-Pinneau tables predict future adult height utilizing the bone age and present height.

C. Instructions: Match each heading with the appropriate word association

A. GnRH dependent precocious puberty
B. GnRH independent precocious puberty

23. heterosexual precocious puberty
24. central precocious puberty
25. peripheral precocious puberty
26. early activation of the hypothalamic-pituitary-gonadal axis
27. true precocious puberty
28. hypothalamic tumor
29. ovarian cyst
30. McCune-Albright

D. Instructions: For each of the following questions choose:

A. if only 1, 2 and 3 are correct
B. if only 1 and 3 are correct
C. if only 2 and 4 are correct
D. if only 4 is correct
E. if all are correct

31. Adrenarche
    1. usually begins 4 years prior to the linear growth spurt
    2. is marked by rising serum DHA, DHAS and androstenedione
    3. is under direct control of ACTH
    4. is considered premature if pubic and axillary hair appear before 8 years of age without other signs of sexual development

32. Sleep-related LH pulses
    1. occur in the early stages of puberty in both sexes
    2. do not correlate with exogenous GnRH pulsility
    3. are also noted in children with idiopathic precocious puberty
    4. become more prominent in late puberty

33. Timing of puberty is determined by
    1. genetics
    2. exposure to light
    3. general health and nutrition
    4. geographic location

34. The growth spurt is associated with an increase in
    1. estrogen
    2. growth hormone
    3. insulin-like growth factor-I
    4. insulin-like growth factor-II

35. Puberty
    1. is initially marked by the development of breast buds
    2. is associated with physical milestones which develop as "bioassays" in response to endogenous estrogen levels
    3. is associated with physical characteristics which occur in a predictable temporarily related fashion
    4. is completed with the development of estrogen positive induced LH surges

36. A workup for precocious puberty should include
    1. thyroid function tests
    2. a nondominant hand-wrist film
    3. an MRI of brain
    4. serum levels of gonadotropins and steroids

37. True precocious puberty can be due to
    1. long-standing hypothyroidism
    2. hamartoma
    3. encephalitis
    4. chorioepithelioma

38. Long-standing hypothyroidism in a young child
    1. can result in short stature
    2. galactorrhea
    3. enlarged sella turcica
    4. ovarian cysts

39. McCune-Albright syndrome is characterized by
    1. by autonomous estrogen production by the ovaries
    2. an association with Cushing's disease, acromegaly, hyperparathyroidism and hyperthyroidism
    3. a basic defect in regulation of the G protein
    4. attenuation of GTPase activity

40. Objectives of management and treatment of precocious puberty include
    1. diagnosis and treat intracranial disease
    2. maximize eventual adult height
    3. diminish established precocious characteristics
    4. decrease incidence of future infertility

41. Delayed puberty
    1. is seldom associated with short stature
    2. which is physiological tends to be familial
    3. is a common problem in girls
    4. can be associated with normal, elevated or decreased gonadotropin levels

42. The laboratory assessment of delayed puberty includes
    1. x-ray for bone age
    2. thyroid function tests
    3. prolactin
    4. gonadotropin levels

43. Hypergonadotropic hypogonadism
    1. is the most frequent etiology classification for delayed puberty
    2. is commonly associated with gonadal dysgenesis
    3. may be present in women with normal karyotypes who have sickle cell disease
    4. may be due to a craniopharyngioma

44. Hypogonadotropic hypogonadism
    1. is more frequently due to a reversible than an irreversible cause
    2. is associated with a physiologic delay
    3. may be associated with pituitary or hypothalamic tumors
    4. is associated with poor nutrition

45. Anabolic-androgenic steroid use
    1. can be associated with impotence and oligospermia in males
    2. is an effective treatment for short stature
    3. prevents individuals from reaching their genetic height potential
    4. is not associated with liver disease

Answers for Chapter 11 — Pre-Test Questions

1. 4.5   p.366

On the average, the pubertal sequence of accelerated growth, breast development, adrenarche, and menarche requires a period of 4.5 years (range 1.5 to 6 years). The largest body of data was accumulated in healthy European girls; current North American standards are approximately 6 months earlier for each stage. Secondary sex characteristics develop slightly earlier in black girls compared to white girls.

2. 11   p.373

Classification and Relative Occurrence of Precocious Puberty

	Female	Male
GnRH-Dependent (True Precocity)		
Idiopathic	74.0%	41.0%
CNS problem	7.0%	26.0%
GnRH-Independent (Precocious Pseudopuberty)		
Ovarian (cyst or tumor)	11.0%	—
Testicular	—	10.0%
McCune-Albright syndrome	5.0%	1.0%
Adrenal feminizing	1.0%	0.0%
Adrenal masculinizing	1.0%	22.0%
Ectopic gonadotropin production	0.5%	0.5%

3. false   p.365

The amplification of peptide-steroid interactions during pubescence is not restricted to the GnRH impact on gonadotropin or steroid feedback on the pituitary and hypothalamus. As pubertal transition advances there is a disproportionate rise of biologically potent LH beyond the increase seen in immunologic LH. This marked increase in the bioactive to immunoactive ratio is due to molecular alterations in the glycosylation pattern of LH.

4. true   p.382

Delayed puberty is a rare condition in girls, and a genetic problem or hypothalamic-pituitary disorder must be suspected. In addition, anatomic abnormalities of the target organ (uterus and endometrium) or outflow tract are unique but important elements to consider in amenorrheic but otherwise normal pubertal adolescents.

5. D   p.380,381

A number of therapies have been used to achieve these goals. These have included medroxyprogesterone acetate, cyproterone acetate, and danazol. In addition to undesirable side effects, bone maturation and growth were not regularly or sufficiently controlled. Major progress has been made with the use of GnRH analogues for the treatment of true precocious puberty.

6. D   p.385

Craniopharyngioma is the most common neoplasm associated with delayed puberty. Craniopharyngioma is a tumor of Rathke's pouch, originating from the pituitary stalk with suprasellar extension. The peak incidence is between ages 6 and 14. Imaging reveals an abnormal sella and calcifications in 70% of cases. Treatment consists of a combination of surgery and irradiation.

Answers for Chapter 11 — Post-Test Questions

1. 5; 11   p.362,364

Low levels of FSH and LH even exist in hypogonadal children (with gonadal dysgenesis) between the ages of 5 and 11 years and are similar to the low levels in normal infants of this age. Because gonadotropin releasing hormone (GnRH) infusion stimulates moderate LH and FSH secretion in these agonadal subjects, a central nonsteroidal suppressor of endogenous GnRH and gonadotropin synthesis appears to be operative. Gonadal dysgenesis patients display marked elevations of gonadotropins for the first 2–3 years of life. Thereafter, a striking decline in concentrations of FSH and LH occurs, reaching a nadir at 6–8 years. By age 10–11 (at the time puberty would have occurred), however, gonadotropins are elevated once again to the postmenopausal range. The overall pattern of basal gonadotropin secretion in agonadal children is qualitatively similar to that observed in normal females.

2. without   p.363,376

Premature adrenarche by itself is occasionally seen; i.e., pubic and axillary hair without any other sign of sexual development. Premature adrenarche is the consequence of an early modest increase in the adrenal androgens, androstenedione, dehydroepiandrosterone and dehydroepiandrosterone sulfate. An adrenal enzyme deficit should be excluded by appropriate laboratory testing, but it is rarely discovered in a prepubertal child who presents only with early growth of pubic hair.

3. suppression; GnRH; estrogen   p.364

Whereas negative feedback inhibition may play the more important role in early childhood, the central intrinsic inhibitor becomes functionally dominant in midchildhood and persists up to prepuberty. Suppression of, or damage to, the neural source of this inhibition has been postulated in the pathogenesis of the precocious puberty secondary to hypothalamic lesions that compress or destroy posterior hypothalamic areas. Thus, normal pubertal timing of gonadarche, with the reactivation of gonadotropin synthesis and secretion, results from the combined reduction in intrinsic suppression of GnRH and decreased sensitivity to the negative feedback of estrogen.

4. pulsatile   p.368

Like the gonadotropins, growth hormone is secreted in pulsatile fashion, and during puberty, the amplitude of the pulses increases, especially during sleep. Your grandmother was right when she said: sleep and you'll grow. The age at which an increase in pulse amplitude first occurs corresponds to the the age of most rapid growth. Slower growing children secrete fewer and smaller pulses of growth hormone. The pulsatile pattern of growth hormone secretion is regulated by stimulation from growth hormone releasing hormone and inhibition from somatropin release-inhibiting hormone, both released into the hypothalmic-pituitary portal circulation from hypothalamic nuclei. This mechanism is influenced at multiple levels by estrogens and androgens. Prior to puberty, the sex steroid hormones are not involved with growth hormone secretion, beyond a low maintenance effect on secretion. At puberty, however, the dynamics of growth hormone secretion are critically dependent on the gonadal sex steroid hormones. Growth hormone secretion must be very sensitive to the stimulatory effect of estrogens because growth hormone levels increase before any signs of sexual development appear.

5. 8; growth   p.371

If one accepts the mean ±2.5 standard deviations as encompassing the normal range, then pubertal changes before the age of 8 are regarded as precocious. Increased growth is often the first change in precocious puberty. This is usually followed by breast development and growth of pubic hair. On occasion, adrenarche, thelarche, and linear growth occur simultaneously. Menarche, however, can be the first sign.

6. hamartoma; MRI p.373

A number of CNS problems, including abnormal skull development due to rickets, can cause true precocious development. Various tumors can induce precocity, including hamartomas in the hypothalamus (the most common lesion in very young girls), craniopharyngioma, astrocytoma, glioma, neurofibroma, ependymoma, and suprasellar teratoma — all usually near the hypothalamus. Pineal tumors, for unknown reasons, have been seen only in male precocious puberty. Nontumorous causes include encephalitis, meningitis, hydrocephalus, and von Recklinghausen's disease. An injury to the skull may stimulate sexual development. The mechanism is unknown, and a latent period of 1–2 months is usually seen. A hamartoma is a hyperplastic congenital malformation in the floor of the third ventricle that usually produces precocity in the first few years of life; magnetic resonance imaging is the most sensitive method for the detection of small tumors like a hamartoma. Patients with true precocious puberty and known CNS lesions or a history of cranial irradiation should be evaluated for growth hormone deficiency because of the recognized association of these defects.

7. CNS; ovary p.376

The cause of precocious development may be obvious by findings in the history or physical examination. Familial occurrence helps to exclude certain disease processes (tumors). Clinically, the nature of precocity dictates certain diagnostic priorities.

1. **Rule out life-threatening disease.** This includes neoplasms of the CNS, ovary, and adrenal.
2. **Define the velocity of the process.** Is it progressing or stabilized? Management decisions hinge on this determination. Isolated, nonendocrine causes of vaginal bleeding (trauma, foreign body, vaginitis, genital neoplasm) must be excluded.

8. Hypergonadotropic p.384
(See table on page 161 in this Study Guide)

9. bone; chronologic p.387

In cases of gonadal failure, estrogen can be used in a female to stimulate epiphyseal growth, bringing the bone age to match the chronologic age. Conjugated estrogens (0.3 mg) or estradiol (0.5 mg) administered daily are effective in hypogonadal individuals (this is a much smaller dose than previously used). Patients should be observed at monthly intervals to document the pattern of growth and development. Hormone treatment may be discontinued when the bone age matches the chronologic age.

10. true p.362

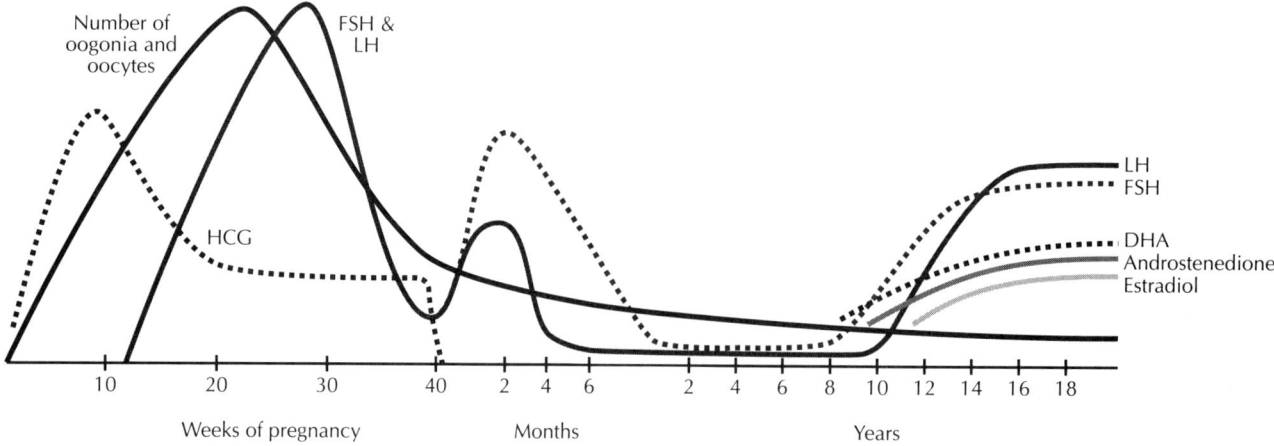

Relative Frequency of Delayed Pubertal Abnormalities

Hypergonadotropic Hypogonadism	**43.0%**
Ovarian failure, abnormal karyotype	26.0%
Ovarian failure, normal karyotype	17.0%
46, XX	15.0%
46, XY	2.0%
Hypogonadotropic Hypogonadism	**31.0%**
Reversible	18.0%
Physiologic delay	10.0%
Weight loss/anorexia	3.0%
Primary hypothyroidism	1.0%
Congenital adrenal hyperplasia	1.0%
Cushing's syndrome	0.5%
Prolactinomas	1.5%
Irreversible	13.0%
GnRH deficiency	7.0%
Hypopituitarism	2.0%
Congenital CNS defects	0.5%
Other pituitary adenomas	0.5%
Craniopharyngioma	1.0%
Malignant pituitary tumor	0.5%
Eugonadism	**26.0%**
Müllerian agenesis	14.0%
Vaginal septum	3.0%
Imperforate hymen	0.5%
Androgen insensitivity syndrome	1.0%
Inappropriate positive feedback	7.0%

11. true   p.363

Considerable evidence, however, supports a *dissociation* of the control mechanisms that initiate adrenarche and those governing GnRH-pituitary-ovarian maturation ("gonadarche"). Premature adrenarche (precocious appearance of pubic and axillary hair before age 8 years) is not associated with a parallel abnormal advancement of gonadarche. In hypergonadotropic hypogonadism (gonadal dysgenesis) or in hypogonadotropic states such as Kallmann's syndrome, adrenarche occurs despite the absence of gonadarche. When adrenarche is absent, as in children with cortisol-treated Addison's disease (hypoadrenalism), gonadarche still occurs. Finally, in true precocious puberty occurring before 6 years of age, gonadarche precedes adrenarche.

12. false   p.364

It has been suggested that the reversal of central intrinsic suppression is due to a reduction in melatonin secretion by the pineal gland. In lower animals affected by photoperiodicity, pineal melatonin appears to inhibit hypothalamic-pituitary gland secretion. While melatonin may play a role in the altered timing of puberty associated with pineal tumors and in the pathophysiology of central precocious puberty, there is no evidence that it is important in the physiologic onset of normal puberty in humans. In two large studies of circadian rhythms of serum melatonin from infancy to adulthood (1–18 years) the decline in the nocturnal surge of melatonin, thought to have been exclusively related to the pubertal conversion, was observed to begin in infancy and progressively decline through pubescence. Pinealectomy in agonadal primates does not prevent the inhibition of FSH and LH seen during transition from infancy to childhood nor the return of gonadotropins with the advent of puberty.

13. false   p.366,369

The normal age range of menarche in U.S. girls is 9.1–17.7 years with a median of 12.8. The final endocrine hallmark of puberty is the development of positive estrogen feedback on the pituitary and hypothalamus. This feedback stimulates the midcycle surge of LH required for ovulation. Thus, the menses following menarche are usually anovulatory, irregular, and occasionally heavy. Anovulation lasts as long as 12–18 months after menarche, but there are reports of pregnancy before menarche. Ovulation increases in frequency as puberty progresses, but it is common for 25–50% of adolescents to still be anovulatory 4 years after menarche.

14. true   p.367

The most abundant hormone produced by the pituitary gland is growth hormone, which is secreted not as a single substance but as one predominant form and one smaller variant. Growth hormone is encoded by 5 genes located on chromosome 17q22-q24. One gene is for the predominant form in the pituitary; 3 of the genes are expressed in the placenta. The pituitary gene is regulated by growth hormone-releasing hormone, thyroid hormone, and glucocorticoids.

15. false   p.371

Precocity occurs in girls 5 times more frequently than boys, and almost three-quarters of precocity in girls is idiopathic. Nevertheless, in the face of any precocious development, the clinician is obligated to rule out a serious disease process in central or peripheral sites. In girls over 4 years old a specific etiology is rarely found. In younger girls, a CNS lesion is usually present.

16. true   p.371,372

While it is true that the most common form of sexual precocity in females is idiopathic or constitutional precocity (true sexual precocity), this must be a diagnosis by exclusion with prolonged follow-up in an effort to detect slowly developing lesions of the brain, ovary, or adrenal gland.

17. false   p.372,382

Sexual precocity is consistent with normal reproductive life and it is not associated with premature menopause. The most serious effect of precocity is the resultant adult short stature. Because the skeleton is very sensitive to even the lowest levels of estrogen, these children are transiently tall for their age, but as a result of early epiphyseal fusion, eventually short stature results. The mean height in adult women is approximately 152 cm (5 feet). Even with prompt GnRH agonist treatment final adult height is likely to be compromised because some stimulation to epiphyseal closure will already have occurred before treatment is initiated. Most women have normal menstrual cycles and fertility, and they do not have premature menopause.

18. true   p.377

When signs of sexual precocity are associated with accelerated growth and skeletal maturation, in the absence of virilization, the etiology may be an ovarian tumor or cyst. A pelvic mass is usually palpable. In this situation, serum FSH and LH are suppressed, while serum estradiol is usually elevated. An elevated serum progesterone suggests an ovarian luteoma. Pelvic ultrasound or imaging can help to confirm the presence of an ovarian mass. Laparotomy is indicated to confirm the diagnosis and carry out surgical resection.

Adrenal hyperplasia or a virilizing adrenal or ovarian tumor must be considered if signs of sexual precocity are accompanied by virilization. With elevation of serum 17-hydroxyprogesterone (17-OHP) and adrenal androgens, the diagnosis of 21-hydroxylase deficient adrenal hyperplasia is established, whereas an elevation of serum 11-deoxycortisol leads to the diagnosis of 11-hydroxylase deficient adrenal hyperplasia. If these two serum hormones are normal, while serum DHAS or androstenedione is elevated, an adrenal tumor or a virilizing ovarian tumor is suspect. Ultrasound examination and abdominal imaging can be utilized to further localize the tumor.

19. true p.377

Breast development usually correlates with a bone age of 11 and menarche with a bone age of 13. If breast and genital development, pubic hair growth, and vaginal bleeding are seen in a short child with a *delayed* bone age, primary hypothyroidism is the most likely diagnosis. This can be confirmed by finding a low serum T_4 and elevated TSH concentration. Serum FSH and LH levels may be in the pubertal range, but these will decrease following thyroid treatment. Galactorrhea may be present along with elevated serum prolactin concentrations. These return to normal with thyroid treatment.

20. false p.381

GnRH agonist treatment is not effective for noncentral forms of precocious puberty such as McCune-Albright syndrome, GnRH-independent sexual precocity, or congenital adrenal hyperplasia. However, should patients with McCune-Albright syndrome or congenital adrenal hyperplasia mature their hypothalamic-pituitary-gonadal axis and develop true sexual precocity, then supplementary GnRH agonist therapy is helpful. Primary treatment in these cases is directed toward suppression of gonadal steroidogenesis. Medroxyprogesterone acetate can be utilized in depot form to suppress LH secretion, or testolactone, an aromatase inhibitor, can be administered.

21. false p.382

With the exception of short stature as an adult, the prognosis for idiopathic sexual precocity remains good if the children enter adult life without psychosexual scars.

22. true p.386

The basic and essential laboratory procedure is a left hand-wrist x-ray for bone age. The Bayley-Pinneau tables predict future adult height, utilizing the bone age and present height.

23. B p.371,372

GnRH-Independent Precocious Puberty. Incomplete, isosexual or heterosexual, peripheral or ***precocious pseudopuberty.*** Sexual maturation in these instances may be due to extra pituitary secretion of human chorionic gonadotropin (HCG) or sex steroid secretion independent of hypothalamic-pituitary gonadotropin stimulation. Thus, this mechanism is GnRH-independent.

24. A p.371,372

GnRH-Dependent Precocious Puberty. Complete, isosexual, central (or specifically GnRH- and gonadotropin-dependent) precocity — also known as ***true precocious puberty.*** These terms all refer to early activation of the hypothalamic-pituitary-gonadal axis.

25. B p.371,372

Peripheral precocious puberty is due to a mechanism separate and independent of GnRH secretion.

26. A p.371,372

27. A p.371,372

Early activation of the hypothalamic-pituitary-gonadal axis is *true precocious puberty,* and is dependent upon GnRH secretion.

28. A p.371,372

29. B p.371,372

30. B p.371,372

Classification and Relative Occurrence of Precocious Puberty

	Female	Male
GnRH-Dependent (True Precocity)		
Idiopathic	74.0%	41.0%
CNS problem	7.0%	26.0%
GnRH-Independent (Precocious Pseudopuberty)		
Ovarian (cyst or tumor)	11.0%	—
Testicular	—	10.0%
McCune-Albright syndrome	5.0%	1.0%
Adrenal feminizing	1.0%	0.0%
Adrenal masculinizing	1.0%	22.0%
Ectopic gonadotropin production	0.5%	0.5%

31. C   p.363,370

The growth of pubic and axillary hair is due to an increased production of adrenal androgens at puberty. Thus, this phase of puberty is often referred to as adrenarche (or pubarche). ***Premature adrenarche*** by itself is occasionally seen; i.e., pubic and axillary hair without any other sign of sexual development. Increased adrenal cortical function, expressed by a rise in circulating dehydroepiandrosterone (DHA), dehydroepiandrosterone sulfate (DHAS), and androstenedione, occurs progressively in late childhood from about age 6–7 to adolescence (13–15 years of age).

32. B   p.365,369

The onset of significant GnRH pulses first occurs during sleep. There is sleep-associated release of LH in both sexes that correlates with the timing (early puberty) of LH responses to exogenous GnRH. The early stages of puberty are associated with a marked nocturnal augmentation of FSH and LH pulses (both amplitude and frequency); this difference between nighttime and daytime switches by late puberty with an increase in daytime and a decrease in sleep pulsatility. Sleep-related LH pulses also are seen in children with idiopathic precocious puberty, in anorexia nervosa patients during intermediate stages of exacerbation and recovery, and also in agonadal patients during the pubertal age period when their gonadotropins are returning from midchildhood reductions. GnRH pulses appear and are maintained independent of steroid feedback.

33. E   p.366

Although the major determinant of the timing of puberty is genetic, other factors appear to influence the time of initiation and the rate of progression of puberty: geographic location, exposure to light, general health and nutrition, and psychologic factors. For example, children with a family history of early puberty start early. Children closer to the equator, at lower altitudes, those in urban areas, and mildly obese children start earlier than those in Northern latitudes, at higher elevations above sea level, in rural areas, and normal weight children, respectively. There is a fairly good correlation between the times of menarche of mothers and daughters and between sisters.

34. A   p.367,368

Hormonal requirements for this increased growth velocity include growth hormone and gonadal estrogen. The pubertal growth spurt is associated with an increase in the circulating levels of growth hormone and insulin-like growth factor-I. Adrenal androgens are not involved because cortisol-repleted Addisonian patients display normal pubertal growth patterns. The amounts of estrogen required to stimulate long-bone cortical growth are incredibly small. Doses of 100 nanograms of estradiol per kilogram body weight per day increase the amplitude of growth hormone pulsatile secretion and produce maximal growth in agonadal recipients. These doses are insufficient to cause breast budding, vaginal cornification, or an increase in sex hormone binding globulin. These low dose effects are consistent with the observation that girls attain peak height velocity early in puberty at a serum estradiol concentration of 20 pg/mL (80 pmol/L) which is one-sixth the mean level of adult women. Furthermore, at low doses, estrogen stimulates growth hormone-induced IGF-I secretion, while high doses suppress IGF-I levels.

35. E p.369,370

Summary of Pubertal Events
1. FSH and then LH levels rise moderately before the age of 10 and are followed by a rise in estradiol. An increase in LH pulses is first seen only in sleep but gradually extends throughout the day. In the adult, they occur at roughly 1.5–2 hourly intervals.
2. As gonadal estrogen increases (gonadarche), breast development, female fat distribution, and vaginal and uterine growth occur. Skeletal growth rapidly increases as a result of initial gonadal secretion of low levels of estrogen, which increases the secretion of growth hormone, which in turn stimulates the production of IGF-I.
3. Adrenal androgen (adrenarche) and, to a lesser degree, gonadal androgen secretion cause pubic and axillary hair growth. Adrenarche plays little if any part in skeletal growth. While temporarily related to gonadarche, adrenarche is an independent, functionally unrelated biological event.
4. At midpuberty, sufficient gonadal estrogen secretion proliferates the endometrium, and the first menses (menarche) occurs.
5. Postmenarchal cycles are initially anovulatory. Sustained, predictable positive LH surge responses to estradiol are late pubertal events.

36. E p.372,376

Laboratory Diagnosis of Precocious Puberty:
Bone age.
Head CT scan or MRI, ultrasonography of abdomen and pelvis.
FSH, LH, HCG assay.
Thyroid function tests (TSH and free T_4).
Steroids (serum DHAS, testosterone, estradiol, progesterone, 17-hydroxyprogesterone).
GnRH testing.

37. A p.373

A number of CNS problems, including abnormal skull development due to rickets, can cause true precocious development. Various tumors can induce precocity, including hamartomas in the hypothalamus (the most common lesion in very young girls), craniopharyngioma, astrocytoma, glioma, neurofibroma, ependymoma, and suprasellar teratoma — all usually near the hypothalamus. Pineal tumors, for unknown reasons, have been seen only in male precocious puberty. Nontumorous causes include encephalitis, meningitis, hydrocephalus, and von Recklinghausen's disease. An injury to the skull may stimulate sexual development. The mechanism is unknown, and a latent period of 1–2 months is usually seen. A hamartoma is a hyperplastic congenital malformation in the floor of the third ventricle that usually produces precocity in the first few years of life; magnetic resonance imaging is the most sensitive method for the detection of small tumors like a hamartoma. Patients with true precocious puberty and known CNS lesions or a history of cranial irradiation should be evaluated for growth hormone deficiency because of the recognized association of these defects. True sexual precocity occurs in a small number of children with long-standing hypothyroidism.

38. E p.373

With hypothyroidism in children, in addition to short stature (but not bone age acceleration), galactorrhea may be present. The sella turcica is frequently enlarged, but with thyroid replacement pubertal development will stop and even regress. The sella films will return to normal. Although reported cases have been severe and therefore clinically obvious, laboratory evaluation of thyroid function is indicated in all cases of sexual precocity.

39. E p.374

McCune-Albright syndrome (polyostotic fibrous dysplasia) accounts for 5% of female precocity and consists of multiple disseminated cystic bone lesions that easily fracture, cafe au lait skin spots of various sizes and shapes, and sexual precocity. In addition, this syndrome can be associated with ovarian cysts, growth hormone and prolactin secreting adenomas, hyperthyroidism, adrenal hypercortisolism, and osteomalacia. Premature menarche may be the first sign of the syndrome. Skeletal abnormalities may become evident following the onset of puberty. The combination of multiple bone fractures, cafe au lait patches, and premature development should lead to the diagnosis

Sexual precocity in McCune Albright syndrome is now demonstrated to be the result of autonomous early production of estrogen by the ovaries. FSH and LH levels are low, respond poorly to GnRH stimulation, and there is an absence of nocturnal gonadotropin pulsations (all unlike central precocity). In addition, Cushing's disease, acromegaly, hyperparathyroidism, and hyperthyroidism have been reported in this syndrome. The protean manifestations of this disorder suggested that the pathophysiology results from a basic defect in cellular regulation at the level of the G protein-cAMP-kinase function in affected tissues. A mutation in the alpha-subunit of the G protein has been identified in all affected tissues in patients with McCune-Albright syndrome. This mutation attenuates GTPase activity which is necessary to terminate adenylate cyclase activation; thus, affected tissues have autonomous activity. Somatic mosaicism of the alpha-subunit accounts for the fact that this mutation is not lethal and for the variation in site and activity throughout the body. This mutation can also occur in nonendocrine tissues in patients with McCune-Albright syndrome, thus explaining the occurrence of hepatitis, intestinal polyps, and cardiac arrhythmias. It is possible that this mechanism is responsible for childhood diseases other than McCune-Albright syndrome.

40. A
p.380,382

The objectives of management and treatment of precocious puberty include:

1. Diagnose and treat intracranial disease.
2. Arrest maturation until normal pubertal age.
3. Attenuate and diminish established precocious characteristics.
4. Maximize eventual adult height.
5. Avoidance of abuse, reduction of emotional problems, and contraception if necessary.

41. C
p.382,383

Delayed puberty is a rare condition in girls. Physiological delayed puberty tends to be familial. The diverse etiologic possibilities for delayed puberty are best classified by the level of gonadotropin encountered: hypergonadotropic hypogonadism, hypogonadotropic hypogonadism and eugonadism.

42. E
p.383

Laboratory work-up of delayed puberty usually includes x-rays for bone age, skull imaging (if hypogonadotropic), gonadotropin and prolactin levels, appropriate adrenal and gonadal steroid measurements, and assessment of thyroid function. In addition, general laboratory screening for systemic disorders is worthwhile. Evaluation according to the program outlined for amenorrhea will lead to the proper diagnosis. Patients with elevated gonadotropins require a karyotype.

43. A
p.384

If gonadotropins are increased into the postmenopausal range (hypergonadotropic hypogonadism), then some type of gonadal deficiency usually is the basis of delayed maturation. In sickle cell disease, approximately 20% of patients have delayed puberty and hypergonadotropism. A 17α-hydroxylase deficiency in steroid synthesis (affecting both adrenals and ovaries) will cause hypergonadotropic delayed puberty **and hypertension.**

The most common disorder of this type is gonadal dysgenesis. In the 45,X patient, the typical phenotypic stigmata of Turner syndrome will be displayed. However, these may be minimal or absent in sex chromosome mosaicism or structural deletions of the X chromosome. A Y-bearing cell line requires gonadal excision as prophylaxis against the risk of gonadal malignancy. Intersex patients can present with delayed puberty.

A hypergonadotropic 46,XX individual presents interesting possibilities. If hypertension, sexual infantilism, and an elevated serum progesterone are found, 17α-hydroxylase deficiency in steroid synthesis is likely. Acquired ovarian damage from torsion or inflammation should be ruled out. Finally, the 46,XX patient may have pure gonadal dysgenesis (gonadal streaks) or the resistant ovary syndrome.

Chapter 11 Abnormal Puberty and Growth Problems

44. E   p.384,385

Decreased secretion of LH (less than 6 IU/L), associated with depressed FSH, is seen in hypothalamic amenorrhea, amenorrhea and anosmia — Kallmann's syndrome, pituitary (tumor) disorders, hyperprolactinemia, or nonpathologic constitutional (physiologic) delay in development. Physiological delayed puberty can be regarded as a physiologic variant in development. The typical patient with physiological delay is short with appropriate bone maturation delay. Physiological delay accounts for only 10% of cases with delayed puberty, emphasizing the need to seek another diagnosis. As previously noted, physiological delay is frequently seen in a familial pattern with the expectation of a late but otherwise normal growth pattern and adult reproductive function.

Poor nutrition (anorexia nervosa, malabsorption, chronic illness, regional ileitis, renal disease) can lead to hypogonadotropic delayed growth and development. Exercise and/or stress-induced amenorrhea can also delay puberty. Unfortunately, illegal drug use (especially marijuana) must be considered.

In the presence of normal olfaction and normal prolactin levels, exclusion of pituitary, parapituitary, or hypothalamic tumor by specialized neuroradiologic procedures is necessary. If tumor or vascular malformation is not found, the diagnosis is (by exclusion) physiological delayed puberty.

45. B   p.387

Anabolic-androgenic steroids are illegally utilized by both adolescent males and females to increase athletic performance and even in an effort to look better. Response to these agents ranges from increased strength and libido (virilization and menstrual dysfunction in women) to liver diseases, impotence, and oligospermia. Excessive androgen use by adolescents can prevent individuals from reaching their genetic height potential. Although not well-studied, most experts believe that there are significant psychological and behavioral effects (such as enhanced aggression), as well as psychological dependence. In addition, adolescents who use anabolic steroids are more likely to use other drugs and to share needles (a major risk factor for human immunodeficiency virus infection).

12 Amenorrhea

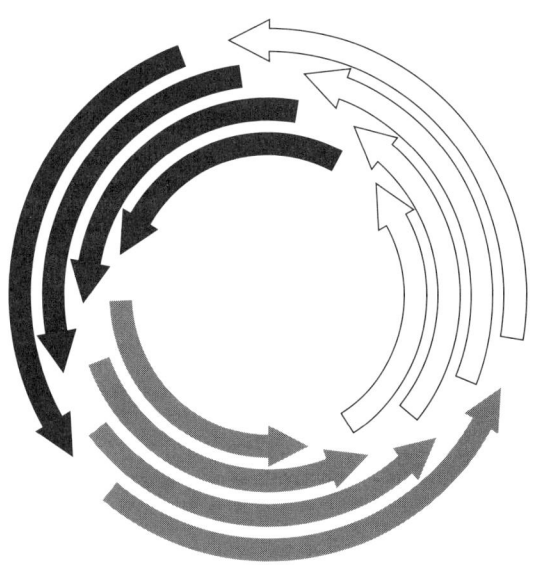

Learning Objectives

Be able to:

1. Detail the differential diagnosis of primary and secondary amenorrhea.

2. Discuss the work-up for amenorrhea and/or galactorrhea.

3. Understand when karyotyping is appropriate in the work-up of amenorrhea.

4. Describe the differential and work-up of premature ovarian failure.

5. Detail the specific disorders of the outflow tract that are responsible for amenorrhea.

6. Discuss the distinguishing clinical and laboratory features between müllerian agenesis and testicular feminization.

7. Detail the work-up and management of a pituitary prolactin secreting adenoma in the pregnant and nonpregnant patient.

8. Discuss the mechanism of action, types available and dosing of dopamine agonists in the treatment of prolactinomas.

9. Discuss the role of transsphenoidal surgery in the treatment of prolactinomas.

10. Describe the work-up and management of hypothalamic amenorrhea.

11. Describe the symptoms and signs associated with anorexia nervosa.

12. Discuss the pathophysiology, workup and treatment of Kallmann's syndrome.

Pre-Test

A. Instructions: Fill in the blanks

1. Amenorrhea should be evaluated in any patient without a period who has an absence of growth or development of secondary sexual characteristics by age _____.

2. The perimenopausal transition is associated with a high _____ but a normal _____.

B. Instructions: True or False

3. A positive withdrawal bleeding response to progestational medication, the absence of galactorrhea and a normal prolactin level do not rule out the presence of a significant pituitary tumor.

4. Selected patients under 30 years old with a diagnosis of ovarian failure should have a karyotype.

C. Instructions: For each of the following questions choose:

A. if only 1, 2 and 3 are correct
B. if only 1 and 3 are correct
C. if only 2 and 4 are correct
D. if only 4 is correct
E. if all are correct

5. Testicular feminization
   1. individuals do not have antimüllerian hormone
   2. is the second most common cause of primary amenorrhea
   3. is caused by an autosomal recessive gene that is responsible for the androgen intracellular receptor
   4. may be distinguished from müllerian agenesis by noting the distribution of sexual hair and the serum testosterone level

6. A clinical response to bromocriptine
   1. can be demonstrated within an average of 2 weeks from the initiation of treatment
   2. usually demonstrates a restoration of ovulation and menses prior to a loss of galactorrhea
   3. will not be noted in the case of a macroadenoma
   4. will often regress with discontinuation of the medication

Post-Test

A. Instructions: Fill in the blanks

1. The initial step in the workup of the amenorrheic patient after excluding _____ begins with a measurement of serum _____ and _____ along with a progestational challenge.

2. The initial step of the patient presenting with galactorrhea regardless of menstrual history also includes _____ and _____ measurement but adds evaluation of the _____ _____.

3. Prolactin levels associated with primary hypothyroidism are usually less than _____ ng/ml.

4. The purpose of the progestational challenge test is to assess the level of endogenous _____ and the competence of the _____.

5. A serum value of less than _____ IU/L for FSH and LH is consistent with a hypogonadotropic state.

6. Approximately _____% of patients with a Y chromosome will not develop signs of virilization.

7. _____ is useful to obtain prior to attempting surgical correction of a müllerian anomaly.

8. The third most common cause of primary amenorrhea is _____ _____.

9. An _____ evaluation should be considered in all 46XX gonadal dysgenesis cases.

10. ____% of individuals who appear to have Turner syndrome are mosaics or have structural aberrations in the X or Y chromosome.

11. Microadenomas less than _____ mm in diameter in an _____ patient, do not require treatment.

12. ____% of women with high prolactin levels have galactorrhea and ____% of women with galactorrhea have normal menses.

B. Instructions: True or False

13. The mechanisms of action responsible for the appearance of galactorrhea in the setting of hypothyroidism are believed to be caused by decreased hypothalamic dopamine.

14. Distortion, expansion or erosion of the sella turcica may be noted on a coned-down view in patients with primary hypothyroidism or premature ovarian failure.

15. A progestational challenge test is positive if 2–7 days following progestin there is bleeding in any amount beyond a few spots.

16. Young women who are anovulatory for relatively long periods of time do not develop endometrial cancer.

17. Anovulation with amenorrhea or oligomenorrhea is a contraindication for use of oral contraception.

18. A negative withdrawal bleeding response to progestational medication should be followed up with 1.25 mg or conjugated estrogen daily for 21 days combined with 10 mg of medroxyprogesterone acetate for the last 5 days.

19. The midcycle surge of LH is approximately three times the baseline level.

20. Galactosemia may be associated with hypogonadal hypogonadism.

21. Genetic evaluation is unnecessary in the context of the presence of mosaicism with a Y chromosome discovered in a young women greater than age 30.

22. A transverse vaginal septum results from failure of canalization of the distal third of the vagina.

23. The most common cause of primary amenorrhea is gonadal dysgenesis.

24. Testicular feminization represents the only exception to the rule that gonads with a Y chromosome should be removed as soon as a diagnosis is made.

25. Women with gonadal dysgenesis do not present with secondary amenorrhea.

26. The presence of mosaicism must be ruled out to detect a Y chromosome because of the potential for malignant transformation and/or heterosexual development.

C. Instructions: For each of the following questions choose:

A. if only 1, 2 and 3 are correct
B. if only 1 and 3 are correct
C. if only 2 and 4 are correct
D. if only 4 is correct
E. if all are correct

27. Microadenomas
    1. are a very uncommon occurrence
    2. very rarely grow during pregnancy
    3. are a contraindication to oral contraception
    4. have a natural course which is unaffected by dopamine agonists

28. Asherman's syndrome
    1. may follow myomectomy or metroplasty
    2. may result in hypomenorrhea or dysmenorrhea
    3. may complicate pregnancy by promoting the occurrence of placenta accreta and/or placenta previa
    4. is not associated with severe pelvic infections

29. Müllerian agenesis
    1. is the second most common cause of primary amenorrhea
    2. is associated with an abnormal karyotype
    3. is associated with spinal skeletal anomalies
    4. requires laparoscopic diagnosis

30. Premature ovarian failure
    1. can result from deletions of portions of the X chromosome
    2. may be characterized by a higher LH than FSH
    3. be associated with low cortisol, high TSH and/or a positive rheumatoid factor
    4. may be associated with rare spontaneous transient remissions

31. Low gonadotropins may be associated with
    1. anorexia nervosa
    2. a negative progestational withdrawal test
    3. large pituitary tumors
    4. ovarian failure

32. The coned-down lateral view of the sella
    1. is a good screening test to detect a craniopharyngioma
    2. will detect suprasellar tumors
    3. when combined with a prolactin assay can determine when to obtain a CT or MRI
    4. can reliably detect a microadenoma

33. The effect of radiation and chemotherapy
    1. upon reproductive function is dependent upon the age, the amount as well as duration of exposure
    2. increases the chances that if a pregnancy does occur, the risk of congenital abnormalities is greater than normal
    3. can cause temporary or permanent premature ovarian failure
    4. is greatest upon young as opposed to older women

34. Pituitary tumors
    1. may cause amenorrhea years before they can be detected with radiologic techniques
    2. may be associated with visual field defects or blurring of vision if they compress upon the optic chiasm
    3. may cause clinical signs of acromegaly or Cushing's disease
    4. may produce free alpha subunit

35. Prolactin secreting adenomas
    1. are the second most common pituitary tumor
    2. are classified according to their staining ability which provides useful clinical information
    3. are encapsulated
    4. depending upon size and symptoms may be managed expectantly, medically or surgically

36. Transsphenoidal neurosurgery for pituitary prolactin secreting adenomas
    1. is associated with complete resolution of hyperprolactinemia with cyclic menses in 40% of patients with microadenomas
    2. may be associated with complications which include panhypopituitarism, cerebrospinal fluid leaks, diabetes insipidus
    3. does not require follow-up for signs of anovulation or hyperprolactinemia
    4. yield the best results in patients with prolactin levels in the 150–500 ng/ml range

37. Bromocriptine
    1. directly mimics dopamine inhibition of pituitary prolactin secretion
    2. when given orally is given in a dose which is 10 times lower than that which improves the symptoms of Parkinson's disease
    3. is associated with side effects which include orthostatic hypotension, nasal congestion and vomiting
    4. has been shown to be harmful to the fetus when ingested during early pregnancy

38. Macroadenomas
    1. may respond to bromocriptine in dosages of 5–10 mg daily
    2. should be treated with transsphenoidal surgery when suprasellar extension persists following bromocriptine
    3. if pretreated with bromocriptine for at least 3 months may make surgical removal more difficult
    4. which do not shrink in size in response to bromocriptine despite normalization of prolactin require early surgery

39. Microadenomas
    1. do not have to be treated
    2. can be treated with bromocriptine but not surgery
    3. should initially be followed with annual prolactin levels and a coned-down view of the sella turcica
    4. are usually not associated with hypoestrogenic amenorrhea

40. Prolactin adenomas during pregnancy
    1. preclude breast-feeding
    2. do not grow or expand 98% of the time if they are initially less than 10 mm in diameter
    3. are associated with an increase risk of abortion
    4. rarely requires neurosurgery

41. The empty sella syndrome
    1. may present on a coned-down view to be indistinguishable from a pituitary tumor
    2. is present in 25% of patients who present with amenorrhea and/or galactorrhea
    3. is a benign condition which does not require treatment
    4. precludes induction of ovulation

42. Hypothalamic amenorrhea
    1. is a diagnosis of exclusion
    2. can be effectively treated depending upon the objective of the patient
    3. should be initially followed up annually with a prolactin and coned-down view of the sella
    4. is usually unrelated to a woman's baseline weight

43. Anorexia nervosa
    1. is associated with a 2% mortality rate
    2. is commonly associated with low blood pressure, rough dry skin, bradycardia and/or amenorrhea
    3. may be associated with diarrhea
    4. is associated with high cortisol levels

44. Extensive exercise
    1. can delay menarche up to 3 years in girls and the onset of puberty in boys up to 2 years
    2. can increase serum testosterone and growth hormone
    3. may cause a decrease in melatonin secretion
    4. can suppress GnRH pulsatility

45. Kallmann's syndrome
    1. may be treated with clomiphene
    2. is associated with hypoplastic or absent olfactory sulci
    3. is not associated with cleft lip and palate
    4. is due to a mutation of a single gene on the short arm of the X chromosome

46. The amenorrheic exerciser
    1. is at greater risk of stress fracture
    2. shows a similar pattern of bone loss as seen in postmenopausal women
    3. requires hormone therapy if she is not a candidate for ovulation induction
    4. would probably have return of menses is she decreased her exercise and gained weight

Answers for Chapter 12 — Pre-Test Questions

1. 14   p.402

Any patient fulfilling the following criteria should be evaluated as having the clinical problem of amenorrhea:

   1. No period by age 14 in the absence of growth or development of secondary sexual characteristics.
   2. No period by age 16 regardless of the presence of normal growth and development with the appearance of secondary sexual characteristics.
   3. In a woman who has been menstruating, the absence of periods for a length of time equivalent to a total of at least 3 of the previous cycle intervals or 6 months of amenorrhea.

2. FSH; LH   p.410

During the perimenopausal period it is normal for FSH levels to begin to rise even before bleeding has ceased. This is true whether the perimenopausal period is premature at age 25–35 or at the usual time. This increase in FSH is associated with a decrease in inhibin. During the perimenopausal period the remaining follicles may be viewed as the least sensitive of all follicles because they have remained in place and failed to respond to gonadotropins for many years. The rise in FSH prior to menopause is due to the declining inhibin production by the less competent ovarian follicles. Attention must be paid to this situation because a period of elevated levels of FSH can be followed by a pregnancy. The value of measuring both FSH and LH is again emphasized because this special perimenopausal condition is associated with a high FSH but a normal LH.

3. false p.407

A positive withdrawal bleeding response to progestational medication, the absence of galactorrhea, and a normal prolactin level together effectively rule out the presence of a significant pituitary tumor.

4. false p.411

All patients under the age of 30 who have been assigned the diagnosis of ovarian failure on the basis of elevated gonadotropins must have a karyotype determination. The presence of mosaicism with a Y chromosome requires excision of the gonadal areas because the presence of any testicular component within the gonad carries with it a significant chance of malignant tumor formation. These are highly malignant secondary tumors from germ cells: gonadoblastomas, dysgerminomas, yolk sac tumors, and choriocarcinoma.

5. D p.421,422

Complete androgen insensitivity (testicular feminization) is the likely diagnosis when a blind vaginal canal is encountered and the uterus is absent (discussed in detail in Chapter 10). This is the third most common cause of primary amenorrhea after gonadal dysgenesis and müllerian agenesis. The male pseudohermaphrodite is a genetic and gonadal male with failure of virilization. Failures in male development can be considered a spectrum with incomplete forms of androgen insensitivity being represented by some androgen response. Transmission of this disorder is by means of an X-linked recessive gene that is responsible for the androgen intracellular. Clinically the diagnosis should be considered in:

1. A female child with inguinal hernias because the testes are frequently partially descended;
2. A patient with primary amenorrhea and an absent uterus;
3. A patient with absent body hair.

Differences between Müllerian Agenesis and Testicular Feminization

	Müllerian Agenesis	Testicular Feminization
Karyotype	46,XX	46,XY
Heredity	Not known	Maternal X-linked recessive; 25% risk of affected child, 25% risk of carrier
Sexual hair	Normal female	Absent to sparse
Testosterone level	Normal female	Normal to slightly elevated male
Other anomalies	Frequent	Rare
Gonadal neoplasia	Normal incidence	5% incidence of malignant tumors

6. C p.430,431

Complete cessation of galactorrhea occurred in 50–60% of patients in an average time of 12.7 weeks, and a 75% reduction of breast secretions was achieved in 6.4 weeks. It is important to advise patients that the loss of galactorrhea is a slower and less certain response compared to restoration of ovulation and menses. There is no question that macroadenomas will regress with bromocriptine treatment. In some there is prompt shrinkage with low dose treatment (5–7.5 mg daily); in others, prolonged treatment is required with higher doses. If a prolactin adenoma fails to shrink with 10 mg daily, further increases in dose are not useful. Visual improvement may be noted within several days. Reduction in tumor size can take place in several days to 6 weeks, but in some cases it is not observed until 6 months or more. In most cases, rapid shrinkage occurs during the first 3 months of therapy, followed by slower reduction.

Answers for Chapter 12 — Post-Test Questions

1. pregnancy; TSH; prolactin　　　　　　　　　　　　　　　　　　　　　　　　　　　　　　p.404
The initial step in the workup of the amenorrheic patient after excluding pregnancy begins with a measurement of thyroid-stimulating hormone (TSH), a prolactin level, and a progestational challenge. (See figure on page 177 in this Study Guide)

2. TSH; prolactin; sella turcica　　　　　　　　　　　　　　　　　　　　　　　　　　　　　p.404
The initial step in the patient presenting with galactorrhea, regardless of menstrual history, also includes TSH and prolactin measurement but adds a coned-down, lateral x-ray view of the sella turcica. The x-ray can be safely omitted in those patients who have galactorrhea, but also have regular, ovulatory menstrual cycles.

3. 100　　　　　　　　　　　　　　　　　　　　　　　　　　　　　　　　　　　　　　　p.405
Only a few patients presenting with amenorrhea and/or galactorrhea will have hypothyroidism which is not clinically apparent. Although it seems rather extravagant to measure TSH in such a large number of patients for such a small return, because treatment for hypothyroidism is so simple and is rewarded by such a prompt return of ovulatory cycles, and, if galactorrhea is present, by a disappearance of the breast secretions (a slower process that can take several months), TSH measurement is warranted. The duration of the hypothyroidism is important with regard to the mechanism of the galactorrhea; the longer the duration the higher the incidence of galactorrhea and the higher the prolactin levels.

4. estrogen; outflow tract　　　　　　　　　　　　　　　　　　　　　　　　　　　　　　　p.405
The purpose of the progestational challenge is to assess the level of endogenous estrogen and the competence of the outflow tract. A course of a progestational agent totally devoid of estrogenic activity is administered. There are two choices: parenteral progesterone in oil (200 mg) or orally active medroxyprogesterone acetate, 10 mg daily for 5 days. The use of an orally active agent avoids an unpleasant intramuscular injection (although this might be necessary when compliance is a concern). Other hormonal preparations, such as oral contraceptives, are not appropriate since they do not exert a purely progestational effect.

5. 5　　p.409

Clinical State	Serum FSH	Serum LH
Normal adult female	5–30 IU/L, with the ovulatory midcycle peak about 2 times the base level	5–20 IU/L, with the ovulatory midcycle peak about 3 times the base level
Hypogonadotropic state: Prepubertal, hypothalamic and pituitary dysfunction	Less than 5 IU/L	Less than 5 IU/L
Hypergonadotropic state: Postmenopausal, castrate and ovarian failure	Greater than 30 IU/L	Greater than 40 IU/L

6. 30　　　　　　　　　　　　　　　　　　　　　　　　　　　　　　　　　　　　　　　p.411,423
Approximately 30% of patients with a Y chromosome will not develop signs of virilization. Therefore, even the normal appearing adult woman with elevated gonadotropin levels must be karyotyped. Even if the karyotype is normal, as an added precaution all patients with ovarian failure should have an annual pelvic examination. Such preventive care is also indicated because these patients will be on hormone therapy. Over the age of 30, amenorrhea with high gonadotropins is best labeled premature menopause. Genetic evaluation is unnecessary because it is essentially unheard of to have a gonadal tumor appear in these patients after the age of 30. These tumors usually appear before age 20.

Chapter 12 Amenorrhea

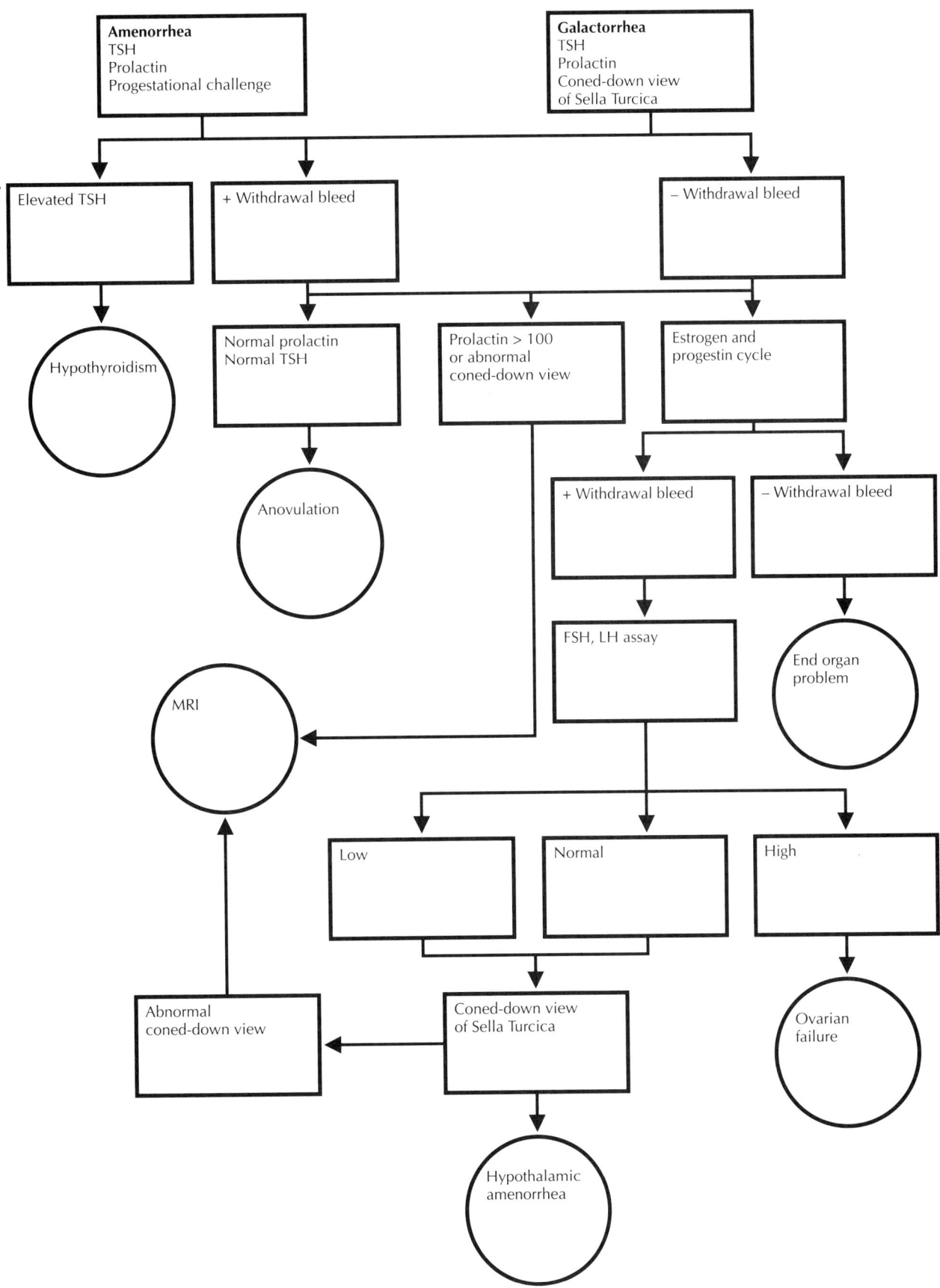

7. MRI　　p.419

Knowing what to expect prior to attempting surgical correction is a great advantage. Magnetic resonance imaging (MRI) can be utilized to accurately delineate the anatomical abnormality. A correct preoperative diagnosis will certainly facilitate the planning and execution of surgery.

8. testicular feminization　　　　　　　　　　　　　　　　　　　　　　　　　　　　　　　　　p.420

Testicular feminization is the third most common cause of primary amenorrhea after gonadal dysgenesis and müllerian agenesis. The patient with testicular feminization is a male pseudohermaphrodite. The adjective male refers to the gonadal sex; thus, the individual has testes and an XY karyotype. Pseudohermaphrodite means that the genitalia are opposite of the gonads; thus, the individual is phenotypically female but with absent or meager pubic and axillary hair.

9. auditory　　　　　　　　　　　　　　　　　　　　　　　　　　　　　　　　　　　　　　　p.423

Gonadal dysgenesis associated with a normal karyotype is also linked to neurosensory deafness (Perrault syndrome). Auditory evaluation should be considered in all 46,XX gonadal dysgenesis cases.

10. 40　　　p.423

A karyotype should be performed on all patients with elevated gonadotropins despite the appearance of a typical case of Turner syndrome. The presence of a pure syndrome, 45,X chromosome single cell line, should be confirmed. This expensive test cannot be viewed just as a step toward academic perfection. Forty percent of individuals who appear to have Turner syndrome are mosaics or have structural aberrations in the X or Y chromosome.

11. 10; asymptomatic　　　　　　　　　　　　　　　　　　　　　　　　　　　　　　　　　　p.426

If imaging discovers a microadenoma (less than 10 mm in diameter) in an asymptomatic patient, no treatment is necessary. These tumors are often incidental findings. A follow-up imaging is recommended in a year or two to be sure there is no growth. If a macroadenoma (greater than 10 mm in diameter) is present, surgery is usually necessary, especially since these tumors are commonly not detected until the onset of symptoms (headaches and visual disturbances).

12. 33;33　　　　　　　　　　　　　　　　　　　　　　　　　　　　　　　　　　　　　　　p.427

A high prolactin level is encountered in about one-third of women with no obvious cause of amenorrhea. Only one-third of women with high prolactin levels will have galactorrhea, probably because the low estrogen environment associated with the amenorrhea prevents a normal response to prolactin. Another possible explanation again focuses on the heterogeneity of peptide hormones. Prolactin circulates in various forms with structural modifications which are the result of glycosylation, phosphorylation, and deletions and additions. The various forms are associated with varying bioactivity (manifested by galactorrhea) and immunoactivity (recognition by immunoassay). The predominant variant is little prolactin (80–85%) which also has more biological activity compared to the larger sized variants. Therefore it is not surprising that big prolactins compose the major form of circulating prolactin in women with normal menses and minimal galactorrhea. This is not always the case, however, because a high blood level (350–400 ng/mL [15,500–17,700 pmol/L]) of prolactin composed predominantly of high molecular weight prolactin has been reported in a woman with oligomenorrhea and galactorrhea but with no evidence of a pituitary tumor. These high levels of relatively inactive prolactin in the absence of a tumor may be due to the creation of macromolecules of prolactin by antiprolactin autoantibodies. Explanations for clinically illogical situations can be found in the variable molecular heterogeneity of the peptide hormones. At any one point in time, the bioactivity and the immunoactivity of prolactin represent the cumulative effect of the circulating family of structural variants.

13. true　　p.405

The galactorrhea associated with hypothyroidism is thought to be due to declining hypothalamic content of dopamine with on-going hypothyroidism. This would lead to an unopposed thyrotropin-releasing hormone (TRH) stimulatory effect on the pituitary cells which secrete prolactin. In our experience, prolactin levels associated with primary hypothyroidism have always been less than 100 ng/mL (4,440 pmol/L).

14. true　　p.405

Constant stimulation by hypothalamic releasing hormones can result in hypertrophy or hyperplasia of the pituitary. The x-ray picture of a tumor (distortion, expansion, or erosion of the sella turcica) can be seen, therefore, with primary hypothyroidism and in patients with elevated GnRH and gonadotropin secretion due to premature ovarian failure. Patients with primary hypothyroidism and hyperprolactinemia can present with either primary or secondary amenorrhea.

15. true   p.406

How much bleeding constitutes a positive withdrawal response? The appearance of only a few blood spots following progestational medication implies marginal levels of endogenous estrogen. Such patients should be followed closely and periodically re-evaluated, since the marginally positive response may progress to a clearly negative response, placing the patient in a new diagnostic category. Bleeding in any amount beyond a few spots is considered a positive withdrawal response.

16. false   p.406,407

All anovulatory patients require therapeutic management, and with this minimal evaluation, therapy can be planned immediately. Because of the short latent period in the progression from normal endometrial tissue to atypia to cancer, clinicians are sensitive to the issue of endometrial cancer. But all too often, the clinician believes that this is a problem limited to older age. The critical feature is the duration of exposure to constant, unopposed estrogen. Therefore even young women, anovulatory for relatively long periods of time, can develop endometrial cancer. If there is any concern, evaluation of the endometrium (with aspiration curettage) is in order. On the other hand, the latent phase for breast cancer is long, perhaps as long as 20 years. It is only recently that data have emerged indicating that women who are anovulatory when they are young may have an increased risk of breast cancer when they are postmenopausal. This could reflect exposure to unopposed estrogen or it could be the consequence of infertility and the absence of the protection against breast cancer that pregnancy early in the reproductive years confers. However, some studies have not observed a link between anovulation and the risk of breast cancer.

17. false   p.407

Minimal therapy of anovulatory women requires the monthly administration of a progestational agent. An easily remembered program is to prescribe 10 mg medroxyprogesterone acetate daily for the first 10 days of each month. Experience with the endometrium in estrogen therapy programs has established the importance of a time period of at least 10 days to provide adequate protection against the growth promoting effects of constant estrogen. When reliable contraception is essential, the use of low dose oral contraceptive pills in the usual cyclic fashion is appropriate. Attempts to demonstrate a relationship between pill use and subsequent postpill amenorrhea have not been successful. Anovulation with amenorrhea or oligomenorrhea should not be viewed as a contraindication to the use of oral contraception.

18. true   p.408

If the course of progestational medication does not produce withdrawal flow, either the target organ outflow tract is inoperative or preliminary estrogen proliferation of the endometrium has not occurred. Step 2 is designed to clarify this situation. Orally active estrogen is administered in quantity and duration certain to stimulate endometrial proliferation and withdrawal bleeding provided that a completely reactive uterus and patent outflow tract exist. An appropriate dose is 1.25 mg conjugated estrogens daily for 21 days. The terminal addition of an orally active progestational agent (medroxyprogesterone acetate 10 mg daily for the last 5 days) is necessary to achieve withdrawal. In this way the capacity of Compartment I is challenged by exogenous estrogen. In the absence of withdrawal flow, a validating second course of estrogen is a wise precaution.

19. true   p.409

One should keep in mind that the midcycle surge of LH is approximately 3 times the baseline level. Therefore, if the patient does not bleed 2 weeks after the blood sample was obtained, a high level can be safely interpreted as abnormal.

20. false   p.411

In patients with galactosemia, an abnormal carbohydrate component of the gonadotropin molecules may render FSH and LH inactive. On the other hand, the problem in patients with galactosemia may be primarily gonadal; fewer oogonia may be the result of a direct effect of galactose on germ cell migration to the genital ridge.

21. true   p.411,412

Over the age of 30, amenorrhea with high gonadotropins is best labeled premature menopause. Genetic evaluation is unnecessary because it is essentially unheard of to have a gonadal tumor appear in these patients after the age of 30. These tumors usually appear before age 20.

The clinician and patient should give consideration to whether it is worth obtaining an expensive karyotype to seek identification of chromosomal abnormalities that have clinical implications for other family members. Deletions of the X chromosome can be responsible for premature ovarian failure. Accurate diagnosis of these deletions is not essential for decision-making regarding the patient; however, the presence of such abnormalities within a family is associated with infertility due to premature ovarian failure. Having this information can influence the family planning decisions of family members. We recommend that women with premature ovarian failure who are less than 63 inches tall (160 cm) be karyotyped because of the close conjunction of the genes responsible for stature and normal ovarian function. Because an individual with a mosaic karyotype (e.g., XX/XO) can experience normal pubertal development, menses, and even pregnancy before the onset of a premature menopause, it is appropriate to consider obtaining a karyotype, regardless of menstrual pattern, in an adolescent or young woman less than 60 inches tall.

22. true   p.420

Patients with a transverse vaginal septum, which is a failure of canalization of the distal third of the vagina, usually present with symptoms of obstruction and urinary frequency. A transverse septum can be differentiated from an imperforate hymen by a lack of distention at the introitus with Valsalva's maneuver.

23. true   p.420,422

Testicular feminization is the third most common cause of primary amenorrhea after gonadal dysgenesis and müllerian agenesis.

24. true   p.421

Therefore, once full development is attained after puberty, the gonads should be removed at about age 16–18, and the patient placed on hormone therapy. This is the only exception to the rule that gonads with a Y chromosome should be removed as soon as a diagnosis is made. There are two reasons: first, the development achieved with hormone treatment does not seem to match the smooth pubertal changes due to endogenous hormones, and second, gonadal tumors in these patients have not been encountered prior to puberty. Removal of gonadal tissue can be accomplished by a skilled operator through the laparoscope, reserving the option of laparotomy if the gonads are inaccessible.

25. false   p.423

Women with gonadal dysgenesis can also present with secondary amenorrhea. The karyotypes associated with this presentation are, in order of decreasing frequency:

    46,XX (most common).
    Mosaics (e.g., 45,X/46,XX).
    Deletions of X short and long arms.
    47,XXX.
    45,X.

26. true   p.423

The presence of mosaicism (multiple cell lines of varying sex chromosome composition) must be ruled out for a very important reason. The presence of a Y chromosome in the karyotype requires excision of the gonadal areas because the presence of any medullary (testicular) component within the gonad is a predisposing factor to tumor formation and to heterosexual development (virilization). Only in the patient with the complete form of androgen insensitivity can laparotomy be deferred until after puberty, because the individual is resistant to androgens and gonadal tumors occur late. In all other patients with a Y chromosome, gonadectomy should be performed as soon as the diagnosis is made to avoid virilization and early tumor formation.

27. C   p.417

Reasons Why the Diagnosis of Microadenoma Is Not Necessary
1. Very common occurrence.
2. Very rarely grow during pregnancy.
3. Significant recurrence rate after surgery.
4. Natural course unaffected by dopamine agonist treatment.
5. No contraindication to hormone therapy or oral contraception.

28. A   p.418,419

Secondary amenorrhea follows destruction of the endometrium (Asherman's syndrome). This condition generally is the result of an overzealous postpartum curettage resulting in intrauterine scarification. A typical pattern of multiple synechiae is seen on a hysterogram. Diagnosis by hysteroscopy is more accurate and will detect minimal adhesions that are not apparent on a hysterogram. In the presence of normal ovarian function, the basal body temperature will be biphasic. The adhesions may partially or completely obliterate the endometrial cavity, the internal cervical os, the cervical canal, or combinations of these areas. Surprisingly, despite stenosis or atresia of the internal os, hematometra does not inevitably occur. The endometrium, perhaps in response to a buildup of pressure, becomes refractory, and simple cervical dilatation cures the problem. Asherman's syndrome also can occur following uterine surgery, including cesarean section, myomectomy, or metroplasty. Very severe adhesions have been noted following postpartum curettage and postpartum hypogonadism, e.g., in Sheehan's syndrome.

Patients with Asherman's syndrome can present with other problems besides amenorrhea, including abortions, dysmenorrhea, or hypomenorrhea. They can even have normal menses. Infertility can be present with mild adhesions, an association not readily explainable. Patients with repeated abortions, infertility, or pregnancy wastage should have investigation of the endometrial cavity by hysterogram or hysteroscopy.

Impairment of the endometrium resulting in amenorrhea can be caused by tuberculosis, a condition that is rare in the United States. Diagnosis is made by culture of the menstrual discharge or tissue obtained by endometrial biopsy. Uterine schistosomiasis is another rare cause of end organ failure, and eggs may be found in urine, feces, rectal scrapings, menstrual discharge, or endometrium. We have seen the syndrome following intrauterine device (IUD)-related infections and severe, generalized pelvic infections.

Pregnancy is frequently complicated, however, by premature labor, placenta accreta, placenta previa, and/or postpartum hemorrhage.

29. B   p.419,420

Lack of müllerian development *(Mayer-Rokitansky-Kuster-Hauser syndrome)* is the diagnosis for the individual with primary amenorrhea and no apparent vagina. This is a relatively common cause of primary amenorrhea, more frequent than congenital androgen insensitivity and second only to gonadal dysgenesis. These patients have an absence or hypoplasia of the vagina. The uterus may be normal, but lacking a conduit to the introitus, or there may only be rudimentary, bicornuate cords present. If a partial endometrial cavity is present, cyclic abdominal pain may be a complaint. Because of the similarity to some types of male pseudohermaphroditism, it is worthwhile to demonstrate the normal female karyotype. Ovarian function is normal and can be documented with basal body temperatures or peripheral levels of progesterone. Growth and development are normal. Although usually sporadic, occasional occurrence may be noted within a family.

Further evaluation should include radiologic studies. Approximately one-third of patients have urinary tract abnormalities, and 12% or more have skeletal anomalies, most involving the spine. Renal tract abnormalities include ectopic kidney, renal agenesis, horseshoe kidney, and abnormal collecting ducts. When the presence of a uterine structure is suspected on examination, ultrasound can be utilized to depict the size and symmetry of the structure. When the anatomic picture on ultrasonography is not certain, MRI is indicated. Laparoscopic visualization of the pelvis is not necessary. MRI is more accurate than ultrasonography and less expensive and invasive than laparoscopy. Extirpation of the müllerian remnants is certainly not necessary unless they are causing a problem such as uterine fibroid growth, hematometra, endometriosis, or symptomatic herniation into the inguinal canal.

30. E p.412,424

Premature ovarian failure (the early depletion of ovarian follicles) is surprisingly common. Approximately 1% of women will experience ovarian failure before the age of 40, and in women with primary amenorrhea, the prevalence ranges from 10% to 28%. The etiology of premature ovarian failure is unknown in most cases. It is useful to explain to the patient that it is probably a genetic disorder with an increased rate of follicle disappearance. Often, specific sex chromosome anomalies can be identified. The most common abnormalities are 45,X and 47,XXY, followed by mosaicism and specific structural abnormalities on the sex chromosomes. Accelerated atresia is most likely because even 45,X (Turner syndrome) patients begin with a full complement of germ cells. In addition, premature ovarian failure can be due to an autoimmune process, or perhaps to destruction of follicles by infections such as mumps, oophoritis or a physical insult such as irradiation or chemotherapy.

31. A p.414

FSH and LH levels in the normal range in a patient with a negative progestational withdrawal test are consistent with pituitary-CNS failure. Indeed, this is the most commonly encountered clinical situation. Extremely low or non-detectable gonadotropins are seldom found, usually only with large pituitary tumors or in patients with anorexia nervosa.

32. B p.415

The initial x-ray evaluation for amenorrheic patients with or without galactorrhea is the coned-down lateral view of the sella turcica. This will detect the presence of a large tumor, although an incredibly rare suprasellar extension might escape this method. The coned-down lateral view of the sella is also a good screen for other lesions, such as a craniopharyngioma. Combining this screening technique with the prolactin assay, we are able to select those few patients who require more sensitive sellar imaging. If the prolactin level is greater than 100 ng/mL (4,440 pmol/L), or if the coned-down view of the sella turcica is abnormal, we recommend CT scan evaluation or MRI.

33. B p.425

The effect of radiation is dependent upon age and the x-ray dose. Steroid levels begin to fall and gonadotropins rise within 2 weeks after irradiation to the ovaries. The higher number of oocytes in younger age is responsible for the resistance to total castration in young women exposed to intense radiation. Function can resume after many years of amenorrhea. On the other hand, the damage may not appear until later in the form of premature ovarian failure. If pregnancy does occur, the risk of congenital abnormalities is no greater than normal.

Alkylating agents are very toxic to the gonads. As with radiation, there is an inverse relationship between the dose required for ovarian failure and age at the start of therapy. Other chemotherapeutic agents have the potential for ovarian damage, but they have been less well studied. The effect of combination chemotherapies is similar to those of the alkylating agents. Resumption of menses and pregnancy can occur, but there is no way to predict which patient will reacquire ovulatory function. As with radiotherapy, damage may present late with premature ovarian failure.

34. E p.425,426

A consideration of the disorders of the hypothalamic-pituitary axis must first focus on the problem of the pituitary tumor. Through the appearance of amenorrhea, the patient with a slowly growing pituitary tumor can present years before the tumor becomes evident by standard radiologic techniques. Growth of a benign tumor can cause problems because it expands in a confined space. The tumor grows upward, compressing the optic chiasm and producing the classic findings of bitemporal hemianopsia. With small tumors, however, abnormal visual fields are rarely encountered. In contrast, other tumors of this region (e.g., craniopharyngioma, usually marked by calcifications on x-ray) may be associated with the early development of blurring of vision and visual field defects because of their close proximity to the optic chiasm. Besides craniopharyngioma, other possible tumors include meningiomas, gliomas, metastatic tumors, and chordomas.

Sometimes the suspicion of a pituitary tumor is increased because of clinical signs of acromegaly caused by excessive secretion of growth hormone, or Cushing's disease due to excessive secretion of ACTH. Rarely, a TSH-secreting tumor will cause secondary hyperthyroidism. Amenorrhea and/or galactorrhea may precede the eventual full clinical expression of a tumor that secretes ACTH or growth hormone. If clinical criteria suggest Cushing's disease, ACTH levels and the 24-hour urinary levels of free cortisol should be measured, and the rapid suppression test (Chapter 14) should be utilized. If acromegaly is suspected, growth hormone should be measured in the fasting state (less than 5 ng/mL [5 mg/L]) and during an oral glucose tolerance test (suppression of growth hormone levels), and the circulating level of IGF-I should be measured. Though usually a problem in adult life, prolactin secreting tumors can be seen in preadolescent and adolescent children, and thus can be a cause of failure of growth and development or of primary amenorrhea.

35. D	p.427,428

Prolactin-secreting adenomas are the most common pituitary tumors, and they account for 50% of all pituitary adenomas identified at autopsy. Classically, pituitary adenomas have been grouped according to their staining ability as eosinophilic, basophilic, or chromophobic. This classification is misleading and of no clinical usefulness. Pituitary adenomas should be classified according to their function, e.g., prolactin-secreting adenoma. The development of transsphenoidal surgery was paralleled by the availability and clinical application of the drug, bromocriptine, that specifically suppresses prolactin secretion. Initially, appropriate decisions between the surgical approach and medical treatment were difficult to make. With increasing experience, clinical perspective has been achieved, and reasonable judgments are now possible.

36. D	p.428,429

Transsphenoidal neurosurgery achieves complete resolution of hyperprolactinemia with resumption of cyclic menses in about 40% of patients with macroadenomas and 80% of patients with microadenomas. Besides an inability to achieve a complete cure, surgery may be followed by recurrence of tumor (long-term cure rate is about 50% overall, ranging from as high as 70% for microadenomas to as low as 10% for macroadenomas) and a still unknown but significant percentage (perhaps as high as 10–30% after surgery for macroadenomas) of development of panhypopituitarism. Other complications of surgery include cerebrospinal fluid leaks, an occasional case of meningitis, and the frequent postoperative problem of diabetes insipidus. The diabetes insipidus is usually a transient problem, rarely lasting as long as 6 months, but it can be permanent. While initial follow-up reports of the results of transsphenoidal adenomectomy were discouraging (high recurrence rates), other authors have argued that surgical techniques improved with time, and recurrent hyperprolactinemia is relatively low. The best results are in patients with prolactin levels in the 150–500 ng/mL (6,660–22,200 pmol/L) range; the higher the prolactin the lower the cure rate.

37. A	p.429,430,433

Bromocriptine is a lysergic acid derivative with a bromine substitute at position 2. It is available as the methanesulfonate (mesylate) in 2.5 mg tablets. It is a dopamine agonist, binding to dopamine receptors and, therefore, directly mimicking dopamine inhibition of pituitary prolactin secretion. The oral dose that suppresses prolactin is 10 times lower than that which improves the symptoms of Parkinson's disease. For some patients, one pill a day (or half a pill bid) will be effective. On the other hand, an occasional patient will require 7.5 mg or 10 mg daily in order to suppress adenoma secretion of prolactin. Nausea, headache, and faintness are the usual initial problems. The faintness is due to orthostatic hypotension that can be attributed to relaxation of smooth muscle in the splanchnic and renal beds, as well as inhibition of transmitter release at noradrenergic nerve endings and central inhibition of sympathetic activity. Neuropsychiatric symptoms, occasionally with hallucinations, occur in less than 1% of patients. Although bromocriptine treatment profoundly lowers both maternal and fetal blood levels of prolactin, no adverse effects on the pregnancy or the newborn have been noted. Fortunately, amniotic fluid prolactin (and its presumed action on regulation of amniotic fluid water and electrolytes) is derived from decidual tissue, and its secretion is controlled by estrogen and progesterone, not dopamine. Therefore, bromocriptine does not affect amniotic fluid levels of prolactin.

38. E	p.431,432

Currently bromocriptine treatment is advocated for the treatment of macroadenomas, utilizing as low a dose as possible. Shrinkage of a tumor may require 5–10 mg bromocriptine daily, but once shrinkage has occurred, the daily dose should be progressively reduced until the lowest maintenance dose is achieved. The serum prolactin level can be utilized as a marker. In many (but not all) patients, control of tumor growth correlates with maintenance of a baseline prolactin level and can be achieved in some patients with as little as one-half a tablet (0.625 mg) daily. Withdrawal of the drug is usually associated with regrowth or re-expansion of the tumor, and therefore treatment must be long-term if not indefinite. Some patients will prefer surgery, and it is certainly a legitimate option. In view of better results claimed in more recent times, this choice should be presented to the patient. Transsphenoidal surgery is recommended when suprasellar extension persists after bromocriptine treatment of a macroadenoma. Because tumor recurrence is high, surgery should be followed by radiotherapy. All patients receiving radiotherapy require on-going surveillance for the development of hypopituitarism. Surgery should be considered as a debulking procedure for very large tumors with or without invasion prior to long-term dopamine agonist therapy.

39. B p.432

The treatment of microadenomas should be directed to alleviating one of two problems: infertility or breast discomfort. Bromocriptine is the method of choice. Again, some patients, deliberately and understandably, choose the surgical approach in hopes of achieving a cure and avoiding the worry and annoyance of continuing surveillance.

The major therapeutic dilemma can be expressed by the following question: should chronic bromocriptine treatment be utilized to retrieve ovarian function in those patients with hypoestrogenic amenorrhea, or should estrogen treatment be offered? Until a clear-cut benefit is demonstrated by clinical studies, we cannot advocate widespread bromocriptine therapy for those patients not interested in becoming pregnant. This conservative approach is supported by documentation of a benign clinical course with spontaneous resolution in many patients. Patients with hypoestrogenic amenorrhea are encouraged to be on an estrogen therapy program to maintain the health of their bones and the vascular system. Low dose oral contraception is recommended for those patients who require contraception.

40. C p.432,433

Approximately 80% of hyperprolactinemic women achieve pregnancy with bromocriptine treatment. Breastfeeding, if desired, can be carried out normally without fear of stimulating tumor growth. Interestingly, some women resume cyclic menses after pregnancy. This spontaneous improvement may be due to tumor infarction brought about by the expansion and shrinkage during and after pregnancy, or there may be a correction of a hypothalamic dysfunction followed by a disappearance of the associated pituitary hyperplasia.

A very small percentage (less than 2%) of women with hyperprolactinemia and microadenomas will develop signs or symptoms suggestive of tumor growth during pregnancy. About 5% of these patients will develop asymptomatic tumor enlargement (determined by radiologic techniques), and essentially none will ever require surgical intervention. The risk is higher with macroadenomas, approximately 15%. Headaches usually precede visual disturbances, and both may occur in any trimester. There is no characteristic headache; they are variable in intensity, location, and character. Bitemporal hemianopsia is the classic visual field finding, but other defects can occur. It has been argued in the past that a desire for pregnancy was a reason for the surgical approach. This argument hinged on the risk of tumor enlargement during pregnancy due to the well-known stimulatory effects of estrogen on the pituitary lactotrophs. Experience has indicated that very few patients develop problems.

41. B p.433,434

An empty sella is found in approximately 5% of autopsies, and approximately 85% are in women, previously thought to be concentrated in middle-aged and obese women. A closer look at the sella turcica, brought about by our pursuit of elevated prolactin levels, has revealed an incidence of empty sellas in 4–16% of patients who present with amenorrhea/galactorrhea. Galactorrhea and elevated prolactins can be seen with an empty sella, and there may be a coexisting prolactin-secreting adenoma. This suggests that the empty sella in these patients may have arisen because of tumor infarction.

This condition is benign; it does not progress to pituitary failure. The chief hazard to the patient is inadvertent treatment for a pituitary tumor. Even though enlargement of the sella turcica with a normal shape is more likely associated with an empty sella than a tumor, all patients should have examination by imaging for confirmation.

42. A p.434

Patients with hypothalamic amenorrhea (hypogonadotropic hypogonadism) have a deficiency in GnRH pulsatile secretion. Hypothalamic problems are usually diagnosed by exclusion of pituitary lesions and are the most common category of hypogonadotropic amenorrhea. Frequently there is an association with a stressful situation, such as in business or in school. There is also a higher proportion of underweight women and a higher occurrence of previous menstrual irregularity. Nevertheless, the clinician is obliged to go through the process of exclusion prior to prescribing hormone therapy or attempting induction of ovulation to achieve pregnancy.

43. C p.435–37

Because the mortality rate associated with this syndrome is significant (5–15%), it warrants close attention. Besides amenorrhea, constipation is a common symptom, often severe and accompanied by abdominal pain. The preoccupation with food may manifest itself by large intakes of lettuce, raw vegetables, and low calorie foods. Hypotension, hypothermia, rough dry skin, soft lanugo-type hair on the back and buttocks, bradycardia, and edema are the most commonly encountered signs. Long-term diuretic and laxative abuse may produce significant hypokalemia. An elevation of the serum carotene is not always associated with a large intake of yellow vegetables, suggesting that a defect in vitamin A utilization is present. The yellowish coloration of the skin is usually seen on the palms. Endocrine studies can be summarized as follows: FSH and LH levels are low, cortisol levels are elevated, prolactin levels are normal, TSH and thyroxine (T_4) levels are normal, but the 3,5,3'-triiodothyronine (T_3) level is low and reverse T_3 is high. Indeed many of the symptoms can be explained by relative hypothyroidism (constipation, cold intolerance, bradycardia, hypotension, dry skin, low metabolic rates, hypercarotenemia). There appears to be a compensation to the state of undernourishment, with diversion from formation of the active T_3 to the inactive metabolite, reverse T_3. With weight gain, all of the metabolic changes revert to normal. Even though normal gonadotropin secretion may be restored with weight gain, 30% of patients remain amenorrheic.

44. C p.440

As many as two-thirds of runners who have menstrual periods have short luteal phases or are anovulatory. When training starts before menarche, menarche can be delayed by as much as 3 years, and the subsequent incidence of menstrual irregularity is higher. In some individuals, secondary amenorrhea is associated with delayed menarche even though training did not begin until after menarche. It is suggested that some girls with these characteristics may be socially influenced to pursue athletic training. Contrary to the female situation, exercise has little effect on the timing of puberty in boys. Although changes in testicular function can be demonstrated in males, the changes are more subtle and less meaningful clinically.

This menstrual disruption is similar to the hypothalamic dysfunction which is more marked in the classic cases of anorexia nervosa. Acute exercise decreases gonadotropins and increases prolactin, growth hormone, testosterone, ACTH, the adrenal steroids, and endorphins as a result of both enhanced secretion and reduced clearance. The prolactin increase is in contrast to the absence of prolactin changes in undernourished women. The prolactin increases are variable, small in amplitude, and exceedingly short in duration. Thus, it is unlikely that the prolactin increase is responsible for the suppression of the menstrual cycle. Most importantly, insignificant differences occur in prolactin when amenorrheic runners are compared to eumenorrheic runners or nonrunners. In addition, women athletes have elevated daytime melatonin levels, and amenorrheic athletes have an exaggerated nocturnal secretion of melatonin. The nocturnal increase in melatonin is also seen in women with hypothalamic amenorrhea and appears to reflect suppression of GnRH pulsatile secretion. Another contrast to undernourished women is found in the thyroid axis. Athletes have relatively low T_4 levels, but amenorrheic athletes have an overall suppression of all circulating thyroid hormones, including reverse T_3.

45. C p.444,445

A rare condition in females is the syndrome of congenital hypogonadotropic hypogonadism associated with anosmia or hyposmia, known as Kallmann's syndrome. There is a chronology of eponyms assigning credit for original descriptions of this syndrome, but with all due respect to the physicians who first recognized this association, it is far easier to remember it in a descriptive way, as a syndrome of amenorrhea and anosmia. In the female, this problem is characterized by primary amenorrhea, infantile sexual development, low gonadotropins, a normal female karyotype, and the inability to perceive odors, e.g., coffee grounds or perfume. Often the affected individuals are not aware of their olfactory defect. The gonads can respond to gonadotropins; therefore induction of ovulation with exogenous gonadotropins is successful. However, clomiphene is ineffective.

Kallmann's syndrome is associated with a specific anatomic defect. Magnetic resonance imaging (as well as postmortem examination) demonstrates hypoplastic or absent olfactory sulci in the rhinencephalon. This defect is a consequence of the failure of both olfactory axonal and GnRH neuronal migration from the olfactory placode in the nose. The cells that produce GnRH originate in the olfactory area and migrate during embryogenesis along cranial nerves which connect the nose and the forebrain. The mutations responsible for this syndrome involve a single gene on the short arm of the X chromosome that encodes a protein responsible for functions necessary for neuronal migration. Location on the X chromosome explains why the syndrome occurs 5–7 times more frequently in males than in females. Other neurologic abnormalities (mirror movements, hearing loss, cerebellar ataxia) can be present, suggesting more widespread neurologic defects. Renal and bone abnormalities and cleft lip and palate also occur in affected individuals, probably reflecting the fact that the gene is expressed in tissues other than the hypothalamus. The syndrome occurs as an inherited or sporadic defect. Three modes of transmission have been documented: X-linked, autosomal dominant, and autosomal recessive. The increased frequency in males indicates that X-linked transmission is the most common. X-linked Kallmann's syndrome can be associated with other disorders due to deletions or translocations of contiguous genes on the distal short arm of the X chromosome (such as X-linked short stature or ichthyosis and sulfatase deficiency).

It is possible that patients with hypothalamic amenorrhea due to isolated deficiency of GnRH secretion (and no other abnormalities) have a defect similar to that of Kallmann's syndrome. With a lesser penetrance, only the GnRH migratory defect is expressed. In some individuals with amenorrhea and a normal sense of smell, family members can be identified with anosmia.

46. E   p.445,446

The patient who is hypoestrogenic and who is not a candidate for induction of ovulation deserves hormone therapy. This includes patients appropriately evaluated and diagnosed as having gonadal failure, patients with hypothalamic amenorrhea, and postgonadectomy patients. The bone density in women is dependent upon normal reproductive age levels of estrogen and progesterone. Even the most strenuous of exercise does not balance the consequences of hypoestrogenism on the bones, especially in adolescents. In the absence of estrogen, the normal response of bone to stress (to become stronger) is impaired. The same arguments that apply to hormone treatment in older women can be convincingly used to encourage these younger women to replace the estrogen they are lacking. The amenorrheic exerciser should be made aware that the hypoestrogenic state is associated with a greater risk of stress fractures. Ballet dancers with delayed menarche are more prone to scoliosis as well as stress fractures. It is not certain, however, whether this greater risk of stress fractures is influenced solely by bone density changes in that some studies fail to correlate fractures with reductions in bone density. It should be noted that bone loss in amenorrheic women shows the same pattern over time as seen in postmenopausal women. The loss is most rapid in the first few years, emphasizing the need for early treatment.

13 Anovulation and the Polycystic Ovary

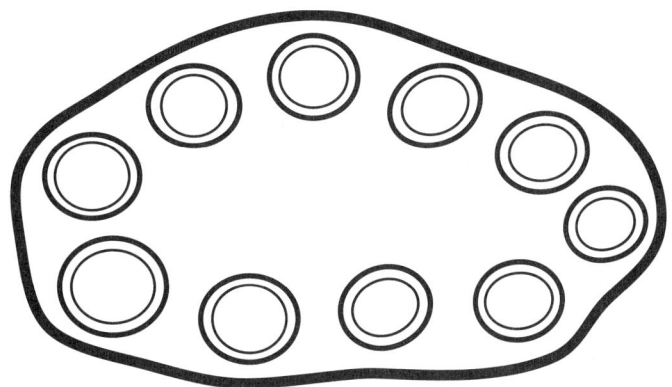

Learning Objectives

Be able to:

1. Describe the association between hyperprolactinemia and menstrual dysfunction.

2. Discuss the role of obesity and weight loss in the regulation of the menstrual cycle.

3. Explain the association between hyperinsulinemia, hyperandrogenism and polycystic ovarian disease.

4. Detail the short- and long-term clinical consequences of persistent anovulation.

Pre-Test

A. Instructions: Fill in the blanks

1. Polycystic ovarian disease is due to a functional derangement associated with accumulated and increased _____ due to a failure to ovulate.

2. _____% of patients with persistent anovulation associated with polycystic ovarian disease do not have elevated LH levels with reversal of the LH:FSH ratio.

B. Instructions: True or False

3. LH stimulation of androgen production in thecal cells is enhanced by IGF-I.

4. The known mechanism explaining the inverse relationship between body weight and circulating levels of SHBG is the increased insulin inhibition of SHBG production by the liver.

5. The lipoprotein profile in androgenized women with polycystic ovaries is similar to the male pattern.

C. Instructions: For each of the following questions choose:

A. if only 1, 2 and 3 are correct
B. if only 1 and 3 are correct
C. if only 2 and 4 are correct
D. if only 4 is correct
E. if all are correct

6. Persistent anovulation
   1. is associated with fluctuating levels of gonadotropins
   2. is associated with an average daily production of estrogen and androgens which are increased and dependent upon LH stimulation
   3. is most commonly due to the presence of hyperprolactinemia
   4. is associated with higher mean concentrations of LH but low or low-normal levels of FSH.

7. Insulin resistance is associated with
   1. hypertension
   2. hyperinsulinemia
   3. decreased HDL-cholesterol levels
   4. increased triglycerides

Post-Test

A. Instructions: Fill in the blanks

1. Ovulation is triggered by the rapid rise in circulating levels of _____.

2. Insulin-like growth factor-I (IGF-I) is produced in _____ cells in response to _____ stimulation and this response is enhanced by _____ and growth hormone.

3. The clinical consequences of uninterrupted estrogen stimulation could be _____ or _____ cancer.

4. _____ refers to patches of luteinized theca-like cells scattered throughout the ovarian stroma.

5. _____ and _____ are the histological characteristics of acanthosis nigricans.

6. Weight loss _____ the levels of both insulin and androgens.

7. IGF-I augments thecal androgen response to _____ and has a receptor with a similar structure to _____.

8. Hyperinsulinemia causes a decrease in _____ and _____ which contribute to increased androgen action.

9. A ratio of fasting glucose to fasting insulin less than _____ defines hyperinsulinemia.

B. Instructions: True or False

10. The dominant follicle is the one that acquires the highest levels of aromatase activity and LH receptors in response to FSH.

11. Examination for galactorrhea and measurement of prolactin are important screening procedures for all women who do not ovulate normally.

12. Hypothyroidism but not hyperthyroidism can cause persistent ovulation.

13. Psychological or physical stress may increase the adrenal contribution of estrogenic precursor thus leading to anovulation.

14. Polycystic ovary is the result of a specific central or local defect not a functional derangement.

15. The ovary of a woman with polycystic ovaries has multiple follicular cysts measuring 2–6 mm in diameter surrounded by luteinized hyperplastic theca cells.

16. The thick sclerotic capsule of the polycystic ovary acts as a mechanical barrier to ovulation.

17. Leprechaunism is a rare syndrome in young girls with a mutation in the insulin receptor gene.

18. Most evidence supports that hyperandrogenism induces hyperinsulinemia.

19. In the typical patient with anovulation evaluation of androgens is not necessary if there are no signs of hirsutism or virilism.

20. In the patient with long-standing anovulation an endometrial biopsy is not recommended.

C. Instructions: For each of the following questions choose:

A. if only 1, 2 and 3 are correct
B. if only 1 and 3 are correct
C. if only 2 and 4 are correct
D. if only 4 is correct
E. if all are correct

21. Activin
    1. in the early follicular phase is produced by granulosa cells and enhances the action of FSH on aromatase activity while suppressing thecal androgen synthesis
    2. exists in two forms
    3. in the late follicular phase decreased activin promotes thecal androgen synthesis in response to LH and IGF-I
    4. is a steroid

22. Weight loss in overweight women promotes normal ovulation by
    1. decreasing peripheral aromatization of androgens
    2. increasing levels of sex hormone binding globulin (SHBG)
    3. decreasing insulin levels that are capable of stimulating ovarian stromal tissue
    4. decreasing insulin-like binding proteins

23. Anovulation can be caused by
    1. pituitary tumor
    2. anorexia nervosa
    3. gonadal dysgenesis
    4. hyperprolactinemia

24. Polycystic ovaries are associated with
    1. decreased SHBG
    2. hyperinsulinemia
    3. increased DHAS
    4. increased testosterone

25. The classic picture of the polycystic ovary includes
    1. follicles at late stage of development
    2. dense stromal tissue
    3. few follicles undergoing atresia
    4. multiple small follicles located at the periphery of the cortex

26. Acanthosis nigricans
    1. is an absolute marker for hyperandrogenism
    2. is a gray-brown velvety discoloration of the skin
    3. frequently progresses to melanoma
    4. is associated with insulin resistance

27. Hyperinsulinemia can contribute to hyperandrogenism by
    1. inhibiting hepatic synthesis of SHBG
    2. decreasing 5-alpha reductase
    3. inhibiting hepatic production of insulin-like growth factors binding protein-I
    4. inhibiting aromatase

28. Clinical consequences of persistent anovulation include
    1. hirsutism and acne
    2. increase risk of endometrial cancer
    3. increase risk of cardiovascular disease
    4. increase risk of diabetes mellitus in patients with hyperinsulinemia

29. In long-term follow-up of women with polycystic ovaries the following problems may persist into the postmenopausal years
    1. hyperinsulinemia
    2. acne
    3. hypertension
    4. hirsutism

30. Treatment options for the patient who does not want to become pregnant and is without hirsutism but anovulatory with irregular bleeding may benefit from
    1. daily medroxyprogesterone acetate for the first 10 days of each month
    2. spironolactone
    3. low dose combination oral contraceptive pills
    4. a GnRH analogue

Answers for Chapter 13 — Pre-Test Questions

1. androgens   p.467
There is no specific pathophysiologic defect. The hypothalamic-pituitary response is entirely appropriate, a response to chronically elevated estrogen feedback. The changes are a functional derangement brought about by accumulated and increased androgen due to a failure of ovulation, whatever the reason. Hence, the polycystic ovary may be associated with extragonadal sources of androgens or with ovarian androgen-producing tumors.

2. 20–40%   p.473
While an elevated LH value in the presence of a low or low-normal FSH may be diagnostic, the diagnosis is easily made by the clinical presentation alone. About 20–40% of patients with this condition do not have elevated LH levels with reversal of the LH:FSH ratio. We do not routinely measure FSH and LH levels in anovulatory patients.

3. true   p.458
The right concentration of androgens in granulosa cells promotes aromatase activity and inhibin production, and, in turn, inhibin promotes LH stimulation of thecal androgen synthesis. LH stimulation of androgen production in thecal cells is further enhanced by the autocrine activity of insulin-like growth factor-I (IGF-I). With development of the follicle, inhibin expression comes under control of LH. A key to successful ovulation and luteal function is conversion of the inhibin production to LH responsiveness, to maintain FSH suppression centrally and enhancement of LH action locally.

4. true   p.472
Independently of any effect on sex steroids, increased insulin will inhibit the hepatic synthesis of sex hormone binding globulin. In vitro studies indicate that both insulin and IGF-I directly inhibit SHBG secretion by human hepatoma cells. This is now known to be the mechanism for the inverse relationship between body weight and the circulating levels of SHBG. In addition, decreased SHBG levels in women represent an independent risk factor for noninsulin-dependent diabetes mellitus, regardless of body weight and fat distribution.

5. true   p.475
The lipoprotein profile in androgenized women with polycystic ovaries is similar to the male pattern. Although the elevated androgens associated with polycystic ovaries and anovulation offer some protection against osteoporosis, the adverse impact on the risk for cardiovascular disease is a more important consideration. Monthly periodic treatment

with a progestational agent has no significant effect on the androgen production by polycystic ovaries. Thus, if contraception is not required and hirsutism is not a complaint, assessment of the lipoprotein profile is a reasonable clinical response, and in the presence of a male pattern, serious consideration should be given to suppression with oral contraceptives. However, a major contributing factor to the abnormal lipid pattern in these patients is the hyperinsulinemia. Therefore, a major effort must be directed to control of body weight.

6. C p.463,464,465

In contrast to the characteristic picture of fluctuating hormone levels in the normal cycle, a "steady state" of gonadotropins and sex steroids can be depicted in association with persistent anovulation. This steady state is only relative, and is being exaggerated here to present a concept of this clinical problem. In patients with persistent anovulation, the average daily production of estrogen and androgens is both increased and dependent upon LH stimulation. This is reflected in higher circulating levels of testosterone, androstenedione, dehydroepiandrosterone (DHA), dehydroepiandrosterone sulfate (DHAS), 17-hydroxyprogesterone (17-OHP), and estrone. The testosterone, androstenedione, and DHA are secreted directly by the ovary, while the DHAS is almost exclusively an adrenal contribution.

The ovary does not secrete increased amounts of estrogen, and estradiol levels are equivalent to early follicular phase concentrations. The increased total estrogen is due to peripheral conversion of the increased amounts of androstenedione to estrone. That is not to say that there is no ovarian secretion of estrogen. Both estrone and estradiol continue to be secreted in significant although low amounts.

When compared to levels found in normal women, patients with persistent anovulation have higher mean concentrations of LH, but low or low-normal levels of FSH. The elevated LH levels are partly due to an increased sensitivity of the pituitary to releasing hormone stimulation, manifested by an increase in LH pulse amplitude and frequency. This is consistent with the concepts discussed in Chapter 5, linking a high estrogen environment with anterior pituitary secretion of LH and suppression of FSH.

7. E p.468

The clinical presentation of patients with insulin resistance (whether they have impaired glucose tolerance or diabetes mellitus) depends on the ability of the pancreas to compensate for the target tissue resistance to insulin. This compensatory response of hyperinsulinemia leads to hypertension; a direct relationship exists between plasma insulin levels and blood pressure. Resistance to insulin is further associated with increased triglycerides and decreased HDL-cholesterol levels.

Answers for Chapter 13 — Post-Test Questions

1. estradiol p.457

Just before and during menses, escape from the negative feedback of estrogen, progesterone, and inhibin results in increased follicle-stimulating hormone (FSH) secretion by the anterior pituitary. This initial increase in FSH is essential for follicular growth and steroidogenesis. With continued growth of the follicle, autocrine/paracrine factors produced within the follicle maintain follicular sensitivity to FSH allowing conversion from a microenvironment dominated by androgens to one dominated by estrogen, a change necessary for a complete and successful follicular lifespan. Continuing and combined action of FSH and activin leads to the appearance of luteinizing hormone (LH) receptors on the granulosa cells, a prerequisite for ovulation and luteinization. Ovulation is triggered by the rapid rise in circulating levels of estradiol. A positive feedback response at the level of the anterior pituitary (and perhaps at the hypothalamus as well) results in the midcycle surge of LH necessary for expulsion of the egg and formation of the corpus luteum. A rise in progesterone follows ovulation along with a second rise in estradiol, producing the 14-day luteal phase characterized by low FSH and LH levels. The demise of the corpus luteum, concomitant with a fall in hormone levels, allows FSH to increase again, thus initiating a new cycle.

Chapter 13 Anovulation and the Polycystic Ovary

2. theca; gonadotropin; estradiol   p.460

Insulin-like growth factor-I (IGF-I) is produced in theca cells in response to gonadotropin stimulation, and this response is enhanced by estradiol and growth hormone.

3. endometrial; breast   p.473

There are potentially severe clinical consequences of the steady state of hormone secretion. Besides the problems of bleeding, amenorrhea, hirsutism, and infertility, the effect of the unopposed and uninterrupted estrogen is to place the patient at considerable risk for cancer of the endometrium and, perhaps, cancer of the breast. The risk of endometrial cancer is increased three-fold, while chronic anovulation during the reproductive years has been reported to be associated with a 3–4 times increased risk of breast cancer appearing in the postmenopausal years. However, the statistical power of these observational studies on breast cancer was limited by small numbers (all fewer than 15 cases). Others have failed to find a link between anovulation and the risk of breast cancer.

4. Hyperthecosis   p.466

Hyperthecosis refers to patches of luteinized theca-like cells scattered throughout the ovarian stroma. It is characterized by the same histologic findings as seen in polycystic ovaries. The clinical picture of more intense androgenization is a result of greater androgen production. This condition is associated with lower LH levels, which is a possible consequence of the higher testosterone levels blocking estrogen action at the hypothalamic-pituitary level. It seems appropriate to view hyperthecosis as a manifestation of the same process, persistent anovulation, but with greater intensity. A greater degree of insulin resistance is correlated with the degree of hyperthecosis.

5. Hyperkeratosis; papillomatosis   p.468

Hyperandrogenism and insulin resistance are commonly associated with acanthosis nigricans. Hyperkeratosis and papillomatosis are the histological characteristics of acanthosis nigricans.

6. decreases   p.475

The only known effective therapy is weight loss. Both the hyperinsulinemia and the hyperandrogenism can be reduced with weight loss which is at least more than 5% of the initial weight. A goal for weight loss that correlates with a good chance of achieving pregnancy (improved menstrual function), a reduction in insulin levels, and a decrease in free testosterone levels is a body mass index of less than 27. Insulin resistance is not detected with a body mass index less than 27.

7. LH; insulin   p.471

There is an impressive correlation between the degree of hyperinsulinemia and hyperandrogenism. At higher concentrations, insulin binds to the IGF-I receptors (which are similar in structure to insulin receptors). Thus, when insulin receptors are blocked or deficient in number, it is to be expected that insulin would bind to the IGF-I receptors.

8. SHBG; IGFBP-1   p.472

(See figure on page 194 in this Study Guide)

9. 3   p.476

It is not certain what levels of insulin in the fasting state or in response to an oral glucose tolerance test are correlated with clinical outcome. A ratio of fasting glucose to fasting insulin less than 3.0 defines hyperinsulinemia, and we recommend the measurement of this ratio in order to provide evidence that lends credence and importance to counseling efforts. When all is said and done, however, concentration on weight loss in overweight, androgenized patients is the most effective therapeutic approach.

10. true   p.458

The successful follicle is the one that acquires the highest level of aromatase activity and LH receptors in response to FSH. The successful follicle is characterized by the highest estrogen (for central feedback action) and the greatest inhibin production (for both local and central actions). This accomplishment occurs in synchrony with the appropriate activin and growth factor expression. The activin proteins (which enhance FSH activity) are produced in greatest amounts early in follicular development to enhance follicle receptivity to FSH.

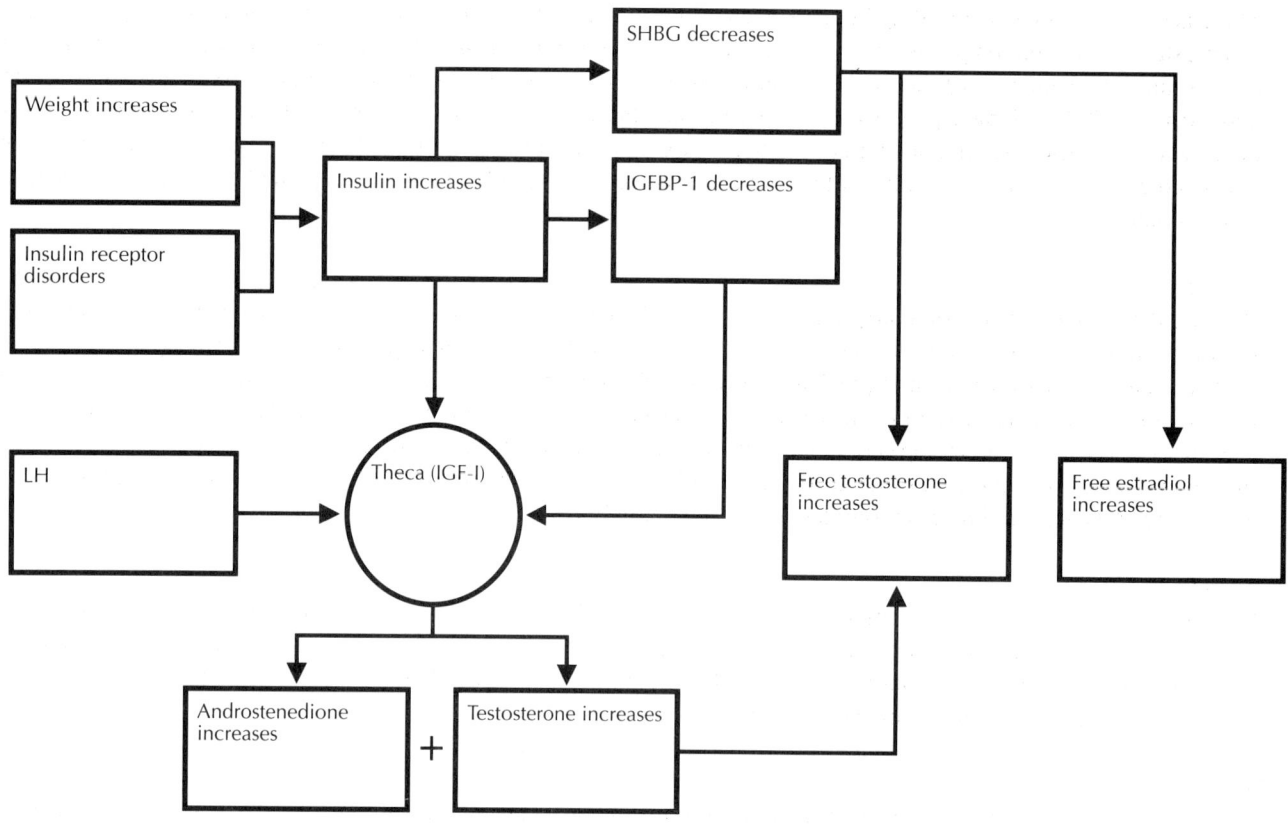

11. true   p.459

At least one specific clinical syndrome of central anovulatory dysfunction has been recognized: hyperprolactinemia. Increasing levels of prolactin can cause a woman to progress through a spectrum, beginning with an inadequate luteal phase to anovulation to the amenorrhea associated with complete GnRH suppression. *A search for galactorrhea and measurement of the prolactin level are important screening procedures for all women who are not ovulating normally.* The presence of galactorrhea or elevated prolactin levels dictates a choice of dopamine agonist treatment for the induction of ovulation.

12. false   p.459,460

The clearance and metabolism of estrogen can be impaired by other pathologic conditions, such as thyroid or hepatic disease. It is for this reason that a careful history and physical examination are important elements in the differential diagnosis of anovulation. Both hyperthyroidism and hypothyroidism can cause persistent anovulation by altering not only metabolic clearance but also the peripheral conversion rates among the various steroids. *The subtle presence of hypothyroidism, which may be associated with elevated prolactin levels, demands screening of anovulatory and amenorrheic women with a thyroid-stimulating hormone (TSH) level.*

13. true   p.460

Extragonadal contribution to the blood estrogen level can reach significant proportions. Although the adrenal gland does not secrete appreciable amounts of estrogen into the circulation, it indirectly contributes to the total estrogen level. This is accomplished by the extragonadal peripheral conversion of C-19 androgenic precursors, mainly androstenedione, to estrogen. In this manner psychological or physical stress may increase the adrenal contribution of estrogenic precursor, and subsequent conversion to estrogen may sustain the blood level of estrogen at a time when a decline is necessary for successful recycling of the menstrual cycle. Adipose tissue is capable of converting androstenedione to estrogen; hence, the percent conversion increases with increasing body weight. This is at least one mechanism for the well-known association between obesity and anovulation.

14. false   p.463

A question which has puzzled gynecologists and endocrinologists for many years is what causes polycystic ovaries.

Chapter 13 Anovulation and the Polycystic Ovary

There is an answer that is appealing in its logic and clinical applicability. The characteristic polycystic ovary emerges when a state of anovulation persists for any length of time. Whether diagnosis is by ultrasonography or by the traditional clinical and biochemical criteria, a cross-section of anovulatory women at any one point of time will reveal that approximately 75% will have polycystic ovaries. Because there are many causes of anovulation, there are many causes of polycystic ovaries. A similar clinical picture and ovarian condition can reflect any of the dysfunctional states discussed above. In other words, the polycystic ovary is the result of a functional derangement, not a specific central or local defect.

15. true   p.465

Because the FSH levels are not totally depressed, new follicular growth is continuously stimulated, but not to the point of full maturation and ovulation. Despite the fact that full growth potential is not realized, follicular lifespan may extend several months in the form of multiple follicular cysts, 2–6 mm in diameter (some can be as large as 15 mm). These follicles are surrounded by hyperplastic theca cells, often luteinized in response to the high LH levels. The accumulation of follicular tissue in various stages of development allows an increased and relatively constant production of steroids in response to the gonadotropin stimulation. This condition is self-sustaining. As various follicles undergo atresia, they are immediately replaced by new follicles of similar limited growth potential.

16. false   p.466

The polycystic ovary is usually enlarged and is characterized by a smooth pearly white capsule. For years, it was erroneously believed that the thick sclerotic capsule acted as a mechanical barrier to ovulation. A more accurate concept is that the polycystic ovary is a consequence of the loss of ovulation and the achievement of the steady state of persistent anovulation. The characteristics of the ovary reflect this dysfunctional state:

17. true   p.469

Peripheral insulin resistance associated with hyperandrogenism can be due to mutations of the insulin receptor gene (which leads to decreased numbers of insulin receptors in target tissue). Leprechaunism is a rare syndrome in young girls with a mutation in the insulin receptor gene; it is associated with severe insulin resistance, polycystic ovaries, hyperandrogenism, and acanthosis nigricans. Another subgroup consists of patients with autoantibodies to insulin receptors. This leaves a large collection of women with neither reduced insulin receptors nor autoantibodies. Possible mechanisms include functional problems in the insulin receptor (which could also be a consequence of insulin receptor gene mutations) and inhibitors which can interfere with insulin-receptor function after binding. Thus, there are at least 3 categories for peripheral target tissue insulin resistance: decreased insulin receptor numbers, decreased insulin binding, and post receptor failures.

18. false   p.470

There are 6 reasons to believe that hyperinsulinism causes hyperandrogenism:

1. The administration of insulin to women with polycystic ovaries increases circulating androgen levels.
2. The administration of glucose to hyperandrogenic women increases the circulating levels of both insulin and androgens.
3. Weight loss decreases the levels of both insulin and androgens.
4. In vitro, insulin stimulates thecal cell androgen production.
5. The experimental reduction of insulin levels in women with polycystic ovaries reduces androgen levels.
6. After normalization of androgens with GnRH agonist treatment, the hyperinsulin response to glucose tolerance testing remains abnormal in obese women with polycystic ovaries.

19. true   p.473

The typical patient presents with anovulation and irregular menses or amenorrhea with withdrawal bleeding after a progestational challenge. If there is no hirsutism or virilism, evaluation of androgen production is not necessary. Documentation of anovulation is usually unnecessary, especially in view of menstrual irregularity with periods of amenorrhea.

20. false p.473

In the patient who has long-standing anovulation, an endometrial biopsy (with extensive sampling) is a wise precaution. The well-known association between this condition and abnormal endometrial changes must be kept in mind. **The decision to perform an endometrial biopsy should not be influenced by the patient's age. It is the duration of exposure to unopposed estrogen that is critical.**

21. B p.458,195

In the early follicular phase, activin produced by granulosa in immature follicles enhances the action of FSH on aromatase activity and FSH and LH receptor formation, while simultaneously suppressing thecal androgen synthesis. In the late follicular phase, increased production of inhibin by the granulosa (and decreased activin) promotes androgen synthesis in the theca in response to LH and insulin-like growth factor-I (IGF-I) to provide substrate for even greater estrogen production in the granulosa. In the mature granulosa, activin serves to prevent premature luteinization and progesterone production.

22. A p.462

Obesity is associated with three alterations that interfere with normal ovulation, and weight loss improves all three:

1. Increased peripheral aromatization of androgens to estrogens.
2. Decreased levels of sex hormone binding globulin (SHBG) resulting in increased levels of free estradiol and testosterone.
3. Increased insulin levels that can stimulate ovarian stromal tissue production of androgens.

23. E p.462

It is usually impossible to reduce the issue of etiology to a single factor of abnormal menstrual function, except in severe states such as pituitary tumors, anorexia nervosa, gonadal dysgenesis, and perhaps hyperprolactinemia and obesity. Not only is it often impossible, but it is usually unnecessary to define the precise etiology. Regardless of the nature of the initial cause of the problem, the final clinical statement of the dysfunction is predictable, and easily diagnosed and managed. In patients who have abnormal or absent menstrual function, but are otherwise medically normal, the diagnosis will fall into one of three categories:

24. E p.465,467

(See figure on page 197 in this Study Guide)

25. C p.466

The classic picture of the polycystic ovary is attained, displaying numerous follicles in the early stages of development and atresia and dense stromal tissue.

1. The surface area is doubled, giving an average volume increase of 2.8 times.
2. The same number of primordial follicles is present, but the number of growing and atretic follicles (up to the secondary follicle stage) is doubled. Each ovary may contain 20–100 cystic follicles.
3. The thickness of the tunica (outermost layer) is increased by 50%.
4. A one-third increase in cortical stromal thickness and a 5-fold increase in subcortical stroma are noted. The increased stroma is due both to hyperplasia of thecal cells and to increased formation subsequent to the excessive follicular maturation and atresia.
5. There are 4 times more ovarian hilus cell nests (hyperplasia).

26. C p.468

The presence of acanthosis nigricans in hyperandrogenic women is dependent upon the presence and severity of hyperinsulinemia. It is most highly correlated with the magnitude of peripheral insulin resistance and less well with the hyperinsulinemia measured by a glucose tolerance test. The mechanism responsible for the development of acanthosis nigricans is uncertain. Conflicting studies suggest mediation through various growth factor receptors, not just insulin or insulin-like growth factor-I. Because acanthosis nigricans can be present in normal women, its presence is not an absolute marker for hyperandrogenism.

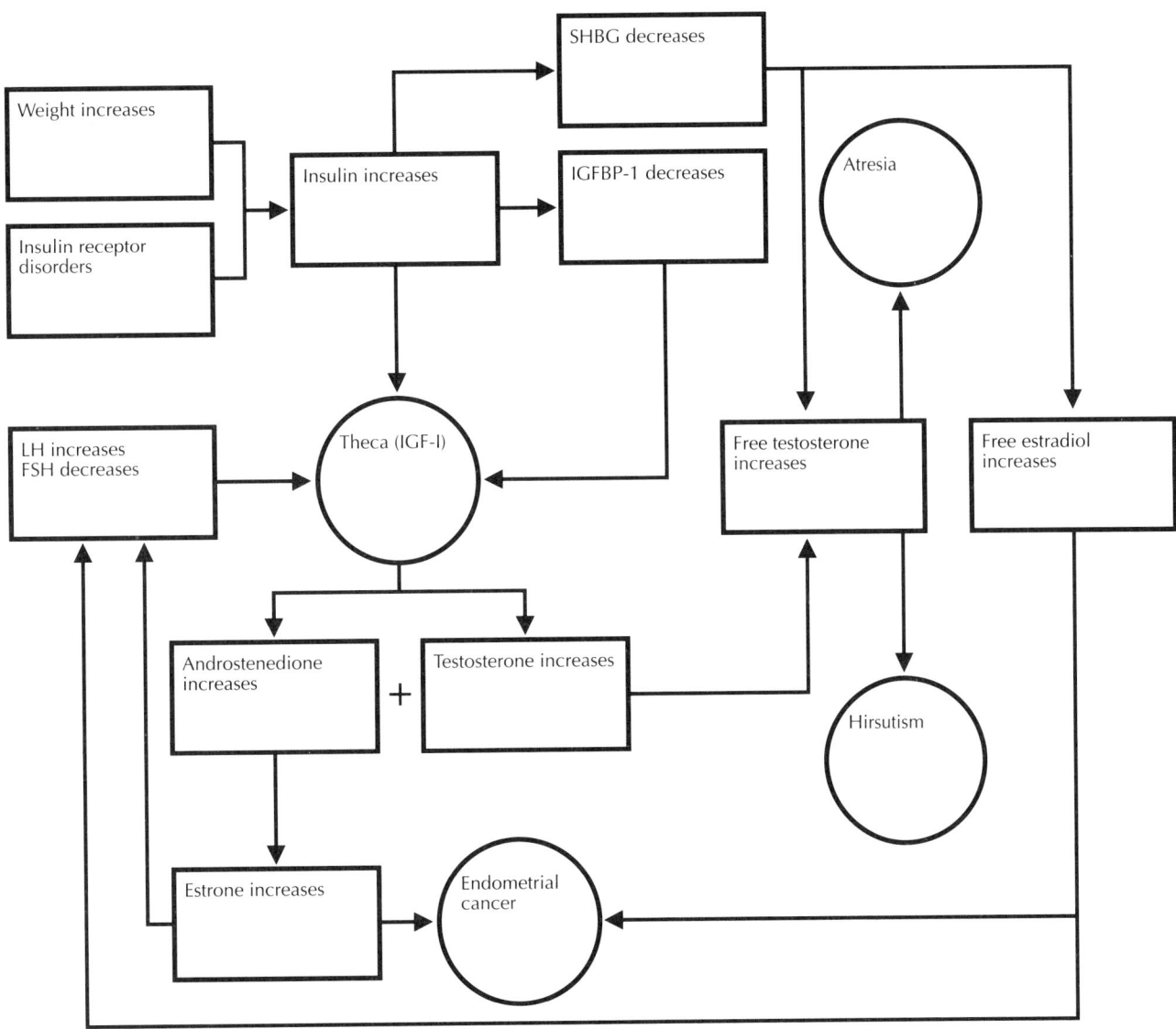

27. B p.471

In view of the known actions of IGF-I in augmenting the thecal androgen response to LH, activation of IGF-I receptors by insulin would lead to increased androgen production in thecal cells. There are two other important actions of insulin which contribute to hyperandrogenism in the presence of hyperinsulinemia: inhibition of hepatic synthesis of sex hormone binding globulin and inhibition of hepatic production of insulin-like growth factor binding protein-1.

28. E p.473

The Clinical Consequences of Persistent Anovulation
1. Infertility.
2. Menstrual bleeding problems, ranging from amenorrhea to dysfunctional uterine bleeding.
3. Hirsutism and acne.
4. An increased risk of endometrial cancer and, perhaps, breast cancer.
5. An increased risk of cardiovascular disease.
6. An increased risk of diabetes mellitus in patients with hyperinsulinemia.

29. B p.473,475

If left unattended, patients with persistent anovulation develop clinical problems, and therefore appropriate therapeutic management is essential for all anovulatory patients. In a long-term follow-up of women with polycystic ovaries, the problems of android obesity, hyperinsulinemia, and hypertension were observed to persist into the postmenopausal years. Overweight, hyperandrogenic and hyperinsulinemic, anovulatory women must be cautioned regarding their increased risk of future diabetes mellitus. In addition, hyperinsulinemia contributes to the increased risk of cardiovascular disease both by means of a direct atherogenic action and indirectly by adversely affecting the lipoprotein profile. Indeed, insulin resistance may be a more significant factor than androgens in determining the abnormal lipoprotein profile in overweight, anovulatory women. It has also been suggested that the increased insulin stimulation of IGF-I could produce bone changes similar to that seen in acromegaly. Hyperinsulinemia may be a factor contributing to the higher risk of endometrial cancer in these patients by increasing IGF-I activity in the endometrium.

30. B p.474,475

For the patient who does not wish to become pregnant and does not complain of hirsutism, but is anovulatory and has irregular bleeding, therapy is directed toward interruption of the steady state effect on the endometrium and breast. The use of medroxyprogesterone acetate (10 mg daily for the first 10 days of every month) is favored to ensure complete withdrawal bleeding and to prevent endometrial hyperplasia and atypia. The monthly 10-day duration has been demonstrated to be essential to protect the endometrium from cancer in women on postmenopausal estrogen therapy. Until specific clinical data are available, it seems logical that young, anovulatory women also require 10 days of progestational exposure every month. The patient will be aware of the onset of ovulatory cycles because bleeding will occur at a time other than the expected withdrawal bleed. In our opinion, when reliable contraception is essential, the use of low dose combination oral contraception in the usual cyclic fashion is appropriate.

Besides contraception, there is another argument in favor of continuous suppression rather than periodic progestational interruption. The lipoprotein profile in androgenized women with polycystic ovaries is similar to the male pattern. Although the elevated androgens associated with polycystic ovaries and anovulation offer some protection against osteoporosis, the adverse impact on the risk for cardiovascular disease is a more important consideration. Monthly periodic treatment with a progestational agent has no significant effect on the androgen production by polycystic ovaries. Thus, if contraception is not required and hirsutism is not a complaint, assessment of the lipoprotein profile is a reasonable clinical response, and in the presence of a male pattern, serious consideration should be given to suppression with oral contraceptives. However, a major contributing factor to the abnormal lipid pattern in these patients is the hyperinsulinemia. Therefore, a major effort must be directed to control of body weight.

14 Hirsutism

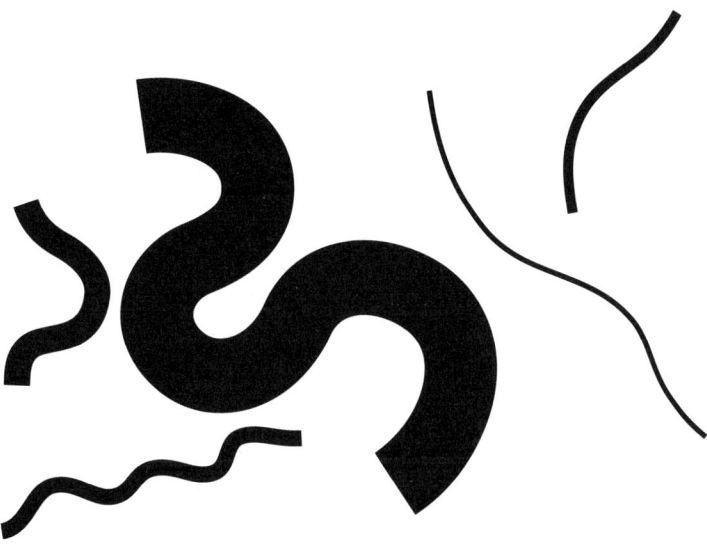

Learning Objectives

Be able to:

1. Describe the basic biology of hair growth and detail how hormones of the menstrual cycle can affect that growth.

2. Detail the differential and diagnostic workup of hirsutism.

3. Discuss the diagnostic and management approaches to androgen-producing tumors.

4. Discuss the various medications and their mechanisms of action for the treatment of hirsutism.

5. Describe some of the basic limitations and pitfalls of the diagnostic workup for hirsute women.

Pre-Test

A. Instructions: Fill in the blanks

1. There are 3 laboratory measurements of potential clinical use for evaluation of androgen excess: _____ — a measure of ovarian and adrenal activity; _____ — a measure of adrenal activity; _____ — a measure of peripheral target tissue activity.

2. Hyperinsulinemia contributes to hyperandrogenism by inhibiting hepatic synthesis of _____ and _____, actions which increase free testosterone levels and augment _____ stimulation of thecal androgen synthesis, respectively.

B. Instructions: True or False

3. Hirsutism implies a vellus to terminal hair transformation.

4. Desogestrel, gestodene and norgestimate are associated with greater increases in SHBG and decreases in free testosterone levels.

C. Instructions: For each of the following questions choose:

A. if only 1, 2 and 3 are correct
B. if only 1 and 3 are correct
C. if only 2 and 4 are correct
D. if only 4 is correct
E. if all are correct

5. Plasma testosterone levels
    1. are elevated in 70% of women with anovulation and hirsutism
    2. if over 200 ng/dl require that an androgen-producing tumor be ruled out
    3. usually reflect total testosterone concentrations
    4. within the normal range are between 20–80 ng/dl

6. Spironolactone
    1. has an effect which is independent of dosage
    2. inhibits ovarian and adrenal biosynthesis of androgens
    3. decreases DHA and DHAS levels
    4. inhibits 5α-reductase activity

Post-Test

A. Instructions: Fill in the blanks

1. The signs of virilism include _____, _____, _____ of the voice and changes in body _____.

2. The _____ _____ determines the events than control hair growth.

3. _____% of testosterone is derived from peripheral conversion of androstenedione while the adrenal gland and ovary contribute equal amounts of _____% to the circulating levels of testosterone.

4. About _____% of anovulatory women develop hirsutism.

5. The initial laboratory evaluation of hirsutism consists of serum levels of _____, _____ and _____ in addition to evaluation of prolactin levels and thyroid function.

6. The most useful measurements in the basal state to detect Cushing's syndrome are _____ and a late evening plasma _____.

7. Hirsutism due to an adrenal enzyme defect usually begins _____ puberty.

8. There are two findings highly suspicious for the presence of an androgen-producing tumor: _____ progressive masculinization and a testosterone level greater than _____ ng/dl.

9. Functioning ovarian tumors are almost all _____.

10. Adrenal masses are discovered incidentally in _____% of patients undergoing abdominal imaging.

11. Oral contraceptives _____ LH and _____ SHBG leading to _____ free testosterone levels.

12. Androgen levels in postmenopausal women are _____.

B. Instructions: True or False

13. Hair growth differences between races probably reflect hair follicle differences in 5α-reductase activity.

14. Hair grows continuously rather than a cyclic fashion with alternating phases of activity and inactivity.

15. About 90% of dehydroepiandrosterone sulfate (DHAS) arises from the adrenal while dehydroepiandrosterone (DHA) is almost exclusively from the adrenal.

16. The only effective treatment for hyperinsulinemia is weight loss.

17. Surgery is rarely indicated for treatment of bilateral adrenal masses.

18. Permanent removal of hair can be accomplished only by electrocoagulation of the dermal papillae.

19. Laparoscopy and ovarian biopsy are indicated in the evaluation of hirsutism.

20. Adrenal androgen secretion is more sensitive to suppression by dexamethasone than is cortisol secretion.

21. The combination of a GnRH agonist and an oral contraceptive should be reserved for the severe case of ovarian hyperandrogenism which has failed to respond to the usual treatment options.

22. Individuals with idiopathic or familial hirsutism probably have increased 5α-reductase activity.

23. Failure of progestin treatment to suppress hair growth and testosterone levels after 6–12 months raises suspicion of adrenal disease or a very small tumor.

C. Instructions: Match the appropriate phrase with each question below

   A. increase rate of growth of hair
   B. decrease rate of growth of hair
   C. minimal effect upon growth of hair

24. progestins
25. estrogens
26. androgens
27. hypopituitarism
28. acromegaly
29. hyperinsulinemia
30. summer
31. Cushing's syndrome

D. Instructions: For each of the following questions choose:

   A. if only 1, 2 and 3 are correct
   B. if only 1 and 3 are correct
   C. if only 2 and 4 are correct
   D. if only 4 is correct
   E. if all are correct

32. Sex steroid hormone binding globulin (SHBG)
    1. is increased by estrogens and thyroid hormone
    2. is decreased by insulin
    3. is produced in the liver
    4. determines the potential action of testosterone

33. Luteoma
    1. may cause virilization during pregnancy
    2. results from an exaggerated reaction of the ovarian stroma to hCG
    3. is unilateral in 4–5% of cases
    4. is often associated with masculinization of the female fetus

34. The workup of Cushing's disease
    1. initially focuses upon making the diagnosis then determining its etiology
    2. may involve a series of a variety of dexamethasone suppression tests
    3. may involve imaging of the adrenal gland
    4. tries to classify its etiology into two broad categories either ACTH-dependent or ACTH-independent

35. DHAS
    1. circulates in lower concentrations than any other steroid
    2. can be obtained as a random sample in the evaluation of hirsutism
    3. increases with aging
    4. provides substrate for the hair follicle synthesis of androgens

36. Late-onset adrenal hyperplasia
    1. is the most common autosomal recessive disorder
    2. is most commonly due to a deficiency P450c11
    3. has a clinical presentation which is extremely variable
    4. can be diagnosed without biochemical testing

37. 3β-hydroxysteroid dehydrogenase deficiency
    1. has no genetic markers currently available
    2. exists solely in the adrenal not the ovary
    3. requires an ACTH stimulation test to make the diagnosis
    4. occurs less often than 11β-hydroxylase deficiency

38. 17-hydroxyprogesterone
    1. is a an effective screening for women presenting with hirsutism
    2. offers a cost-effective means of determining if an ACTH stimulation test is indicated
    3. must be measured first thing in the morning
    4. if over 200 ng/dL is diagnostic of 21-hydroxylase deficiency

39. The ACTH stimulation test
    1. can be done any time during the day or during the menstrual cycle
    2. will yield a one-hour value that is plotted on a nomogram and predicts the genotype of forms of 21-hydroxylase deficiency
    3. can detect 21-hydroxylase and 3β-hydroxysteroid dehydrogenase deficiencies but not 11β-hydroxylase deficiencies
    4. is administered intravenously as a dose of 250 μg

40. When an androgen-producing tumor is suspected and an adnexal mass is not palpable the following diagnostic tests are indicated
    1. suppression tests
    2. selective angiography of adrenal and ovaries
    3. stimulation tests
    4. imaging of the adrenal glands and ovaries

41. Hyperthecosis
    1. can be stimulated by hyperinsulinemia
    2. can occur in postmenopausal women
    3. can simulate an androgen-producing tumor
    4. can be treated with a GnRH agonist

42. Adrenal masses
    1. which are bilateral are more serious than unilateral adrenal masses
    2. which are a primary malignancy are associated with excess androgens
    3. are more likely to be malignant if the diameter is larger
    4. which are stable, no growth from their initial discovery, for more than 18 months can be left in place

43. An adrenal mass accompanied by hypertension could be due to
    1. hyperaldosteronism
    2. pheochromocytoma
    3. Cushing's syndrome
    4. 21-hydroxylase deficiency

44. Long-term treatment options for hirsutism include
    1. ovulation induction for those wanting to become pregnant
    2. oral contraceptives
    3. progestational agents
    4. the use of long-term GnRH agonist alone

45. Side effects of spironolactone include
    1. dysfunctional uterine bleeding
    2. endometrial hyperplasia
    3. fatigue
    4. acne

46. Alternative treatment options for the long-term treatment of hirsutism include
    1. flutamide and oral contraceptives
    2. GnRH agonists and oral contraceptives
    3. cyproterone acetate
    4. GnRH agonists and clomiphene

Answers for Chapter 14 — Pre-Test Questions

1. testosterone; DHAS; 3α-AG   p.4,

There are are 3 principal laboratory measurements of *potential* clinical use for the evaluation of androgen excess:

   1. Testosterone — a measure of ovarian and adrenal activity.
   2. DHAS — a measure of adrenal activity.
   3. 3α-AG — a measure of peripheral target tissue activity.

2. SHBG; IGFBP-I; IGF-I   p.493

In many patients, a disorder in insulin action precedes the increase in androgens. Because of similarity between the receptors for insulin and insulin-like growth factor-I (IGF-I), hyperinsulinemia can augment thecal cell androgen production in the ovary. In addition, hyperinsulinemia contributes to the hyperandrogenism by inhibiting hepatic synthesis of sex hormone binding globulin and insulin-like growth factor binding protein-1, actions which increase free testosterone levels and augment IGF-I stimulation of thecal androgen synthesis, respectively.

3. true   p.485

Hypertrichosis is a generalized increase in hair of the fetal lanugo type, associated with the use of drugs or malignancy. *Vellus hair* is the downy hair associated with the prepubertal years. *Terminal hair* is the coarse hair that grows on various parts of the body during the adult years. Hirsutism implies a vellus to terminal hair transformation.

4. true   p.502

The low dose oral contraceptives are effective in treating acne and hirsutism. Suppression of free testosterone levels is comparable to that achieved with higher dosage. Multiphasic formulations appear to be equally effective. The beneficial clinical effect is the same with low dose preparations containing levonorgestrel, previously recognized to cause acne at high dosage. Formulations with desogestrel, gestodene, and norgestimate are associated with greater increases in sex hormone binding globulin and decreases in free testosterone levels. Theoretically these products would be more effective in the treatment of acne and hirsutism; however, this is yet to be documented by clinical studies.

5. E   p.499

Plasma testosterone levels (normal 20–80 ng/dL [0.69–2.8 nmol/L]) are elevated in the majority of women (70%) with anovulation and hirsutism. Individual variation is great, however, largely because of the changes in the testosterone binding capacity of the sex hormone binding globulin in the blood. Because the binding globulin levels are depressed by androgen and insulin, the total testosterone concentration can be in the normal range in a woman who is hirsute even though the percent unbound and active testosterone is elevated. Indeed, the unbound or free testosterone is approximately twice normal (an increase from 1% to 2%) in women with anovulation and polycystic ovaries. Therefore a normal total testosterone level in hirsute women is still consistent with elevated androgen production rates.

It is not necessary to measure the free testosterone (a technically difficult and expensive assay) because a routine total testosterone assay adequately serves the purpose of screening for testosterone-secreting tumors. Such tumors are associated with testosterone levels that are usually in the male range, and therefore the fine discrimination of the free testosterone level is unnecessary. *If the testosterone level exceeds 200 ng/dL (7 nmol/L), an androgen-producing tumor must be suspected.*

6. C p.504

Spironolactone is an aldosterone-antagonist diuretic. In the treatment of hirsutism, spironolactone has multiple actions, inhibiting the ovarian and adrenal biosynthesis of androgens, competing for the androgen receptor in the hair follicle, and directly inhibiting 5α-reductase activity. The inhibition of steroidogenesis is achieved through an effect on the cytochrome p450 system, but the steroid suppressive effects are so variable that the receptor-blocking action is the most important mechanism. It is probably for this reason that cortisol, DHA, and DHAS levels are not significantly changed with spironolactone treatment, even though androstenedione levels are decreased. The impact of spironolactone treatment on hirsutism is related to dosage, and a better effect is seen with a dose of 200 mg daily.

Answers for Chapter 14 — Post-Test Questions

1. clitoromegaly; balding; deepening; habitus p.483,489

The most sensitive marker for increased androgen production is hirsutism. This is followed in order by acne and increased oiliness of the skin, increased libido, clitoromegaly, and, finally, masculinization. Masculinization and virilization are terms reserved for extreme androgen effects (usually, but not always, associated with a tumor) leading to the development of a male hair pattern, clitoromegaly, deepening of the voice, increased muscle mass, and general male body habitus.

2. dermal papilla p.485

The dermal papilla is the director of the events that control hair growth. Despite major injury to the epithelial component of the follicle (such as freezing, x-rays, or a skin graft), if the dermal papilla survives, the hair follicle will regenerate and regrow hair. Injury to, or degeneration of, the dermal papilla is the crucial factor in permanent hair loss.

3. 50%; 25% p.486

The production rate of testosterone in the normal female is 0.2 to 0.3 mg/day. Approximately 50% of testosterone is derived from peripheral conversion of androstenedione, while the adrenal gland and ovary contribute approximately equal amounts (25%) to the circulating levels of testosterone, except at midcycle when the ovarian contribution increases by 10–15%.

4. 70% p.489

The most common clinical problem is the hirsute woman with irregular menses, with the onset of hirsutism during teenage years or in the early 20s, and long, gradual worsening of the condition. About 70% of anovulatory women develop hirsutism. The picture is so characteristic that a careful history may be sufficient for the diagnosis.

5. testosterone; DHAS; 17-hydroxyprogesterone p.490

The initial laboratory evaluation of hirsutism consists of immunoassays for the blood levels of testosterone, DHAS, and 17-hydroxyprogesterone (17-OHP). As part of the evaluation for anovulation, prolactin levels and thyroid function should be assessed, careful examination of the breasts for the presence of galactorrhea is important, and an aspiration endometrial biopsy should be considered. In addition, consideration should be directed to the possible presence of hyperinsulinemia.

6. 24-hour urinary free cortisol (UFC); cortisol p.490

The most useful measurements in the basal state to detect Cushing's syndrome are the 24-hour urinary free cortisol excretion (10–90 mg [280–2,500 nmol]) and the late evening plasma cortisol level (< 15 mg/dL [418 nmol/L]). The urinary excretion of 17-ketosteroids and 17-hydroxysteroids and measurement of morning and afternoon plasma cortisol levels are less reliable because of a significant overlap between normal and abnormal patients.

7. at   p.496

Besides using the 17-OHP screen to make a cost-effective decision regarding ACTH stimulation, one can be swayed by pertinent clinical findings. A strong family history of androgen excess suggests the presence of an inherited disorder. Hirsutism due to an adrenal enzyme defect usually is more severe and begins at a young age, typically at puberty. Short stature and very high blood levels of androgens also signify a more severe problem. Finally, it is worth considering the following: **With normal baseline steroid levels, even if a woman has a subtle enzyme defect, the management *of the problem does not require its discovery.***

8. rapidly; 200   p.500

There are two findings that should stimulate the clinician to suspect the presence of an androgen-producing tumor. One is a history of rapidly progressive masculinization. Hirsutism associated with anovulation is generally slow to develop, usually covering a time period of at least several years. Tumors are associated with a short time course, measured in months. The second finding that should arouse suspicion is a testosterone level greater than 200 ng/dL (7 nmol/L).

9. palpable   p.501

Functioning ovarian tumors are almost all palpable, and like any ovarian mass, rapid laparotomy and surgical removal are in order. It is well recognized, however, that very small ovarian tumors (usually in the hilus of the ovary) can secrete testosterone.

10. 2   p.501

Adrenal masses will be discovered incidentally in approximately 2% of patients undergoing abdominal imaging. A primary malignancy of the adrenal is usually associated with excess secretion of glucocorticoids and androgens.

11. decrease; increase; decreased   p.502

Androgen production in hirsute women is usually an LH-dependent process. Suppression of ovarian steroidogenesis depends upon adequate LH suppression. In addition to the inhibitory action of the progestational component, oral contraceptives provide a further benefit because of the increase in SHBG levels induced by the estrogen component. The increase in SHBG results in a greater androgen binding capacity with a decrease in free testosterone levels. The progestins in oral contraceptives also inhibit 5α-reductase activity in skin, further contributing to the clinical impact of oral contraceptives on hirsutism.

12. lower   p.507

Androgen levels in postmenopausal women are lower. A testosterone level greater than 100 ng/dL (3.7 nmol/L) is suspicious for a tumor.

13. true   p.484

The concentration of hair follicles laid down per unit area of facial skin does not differ materially between sexes but does differ between races and ethnic groups (Caucasian > Oriental; Mediterranean > Nordic). In addition, hair growth differences between races probably reflect hair follicle differences in 5α-reductase activity (the production of the active androgen, dihydrotestosterone). The pattern of hair growth is genetically predetermined.

14. false   p.484

Hair does not grow continuously but rather in a cyclic fashion with alternating phases of activity and inactivity. The cycles are referred to by the following terms:

> **Anagen — the growing phase.**
> **Catagen — rapid involution phase.**
> **Telogen — quiescent phase.**

15. false   p.486

Dehydroepiandrosterone sulfate (DHAS) arises almost exclusively from the adrenal gland, while 90% of dehydroepiandrosterone (DHA) is from the adrenal.

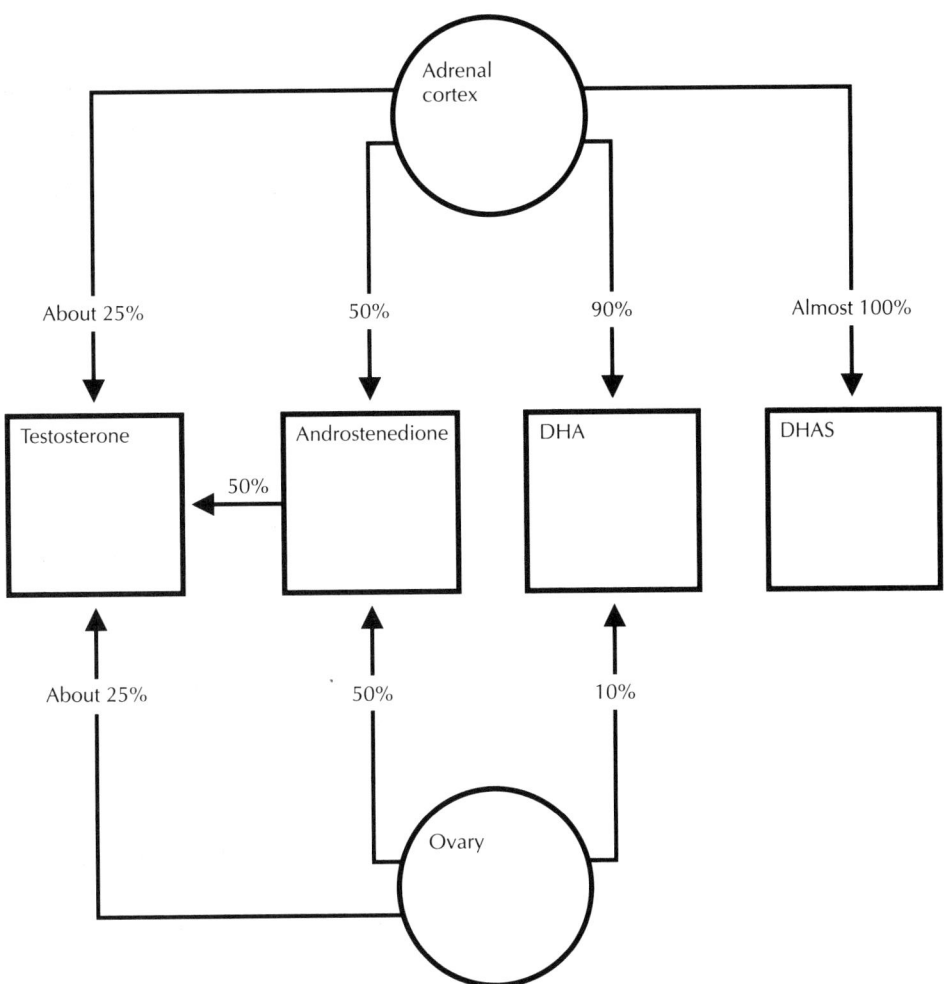

16. true   p.493

The only effective treatment for the hyperinsulinemia is weight loss. In addition, hyperandrogenic and hyperinsulinemic women must be counseled regarding the risk of future diabetes mellitus and cardiovascular disease. The mechanism of hyperandrogenism can be attributed to hyperinsulinemia in an occasional case where the circumstances are hard to understand, for example, the onset of hirsutism in an elderly woman who is found to have hyperthecosis in the ovaries. For these reasons, we recommend that testing for hyperinsulinemia be considered in all patients with android obesity as well as in individuals who remain anovulatory from their teenage years.

17. true   p.501

Bilateral lesions are more serious. Common causes of bilateral lesions are metastatic cancer, infection (tuberculous and fungal), and adrenal hyperplasia; hence, surgery is rarely indicated.

18. true   p.503

New hair follicles will no longer be stimulated to grow but hair growth which has been previously established will not disappear with hormone treatment alone. This can be affected temporarily by shaving, tweezing, waxing, or the use of depilatories. None of these tactics alters the inherent growth of the hair; therefore, they must be reapplied at frequent intervals. Permanent removal of hair can be accomplished only by electrocoagulation of dermal papillae.

19. false   p.507

Laparoscopy and ovarian biopsy are not indicated procedures in the evaluation of hirsutism.

20. true   p.506

If dexamethasone treatment suppresses the morning plasma cortisol level below 2.0 mg/dL (60 nmol/L), the dose should be reduced to avoid an inability to react to stress. Fortunately, adrenal androgen secretion is more sensitive to suppression by dexamethasone than is cortisol secretion. Patients with adrenal hyperplasia may require higher doses to normalize the steroid blood levels. With higher doses, alternate day therapy can still accomplish significant adrenal androgen suppression without affecting cortisol secretion.

21. true p.506

A greater dose of GnRH agonist is required to suppress ovarian androgen secretion compared to estradiol secretion. Therefore we recommend monitoring treatment with testosterone levels. Leuprolide in a dose of 3.75 mg monthly is effective. To avoid the problems associated with estrogen deficiency, estrogen-progestin add back should be initiated after the maintenance dose of a long-acting GnRH agonist has been established. We recommend the daily administration of 0.625 mg conjugated estrogens or 1.0 mg estradiol combined with 2.5 mg medroxyprogesterone acetate or 0.35 mg norethindrone, or, even better, an oral contraceptive. This method of treatment is relatively complicated and expensive and should be reserved for the severe case of ovarian hyperandrogenism which is usually due to significant hyperthecosis and marked hyperinsulinemia (a condition that responds poorly to the usual methods of treatment).

22. true p.507

There are some patients who present with hirsutism, but ovulate regularly. This category of patients has in the past been labeled idiopathic or familial hirsutism and is more pronounced in certain geographic areas and among certain ethnic groups. The only satisfactory explanation for this distressing problem is hypersensitivity of the skin's hair apparatus to normal levels of androgens, probably due to increased 5α-reductase activity. Because of this excessive sensitivity, normal levels of androgen stimulate hair growth.

23. true p.507

Failure of progestin treatment to suppress hair growth and testosterone levels after 6–12 months raises the suspicion of adrenal disease or a very small ovarian tumor.

24. C p.485

25. B p.485

26. A p.485

From animal studies and human disease patterns, the following list of hormonal effects can be compiled:

1. Androgens, particularly testosterone, initiate growth, increase the diameter and pigmentation of the keratin column, and probably increase the rate of matrix cell mitoses in all but scalp hair.
2. Estrogens act essentially opposite from androgens, retarding the rate and initiation of growth, and leading to finer, less pigmented and slower growing hair.
3. Progestins have minimal direct effect on hair.
4. Pregnancy (high estrogen and progesterone) can increase the synchrony of hair growth, leading to periods of growth or shedding.

27. B p.485

28. A p.485

Sexual and nonsexual hair growth can be affected by endocrine problems. In hypopituitarism, there is marked reduction of hair growth. Acromegaly will be associated with hirsutism in 10–15% of patients. While the impact of thyroid hormone is not clear, hypothyroid individuals sometimes display less axillary, pubic, and curiously, lateral eyebrow hair.

29. A p.486

5α-Reductase activity is stimulated by insulin-like growth factor-I (IGF-I). Increased IGF-I activity in anovulatory patients with insulin resistance and hyperinsulinemia can intensify the hirsute response in these hyperandrogenic patients.

30. A p.486

Hair growth can be influenced by nonhormonal factors, such as local skin temperature, blood flow, and edema. Hair grows faster in the summer than in the winter. Hair growth can be seen with central nervous system (CNS) problems such as encephalitis, cranial trauma, multiple sclerosis, and with certain drugs.

31. A p.490

Cushing's syndrome can present with hirsutism, and later, masculinization. Remember that one of the most common referral diagnoses is Cushing's syndrome, but this is one of the least common final diagnoses. When clinical suspicion is high, a screen for Cushing's syndrome is indicated.

32. E p.486,487

About 80% of circulating testosterone is bound to a beta-globulin known as sex steroid hormone binding globulin (SHBG). In women, approximately 19% is loosely bound to albumin, leaving about 1% unbound. Androgenicity is dependent mainly upon the unbound fraction and partly upon the fraction associated with albumin. DHA, DHAS, and androstenedione are not significantly protein bound, and routine immunoassay reflects their biologically available hormone activity. This is not the case with testosterone because routine assays measure the total testosterone concentration, bound and unbound.

SHBG production in the liver is decreased by androgens. Hence, the binding capacity in men is lower than in normal women, and 2–3% of testosterone circulates in the free, active form in men. SHBG is decreased by insulin, and increased by estrogens and thyroid hormone. Therefore, binding capacity is increased in women with hyperthyroidism, in pregnancy, and by estrogen-containing medication. In a hirsute woman, the SHBG level is depressed by the excess androgen (and, when present, by hyperinsulinemia), and the percent free and active testosterone is elevated as is the metabolic clearance rate of testosterone. The total testosterone concentration, therefore, can be in the normal range in a woman who is hirsute. However, there is no clinical need for a specific assay for the free portion of testosterone. The very presence of hirsutism or masculinization indicates increased androgen effects. One can reliably interpret a normal total testosterone level in these circumstances as being compatible with decreased binding capacity and increased free testosterone.

33. A p.490

Virilization during pregnancy raises the suspicion of a luteoma which is not a true tumor but an exaggerated reaction of the ovarian stroma to chorionic gonadotropin. The solid luteoma is unilateral in 45% of cases and associated with a normal pregnancy. Theca-lutein cysts seen with trophoblastic disease are virtually always bilateral. Virilization due to theca-lutein cysts can also be seen with the high human chorionic gonadotropin (HCG) titers associated with multiple gestation. Since a luteoma regresses postpartum, the only risk is masculinization of a female fetus; a risk not reported with theca-lutein cysts. Subsequent pregnancies are usually normal, but maternal virilization is occasionally recurrent. Androgen-secreting ovarian tumors are very rarely encountered during pregnancy, probably because the excess androgen usually suppresses ovulation. Ultrasonographic evaluation of the pelvis in women experiencing virilization in pregnancy is very helpful. Malignancy is frequently encountered when a unilateral ovarian lesion is present.

34. E p.491,492

(See figure on page 210 in this Study Guide)

35. C p.493,494

A random sample of DHAS is sufficient for the evaluation of hirsutism, needing no corrections for body weight, creatinine excretion, or episodic variation. Variations are minimized because of its high circulating concentration and its long half-life. A slow turnover rate results in a large and stable pool in the blood with insignificant variation. Elevated levels of DHAS contribute to the clinical problem of hirsutism because DHAS serves as a prehormone in hair follicles, providing substrate for the hair follicle synthesis of androgens.

36. B p.494,495

Congenital adrenal hyperplasia is due to an enzyme defect leading to excessive androgen production. This severe condition, with its prenatal onset, is inherited in an autosomal recessive fashion. A more mild form of the disease, appearing later in life, has been designated by a variety of adjectives, including late-onset, partial, nonclassical,

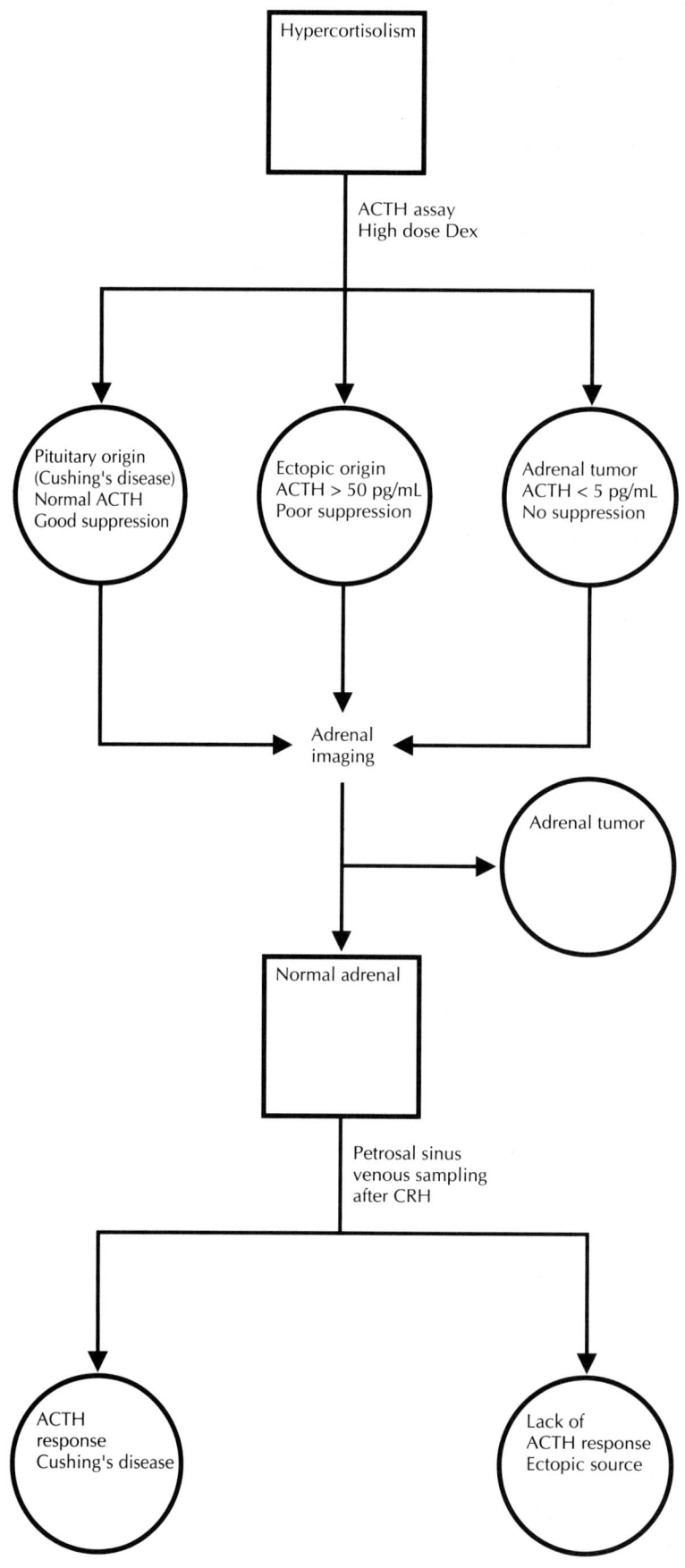

attenuated, and acquired adrenal hyperplasia. An asymptomatic form, cryptic adrenal hyperplasia, is revealed only with biochemical testing. Although each of the enzymatic steps from cholesterol to cortisol can be expressed in specific clinical disease, the most common enzymes to be deficient are 21-hydroxylase (p450c21), 11β-hydroxylase (p450c11), and 3β-hydroxysteroid dehydrogenase.

Women with late-onset adrenal hyperplasia due to a 21-hydroxylase deficiency respond to ACTH stimulation in a moderate fashion, between the classical homozygote response and the mild heterozygote reaction.

This condition is now recognized to be the most common autosomal recessive disorder, surpassing cystic fibrosis and sickle cell anemia. The clinical presentation is extremely variable, and the symptoms may appear and disappear over time.

37. B p.495

The 3β-hydroxysteroid dehydrogenase deficiency exists in both the ovaries and adrenals. This defect precludes significant androgen production; however, this enzyme activity appears to remain intact in peripheral tissues. Therefore, hirsutism seen with this deficiency is probably due to target tissue conversion of the increased secretion of precursors. Unlike 21-hydroxylase deficiency, no genetic markers are currently available; diagnosis requires ACTH stimulation and demonstration of an altered 17-hydroxypregnenolone to 17-OHP ratio. Some argue that late-onset 3β-hydroxysteroid dehydrogenase deficiency is encountered more frequently than 21-hydroxylase deficiency. However, although an exaggerated 17-hydroxypregnenolone response to ACTH stimulation is common in women with hyperandrogenism, the response is consistent with adrenal hyperactivity and not an enzyme deficiency. We believe that this deficiency is so subtle that accurate diagnosis is not essential. Our usual therapeutic approach to hirsutism will be effective.

38. A p.496, 497

From 1 to 5% of women who complain of hirsutism display a biochemical response which is consistent with the less severe form of adrenal hyperplasia. This relative frequency of late-onset adrenal hyperplasia dictates routine 17-OHP screening of women who complain of hirsutism. On the other hand, the routine use of the ACTH stimulation test is not warranted. 17-OHP must be measured first thing in the morning to avoid later elevations due to the diurnal pattern of ACTH secretion. The baseline 17-OHP level should be less than 200 ng/dL (6 nmol/L). Levels greater than 200 ng/dL, but less than 800 ng/dL (24 nmol/L), require ACTH testing. Levels over 800 ng/dL are virtually diagnostic of the 21-hydroxylase deficiency.

39. C p.497

Synthetic ACTH (Cortrosyn) is administered intravenously in a dose of 250 μg. Blood samples for the measurement of 17-OHP are obtained at time 0 and again at 1 hour. The testing must be performed in the morning (8 A.M.), but it can be scheduled at any time during the menstrual cycle. The 1-hour value is plotted on the nomogram which predicts the genotype of homozygote and heterozygote forms of the 21-hydroxylase deficiency. Dexamethasone pretreatment the night before is not necessary. Heterozygote carriers for 21-hydroxylase deficiency have ACTH-stimulated levels of 17-OHP up to 1,000 ng/dL (30 nmol/L); patients with late-onset deficiency have stimulated levels above 1,200 ng/dL (36 nmol/L).

For the diagnosis of the 3β-hydroxysteroid dehydrogenase deficiency, the same ACTH stimulation test is utilized, measuring 17-OHP and 17-hydroxypregnenolone. An abnormal 17-hydroxypregnenolone/17-OHP ratio is usually greater than 6.0. This deficiency is also usually marked by a significant elevation of DHAS in the face of normal or mildly elevated testosterone levels. In the 11β-hydroxylase deficiency, the level of 11-deoxycortisol will be increased; it is normal with the 21-hydroxylase defect.

40. D p.501

The only diagnostic dilemma is when to explore the patient in whom a mass is not palpable. Suppression and stimulation tests are known to falsely lead to oophorectomy in the presence of a virilizing adrenal adenoma. In addition, suppression and stimulation methods do not specifically isolate ovarian or adrenal function. Ovarian androgen-producing tumors are usually responsive to LH and, therefore, will respond to ovarian suppression and stimulation.

Selective angiography with venous sampling and measurement of adrenal and ovarian steroids is not without problems. It is technically difficult to achieve bilateral catheterization of the ovaries, steroid secretion is episodic (especially by the adrenal glands), and the technique is not without risk. Selective retrograde catheterization of ovarian and adrenal veins by an expert should be reserved for those few patients who have been imaged with negative findings. Surgical exploration and bivalving of the ovaries may be necessary if the catheterization studies are negative.

When an androgen-producing tumor is suspected and an adnexal mass is not palpable, imaging of the adrenal glands and ovaries should be obtained. Imaging of the adrenal is a sensitive diagnostic technique for small tumors which produce Cushing's syndrome as well as for virilizing adrenal adenomas. (See figure on page 213 in this Study Guide)

41. E   p.501

In postmenopausal women with hyperandrogenism, it is usually appropriate to be more aggressive surgically; however, keep in mind that hyperinsulinemia in the postmenopausal years can stimulate hyperthecosis which would simulate the presentation of a tumor. GnRH agonist treatment can avoid surgery in these patients because insulin-induced steroidogenic activity in the ovary is still LH-dependent.

42. E   p.501

The size of an adrenal lesion is significant. The probability of malignancy roughly parallels the diameter of the lesion; a 2 cm lesion has a 20% chance of being malignant, an 8 cm lesion has an 80% probability. Bilateral lesions less than 3 cm usually are due to metastatic disease. Thus, the current recommendation is to excise unilateral masses if they are greater than 3 cm in diameter. Fine needle aspiration is also recommended for all unilateral adrenal lesions. When following a mass, imaging should be performed at 3, 9, and 18 months. Any mass which is stable after 18 months can be left in place.

43. A   p.501

Incidental adrenal masses require evaluation for biochemical function. The presence of hypertension raises the suspicion of Cushing's syndrome, hyperaldosteronism, or pheochromocytoma. The evaluation should include a screening test for pheochromocytoma (plasma catecholamines after clonidine), electrolyte and renin activity assessment for aldosteronism, a 24-hour urinary free cortisol, and a testosterone level. A relatively high incidence of cortisol-secreting tumors in the presence of normal 24-hour urinary free cortisol excretion indicates the need to perform an overnight dexamethasone suppression test in patients with asymptomatic incidental adrenal masses. There appears to be a high incidence of adrenal masses in patients with adrenal hyperplasia. These need not be removed surgically, but a laboratory evaluation for adrenal hyperplasia is, therefore, indicated in patients with incidental adrenal masses.

44. A   p.502

Almost all patients presenting with hirsutism represent excess androgen production in association with the steady state of persistent anovulation. Treatment is directed toward interruption of the steady state. In those patients who wish to become pregnant, ovulation can be induced. In patients in whom pregnancy is not desired, the steady state can be interrupted by suppression of ovarian steroidogenesis by utilizing the potent inhibitory action of progestational agents on LH.

45. B   p.505

Side effects are minimal, including diuresis in the first few days of use, occasional complaints of fatigue, and dysfunctional uterine bleeding. Remember that the anovulatory state requires progestational management in order to avoid abnormal uterine bleeding (and endometrial hyperplasia).

46. A   p.506

Cyproterone is a potent progestational agent that both inhibits gonadotropin secretion and blocks androgen action by binding to the androgen receptor. Because ovarian androgen production is LH-dependent, suppression of the pituitary with chronic GnRH agonist treatment improves hirsutism. However, inconsistent results in the literature attest to the fact that sufficient dosage must be administered to achieve effective suppression and clinical response. Therefore, monitoring dosage and response is recommended. We recommend the daily administration of 0.625 mg conjugated estrogens or 1.0 mg estradiol combined with 2.5 mg medroxyprogesterone acetate or 0.35 mg norethindrone, or, even better, an oral contraceptive. This method of treatment is relatively complicated and expensive and should be reserved

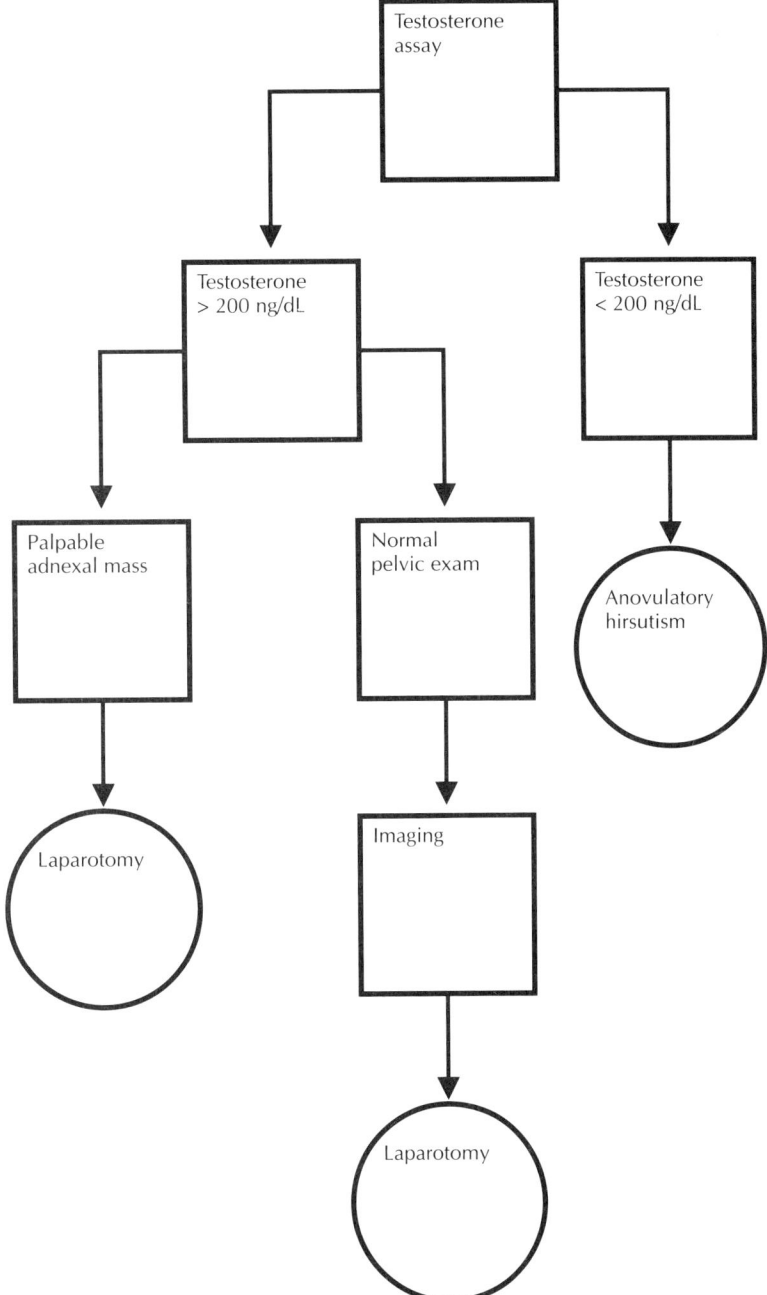

for the severe case of ovarian hyperandrogenism which is usually due to significant hyperthecosis and marked hyperinsulinemia (a condition that responds poorly to the usual methods of treatment).

Flutamide is a nonsteroidal antiandrogen that can be administered in a dose of 250 mg tid. Flutamide directly inhibits hair growth without significant side effects. Comparison studies with other treatments for hirsutism are not available. Treatment with flutamide should be combined with a method of contraception.

15 Menstrual Disorders

Learning Objectives

Be able to:

1. Define the premenstrual syndrome.

2. Understand the potential limitations and pitfalls of clinical research in the field of PMS.

3. Detail some of the ineffective and effective treatments of PMS.

Pre-Test

A. Instructions: Fill in the blanks

1. In treating PMS the patient and physician must be convinced the problem is _____ in timing.

2. About _____% of dysmenorrheic women are relieved by prostaglandin inhibitors.

B. Instructions: True or False

3. Spironolactone has not been shown to be effective treatment in PMS in double-blinded, placebo-controlled trials.

4. Many treatments for PMS are empiric and subject to a placebo response.

C. Instructions: For the following question choose:
   A. if only 1, 2 and 3 are correct
   B. if only 1 and 3 are correct
   C. if only 2 and 4 are correct
   D. if only 4 is correct
   E. if all are correct

5. Each of the following have failed to demonstrate any benefit over placebo
   1. oral contraceptives
   2. vitamin B_6
   3. bromocriptine
   4. synthetic progestational agents

Post-Test

A. Instructions: Fill in the blanks

1. The American Psychiatric Association refers to premenstrual syndrome (PMS) as the _____ _____ _____ disorder.

2. In PMS, symptoms are temporarily related to the menstrual cycle, beginning during the last week of the _____ phase and remitting after the _____ of menses.

3. PMS studies prior to 1983 did not incorporate appropriate diagnostic _____ and therefore, suffer from inaccuracy and heterogeneity.

4. The only instrument of diagnosis for PMS available at present is the _____ _____.

5. Exacerbation of seizure activity with menses occurs in _____% of epileptic women.

6. Intramuscular injections of _____ can decrease catamenial seizures.

B. Instructions: True or False

7. Using the National Institute of Mental Health and the American Psychiatric Association criteria, it is estimated that about 15% of women of reproductive age can be diagnosed with PMS.

8. Studies on premenstrual symptoms which have appropriate controls and statistical treatment find no significant variation associated with the menstrual cycle for cognitive or motor behavior.

9. In general, thyroid function is normal in patients with PMS.

10. The only effective treatments presently available for PMS are medical and/or surgical oophorectomy, and antidepressant therapy.

11. If dysmenorrhea is not relieved by one of the nonsteroidal anti-inflammatory analgesics, laparoscopy should be seriously considered to determine the cause of the symptoms.

12. Migraine headaches have a peak incidence at age 39–45 and are common after menopause.

13. True severe vascular headaches are an indication to discontinue oral contraception.

C. Instructions: Match each phrase with the appropriate item.

A. vascular headaches
B. secondary headaches
C. tension headaches

14. pain is dull, steady, bilateral, worsens throughout the day
15. due to underlying organic disease
16. acute and throbbing, may be precipitated by tyramine- or tryptophan-rich foods
17. cyclic

D. Instructions: For each of the following questions choose:

A. if only 1, 2 and 3 are correct
B. if only 1 and 3 are correct
C. if only 2 and 4 are correct
D. if only 4 is correct
E. if all are correct

18. The following may have benefit in the treatment of PMS
    1. GnRH agonist plus add back therapy
    2. fluoxetine and alprazolam
    3. oophorectomy
    4. lithium

19. The problems and challenges regarding research done in the field of PMS include
    1. the fact that clinical symptoms are variable, difficult to quantitate and many in number
    2. a discrepancy between retrospective and prospective accounts of symptoms by study subjects
    3. the fact that experimenter expectancy effect has to be properly controlled
    4. a high placebo response

20. Dysmenorrhea
    1. has been shown to be present in over 70% of a random sample of 19-year-old women
    2. may be due to prostaglandin E
    3. is accompanied by an increase in endometrial production of prostaglandins
    4. is usually not associated with headaches, nausea, backache or diarrhea

21. Treatment options for dysmenorrhea include
    1. alprazolam
    2. nonsteroidal anti-inflammatory agents
    3. GnRH-agonist
    4. oral contraceptives

22. Prostaglandin inhibitors
    1. relieve symptoms associated with menses specifically backache, dizziness, headache
    2. should be attempted up to 3 months before abandoning because of lack of a response
    3. are just as effective if begun at the sign of first bleeding rather than 3 days before menses
    4. have a minimal benefit with regard to amount of blood lost

23. Conditions associated with dysmenorrhea include
    1. pelvic inflammatory disease
    2. müllerian duct anomalies
    3. endometriosis
    4. adenomyosis

Answers for Chapter 15 — Pre-Test Questions

1. cyclic   p.522
The first step is to be convinced (both patient and physician) that the problem is cyclic.

2. 80   p.524
About 80% of dysmenorrheic women are relieved by prostaglandin inhibitors. Improvement is noted in the symptoms associated with menses, specifically cramping, backache, nausea, vomiting, dizziness, leg pain, insomnia, and headache.

3. true   p.520
The use of spironolactone has many advocates, especially for women with a major complaint of bloating; however, appropriate double-blind, placebo-controlled trials have failed to demonstrate a clinical impact greater than placebo.

4. true   p.523
Studies are complicated by high placebo responses. Clinical studies of premenstrual syndrome typically demonstrate a 30–50% response to placebo and, if a positive effect is anticipated by the subjects, up to 80%. Only well-designed, double-blind, placebo-controlled, randomized trials yield reliable data.

5. E   p.520
Various methods of treatment have been proposed, each championing a presumed etiology. All of the following have

failed to demonstrate any clear-cut benefits over placebo: oral contraceptives, vitamin B_6, bromocriptine, monoamine oxidase inhibitors, and synthetic progestational agents.

Answers for Chapter 15 — Post-Test Questions

1. luteal phase dysphoric   p.516

There are two established guidelines for the diagnosis of PMS. The first is from the American Psychiatric Association (APA) and consists of the criteria for what the APA has designated as the luteal phase dysphoric disorder.

2. luteal; onset   p.516

   A. Symptoms are temporally related to the menstrual cycle, beginning during the last week of the luteal phase and remitting after the onset of menses.

   B. The diagnosis requires at least 5 of the following, and one of the symptoms must be either one of the first 4:

      1. Affective lability, e.g., sudden onset of being sad, tearful, irritable, or angry.
      2. Persistent and marked anger or irritability.
      3. Marked anxiety or tension.
      4. Markedly depressed mood, feelings of hopelessness.
      5. Decreased interest in usual activities.
      6. Easy fatigability or marked lack of energy.
      7. Subjective sense of difficulty in concentrating.
      8. Marked change in appetite, overeating, or food craving.
      9. Hyersomnia or insomnia.
      10. Physical symptoms such as breast tenderness, headaches, edema, joint or muscle pain, weight gain.

   C. The symptoms interfere with work or usual activities or relationships.

   D. The symptoms are not an exacerbation of another psychiatric disorder.

3. criteria   p.519

Studies prior to 1983 did not incorporate appropriate diagnostic criteria and, therefore, suffer from inaccuracy and heterogeneity. Since 1983, efforts to isolate a specific pathophysiologic mechanism have failed to demonstrate differences between women with and without symptoms for all hormone levels throughout the menstrual cycle (including estrogens, progesterone, testosterone, follicle-stimulating hormone [FSH], luteinizing hormone [LH], prolactin, and sex hormone binding globulin) or weight gain and measurements of substances involved in fluid regulation, such as aldosterone. This further includes both the circulating levels as well as the pattern of secretion over the menstrual cycle. Dynamic testing has revealed no abnormalities in the hypothalamic-pituitary axis and its relationships with the adrenal glands, the thyroid gland, and the ovaries. No differences can be detected in magnesium, zinc, vitamin A, vitamin E, thiamin, or vitamin B_6. Some have argued for a greater change in endorphins, proposing that the luteal phase symptom complex is due to a greater withdrawal from endogenous opioids (in effect, an autoaddiction and withdrawal), but others have been unable to detect a difference in circulating endorphins in symptomatic patients.

4. menstrual calendar   p.522

The only instrument of diagnosis available at the present time is the menstrual calendar. At least 3 months of prospective recording, aided if possible by other observers (such as family members), are necessary in order to document a recurring problem in the luteal phase of the cycle, interfering with work or lifestyle, and followed by a period entirely free of symptoms. This time period should be utilized to develop a solid patient-physician relationship and, in so doing, to provide as much education as possible for the patient.

5. 50   p.527

Catemenial epilepsy in ancient times was attributed to the moon, giving rise to the word, "lunatic." Epileptic seizures increase in frequency during menstruation and decrease during the luteal phase. Exacerbation of seizure activity with menses occurs in 50% of epileptic women. In addition, seizure frequency increases at the time of the midcycle peak in estrogen and during anovulatory cycles. In animal experiments, estrogen increases seizure activity and progesterone is antiepileptic. These observations suggest an antiepileptic effect of progesterone.

6. depot-medroxyprogesterone acetate   p.527

The administration of oral medroxyprogesterone acetate has little impact, but intramuscular injections of depot-medroxyprogesterone acetate can improve seizure control. Depot-medroxyprogesterone acetate, 150 mg im every 1–2 months, can decrease seizure frequency by approximately 50%. In a case report of an 8-year-old girl, 150 mg administered every 2 weeks abolished seizure activity. Intravenous progesterone (producing luteal phase levels) can produce a significant decrease in spike frequency.

7. false   p.516

The guidelines from the National Institute of Mental Health (NIMH) state that the diagnosis of PMS requires the documentation of at least a 30% increase in severity of symptoms in the 5 days prior to menses compared with the 5 days following menses. Using the NIMH and APA criteria, it is estimated that about 5% of women of reproductive age can be diagnosed with PMS.

8. true   p.518

Dalton has argued that PMS is responsible for an increased incidence of crime, jailing for alcoholism, school misdemeanors, sickness in industry, hospitalization for accidents, and general hospital admissions. However studies on premenstrual symptoms which have appropriate controls and statistical treatment find no significant variation associated with the menstrual cycle for cognitive or motor behavior. Social behavior (including crime and suicide) reveals effects similar to all others seen in self-report studies. When social or psychological expectations are altered, the effect disappears. PMS is likely to be accepted by courts in the same manner that factors related to social and psychological stress or physical illness are accepted, and such factors do not absolve the accused of criminal responsibility.

9. true   p.519

There have been reported differences in various biologic factors, but these differences are not always confined to the luteal phases. Some of these factors, besides the endorphins, include the response to thyrotropin releasing hormone (TRH), melatonin secretion, red blood cell magnesium levels, growth hormone and cortisol responses to tryptophan, cortisol response to corticotropin releasing hormone, free cortisol secretion, and cortisol secretion patterns.

10. true   p.520

A lasting response to surgical hysterectomy and oophorectomy was reported in women unresponsive to medical therapy. Gonadotropin-releasing hormone (GnRH) agonist treatment can produce hypogonadotropic hypogonadism, in effect, a medical oophorectomy. GnRH agonist treatment has been effective; adding estrogen-progestin to avoid the side effects of the GnRH agonist diminished somewhat the improvement in symptoms. However, the beneficial impact was still considerable. While medical and surgical oophorectomy is undoubtedly effective, it is impossible to blind such treatment, and the mechanism is therefore uncertain. In the GnRH agonist-steroid addback study, patients receiving a placebo instead of estrogen-progestin had a return of symptoms (despite continued GnRH agonist treatment), probably in anticipation of a negative reaction to estrogen-progestin. This experience is a strong statement of the power of the placebo response (in this case, a negative response).

The only randomized trials, double-blinded and placebo-controlled, which have had consistent, excellent results are those with the antidepressants, fluoxetine (Prozac) and alprazolam (Xanax).

11. true   p.525

If dysmenorrhea is not relieved by one of the nonsteroidal, anti-inflammatory analgesics, laparoscopy should be seriously considered to determine the cause of the symptoms. Conditions associated with dysmenorrhea include müllerian duct anomalies, endometriosis, and pelvic inflammatory disease.

12. false   p.525

Migraine headaches have a peak incidence of first occurrence at age 15–19, and they are rare after menopause. An association with menses is observed by 60% of women with migraine headaches. In 14% of women with migraine, headaches occur exclusively with menses. Because menstrual migraine improves in two-thirds of migraineurs with pregnancy, this type of migraine seems to be due to falling levels of estrogen and progesterone.

13. true   p.526

A problem of severe headaches on oral contraception requires an immediate response. The conservative reaction is to discontinue the oral contraceptives. On the other hand, the headache can be due to stress or some other reversible condition. We would argue that automatic discontinuation of oral contraception is not necessary with the low dose preparations. It would be better to evaluate the patient and find out if the patient can continue her contraceptive protection, by discovering an explanation for the headaches. Case-control studies with the old higher dose oral contraceptives indicated that migraine headaches were linked to a risk of stroke. Strokes are essentially no longer seen with low dose oral contraception. This probably reflects both lower dosage as well as the reluctance of clinicians to prescribe oral contraception to women with severe headaches.

14. C   p.525

The common tension headache is due to prolonged and excessive muscle contraction. The pain is dull, steady, bilateral, and worsens throughout the day.

15. B   p.525

Secondary headaches are due to underlying organic disease. The pain is usually due to pressure or pulling of structures. Headaches associated with brain tumors are usually accompanied by neurologic abnormalities. Other causes are brain abscesses, subdural hematomas, hypertension, drug-use, and concussions. The main cause of inflammatory headaches is meningitis.

16. A   p.525

Acute and throbbing headaches are due to abnormal vasodilatation. The vasodilatation associated with migraine headaches is believed to follow a period of vasoconstriction. Migraine headaches are usually, but not always, preceded by prodromal symptoms (which may reflect the period of vasoconstriction). Significant vascular headaches can be precipitated by stress, alcohol, or tyramine- and tryptophan-rich foods (red wine, chocolate, ripe cheeses). Vascular headaches can accompany other problems, such as systemic viral infections, fever, or hypertension. Common migraine headaches are known as "migraine without aura." Classic migraine is referred to as "migraine with aura."

17. A   p.525

An association with menses is observed by 60% of women with migraine headaches. In 14% of women with migraine, headaches occur exclusively with menses.

18. A   p.520,521

Medical and surgical oophorectomy has been described to have dramatic success. A dose (20–60 mg daily) of fluoxetine (which inhibits neuronal uptake of serotonin) effectively abolished symptoms without side effects. Alprazolam is a short-acting benzodiazepine with anxiolytic, antidepressant, and smooth muscle relaxant properties. A dose of 0.25 mg bid-tid during the luteal phase is very effective. In contrast, lithium has no effect.

19. E   p.521,522

The problems and questions are many:

1. The clinical symptoms are variable, difficult to quantitate, and enormous in number. The symptoms cover emotions, sexual feelings, mood states, behavioral changes, and somatic complaints. Despite multiple questionnaires, we are still not convinced that there exists a reliable, objective method for observing and measuring symptoms that are experienced internally, rather than manifested via external behavior.
2. The discrepancy between retrospective and prospective accounts regarding cyclic changes is now well-documented and recognized. Women use menses as a marker of time, and unpleasant, easily

remembered experiences are attributed to an easily recognized signpost. If women in our culture have been conditioned to expect symptoms in the premenstrual phase and have been taught to expect fluid retention, pain, and emotional reactions, that is precisely what will be reported. Our lives are rhythmical. Day alternates with night. There are sleeping and waking, being hungry and being full, the circadian rhythms of our glands, and the ultimate rhythm: the sexual cycle. It is the most natural thing to seek a rhythm for our behavior.

The Ruble study is now a classic. In this study, 44 undergraduates at Princeton University were deliberately deceived about which phase of the menstrual cycle they were experiencing. A bogus electroencephalogram, complete with electrodes attached to the head, was heralded as a new technique capable of predicting the date of menstruation. Subjects were told they were either premenstrual (due in 1–2 days) or intermenstrual (due in 7–10 days). Only those women who were led to believe that their period would begin in 2 days reported significantly higher symptom ratings on pain, water retention, and eating habit changes. This was interpreted as a reflection of stereotypic expectations.

3. Is there a specific syndrome? A syndrome must have a specific pathophysiology; specific signs and symptoms can be documented; and a specific treatment achieves a beneficial response. Not a single one of these criteria can be met. One of the basic problems is that we have lumped everything into PMS, including behavioral changes, somatic complaints, and psychological problems, implying the existence of a specific syndrome. Part of the problem is that all the tools of research reflect the way the author of the tool conceptualizes PMS, which in turn is based upon the background and training of the author.

4. The experimenter expectancy effect has to be properly controlled. Subjects tend to comply with what they deem to be the experimenter's hypothesis. This has been studied in regard to PMS, and no significant difference in PMS symptomatology can be demonstrated when the purpose of the study is disguised, and in addition the responses can be influenced by positive or negative manipulations. This relates to findings of negative mood changes when subjects are asked to assess their menstrual distress retrospectively.

5. Studies are complicated by high placebo responses. Clinical studies of premenstrual syndrome typically demonstrate a 30–50% response to placebo and, if a positive effect is anticipated by the subjects, up to 80%. Only well-designed, double-blind, placebo-controlled, randomized trials yield reliable data.

20. B p.524

Dysmenorrhea is pain with menstruation, usually cramping in nature and centered in the lower abdomen. Studies on the prevalence of dysmenorrhea are few. In a random sample of 19-year-old women in Gothenburg, Sweden, 72% reported dysmenorrhea, 15% had to limit their daily activity and the severity was unimproved by analgesics, 8% missed school or work at every menses, and 38.2% regularly used medical treatment. Primary dysmenorrhea, a condition associated with ovulatory cycles, is due to myometrial contractions induced by prostaglandins originating in secretory endometrium, while secondary dysmenorrhea is associated with a variety of pathological conditons. Other symptoms associated with menstrual flow, such as headache, nausea and vomiting, backache, and diarrhea, can be explained by entry of the prostaglandins and prostaglandin metabolites into the systemic circulation. There is a 3-fold increase in prostaglandin levels in the endometrium from the follicular phase to the luteal phase, with a further increase during menstruation. Women with primary dysmenorrhea have greater endometrial production of prostaglandins compared to asymptomatic women. Most of the release of prostaglandins during menstruation occurs during the first 48 hours, which coincides with the greatest intensity of the symptoms.

Prostaglandin $F_{2\alpha}$ ($PGF_{2\alpha}$) is the agent responsible for dysmenorrhea. It always stimulates uterine contractions, while the E prostaglandins inhibit contractions in the nonpregnant uterus. Uterine muscle from both normal and dysmenorrheic women is sensitive to $PGF_{2\alpha}$, but the amount of $PGF_{2\alpha}$ produced is the major differentiating factor.

21. C p.524

The clinical benefit derived from the pharmacologic use of inhibitors of prostaglandin synthesis depends upon a significant decrease in prostaglandin production in the endometrium. An additional role may be attributed to decreased prostaglandins from the platelets participating in the clotting of menstrual blood. The explanation for the benefit seen with oral contraceptives is decreased prostaglandin synthesis associated with the atrophic decidualized endometrium. Oral contraception is a good choice for therapy, combining contraception with a beneficial impact on dysmenorrhea, menstrual flow, and menstrual irregularity. In women who do not desire hormonal contraception, the best therapy is one of the agents that inhibit prostaglandin synthesis.

22. B p.524

About 80% of dysmenorrheic women are relieved by prostaglandin inhibitors. Improvement is noted in the symptoms associated with menses, specifically cramping, backache, nausea, vomiting, dizziness, leg pain, insomnia, and headache. A trial of up to 6 months is warranted, with necessary changes in dosage and inhibitors, before abandoning this therapy. Initially it was felt that better relief was achieved if treatment was started 2–3 days before menses in order to lower the tissue level of prostaglandins before breakdown of the endometrium. Fortunately, studies have indicated that treatment is just as effective if begun at the sign of first bleeding, thus decreasing the possibility of taking one of these agents early in pregnancy. Another benefit of prostaglandin inhibition is a reduction in the amount of blood lost with periods. Indeed the agents may be used to treat idiopathic menorrhagia, or the excess flow associated with an intrauterine device (IUD). Most women do not need to take the medication more than 2–3 days.

23. E p.525

If dysmenorrhea is not relieved by one of the nonsteroidal, anti-inflammatory analgesics, laparoscopy should be seriously considered to determine the cause of the symptoms. Conditions associated with dysmenorrhea include müllerian duct anomalies, endometriosis, and pelvic inflammatory disease. We should especially be aware that endometriosis occurs in adolescents; dysmenorrhea caused by endometriosis in adolescents usually begins 3 or more years after menarche.

16 Dysfunctional Uterine Bleeding

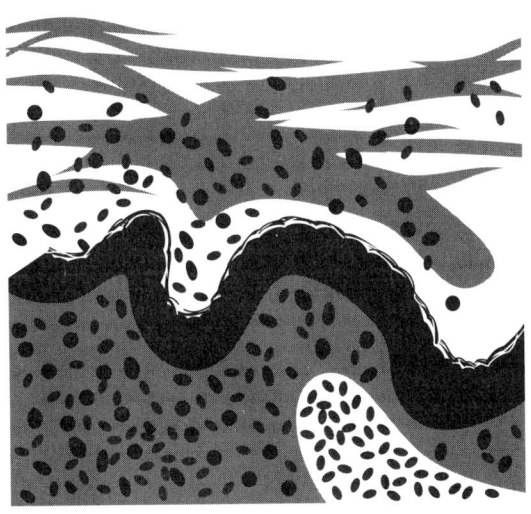

Learning Objectives

Be able to:

1. Describe the major categories of dysfunctional uterine bleeding and provide clinical examples of each.

2. Discuss the appropriate diagnostic tests in the workup of dysfunctional uterine bleeding.

3. Detail medical and surgical treatment options for dysfunctional uterine bleeding.

Clinical Gynecologic Endocrinology and Infertility: Self Assessment and Study Guide

Pre-Test

A. Instructions: Fill in the blank

1. Oral contraceptives can reduce menstrual flow by at least _____% in normal uteri.

B. Instructions: True or False

2. Most instances of anovulatory bleeding are examples of estrogen withdrawal or estrogen breakthrough bleeding.

C. Instructions: For the following question choose:

   A. if only 1, 2 and 3 are correct
   B. if only 1 and 3 are correct
   C. if only 2 and 4 are correct
   D. if only 4 is correct
   E. if all are correct

3. Treatment options for dysfunctional uterine bleeding in patients with chronic illnesses such as renal failure or blood dyscrasias include
   1. a GnRH agonist
   2. a levonorgestrel-releasing IUD
   3. desmopressin
   4. antiprostaglandins

Post-Test

A. Instructions: Fill in the blanks

1. Dysfunctional uterine bleeding is defined as a variety of bleeding manifestations of _____ cycles in the absence of pathology or medical illness.

2. The normal volume of menstrual blood loss is ___ml; greater than ___ml is abnormal.

3. _____ and _____ play a direct part in the hemostasis achieved in a bleeding menstrual endometrium.

4. The mechanisms of tissue breakdown as well as clearance of debris and restructuring of the endometrium are thought to proceed via sex steroid effects on the endometrial cell _____.

5. Dysfunctional uterine bleeding is a diagnosis made by _____.

6. Abnormal menstrual cycles are occasionally the first sign of either _____ or _____.

7. As many as _____% of adolescents with dysfunctional uterine bleeding have a coagulation defect.

8. Progesterone and progestins are powerful _____ when given in pharmacologic doses.

9. Excessive bleeding in women with menorrhagia can be reduced 40–50% using prostaglandin synthetase _____ .

B. Instructions: True or False

10. Bleeding secondary to a blood dyscrasia is usually a heavy flow with menorrhagia.

11. Irregular, serious bleeding is often associated with severe organ disease such as renal failure.

12. Clinical studies consistently support the concept of poststerilization menstrual changes.

13. Progestins have an antimitotic, antigrowth impact on the endometrium.

14. The concentrations of PGE_2 and $PGF_{2\alpha}$ decrease in human endometrium during the menstrual cycle.

15. Curettage is not the first line of defense, but rather the last for treatment of dysfunctional uterine bleeding.

C. Match each phrase with the appropriate clinical situation

A. estrogen withdrawal bleeding
B. estrogen breakthrough bleeding
C. progesterone withdrawal bleeding
D. progesterone breakthrough bleeding

16. removal of the corpus luteum
17. relatively low doses of estrogen yield spotting
18. occurs after bilateral oophorectomy
19. Norplant and Depo-Provera
20. radiation of mature follicles

D. Instructions: For each of the following questions choose:

A. if only 1, 2 and 3 are correct
B. if only 1 and 3 are correct
C. if only 2 and 4 are correct
D. if only 4 is correct
E. if all are correct

21. Endometrial intraepithelial neoplasm (EIN)
    1. is defined as hyperplasia with cytologic atypia
    2. is persistent after curettings on high dose progestin therapy in less than 50% of the cases
    3. is best treated surgically
    4. is not the same as atypical adenomatous hyperplasia

22. The heaviest bleeding is secondary to high sustained levels of estrogen associated with
    1. polycystic ovaries
    2. obesity
    3. immaturity of the hypothalamic-pituitary-ovarian axis
    4. late anovulation

23. Well tested treatment regimens for control of anovulatory bleeding include
    1. spironolactone
    2. medroxyprogesterone acetate 10 mg QD for 10 days each month
    3. danocrine
    4. oral contraceptives twice a day for 5–7 days followed by daily use in subsequent months beginning day 5

24. Depo-Provera may be used for
    1. endometriosis
    2. contraception
    3. prevention of menses during chemotherapy
    4. leiomyomata

25. Options for estrogen therapy in the treatment of dysfunctional uterine bleeding include
    1. 25 mg conjugated estrogens intravenously every 4 hours for acute and heavy bleeding
    2. 1.25 mg of conjugated estrogens daily for 7–10 days for mild bleeding
    3. 1.25 mg conjugated estrogens every 4 hours for 24 hours, followed by the single daily dose for 7–10 days for moderately heavy bleeding
    4. follow-up with progestin coverage to induce a withdrawal bleed

26. Estrogen therapy is useful in clinical situations associated with
    1. bleeding associated with polycystic ovarian disease
    2. breakthrough bleeding occurring with use of oral contraceptives
    3. bleeding associated with residual polyps
    4. breakthrough bleeding associated with depo-progestational agents

27. Ablation of the endometrium
    1. may be indicated if previous medical therapy has failed
    2. achieves improvement in 90% of women
    3. achieves amenorrhea in only 50% of women
    4. is accompanied by the long-term risk of the development of occult endometrial carcinoma

28. Workup for dysfunctional uterine bleeding includes
    1. a physical exam with attention to the appearance of acne, hirsutism, galactorrhea
    2. laboratory tests such as coagulation studies, HCG, thyroid function tests, prolactin
    3. endometrial biopsy
    4. MRI

29. Women who are ovulating but have menorrhagia can be treated with
    1. prostaglandin inhibitions
    2. progestins
    3. oral contraceptives
    4. danocrine

Answers for Chapter 16 — Pre-Test Questions

1. 60 p.538
In young women, anovulatory bleeding may be associated with prolonged endometrial buildup, delayed diagnosis, and heavy blood loss. In these cases, combined progestin-estrogen therapy is used in the form of oral contraceptives. Any of the low dose oral combination monophasic tablets are useful. Whatever formulation is available or chosen, therapy is administered as one pill twice a day for 5–7 days. This therapy is maintained despite cessation of flow within 12–

24 hours. If flow does not abate, other diagnostic possibilities (polyps, incomplete abortion, and neoplasia) should be reevaluated.

If flow does diminish rapidly, the remainder of the week of treatment can be given over to the evaluation of causes of anovulation, investigation of hemorrhagic tendencies, and blood replacement or initiation of iron therapy. In addition, the week provides time to prepare the patient for the estrogen-progestin withdrawal flow that will soon be induced. For the moment, therapy has produced the structural rigidity intrinsic to the compact pseudodecidual reaction. Continued random breakdown of formerly fragile tissue is avoided and blood loss stopped. However, a large amount of tissue remains to react to estrogen-progestin withdrawal. The patient must be warned to anticipate a heavy and severely cramping flow 2–4 days after stopping therapy. If not prepared in this way, it is certain that the patient will view the problem as recurrent disease or failure of hormonal therapy.

In successful therapy, on the 5th day of flow, a low dose combination oral contraceptive medication (one pill a day) is started. This will be repeated for several (usually three) 3-week treatments, punctuated by 1-week withdrawal flow intervals. A decrease in volume and pain with each successive cycle is reassuring. Birth control pills reduce menstrual flow by at least 60% in normal uteri. Early application of the estrogen-progestin combination limits growth and allows orderly regression of excessive endometrial height to normal controllable levels. If the estrogen-progestin combination is not applied, abnormal endometrial height and persistent excessive flow will recur.

2. true   p.535

Most instances of anovulatory bleeding are examples of estrogen withdrawal or estrogen breakthrough bleeding. The heaviest bleeding is secondary to high sustained levels of estrogen associated with polycystic ovaries, obesity, immaturity of the hypothalamic-pituitary-ovarian axis as in postpubertal teenagers, and late anovulation, usually involving women in their late 30s and early 40s. In the absence of growth limiting progesterone and periodic desquamation, the endometrium attains an abnormal height without concomitant structural support. The tissue increasingly displays intense vascularity, back to back glandularity, but without an intervening stromal support matrix. This tissue is fragile and will suffer spontaneous superficial breakage and bleeding. As one site heals, another, and yet another new site of breakdown will appear. The typical clinical picture is that of a pale frightened teenager who has bled for weeks. Also frequently encountered is the older woman with prolonged bleeding who is deeply concerned over this experience as a manifestation of cancer.

3. A   p.539,540

Whatever the exact mechanism, prostaglandin synthetase inhibitors diminish menstrual bleeding in normal women as well as in the bleeding secondary to intrauterine device (IUD) use. This approach should be considered as a first line of defense in the absence of pathology in those women who are ovulatory but bleed heavily. Side effects are unusual because treatment is limited, usually beginning with the onset of bleeding and continuing for 3–4 days. This treatment will also relieve the other symptoms of menstrual molimina.

The delivery of a progestational agent directly to the endometrium in a local fashion is possible with an intrauterine device which releases progesterone or levonorgestrel. In a comparison trial with a prostaglandin synthetase inhibitor and an antifibrinolytic agent, the levonorgestrel-releasing IUD outperformed the medical treatment dramatically. The reduction in menstrual flow reached 96% after 12 months, and some patients even become amenorrheic. This is an attractive option in patients with intractable bleeding associated with chronic illnesses (such as renal failure).

Treatment with a GnRH agonist can achieve short-term relief from a bleeding problem, for example, in a patient with renal failure or a blood dyscrasia. This choice is a good one for patients who experience menstrual bleeding problems after organ transplantation (especially after liver transplantation) where the toxicity of immunosuppressive drugs makes the use of sex steroids less desirable. However, the expense and long-term side effects make this an unlikely choice for chronic therapy. If long-term GnRH agonist therapy is chosen, after gonadal suppression is achieved (2–4 weeks), we recommend addback treatment with a daily combination of 0.625 mg conjugated estrogens or 1.0 mg estradiol and 2.5 mg medroxyprogesterone acetate or 0.35 mg norethindrone.

Desmopressin is a synthetic analogue of arginine vasopressin. It has been used to treat abnormal uterine bleeding in patients with coagulation disorders. It can be administered intranasally, but the intravenous route (0.3 mg/kg diluted in 50 mL saline and administered over 15–30 minutes) is more effective. Treatment is followed by a rapid increase in coagulation factor VIII which lasts approximately 6 hours. This treatment should be regarded as a last resort for selected patients with coagulation problems.

Answers for Chapter 16 — Post-Test Questions

1. anovulatory p.531

Dysfunctional uterine bleeding is defined as a variety of bleeding manifestations of anovulatory cycles (in the absence of pathology or medical illness). It can be confidently managed without surgical intervention by therapeutic regimens founded on sound physiologic principles. Our formulation is based on knowledge of how the postovulatory menstrual function is naturally controlled, and utilizes pharmacologic application of sex steroids to reverse the abnormal tissue factors that lead to the excessive and prolonged flow typical of anovulatory cycles.

2. 30; 80 p.532

Of all the types of hormonal-endometrial relationships, the most stable endometrium and the most reproducible menstrual function in terms of quantity and duration occurs with postovulatory estrogen-progesterone withdrawal bleeding. It is so controlling that many women over the years come to expect a certain characteristic flow pattern. Any slight deviations, such as plus or minus 1 day in duration or minor deviation from expected napkin or tampon utilization, are causes for major concern in the patient. So ingrained is the expected flow that considerable physician reassurance may be required in some instances of minor variability. The usual duration of flow is 4–6 days, but many women flow as little as 2 days, and as much as 8 days. The normal volume of menstrual blood loss is 30 mL. Greater than 80 mL is abnormal. Most of the blood loss occurs during the first 3 days of a period, so excessive flow may exist without prolongation of flow.

While the postovulatory phase averages 14 days, greater variability in the proliferative phase produces a distribution in the duration of a menstrual cycle. Based on the normal experience, menstrual bleeding more often than every 24 days or less often than every 35 days deserves evaluation. Flow which lasts 7 or more days also deserves evaluation. A flow that totals more than 80 mL per month usually leads to anemia and should be treated. In general, however, an effort to quantitate menstrual flow beyond historical information is not necessary because evaluation and treatment are responses to a patient's own perceptions regarding duration, amount, and timing of her menstrual bleeding. Midcycle bleeding can be a consequence of the preovulatory fall in estrogen; however, intermenstrual bleeding is often due to pathology.

3. Platelets; fibrin p.533

Platelets and fibrin play a direct part in the hemostasis achieved in a bleeding menstrual endometrium. Deficiencies in these constituents cause the increased blood loss seen in von Willebrand's disease and in thrombocytopenia. The blood loss at menses in afibrinogenemia indicates the importance of fibrin-generating and fibrinolytic factors in the menstrual process. Intravascular thrombi are observed in the functional layers and are localized to the shedding surface of the tissue. These are known as impeding "plugs" in that blood may flow past these only partially occlusive barriers. Therefore, thrombi continue to develop within the menstrual blood, accounting for the platelets and large amounts of fibrin found in this effluent. Fibrinolysis occurs in the endometrial tissue, limiting fibrin deposition in the proximal, still unshed layer. Despite large holes in vessel walls, with blood exposed to collagen surfaces, no occlusive surface thrombus is formed. After early dependence on thrombin plugs to restrain blood loss, later generalized vasoconstrictive hemostasis without thrombin plugs occur. The healing endometrium is pale, collapsed, and disorderly, but no thrombi and no fibrin deposits are seen.

4. lysosomes p.533

The mechanisms of tissue breakdown, as well as clearance of debris and restructuring of the endometrium, are thought to proceed via sex steroid effects on the endometrial cell lysosomes. With reduced steroids, lysosomal membrane destabilization and leakage of lysosomal prostaglandin synthetase enzymes, proteases, and collagenases occur. These cause breakdown of endometrial structures, dissolution of ground substance and cell walls, and vasoconstriction.

Further "liquefaction" permits efficient absorption and possible recycling of protein components.

5. exclusion p.536
Dysfunctional uterine bleeding is a diagnosis made by exclusion. A very common cause of abnormal uterine bleeding is pregnancy and pregnancy-related problems such as ectopic pregnancy or spontaneous abortion. This category of problems should always receive diagnostic consideration. Patients may be using medications unknowingly with an impact on the endometrium. For example, the use of ginseng, an herbal root, has been associated with estrogenic activity and abnormal bleeding. Pathology of the menstrual outflow tract includes cancers of the cervix and endometrium, endometrial polyps, and leiomyomata uteri. While uterine bleeding is a common problem with various contraceptive methods and postmenopausal hormonal therapy, the clinician should always be confident no pathology is present.

6. hypothyroidism; hyperthyroidism p.536
Abnormal menstrual cycles are occasionally the first sign of either hypothyroidism or hyperthyroidism.

7. 20 p.536
One should keep in mind that as many as 20% of adolescents with dysfunctional uterine bleeding will have a coagulation defect, although the most common cause is anovulation.

8. antiestrogens p.537
Progesterone and progestins are powerful antiestrogens when given in pharmacologic doses. Progestins stimulate 17β-hydroxysteroid dehydrogenase and sulfotransferase activity, which convert estradiol to estrone sulfate (which is rapidly excreted from the cell). Progestins also diminish estrogen effects on target cells by inhibiting the augmentation of estrogen receptors that ordinarily accompanies estrogen action (receptor replenishment inhibition). In addition, progestins suppress estrogen-mediated transcription of oncogenes.

9. inhibitors p.539,540
Excessive bleeding in women with menorrhagia can be reduced by approximately 40–50%. In a comparison study of ovulating women with menorrhagia, treatment during menses with a prostaglandin synthetase inhibitor was no more effective than high dose progestin supplementation during the 7 days preceding menstruation, but both treatments were effective. Occasionally a woman will demonstrate, for unknown reasons, an anomalous response to this treatment, with an increase in menstrual bleeding. A study of postoperative surgical specimens after mefenamic acid treatment revealed evidence of vasoconstriction and improved platelet aggregation.

10. true p.536
Bleeding secondary to a blood dyscrasia is usually a heavy flow with regular, cyclic menses (menorrhagia), and this same pattern can be seen in patients being treated with anticoagulants.

11. true p.536
Irregular, serious bleeding is often associated with severe organ disease, such as renal failure and liver failure. Finally, careful examination is worthwhile to discover genital injury or a foreign object.

12. false p.536
The effects of tubal ligation are still not certain. The first well-controlled studies of this issue demonstrated no change in menstrual patterns, volume, or pain. Subsequently, these same authors reported an increase in dysmenorrhea and changes in menstrual bleeding. However, these authors failed to agree in their findings (a change found by one group was not confirmed by the other). Adding to the confusion, the incidence of hysterectomy for bleeding disorders in women after tubal sterilization was reported to be increased by some, but not by others. In a large cohort of women in a group health plan, hospitalization for menstrual disorders was significantly increased; however, the authors believed this reflected bias by patient and physician preference for surgical treatment. It is possible that extensive electrocoagulation of the fallopian tubes can change ovarian steroid production. Perhaps this is why menstrual changes have been detected with longer (4 years) follow-up, while no changes have been noted with the use of rings or clips. However, attempts to relate poststerilization menstrual changes with extent of tissue destruction fail to find a correlation, and an increase in hospitalization for menstrual disorders after unipolar cautery cannot be documented. Still another long-term follow-up study (3–4.5 years) failed to document any significant changes in menstrual cycles. This inconsistency can

reflect differences in sterilization techniques, as well as the fact that a surgical solution is more likely to be chosen if continuing fertility is no longer an issue. The best answer for now is that some women experience menstrual changes, but most do not.

13. true   p.537

The cellular actions of progestins account for the antimitotic, antigrowth impact of progestins on the endometrium (prevention and reversal of hyperplasia, limitation of growth postovulation, and the marked atrophy during pregnancy or in response to combined oral contraceptives).

14. false   p.539

There seems little doubt that prostaglandins (PG) have important actions on the endometrial vasculature and presumably on endometrial hemostasis. The concentrations of PGE_2 and $PGF_{2\alpha}$ increase progressively in human endometrium during the menstrual cycle, and nonsteroidal eicosanoid synthesis inhibitors decrease menstrual blood loss perhaps by also altering the balance between the platelet proaggregating vasoconstrictor thromboxane A_2 (TXA_2) and the antiaggregating vasodilator prostacyclin (PGI_2).

15. true   p.542

Curettage is *not* the first line of defense, but rather the last. The utilization of appropriate steroids for the clinical management of dysfunctional bleeding is based upon a physiologic understanding of the endometrium and its responses to hormones. Adherence to this program will avoid D and C except in a rare case of dysfunctional bleeding and except in those cases where bleeding is due to a pathologic entity within the reproductive tract where D and C is truly indicated and necessary.

16. C   p.534

Removal of the corpus luteum will lead to endometrial desquamation. Pharmacologically, a similar event can be achieved by administration and discontinuation of progesterone or a nonestrogenic synthetic progestin. Progesterone withdrawal bleeding occurs only if the endometrium is initially proliferated by endogenous or exogenous estrogen. If estrogen therapy is continued as progesterone is withdrawn, the progesterone withdrawal bleeding still occurs. Only if estrogen levels are increased 10–20-fold will progesterone withdrawal bleeding be delayed.

17. B   p.534

A semiquantitative relationship exists between the amount of estrogen stimulating the endometrium and the type of bleeding that can ensue. Relatively low doses of estrogen yield intermittent spotting that may be prolonged, but is generally light in quantity of flow. On the other hand, high levels of estrogen and sustained availability lead to prolonged periods of amenorrhea followed by acute, often profuse bleeds with excessive loss of blood.

18. A   p.534

Estrogen withdrawal bleeding can occur after bilateral oophorectomy, radiation of mature follicles, or administration of estrogen to a castrate and then discontinuation of therapy. Similarly, the bleeding that occurs postcastration can be delayed by concomitant estrogen therapy. Flow will occur on discontinuation of exogenous estrogen. Midcycle bleeding can occur secondary to the decrease in estrogen which immediately precedes ovulation.

19. D   p.534

Progesterone breakthrough bleeding occurs only in the presence of an unfavorably high ratio of progesterone to estrogen. In the absence of sufficient estrogen, continuous progesterone therapy will yield intermittent bleeding of variable duration, similar to low dose estrogen breakthrough bleeding noted above. This is the type of bleeding associated with the long-acting progestin-only contraceptive methods, Norplant and Depo-Provera.

20. A   p.534

Radiation of mature ovarian follicles can cause an abrupt loss of estrogen, followed by estrogen withdrawal bleeding.

21. B   p.534

Hyperplasia without atypia can be referred to as *endometrial hyperplasia*, and this is usually not a precursor of carcinoma. Lesions with cytologic atypia should be referred to as *endometrial intraepithelial neoplasia (EIN)*. In these cases, persistence after multiple curettings or high dose progestin therapy is approximately 75%. EIN would replace the following terms: atypical adenomatous hyperplasia and carcinoma in situ of the endometrium. This lesion is characterized by nuclear atypia of the cells lining the endometrial glands (enlargement, rounding, and pleomorphism of the nuclei with aneuploid DNA content). Invasive carcinoma is distinguished from EIN by stromal invasion.

22. E p.535

Most instances of anovulatory bleeding are examples of estrogen withdrawal or estrogen breakthrough bleeding. The heaviest bleeding is secondary to high sustained levels of estrogen associated with polycystic ovaries, obesity, immaturity of the hypothalamic-pituitary-ovarian axis as in postpubertal teenagers, and late anovulation, usually involving women in their late 30s and early 40s. In the absence of growth limiting progesterone and periodic desquamation, the endometrium attains an abnormal height without concomitant structural support. The tissue increasingly displays intense vascularity, back to back glandularity, but without an intervening stromal support matrix. This tissue is fragile and will suffer spontaneous superficial breakage and bleeding. As one site heals, another, and yet another new site of breakdown will appear. The typical clinical picture is that of a pale frightened teenager who has bled for weeks. Also frequently encountered is the older woman with prolonged bleeding who is deeply concerned over this experience as a manifestation of cancer.

23. C p.537

In the treatment of oligomenorrhea, orderly limited withdrawal bleeding can be accomplished by administration of a progestin such as medroxyprogesterone acetate, 10 mg daily for 10 days every month. Absence of induced bleeding requires workup. In the treatment of dysfunctional menometrorrhagia or polymenorrhea, progestins are prescribed for 10 days to 2 weeks (to induce stabilizing predecidual stromal changes) followed by a withdrawal flow — the so-called "medical curettage." Thereafter, repeat progestin is offered cyclically the first 10 days of each month to ensure therapeutic effect. Failure of progestin to correct irregular bleeding requires diagnostic reevaluation. *If contraception is desired, the use of an oral contraceptive is a better choice.*

24. A p.539

Depo-Provera is used not only for contraception, but also in the treatment of endometriosis and the prevention of menses during chemotherapy. In 75% of recipients, continuous therapy is not associated with abnormal menstrual bleeding. In the remainder, breakthrough progestin bleeding occurs. Judicious use of estrogen is the appropriate and effective therapy in these instances.

25. E p.538,539,541

When bleeding is acute and heavy, high dose estrogen therapy is applied using as much as 25 mg conjugated estrogen intravenously every 4 hours until bleeding abates or for 24 hours. This is the sign that the "healing" events are initiated to a sufficient degree. The mechanism of action for estrogen is believed to be a stimulus to clotting at the capillary level. Progestin treatment (usually an oral contraceptive) is started at the same time. Where bleeding is less, lower oral doses of estrogen (1.25 mg of conjugated estrogens or 2.0 mg estradiol daily for 7–10 days) can be prescribed initially. When bleeding is moderately heavy, a more intensive oral program can be utilized, 1.25 mg conjugated estrogens or 2 mg estradiol every 4 hours for 24 hours, followed by the single daily dose for 7–10 days. All estrogen therapy must be followed by progestin coverage and a withdrawal bleed.

If bleeding has been prolonged, if biopsy yields minimal tissue, if the patient is on progestin medication, if follow-up is uncertain:

Conjugated estrogens (1.25 mg) or estradiol (2.0 mg) daily for 7–10 days, followed by the daily estrogen combined with 10 mg medroxyprogesterone acetate for 7 days. If acute bleeding is moderately heavy, the oral estrogen dose can be administered every 4 hours during the first 24 hours. For very heavy, acute bleeding, conjugated estrogen, 25 mg intravenously every 4 hours until bleeding stops or significantly slows. If no response in 12–24 hours, proceed to D and C.

26. C p.539,542

Estrogen therapy is useful in two examples of problems associated with progestin breakthrough bleeding. These are the breakthrough bleeding episodes occurring with use of oral contraception or with depot forms of progestational agents.

In the absence of sufficient endogenous and exogenous estrogen, the endometrium shrinks by pharmacologically induced pseudoatrophy. Furthermore, it is composed almost exclusively of pseudodecidual stroma and blood vessels with minimal glands. Peculiarly, experience has shown that this type of endometrium also leads to the fragility bleeding more typical of pure estrogen stimulation.

The initial choice of therapy should be estrogen in the following situations:

1. When bleeding has been heavy for many days and it is likely that the uterine cavity is now lined only by a raw basalis layer.
2. When the endometrial curet yields minimal tissue.
3. When the patient has been on progestin medication (oral contraceptives, intramuscular progestins) and the endometrium is shallow and atrophic.
4. When follow-up is uncertain, because estrogen therapy will temporarily stop all categories of dysfunctional bleeding.

27. E p.540,541

Persistent bleeding despite treatment is both aggravating and concerning. Hysterectomy is an appropriate choice for some of these patients. Others would prefer to avoid a major operation, and still others have conditions that make major surgery a high risk procedure. Patients and clinicians should consider the option of endometrial ablation. Ablation of the endometrium can be accomplished with either a laser, a resectoscope with a loop or rolling ball electrode, or radio frequency-induced thermal destruction. Success with these methods is not 100%. Approximately 90% of women with menorrhagia will have an improvement following an ablation procedure; only 50% will become amenorrheic. The best results are obtained if the endometrium is first suppressed for 4–6 weeks with either a high dose of a progestin, GnRH agonist treatment, or danazol. Caution must be exercised regarding the possiblity of excessive absorption of irrigating fluid with subsequent fluid overload.

There is concern that obliteration of segments of the uterine cavity can allow isolated, residual endometrium to progress to carcinoma without recognition. Long-term follow-up will be necessary before we know if this is a real risk.

28. A p.542

Laboratory tests which are often helpful (but not always necessary) are coagulation studies (prothrombin time, partial thromboplastin time, platelet count, bleeding time), quantitative human chorionic gonadotropin (HCG), prolactin, thyroid function tests, liver function tests, and appropriate cervical cultures.

Office aspiration biopsy of the endometrium should always be performed in patients considered to be at high risk for endometrial hyperplasia and cancer. Texts and review articles continue to emphasize that endometrial biopsy is in order if the patient is older, e.g., greater than 35 or 40 years old. *It is not the age of the patient that is critical; it is the duration of exposure to unopposed estrogen. Women in their 20s and even teenagers can develop endometrial cancer.* The small flexible suction canulas are preferred for greater patient comfort, and results are comparable to the older, traditional methods. Office hysteroscopy is also useful for the direction of biopsies and the detection of polyps and submucous myomas.

29. A p.543

Patients who are ovulating but have a heavy menstrual flow (menorrhagia) can be effectively treated with prostaglandin inhibitors, progestins administered daily for the 7 days preceding menses, or oral contraceptives in the routine manner. If contraception is not required, we prefer the use of one of the fenamate prostaglandin inhibitors (which block both synthesis and prostaglandin receptors). The IUD which releases progesterone or a progestin should be considered in patients with chronic illnesses.

17 The Breast

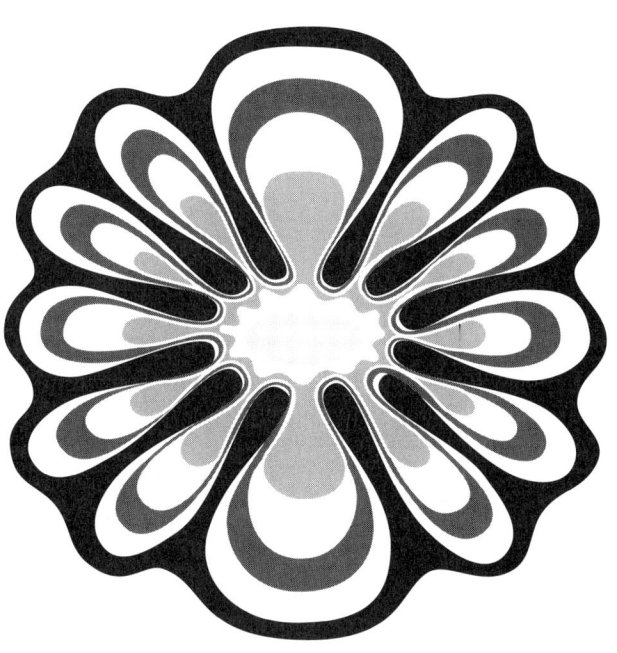

Learning Objectives

Be able to:

1. Describe the physiology and secretion pattern of prolactin during pregnancy, postpartum and during lactation.

2. Define galactorrhea and discuss the differential diagnosis, workup and management of this clinical problem.

3. Discuss the epidemiology, risk factors and current treatment recommendations for breast cancer.

Pre-Test

A. Instructions: Fill in the blanks

1. During pregnancy, prolactin levels arise from the normal level of _____ ng/ml to high concentrations beginning about 8 weeks and reaching a peak of _____ ng/ml at term.

2. Breast cancer is now viewed as a _____ disease, with spread to local and distant sites at the same time.

B. Instructions: True or False

3. Maternal prolactin does not pass to the fetus.

4. Medical therapy with dopamine agonists shrinks tumors, prevents growth and can completely eliminate microadenomas.

C. Instructions: For each of the following questions choose:

A. if only 1, 2 and 3 are correct
B. if only 1 and 3 are correct
C. if only 2 and 4 are correct
D. if only 4 is correct
E. if all are correct

5. A variety of drugs can inhibit hypothalamic prolactin inhibiting factor including
   1. tricyclic antidepressants
   2. amphetamines
   3. opiates
   4. spironolactone

6. Risk status for recurrence following treatment of breast cancer is determined by
   1. estrogen receptor status
   2. ploidy of tumor
   3. percent of cells in the S-phase fraction
   4. duration of initial chemotherapy

Post-Test

A. Instructions: Fill in the blanks

1. The failure to lactate within the first 7 days postpartum may be the first sign of _____ _____.

2. As a general rule approximately ____% of any drug ingested by the mother appears in the breast milk.

3. Prolactin is uniformly elevated in patients on therapeutic amounts of phenothiazines but never as high as _____ ng/ml.

4. If galactorrhea has been present for _____ months or hyperprolactinemia is noted in the process of working up menstrual disturbances, infertility or hirsutism, the probability of a pituitary tumor must be recognized.

5. For pregnancy to be protective of breast cancer it must occur before the age of_____.

6. In general, the increased risk of developing breast cancer with a positive family history is approximately _____ times the normal incidence.

7. When needle aspiration of a breast lump yields _____ or _____ fluid and the mass disappears, the procedure is both diagnostic and therapeutic.

8. All women over the age of _____ should have an annual breast examination.

9. Breast examination is most effective during the _____ phase of the cycle.

B. Instructions: True or False

10. There is marked variability in maternal prolactin levels in pregnancy, with a diurnal variation similar to that found in nonpregnant women.

11. Thyrotropin releasing hormone or dopamine receptor blockers can augment prolactin.

12. Secretion of calcium into the milk of lactating women is double the daily loss of calcium.

13. Suckling stimulates the formation of dopamine.

14. Routine use of a dopamine agonist for suppression of lactation is not recommended because of reports of hypertension, seizure and strokes associated with its postpartum use.

15. Galactorrhea refers to the mammary secretion of a milky fluid which is nonphysiologic, persistent and sometimes excessive.

16. Galactorrhea caused by excessive estrogens disappears within 2 months after discontinuing medication.

17. Stress can stimulate hypothalamic PIF.

18. Increased prolactin concentrations do not result from nonpituitary sources.

19. Microadenomas, if exclusively prolactin producing, rarely progress to macroadenoma size.

20. Danazol 200 mg/day is effective in relieving breast discomfort as well as decreasing nodularity of the breast.

21. Breast cancer is the leading cause of death from cancer in women.

22. At the present time there is no conclusive evidence that estrogen doses known to protect against osteoporosis and cardiovascular disease increase the risk of breast cancer.

23. Exposure to DES is not associated with an increase risk of breast cancer.

24. The presence of progesterone receptors has a correlation with disease free survival of patients only second to the number of positive nodes.

C. Instructions: For each of the following questions choose:

- A. if only 1, 2 and 3 are correct
- B. if only 1 and 3 are correct
- C. if only 2 and 4 are correct
- D. if only 4 is correct
- E. if all are correct

25. Hyperprolactinemia may be associated with a variety of menstrual cycle disturbances which include
    1. luteal phase defect
    2. amenorrhea
    3. oligoovulation
    4. anovulation

26. Risk factors associated with breast cancer include
    1. lactation
    2. amount of fat in diet
    3. age at which a woman bears her last full-term child
    4. amount of alcohol in diet

27. The "open window hypothesis" regarding breast cancer
    1. states that unopposed estrogen stimulation is the most favorable state for tumor induction
    2. is associated with two main open window periods which are puberty and time of the first pregnancy
    3. has not always been confirmed by clinical research
    4. explains the increase risk of breast cancer associated with a late onset of menarche

28. The presence of positive estrogen receptors
    1. are less likely in premenopausal and younger patients
    2. is associated with longer survival and longer disease-free intervals following mastectomy than those with receptor negative tumors
    3. correlate with increased disease free interval regardless of the presence of axillary nodes
    4. is associated with a more likely response to endocrine treatment

29. Adjuvant treatment for breast cancer includes
    1. chemotherapy
    2. ovarian ablation
    3. tamoxifen
    4. radiation

30. Tamoxifen
    1. is useful in postmenopausal women with estrogen receptor positive disease
    2. is useful often in patients who have been unresponsive to other endocrine treatment
    3. 20 mg is the standard daily dose
    4. is responsible for a 75% response rate for patients with ER positive tumors

31. Problems associated with tamoxifen include
    1. endometrial polyps
    2. endometrial hyperplasia
    3. symptomatic growth of endometriosis
    4. increase leiomyomata growth

32. Screening for breast cancer using a mammogram
    1. is associated with a false negative rate of 5–10%
    2. is associated with a 25% chance of cancer if more than 5 calcifications are clustered
    3. should be initiated at age 40 or earlier if high risk factors are present
    4. should be performed annually in all women over the age of 50

Answers for Chapter 17 — Pre-Test Questions

1. 10–25; 200–400   p.550,551

During pregnancy, prolactin levels rise from the normal level of 10–25 ng/mL (444–1,100 pmol/L) to high concentrations, beginning about 8 weeks and reaching a peak of 200–400 ng/mL (8,800–17,600 pmol/L) at term. The increase in prolactin parallels the increase in estrogen beginning at 7–8 weeks gestation, and the mechanism for increasing prolactin secretion is believed to be estrogen suppression of the hypothalamic prolactin inhibiting factor, dopamine, and direct stimulation of prolactin gene transcription in the pituitary.

2. systemic   p.563

Over the years breast cancer has continued a deadly impact despite advances in surgical and diagnostic techniques. Classically, the single most useful prognostic information in women with operable breast cancer has been the histologic status of the axillary lymph nodes. At 10 years only 25% of patients with positive nodes are free of disease compared to 75% of patients with negative nodes. If more than 3 nodes are involved, the 10-year survival rate drops from about 38% to 13%. Because of this recognition for the importance of the axillary nodes, the traditional approach to breast cancer (the Halsted surgical approach) was based on the concept that breast cancer is a disease of stepwise progression. ***There is an important change in concept. Breast cancer is now viewed as a systemic disease, with spread to local and distant sites at the same time. Breast cancer is best viewed as occultly metastatic at the time of presentation.*** Therefore, dissemination of tumor cells has occurred by the time of surgery in many patients.

3. true   p.551

Amniotic fluid concentrations of prolactin parallel maternal serum concentration until the 10th week of pregnancy, rise markedly until the 20th week, and then decrease. Maternal prolactin does not pass to the fetus in significant amounts. Indeed the source of amniotic fluid prolactin is neither the maternal pituitary nor the fetal pituitary. The failure of dopamine agonist treatment to suppress amniotic fluid prolactin levels, and studies with in vitro culture systems, indicate a primary decidual source with transfer via amnion receptors to the amniotic fluid, requiring the intactness of amnion, chorion, and adherent decidua. This decidual synthesis of prolactin is initiated by progesterone, but once decidualization is established, prolactin secretion continues in the absence of both progesterone and estradiol. Various decidual factors regulate prolactin synthesis and release, including relaxin, insulin, and insulin-like growth factor-I. It is hypothesized that amniotic fluid prolactin plays a role similar to its regulation of sodium transport and water movement across the gills in fish (allowing the ocean dwelling salmon and steelhead to return to freshwater streams for reproduction). Thus prolactin would protect the human fetus from dehydration by control of salt and water transport across the amnion. Prolactin reduces the permeability of the human amnion in the fetal to maternal direction by a receptor-mediated action on the epithelium lining the fetal surface.

4. false   p.560

Some tumors regress spontaneously. Medical therapy with dopamine agonists shrinks tumors and can prevent growth, although complete elimination of a tumor by dopamine agonist treatment does not occur, and rapid regrowth usually follows discontinuation of the drug.

5. A   p.556

A variety of drugs can inhibit hypothalamic PIF. There are nearly 100 phenothiazine derivatives with indirect mammotropic activity. In addition, there are many phenothiazine-like compounds, reserpine derivatives, amphetamines, and an unknown variety of other drugs (opiates, diazepams, butyrophenones, α-methyldopa, and tricyclic antidepressants) which can initiate galactorrhea via hypothalamic suppression. The final action of these compounds is either to deplete dopamine levels or to block dopamine receptors. Chemical features common to many of these drugs are an aromatic ring with a polar substituent as in estrogen and at least two additional rings or structural attributes making spatial arrangements similar to estrogen. Thus, these compounds may act in a manner similar to estrogens to decrease PIF or to act directly on the pituitary. In support of this conclusion, it has been demonstrated that estrogen and phenothiazine derivatives compete for the same receptors in the median eminence.

6. A   p.571

Definition of Low Risk (Less than a 10% chance of recurrence at 10 years):
    Noninvasive tumors (ductal ca-in-situ).
    Pure (not mixed) tubular, papillary, or medullary types of cancer.
    Tumor size less than 1 cm.
    Diploid tumor (normal amount of DNA) with low S-phase fractions (low proliferation).
    Nuclear grade 1 (score according to nuclear size and shape, mitotic figures, and other histologic characteristics).

Definition of Good Risk (85–90% chance of being disease free at 5 years):
    Estrogen receptor positive tumors 1–2 cm in size.
    No high risk histologic features.
    Low nuclear grade.

Definition of High Risk:
    Receptor negative tumors that are 1 cm or greater in size or receptor positive tumors greater than 2 cm and with poor nuclear grade.
    Aneuploid tumor (abnormal amount of DNA).
    High S-phase fractions (high proliferation).
    High cathepsin D levels (a lysomal enzyme oversecreted in invasive and metastatic breast cancers).

Answers for Chapter 17 — Post-Test Questions

1. Sheehan's syndrome   p.552
Suckling elicits increases in prolactin, which are important in initiating milk production. Until 2–3 months postpartum, basal levels are approximately 40–50 ng/mL (1,760–2,200 pmol/L), and there are large (about 10–20-fold) increases after suckling. Throughout breastfeeding baseline prolactin levels remain elevated, and suckling produces a two-fold increase that is essential for continuing milk production. The failure to lactate within the first 7 days postpartum may be the first sign of Sheehan's syndrome (hypopituitarism following intrapartum infarction of the pituitary gland).

2. 1   p.552
Antibodies are present in breast milk and contribute to the health of an infant. Human milk prevents infections in infants both by transmission of immunoglobulins and by modifying the bacterial flora of the infant's gastrointestinal tract. Viruses are transmitted in breast milk, and although the actual risks are unknown, women infected with cytomegalovirus, hepatitis B, or human immunodeficiency virus are advised not to breastfeed. Vitamin A, vitamin B_{12}, and folic acid are significantly reduced in the breast milk of women with poor dietary intake. As a general rule approximately 1% of any drug ingested by the mother appears in breast milk.

3. 100   p.556
Prolactin is uniformly elevated in patients on therapeutic amounts of phenothiazines, but essentially never as high as 100 ng/mL (4,400 pmol/L). Approximately 30% will exhibit galactorrhea that should not persist beyond 3–6 months after drug treatment is discontinued.

4. 6 to 12   p.559
If galactorrhea has been present for 6 months to 1 year, or hyperprolactinemia is noted in the process of working up

menstrual disturbances, infertility, or hirsutism, the probability of a pituitary tumor must be recognized.

With the current diagnostic techniques there is no difficulty in discovering and monitoring the size and function of a pituitary prolactin secreting "tumor." With few exceptions the combination of elevation in basal levels of prolactin and radiographic imaging offers complete confidence in diagnosing sellar pathology. The major concern remains in determining management — medical, surgical, or expectant?

5. 30 p.564

The risk of breast cancer increases with the increase in age at which a woman bears her first full-term child. A woman pregnant before the age of 18 has about one-third the risk of one who first delivers after the age of 35. To be protective, pregnancy must occur before the age of 30. In fact, women over the age of 30 years at the time of their first birth have a greater risk than women who never become pregnant. There is, however, a significant protective effect with increasing parity, present even when adjusted for age at first birth and other risk factors. Delayed childbearing in modern society probably has contributed significantly to the increased incidence of breast cancer observed over the last decades.

6. 2 p.564

Female relatives of women with breast cancer have 2–3 times the rate of the general population. There is an excess of bilateral disease among patients with a family history of breast cancer. Relatives of women with bilateral disease have about a 45% lifetime chance of developing breast cancer. In data from the Centers for Disease Control and Prevention (CDC), these relative risks were observed:

Affected mother or sister:	**2.3 relative risk.**
Affected aunt or grandmother:	**1.5 relative risk.**
Affected mother and sister:	**14.0 relative risk**

Results from the Nurses' Health Study indicate that the magnitude of risk associations with a positive family history is smaller than previously believed, comparable to the CDC data above, except for a relative risk of only 2.3 when both mother and sister had breast cancer. In general the size of the increased risk with a positive family history is approximately 2 times the normal incidence. In the Nurses' Health data, there was no interaction between family history and alcohol intake.

7. clear; yellow p.573

When aspiration yields clear or yellow fluid and the mass disappears, the procedure is both diagnostic and therapeutic. Fluid of any other nature requires cytologic assessment. Failure to obtain material for cytologic evaluation or the persistence of a mass requires biopsy. Locally recurrent cysts should be surgically removed.

8. 35 p.576

Screening for Breast Cancer
    All women should be taught self-breast examination by age 20.
    All women over the age of 35 should have an annual breast examination.
    A baseline mammogram should be obtained by age 40, or earlier if high risk factors are present.
    From ages 40 to 50, mammography should be performed every 2 years in low risk women and every year
        in women with significant risk factors.
    Annual mammography should be performed in all women over age 50.

9. follicular p.576

Because of the changes which occur routinely in response to the hormonal sequence of a normal menstrual cycle, breast examination is most effective during the follicular phase of the cycle and should be performed monthly.

10. true p.550

There is marked variability in maternal prolactin levels in pregnancy, with a diurnal variation similar to that found in nonpregnant persons. The peak level occurs 4–5 hours after the onset of sleep.

11. true   p.552

Breast engorgement and milk secretion begin 3–4 days postpartum when steroids have been sufficiently cleared. Maintenance of steroidal inhibition or rapid reduction of prolactin secretion (bromocriptine, 2.5 mg bid for 2 weeks) are effective in preventing postpartum milk synthesis and secretion. Augmentation of prolactin (by thyrotropin releasing hormone or sulpiride, a dopamine receptor blocker) results in increased milk yield.

12. true   p.552

Secretion of calcium into the milk of lactating women approximately doubles the daily loss of calcium. In women who breastfeed for 6 months or more, this is accompanied by significant bone loss even in the presence of a high calcium intake. However, bone density rapidly returns to baseline levels in the 6 months after weaning. The bone loss is due to increased bone resorption, probably secondary to the relatively low estrogen levels associated with lactation. It is possible that recovery is impaired in women with inadequate calcium intake; total calcium intake during lactation should be at least 1500 mg per day.

13. false   p.553

Suckling suppresses the formation of a hypothalamic substance, prolactin inhibiting factor (PIF). This intrahypothalamic effect is either mediated by dopamine, or most likely, in contrast to the peptide nature of other hypothalamic hormones, PIF is dopamine itself. Dopamine is secreted by the basal hypothalamus into the portal system and conducted to the anterior pituitary. Dopamine binds specifically to lactotroph cells and suppresses the secretion of prolactin into the general circulation; in its absence, prolactin is secreted. Suckling, therefore, acts to refill the breast by activating both portions of the pituitary (anterior and posterior) causing the breast to produce new milk and to eject milk.

14. true   p.554

Lactation can be terminated by discontinuing suckling. The primary effect of this cessation is loss of milk letdown via the neural evocation of oxytocin. With passage of a few days, the swollen alveoli depress milk formation probably via a local pressure effect. With resorption of fluid and solute, the swollen engorged breast diminishes in size in a few days. In addition to the loss of milk letdown the absence of suckling reactivates dopamine (PIF) production so that there is less prolactin stimulation of milk secretion. Routine use of a dopamine agonist for suppression of lactation is not recommended because of reports of hypertension, seizure, myocardial infarctions, and strokes associated with its postpartum use.

15. true   p.555

Galactorrhea refers to the mammary secretion of a milky fluid which is nonphysiologic in that it is inappropriate (not immediately related to pregnancy or the needs of a child), persistent, and sometimes excessive. Although usually white or clear, the color may be yellow or even green. In the latter circumstance, local breast disease should be considered. To elicit breast secretion, pressure should be applied to all sections of the breast beginning at the base of the breast and working up toward the nipple. ***Hormonal secretions usually come from multiple duct openings in contrast to pathologic discharge that usually comes from a single duct.*** The quantity of secretion is not an important criterion. Any galactorrhea demands evaluation in a nulliparous woman and if at least 12 months have elapsed since the last pregnancy or weaning in a parous woman. Galactorrhea can involve both breasts or just one breast. Amenorrhea does not necessarily accompany galactorrhea, even in the most serious provocative disorders.

16. false   p.555

Excessive estrogen (e.g., oral contraceptives) can lead to milk secretion via hypothalamic suppression, causing reduction of PIF and release of pituitary prolactin and direct stimulation of the pituitary lactotrophs. Galactorrhea developing during oral contraceptive administration may be most noticeable during the days free of medication (when the steroids are cleared from the body and the prolactin interfering action of the estrogen and progestin on the breast wanes). Galactorrhea caused by excessive estrogen disappears within 3–6 months after discontinuing medication. This is now a rare occurrence with the lower dose pills.

17. false   p.556

Stresses can inhibit hypothalamic PIF, thereby inducing prolactin secretion and galactorrhea. Trauma, surgical procedures, and anesthesia can be seen in temporal relation to the onset of galactorrhea.

18. false   p.556

Increased prolactin concentrations can result from nonpituitary sources such as lung and renal tumors and even a uterine leiomyoma. Severe renal disease requiring hemodialysis is associated with elevated prolactin levels due to the decreased glomerular filtration rate.

19. true   p.560

Microadenomas, if exclusively prolactin producing, rarely progress to macroadenoma size. Most are exceedingly slow growing or stable.

20. true   p.561

Danazol in a dose of 200 mg/day is effective in relieving discomfort as well as decreasing nodularity of the breast. A daily dose is recommended for a period of 6 months. This treatment may achieve long-term resolution of the histologic changes in addition to the clinical improvement. Doses below 400 mg daily do not assure inhibition of ovulation, and a method of effective contraception is necessary because of possible teratologic effects of the drug. Significant improvement has been noted with vitamin E, 600 units/day of the synthetic tocopheral acetate. No side effects have been noted, and the mechanism of action is unknown. Bromocriptine (2.5–5.0 mg/day) and antiestrogens such as tamoxifen (20 mg daily) are also effective for treating mammary discomfort and benign disease.

Clinical observations had suggested that abstinence from methylxanthines leads to resolution of symptoms. Methylxanthines are present in coffee, tea, chocolate, and cola drinks. In controlled studies, however, a significant placebo response rate (30–40%) has been observed. Careful assessments of this relationship have failed to demonstrate a link between methylxanthine use and mastalgia, mammographic changes, or atypia (premalignant tissue changes).

21. false   p.563

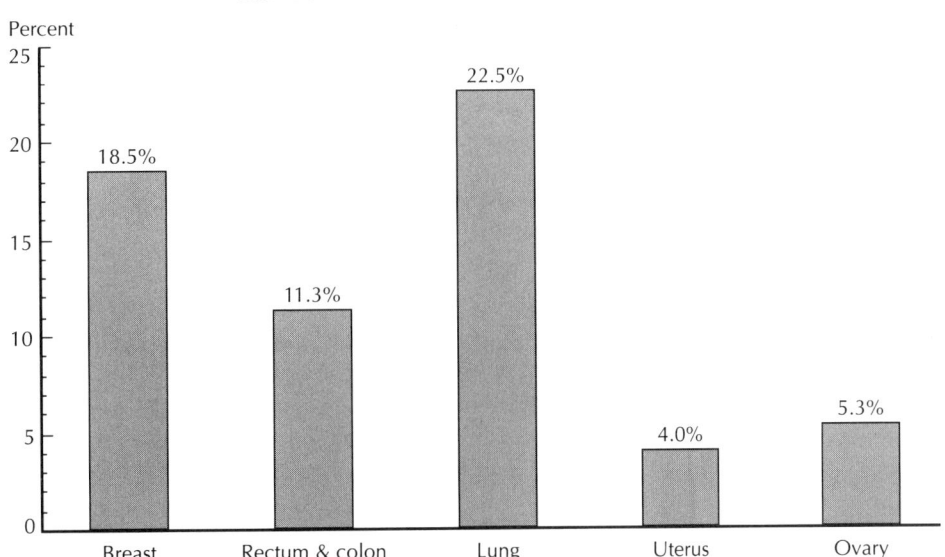

22. true   p.568

The relationship between the use of exogeneous estrogens and the risk of breast cancer has been intensively studied. At the present time there is no conclusive evidence that estrogen doses known to protect against osteoporosis and cardiovascular disease (0.625 mg conjugated estrogens and 1.0 mg estradiol) increase the risk of breast cancer. Some have concluded that a slight increase is noted with long durations of use. However, notable studies (e.g., the Nurses' Health study and the CDC study) have failed to document such an increase. There certainly is no evidence that women who have used estrogen have an increased mortality rate from breast cancer.

The use of regimens that combine estrogen with a progestin is relatively recent (in the time frame of epidemiology), and thus far neither a protective effect nor a detrimental effect has been demonstrated with the addition of a progestational agent.

23. false p.569

Exposure to DES occurred in association with 2 million live births; therefore, the risk for induction of breast cancer during a period of breast differentiation could be significant if DES were a true breast carcinogen. The first study on this subject reported on the follow-up of women who participated in a controlled trial of DES in pregnancy between 1950 and 1952 at the University of Chicago. In this study, an increase which did not reach significance was observed between breast cancer risk and DES exposure. A large collaborative study, involving approximately 6000 women, concluded that there is a small but significant increase in the risk of breast cancer many years later in life in women exposed to DES during pregnancy. A longer follow-up (more than 30 years) of this large cohort of DES-exposed women is now available. Exposure to DES is associated with a significant, but modest (less than two-fold), increase in the risk of breast cancer. Importantly, the relative risk did not increase with duration of follow-up and remained stable over time. Certainly it is wise to recommend to DES-exposed women that they adhere religiously to screening for breast cancer, including mammography.

24. true p.569

Therefore the presence of progesterone receptors proves that the estrogen receptor in the tumor is biologically active. Thus, the presence of progesterone receptors has a correlation with disease free survival of patients only second to the number of positive nodes. The best prognosis is seen in patients with positive progesterone receptors, even with subsequent disease if the recurrent disease is still progesterone receptor positive. The loss of progesterone receptors is an ominous sign.

25. E p.559

Hyperprolactinemia may be associated with a variety of menstrual cycle disturbances: oligoovulation, corpus luteum insufficiency, as well as amenorrhea. About one-third of women with secondary amenorrhea will have elevated prolactin concentrations. Pathologic hyperprolactinemia inhibits the pulsatile secretion of GnRH, and the reduction of circulating prolactin levels restores menstrual function.

26. C p.564,565

A constellation of factors influences the risk for breast cancer. These include reproductive experience, ovarian activity, benign breast disease, familial tendency, genetic differences, dietary considerations, and specific endocrine factors.

27. B p.567

Called the "Open Window Hypothesis," Korenman argued that unopposed estrogen stimulation is the most favorable state for tumor induction (the "open" window). Susceptibility to breast cancer declines with the establishment of normal luteal phase progesterone secretion and becomes very low during pregnancy; the open window is closed.

The two main open window periods are the pubertal years prior to the establishment of regular ovulatory menstrual cycles and the perimenopausal period of waning follicle maturation and ovulation. The prolongation of these open windows by obesity, infertility, delayed pregnancy, earlier menarche, and later menopause would be associated with greater susceptibility. This argument is supported by observational studies indicating that anovulatory and infertile women (exposed to less progesterone) have an increased risk of breast cancer later in life. However, the statistical power of these observational studies was limited by small numbers (all fewer than 15 cases).

Although theoretically appealing on the basis of presumed correlation with epidemiologic risks (infertility, late menopause) clinical research has not always confirmed the thesis. Young women at high genetic risk for breast cancer had normal luteal phases, and a group of premenopausal women with breast cancer also had normal luteal phases. Others have failed to find a link between anovulation and the risk of breast cancer. Another attempt to link the risk of breast cancer to the endogenous estrogen level focused on prenatal exposure. A reduced risk for breast cancer is observed for women born to mothers with pregnancy-induced hypertension, suggesting that this finding is due to the lower estrogen levels associated with preeclampsia.

The logic and epidemiologic support for an estrogen link are impressive arguments. Whether the important factor is the total amount of estrogen, the amount of estrogen unopposed by progesterone, or some other combination is not known. Biologically available estrogen may be the more important factor. Women who develop breast cancer have higher levels of nonbound estradiol and lower levels of sex hormone binding globulin (SHBG).

28. E   p.569

There is an excellent correlation between the presence of estrogen receptors and certain clinical characteristics of breast cancer, including response to endocrine therapy. Premenopausal and younger patients are more frequently receptor negative. Patients with receptor positive tumors survive longer and have longer disease-free intervals after mastectomy than those with receptor negative tumors. The presence of estrogen receptors correlates with increased disease-free interval regardless of the presence of axillary nodes or the size and location of the tumors. Similarly, patients without axillary lymph node metastases, but with estradiol receptor negative tumors, have the same high rate of recurrence as do patients with axillary lymph node metastases. Patients with tumors that are positive for estrogen receptors are more likely to respond to endocrine treatment.

29. A   p.569

Adjuvant treatment with the antiestrogen, tamoxifen, achieves highly significant reductions in recurrence and increases in survival. The beneficial effect of tamoxifen is evident no matter what the age of the patient, in both premenopausal and postmenopausal women, in node positive and node negative disease, and in both estrogen receptor positive and negative tumors. The benefit of tamoxifen is of course more concentrated in estrogen receptor positive disease. The impact on recurrence occurs in the first 5 years, but continued impact on survival occurs throughout 10 years (and this was achieved with a median duration of treatment of only 2 years). The 10-year survival difference is even greater than that at 5 years. Adjuvant treatment (which is either tamoxifen, chemotherapy, or ovarian ablation) yields world-wide an extra 100,000 10-year survivors.

30. B   p.570

Tamoxifen therapy is definitely justified for postmenopausal women with estrogen receptor positive disease, and a benefit with tamoxifen alone can be demonstrated with early breast cancer regardless of receptor status. The disease-free interval is consistently prolonged with postsurgical tamoxifen treatment of early breast cancer. In addition, there is a reduced rate of recurrence. The ideal duration of therapy remains unsettled. Certainly the data support a duration of at least 5 years, but there is reason to believe that longer treatment with tamoxifen will be worthwhile. Longer, even lifelong, durations are now being studied. Dose-response studies with tamoxifen have failed to demonstrate an increase in activity with doses larger than the standard, 20 mg daily.

31. A   p.572

Tamoxifen is both an estrogen antagonist and an estrogen agonist. There have been many reports of endometrial hyperplasia, endometrial polyps, rapid and symptomatic growth of endometriosis, and endometrial cancer occurring in women receiving tamoxifen treatment. A tissue that is highly sensitive to estrogen, the endometrium, responds to the weak estrogenic action of tamoxifen, which is present in high doses for long durations in women receiving adjuvant treatment for breast cancer. The development of endometrial cancer in women receiving tamoxifen should not be so surprising. We know that duration of exposure to estrogen is more important than the dose of estrogen in influencing progression from proliferative endometrium through hyperplasia to cancer. The proper surveillance and management of women being treated with tamoxifen are critical problems.

32. E   p.575

Mammography is the only method that detects clustered microcalcifications. These calcifications are less than 1 mm in diameter and are frequently associated with malignant lesions. More than 5 calcifications in a cluster are associated with cancer 25% of the time and require biopsy.

Mammography has a false negative rate of 5–10%. This means that masses are palpable but not visible. Mammography cannot and should not replace examination by patient and physician. Cancer commonly presents as a solitary, solid, painless (but not always), hard, unilateral, irregular nonmobile mass. A mass requires biopsy regardless of the mammographic picture.

A baseline mammogram should be obtained by age 40, or earlier if high risk factors are present.
From ages 40 to 50, mammography should be performed every 2 years in low risk women and every year in women with significant risk factors.
Annual mammography should be performed in all women over age 50.

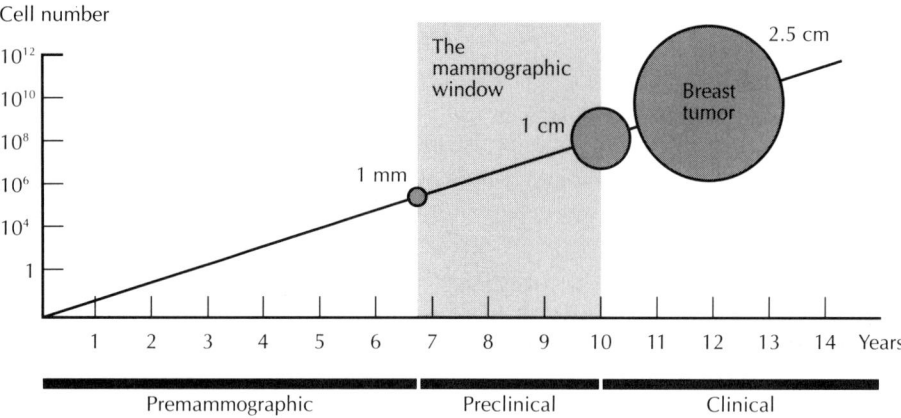

After Wertheimer, et al.[106]

18 Menopause and Postmenopausal Hormone Therapy

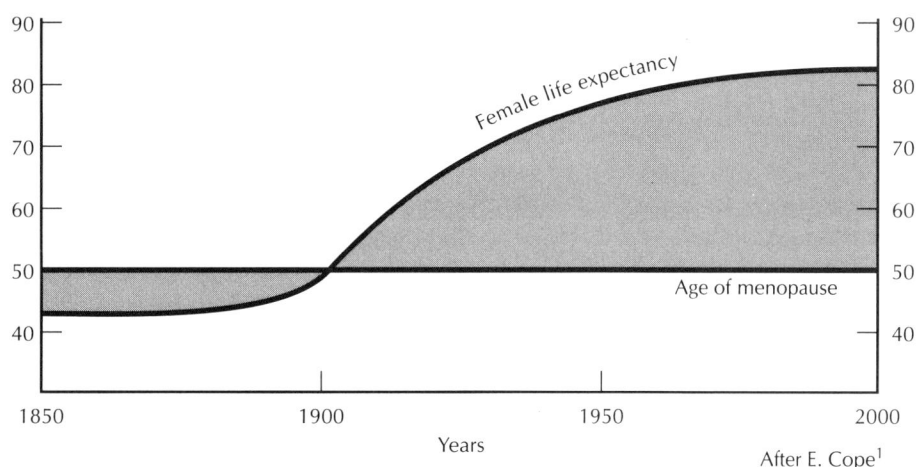

After E. Cope[1]

Learning Objectives

Be able to:

1. Describe the endocrine changes which occur in the perimenopause, menopause and postmenopause.

2. Describe the changes in sexuality in the postmenopausal woman.

3. Detail the differential diagnosis and workup for perimenopausal, menopausal and postmenopausal uterine bleeding.

4. Describe the symptoms and signs of the perimenopause and menopause.

5. Explain the long-term effects of estrogen deprivation.

6. Describe the calcium requirements in menopausal women on and off hormone therapy.

7. Describe the possible mechanisms by which estrogen may be cardioprotective and protective against osteoporosis in menopausal women.

8. Detail possible options and discuss the benefits and potential disadvantages of different hormone therapy regimens.

9. Describe the contraindications and detail alternatives to hormone therapy.

Pre-Test

A. Instructions: Fill in the blanks

1. The inability to suppress gonadotropins with postmenopausal hormone therapy is a consequence of the loss of _____.

2. The average nontreated postmenopausal white woman can expect to shrink _____ inches.

B. Instructions: True or False

3. An earlier menopause is associated with living at high altitudes and cigarette smoking.

4. In general, cortical bone resorption and formation occur four to eight times as fast as trabecular bone.

C. Instructions: For each of the following questions choose:

A. if only 1, 2 and 3 are correct
B. if only 1 and 3 are correct
C. if only 2 and 4 are correct
D. if only 4 is correct
E. if all are correct

5. Menstrual cycle changes immediately prior to menopause are marked by
   1. elevated FSH
   2. decreasing levels of inhibin
   3. normal levels of estradiol
   4. normal levels of LH

6. Purposed mechanisms for the action of sex steroid protection of bones include
   1. increased efficiency of calcium absorption
   2. promoting the synthesis of calcitonin
   3. a direct role for the estrogen receptors in osteoblasts
   4. the modulation of cytokines and growth factors in the remodeling process

Post-Test

A. Instructions: Fill in the blanks

1. The perimenopausal transition, for most women, is approximately _____ years in duration.

2. Undernourished women experience menopause _____ than do nourished women.

3. When women are in their forties, anovulation becomes more prevalent, and prior to anovulation, menstrual cycle length _____, beginning 2 to 8 years before menopause.

4. Following the onset of menopause there is eventually a _____ fold increase in FSH and approximately a _____ fold increase in LH, reaching a maximal level 1–3 years after menopause.

5. The hot flush coincides with a surge of _____ and is preceded by a subjective prodromal awareness that a flush is beginning.

6. Estrogen therapy in the menopausal woman improves the quality of sleep, _____ the time to onset of sleep and _____ the rapid eye movement (REM) sleep time.

7. _____ bone is responsible for 80% of total bone, while _____ bone constitutes a honeycomb structure.

8. The critical blood level of estradiol that is necessary to maintain bone is _____ pg/ml.

9. In women, data from two large prospective studies indicate that _____-cholesterol is more closely related to cardiovascular disease than is _____-cholesterol.

10. Sufficient evidence exists to indicate the possibility of a slightly _____ risk of breast cancer associated with _____ years or more of postmenopausal estrogen use.

11. The purpose of a meta-analysis is to gain the statistical _____ that is lacking in individual studies.

12. The dose equivalent to 0.625 mg of conjugated estrogen is approximately ___ µg of ethinyl estradiol with respect to comparable effects upon bone.

B. Instructions: True or False

13. In the Massachusetts Women's Health Study, the median age for the onset of the perimenopause was 47.5 years. The median age for menopause was 51.3 years.

14. There is a correlation between age of menarche and age of menopause.

15. The association between obesity and endometrial cancer is attributed to increased estrogen production from androstenedione and decreased levels of SHBG.

16. Women with gonadal dysgenesis have hot flashes only after they have received estrogen which is withdrawn.

17. Vaginal relaxation with cystocele, rectocele and uterine prolapse and vulvar dystrophies result from estrogen deprivation.

18. Estrogen therapy does little to improve a woman's muscular strength.

19. Menopause has a deleterious effect on mental health.

20. 0.3 mg daily of conjugated estrogens or 0.5 mg estradiol prevents loss of vertebral trabecular bone when combined with a total intake of 1500 mg calcium daily.

21. The average postmenopausal woman on estrogen therapy requires a minimal daily supplement of an additional 1000 mg.

22. Side effects related to high oral calcium supplementation include constipation and flatulence.

C. Instructions: For each of the following questions choose:

   A. if only 1, 2 and 3 are correct
   B. if only 1 and 3 are correct
   C. if only 2 and 4 are correct
   D. if only 4 is correct
   E. if all are correct

23. In the Massachusetts Women's Health Study the following factors were associated with the onset of earlier menopause
    1. oral contraceptives
    2. marital status
    3. socioeconomic status
    4. current smoking

24. The main sexual changes which occur in the aging woman include
    1. loss of vaginal elasticity
    2. diminished libido
    3. reduction in the rate of production and volume of vaginal lubricating fluid
    4. diminished ability to have orgasm

25. Following menopause
    1. FSH is elevated
    2. DHAS is decreased
    3. LH is elevated
    4. androstenedione is decreased

26. The symptoms frequently seen and related to estrogen loss include
    1. vasomotor instability
    2. urgency and cystitis
    3. osteoporosis and cardiovascular disease
    4. decreased libido

27. Perimenopausal women may have dysfunctional uterine bleeding but may require endometrial sampling to rule out organic disease. Biopsies show
    1. normal endometrium in greater than 50% of cases
    2. endometrial cancer in 2% of cases
    3. polyps in 3% of cases
    4. endometrial hyperplasia in 15% of cases

28. Hot flushes
    1. are more frequent and severe at night
    2. are a major feature of perimenopause
    3. are a major feature of postmenopause
    4. present a clear inherent health hazard

29. Bone loss following menopause
    1. is accelerated in blacks versus whites
    2. is up to 5% of trabecular bone and 1.5% of total bone mass per year
    3. is more due to aging itself than estrogen loss
    4. for the first 20 years results in a 50% reduction in trabecular bone and a 30% reduction in cortical bone

30. Hip fractures
    1. occur in 100,000 women per year in the US
    2. begin to occur 10–15 years following menopause
    3. can be reduced by 15% with estrogen therapy
    4. will occur in 20% of all white women by age 90

31. Progestational agents
    1. reduce bone resorption independent of estrogen
    2. are cardioprotective
    3. when added to estrogen lead to a synergetic increase in bone formation
    4. when given in continuous combination with estrogen is not as efficacious in maintaining bone density as the standard sequential regimens.

32. In order to remain in zero calcium balance women
    1. require supplementation in addition to the 500 mg of calcium present in their daily diet
    2. not on estrogen require a daily supplement of at least 1000 mg of calcium
    3. on estrogen therapy requires a minimal daily supplement of 500 mg of calcium
    4. should receive vitamin D supplementation of 800 units daily

33. Alternatives to estrogen therapy for protection against osteoporosis in menopausal women include
    1. calcitonin
    2. exercise
    3. etidronate disodium
    4. calcium and vitamin D

34. Increased risk of osteoporosis is associated with excessive
    1. cigarette smoking
    2. alcohol
    3. thyroid replacement
    4. glucocorticoids

35. Conditions other than menopause which can be responsible for osteoporosis include
    1. hyperparathyroidism
    2. multiple myeloma
    3. hyperthyroidism
    4. Cushing's disease

36. Dual energy x-ray absorptiometry (DEXA) is the state of the art in accessing bone mineral density because
    1. it has the greatest precision compared to other methods
    2. it uses low amounts of radiation
    3. it can access three sites of greatest interest the radius, hip and spine
    4. it can yield meaningful data with serial measurements one year apart

37. Reasons to obtain a DEXA are
    1. to improve compliance
    2. to access response to selected therapies
    3. to establish a baseline in those receiving corticosteroids or thyroxine
    4. to consider stopping therapy

38. The following prospective studies support a cardioprotective effect of estrogen
    1. The Leisure World Study
    2. The Nurses Health Study
    3. The Lipid Research Clinics Follow-up Study
    4. The Framingham Heart Study

39. The possible beneficial actions of estrogens on cardiovascular disease include
    1. a direct inotropic action on the heart
    2. the augmentation of vasodilating factors
    3. the inhibition of lipoprotein oxidation
    4. the decrease in circulating insulin levels

40. Endometrial hyperplasia
    1. risk ends immediately upon discontinuing estrogen
    2. will result in 20% of cases treated with unopposed 0.625 mg of conjugated estrogen taken for 1 year
    3. if accompanied by atypia 50% will develop into carcinoma within a year
    4. will develop into carcinoma in an average time of approximately 5 years

41. When assessing the relative potencies of commercially available estrogens it is important to keep in mind which end organ effect is being examined. The relative estrogen potencies are compared between
    1. FSH levels
    2. liver proteins
    3. bone density
    4. maturation index

42. Effective continuous daily use of estrogen-progestin combinations should include
    1. 0.5 mg micronized estradiol and 0.35 mg norethindrone
    2. 0.625 mg estrone sulfate and 0.35 mg norethindrone
    3. 1.0 mg micronized estradiol and 5.0 mg medroxyprogesterone acetate
    4. 250 mg bid of calcium with meals and vitamin D supplementation

43. Common reasons why women discontinue or do not start hormone treatment
    1. inconvenience
    2. fear of cancer
    3. cost
    4. vaginal bleeding

44. Breakthrough bleeding with continuous therapy
    1. occurs in 40–60% of patients during the first 6 months of treatment but is approximately 20% after 1 year
    2. is similar in mechanism to that seen with oral contraceptives
    3. may require switching a patient to a sequential program if it persists beyond a year
    4. can be stopped by prescribing a higher dose of progestin

45. In the context of postmenopausal hormone therapy endometrial biopsy is indicated
    1. in women with endometrial thickens less than 5 mm on transvaginal ultrasound
    2. in those at high risk for endometrial changes (i.e., obesity)
    3. in those with breakthrough bleeding on continuous therapy for less than 6 months
    4. in those previous treated for a period of time with unopposed estrogen

46. Typical side effects of progestational hormones include
    1. breast tenderness
    2. bloating
    3. depression
    4. palpitations

47. Androgens added to the hormone therapy regimens
    1. may have a negative impact on the cholesterol-lipoprotein profile
    2. may substitute for progestin in protecting the endometrium if given with estrogen
    3. may increase libido
    4. should be considered in any woman with a serum testosterone below normal

48. The following clinical situations have not been shown to have an adverse impact on the prognosis of breast cancer
    1. pregnancy
    2. oral contraception
    3. depo-provera
    4. pregnancy after diagnosis and treatment of breast cancer

49. Tamoxifen
    1. decreases total cholesterol and LDL cholesterol with an increase in triglycerides and HDL cholesterol
    2. stimulates the endometrium and vaginal mucosa
    3. provides limited protection of bone
    4. is effective in the treatment of hot flushing

50. Contraindications to estrogen hormone therapy include
    1. impaired liver function
    2. acute vascular disease
    3. familial hyperlipidemias
    4. controlled hypertension

51. Effective alternative treatments to estrogen for hot flushes associated with minimal side effects include
    1. propranolol
    2. oral bromocriptine
    3. veralipride
    4. transdermal clonidine

Answers for Chapter 18 — Pre-Test Questions

1. inhibin   p.589
The changes in the later reproductive years (the decline in inhibin allowing a rise in FSH) reflect lesser follicular competence because the better follicles respond early in life, leaving the lesser follicles for later. The decrease in inhibin secretion by the ovarian follicles begins early (around age 35), but accelerates after 40 years of age. This is reflected in the decrease in fecundability that occurs with aging. Furthermore, the ineffective ability to suppress gonadotropins with postmenopausal hormone therapy is a consequence of the loss of inhibin, and for this reason **FSH cannot be used clinically to titer estrogen dosage.**

2. 2.5   p.598
The risk of fracture from osteoporosis will depend upon bone mass at the time of menopause and the rate of bone loss following menopause. In general, bone mass is increased in black and obese women and decreased in white, Asian, thin and sedentary women. Vertebral bone is especially vulnerable, with a bone density threshold for fracture only slightly below the lower limit of normal for premenopausal women. It is no surprise that vertebral fractures account for 50% of all fractures. Indeed 25% of individuals over 70 years of age show radiographic evidence of these crush type fractures that lead to dorsal kyphosis (dowager's hump). The average nontreated postmenopausal white woman can expect to shrink 2.5 inches (6.4 cm).

3. true   p.588

An earlier menopause is associated with living at high altitudes and, as mentioned previously, with cigarette smoking. There is a dose-response relationship with the number of cigarettes smoked and the duration of smoking. Even former smokers show evidence of an impact. There is reason to believe that premature ovarian failure can occur in women who have previously undergone abdominal hysterectomy, presumably because ovarian vasculature has been compromised. About 1% of women will experience menopause before the age of 40.

4. false   p.597

In general, trabecular bone resorption and formation occur four to eight times as fast as cortical bone. Beyond age 40 resorption begins to exceed formation by about 0.5% per year. This adverse relationship accelerates after menopause and up to 5% of trabecular bone and 1–1.5% of total bone mass loss will occur per year after menopause. This accelerated loss will continue for 10–15 years, after which bone loss is considerably diminished but continues as the aging-related loss. For the first 20 years following cessation of menses, menopause-related bone loss results in a 50% reduction in trabecular bone and a 30% reduction in cortical bone. The process is slower in blacks.

5. E   p.589

The duration of the follicular phase is the major determinant of cycle length. This menstrual cycle change prior to menopause is marked by elevated follicle-stimulating hormone (FSH) levels and decreased levels of inhibin, but normal levels of estradiol and luteinizing hormone (LH). We now know that estradiol levels do not gradually wane in the years before menopause, but remain in the normal range until follicular growth and development cease. The FSH and inhibin change and inverse relationship indicate that inhibin is a more sensitive marker of ovarian follicular competence and, in turn, that FSH measurement is a clinical assessment of inhibin.

6. E   p.599

Bone mass is determined by the balance present in the constant process of remodeling. Each remodeling unit is initiated by osteoclast excavation followed by osteoblast refilling. Estrogen exerts a tonic suppression of remodeling and maintains a balance between osteoclastic and osteoblastic activity. The precise mechanism of action for sex steroid protection of bones remains unknown; however a growing body of knowledge indicates complex interactions at the molecular level. Increased efficiency of calcium absorption (probably secondary to estrogen-induced enhancement of the availability of the active metabolite of vitamin D, 1,25-dihydroxyvitamin D) and a direct role for the estrogen receptors in the osteoblasts are likely important factors. Many estrogen-dependent growth factors and cytokines are involved in bone remodeling. Estrogen modulates the production of bone resorbing cytokines such as interleukin-1 and -6, bone stimulating factors such as insulin-like growth factors I and II, and transforming growth factor-β. Estrogen increases vitamin D receptors in osteoblasts, and this may be a method by which estrogen modulates 1,25-dihydroxyvitamin D activity in bone. There is little evidence that estrogen affects bone by altering the circulating calcitropic hormones. Thus, the actions of estrogen are primarily direct effects on bone and important effects on renal and intestinal handling of calcium.

Answers for Chapter 18 — Post-Test Questions

1. 4   p.587

In the longitudinal Massachusetts Women's Health Study, women who reported the onset of menstrual irregularity were considered to be perimenopausal. The median age for the onset of the perimenopause was 47.5 years. Only 10% of women ceased menstruating abruptly with no period of prolonged irregularity. The perimenopausal transition from reproductive to postreproductive status was, for most women, approximately 4 years in duration. In the extensive study of over 2,700 women by Treloar, most women experienced a perimenopausal transition between 2 and 7 years in length.

2. earlier   p.588

Although clinical impression has suggested that mothers and daughters tend to experience menopause at the same age, what little data that exist are derived from retrospective, cross-sectional studies. The existence of a familial (inherited) effect must await longitudinal data. Ethnic differences suffer from the same methodologic problems. There is sufficient evidence to believe that undernourished women experience an earlier menopause. Because of the contribution of body fat to estrogen production, thinner women experience a slightly earlier menopause. Race, parity, and height have no influence on the age of menopause.

3. increases   p.589

When women are in their forties, anovulation becomes more prevalent, and prior to anovulation, menstrual cycle length increases, beginning 2 to 8 years before menopause. At the same time fewer follicles grow during each cycle until eventually the supply of follicles is depleted.

4. 10–20; 3   p.589

As cycles become irregular, vaginal bleeding occurs at the end of an inadequate luteal phase or after a peak of estradiol without subsequent ovulation or corpus luteum formation. But shortly after the menopause, one can safely say that there are no remaining ovarian follicles. Eventually there is a 10–20-fold increase in FSH and approximately a 3-fold increase in LH, reaching a maximal level 1–3 years after menopause, after which there is a gradual, but slight, decline in both gonadotropins. Elevated levels of both FSH and LH at this time in life are conclusive evidence of ovarian failure. FSH levels are higher than LH because LH is cleared from the blood so much faster (half-lives are about 30 minutes for LH and 4 hours for FSH).

5. LH   p.595

The flush is accompanied by a discrete and reliable pattern of physiologic changes. The flush coincides with a surge of LH (not FSH) and is preceded by a subjective prodromal awareness that a flush is beginning. This aura is followed by measurable increased heat over the entire body surface. The body surface experiences an increase in temperature, accompanied by changes in skin conductance, and followed by a fall in core temperature — all of which can be objectively measured. In short, the flush is not a release of accumulated body heat but is a sudden inappropriate excitation of heat release mechanisms. Its relationship to the LH surge and temperature change within the brain is not understood. The observation that flushes occur after hypophysectomy indicates that the mechanism is not dependent on or due directly to LH release. In other words, the same hypothalamic event that causes flushes also stimulates gonadotropin releasing hormone (GnRH) secretion and elevates LH.

6. decreases; increases   p.597

Emotional stability during the perimenopausal period can be disrupted by poor sleep patterns. Estrogen therapy improves the quality of sleep, decreasing the time to onset of sleep and increasing the rapid eye movement (REM) sleep time. Perhaps flushing may be insufficient to awaken a woman but sufficient to affect the quality of sleep, thereby diminishing the ability to handle the next day's problems and stresses.

7. Cortical; trabecular   p.597

Osteoporosis is characterized by microarchitectural deterioration of bone tissue, leading to enhanced bone fragility and a consequent increase in the risk of fractures with little or no trauma. The skeleton consists of two bone types. Cortical bone is responsible for 80% of total bone, while trabecular bone, the bone of the spinal column, constitutes a honeycomb structure providing greater surface area per unit volume. The onset of spinal bone loss begins in the 20s, but the overall change is small until menopause. Bone density in the femur peaks in the mid to late 20s and begins to decrease around age 30.

8. 40–50   p.598

Estrogen therapy will stabilize the process of osteoporosis or prevent it from occurring. *The critical blood level of estradiol that is necessary to maintain bone is 40–50 pg/mL (146–184 fmol/L).* With estrogen therapy one can expect a 50–60% decrease in fractures of the arm and hip, and when estrogen is supplemented with calcium, an 80% reduction in vertebral compression fractures can be observed. This reduction is seen primarily in patients who have taken estrogen for more than 5 years. If bone loss can be delayed with estrogen therapy for 8 years, fracture incidence can be reduced by 75%.

9. HDL; LDL   p.604

The higher HDL levels in women compared to men represent the net effect of estrogen (HDL elevating) in women and androgens (HDL lowering) in men. While the exact mechanism of protection provided by HDL is not totally understood, it is fair to say that HDL promotes the efflux of cholesterol from macrophages and the intimal wall of the arteries. At roughly the age of menopause (48–55) the average cholesterol level in women rises higher than the average level in men as the HDL declines and LDL increases. In women, data from two large prospective studies indicate that HDL-cholesterol is more closely related to cardiovascular disease than is LDL-cholesterol.

10. increased; 10 p.612

Sufficient evidence exists to indicate the possibility of a slightly increased risk of breast cancer associated with long durations (10 or more years) of postmenopausal estrogen use. However, the epidemiologic data on this relationship are by no means consistent and uniform. A review of the epidemiologic studies on postmenopausal hormone therapy and the risk of breast cancer fails to provide definitive evidence regarding this issue. Nevertheless, we believe that patients must consider this possibility in their informed decision-making.

11. power p.614

Meta-analysis is an increasingly popular statistical method in which many studies are combined and undergo rigorous analysis. Simply put, the purpose of a meta-analysis is to gain the statistical power that is lacking in individual studies.

12. 5–10 p.618

Relative Estrogen Potencies

Estrogen	FSH levels	Liver proteins	Bone density
Piperazine estrone sulfate	1.0 mg	2.0 mg	0.625 mg
Micronized estradiol	1.0 mg	1.0 mg	1.0 mg
Conjugated estrogens	1.0 mg	0.625 mg	0.625 mg
Ethinyl estradiol	5.0 µg	2–10 µg	5–10 µg
Transdermal estradiol	—	—	50 µg

13. true p.587

The median age for menopause in the Massachusetts Study was 51.3 years. Only current smoking could be identified as a cause of earlier menopause, a shift of approximately 1.5 years. Those factors that did not affect the age of menopause included the use of oral contraception, socioeconomic status, and marital status. Keep in mind that a median age of menopause means that only half the women have reached menopause at this age. Thus, it is more useful clinically to remember the range for the age of menopause, approximately age 48 to age 55.

14. false p.588

There is no correlation between age of menarche and age of menopause.

15. true p.590

The percent conversion of androstenedione to estrogen correlates with body weight. Increased production of estrogen from androstenedione with increasing body weight is probably due to the ability of fat to aromatize androgens. This fact and a decrease in the levels of sex hormone binding globulin (which results in increased free estrogen concentrations) contribute to the well-known association between obesity and the development of endometrial cancer. Body weight, therefore, has a positive correlation with the circulating levels of estrone and estradiol. Aromatization of androgens to estrogens is not limited to adipose tissue, however, because almost every tissue tested has this activity.

16. true p.595

The correlation between the onset of flushes and estrogen reduction is clinically supported by the effectiveness of estrogen therapy and the absence of flushes in hypoestrogen states, such as gonadal dysgenesis. Only after estrogen is administered and withdrawn do hypogonadal women experience the hot flush. Although the clinical impression that premenopausal surgical castrates suffer more severe vasomotor reactions is widely held, this is not borne out in objective study.

17. false   p.595
With extremely low estrogen production in the late postmenopausal age, or many years after castration, atrophy of mucosal surfaces takes place, accompanied by vaginitis, pruritus, dyspareunia, and stenosis. Genitourinary atrophy leads to a variety of symptoms which affect the ease and quality of living. Urethritis with dysuria, urgency incontinence, and urinary frequency are further results of mucosal thinning, in this instance, of the urethra and bladder. Recurrent urinary tract infections are effectively prevented by postmenopausal estrogen treatment. Vaginal relaxation with cystocele, rectocele, and uterine prolapse, and vulvar dystrophies are not a consequence of estrogen deprivation. Although it is argued that genuine stress incontinence will not be affected by treatment with estrogen, others contend that estrogen treatment improves or cures genuine stress incontinence in over 50% of patients due to a direct effect on the urethral mucosa. Most cases of urinary incontinence in elderly women are a mixed problem with a significant component of urge incontinence that definitely can be improved by estrogen therapy.

18. false   p.596
One of the features of aging in men and women is a steady reduction in muscular strength. Many factors affect this decline, including height, weight, and level of physical activity. However, women currently using estrogen do not demonstrate this age-related decline in muscular competence (as measured by handgrip strength). This can be viewed as another substantial benefit of estrogen, with potential protective consequences against fractures, as well as a benefit due to the ability to maintain vigorous physical exercise. In addition, there is some evidence that estrogen treatment before the onset of joint disease is associated with protection against rheumatoid arthritis, however this protective effect is debatable.

19. false   p.596
The view that menopause has a deleterious effect on mental health is not supported in the psychiatric literature, or in surveys of the general population. The concept of a specific psychiatric disorder (involutional melancholia) has been abandoned. Indeed, depression is less common, not more common, among middle-aged women. A negative view of mental health at the time of the menopause is not justified; many of the problems reported at the menopause are due to the vicissitudes of life. Thus, there are problems encountered in the early postmenopause that are seen frequently, but their causal relation with estrogen is uncertain. These problems include fatigue, nervousness, headaches, insomnia, depression, irritability, joint and muscle pain, dizziness, and palpitations.

20. true   p.598
Studies have demonstrated that a dose of 0.625 mg of conjugated estrogens is necessary to preserve bone density. A lower dose of 0.3 mg daily of conjugated estrogens or 0.5 mg estradiol prevented loss of vertebral trabecular bone when combined with calcium supplementation (to achieve a total intake of 1,500 mg daily). A study of women randomized to treatment either with continuous transdermal delivery of estradiol 50 mg daily or oral estrogen demonstrated that both equally prevented postmenopausal bone loss. The positive impact of estrogen increases with increasing dose; thus, whether fracture protection with either the lower oral dose regimens or via a transdermal route of administration is equal to the standard oral program awaits further epidemiologic study. Furthermore, some decrease in cardiovascular protection occurs with the use of lower doses of estrogen.

21. false   p.600
Calcium absorption decreases with age and becomes significantly impaired after menopause. A positive calcium balance is mandatory to achieve adequate prevention against osteoporosis. Calcium supplementation (1,000 mg per day) reduces bone loss and decreases fractures, especially in individuals with low daily intakes. However, estrogen acts to improve calcium absorption and makes it possible to utilize effective supplemental calcium in lower doses. In order to remain in zero calcium balance, women on estrogen therapy require a total of 1,000 mg elemental calcium per day. Since the average woman receives only 500 mg of calcium in her diet, the minimal daily supplement equals an additional 500 mg. Women not on estrogen require a daily supplement of at least 1,000 mg calcium. Even with the commonly used therapeutic doses of calcium, nearly 40% of postmenopausal women will have inefficient absorption.

22. true
p.600

Estrogen improves calcium absorption and makes it possible to utilize supplemental calcium in effective doses without the side effects associated with higher doses (constipation and flatulence) that diminish compliance. Nevertheless, the calcium supplementation should be administered in divided doses with meals. We must emphasize that although calcium supplementation is important, it cannot provide the same degree of protection against osteoporosis as that achieved by hormonal therapy.

23. D
p.587

The median age for menopause in the Massachusetts Study was 51.3 years. Only current smoking could be identified as a cause of earlier menopause, a shift of approximately 1.5 years. Those factors that did not affect the age of menopause included the use of oral contraception, socioeconomic status, and marital status. Keep in mind that a median age of menopause means that only half the women have reached menopause at this age. Thus, it is more useful clinically to remember the range for the age of menopause, approximately age 48 to age 55.

24. B
p.588

There are two main sexual changes in the aging woman. There is a reduction in the rate of production and volume of vaginal lubricating fluid, and there is some loss of vaginal elasticity. The dyspareunia associated with postmenopausal urogenital atrophy includes a feeling of dryness and tightness, vaginal irritation and burning with coitus, and postcoital spotting and soreness. Less vaginal atrophy is noted in sexually active women compared to inactive women; presumably the activity maintains vaginal vasculature and circulation.

25. E
p.589,590

Eventually there is a 10–20-fold increase in FSH and approximately a 3-fold increase in LH, reaching a maximal level 1–3 years after menopause, after which there is a gradual, but slight, decline in both gonadotropins. Elevated levels of both FSH and LH at this time in life are conclusive evidence of ovarian failure. After menopause, the circulating level of androstenedione is about one-half that seen prior to menopause. Most of this postmenopausal androstenedione is derived from the adrenal gland, with only a small amount secreted from the ovary. Testosterone levels do not fall appreciably, and, in fact, the postmenopausal ovary in most women, but not all, secretes more testosterone than the premenopausal ovary. With the disappearance of follicles and estrogen, the elevated gonadotropins drive the remaining stromal tissue in the ovary to a level of increased testosterone secretion. Suppression of gonadotropins with gonadotropin releasing hormone (GnRH) agonist or antagonist treatment of postmenopausal women results in a significant decrease in circulating levels of testosterone, indicating the gonadotropin-dependent postmenopausal ovarian origin. The total amount of testosterone produced after menopause, however, is decreased because the amount of the primary source, peripheral conversion of androstenedione, is reduced.

The circulating estradiol level after menopause is approximately 10–20 pg/mL (37–74 fmol/L), most of which is derived from peripheral conversion of estrone. The circulating level of estrone in postmenopausal women is higher than that of estradiol, the mean level being approximately 30–70 pg/mL (111–260 fmol/L). The average postmenopausal production rate of estrogen is approximately 45 mg/24 hours, almost all, if not all, being estrogen derived from the peripheral conversion of androstenedione. The androgen:estrogen ratio changes drastically after menopause because of the more marked decline in estrogen, and an onset of mild hirsutism is common, reflecting this marked shift in the sex hormone ratio. With increasing age, a decrease can be measured in the circulating levels of dehydroepiandrosterone (DHA) and its sulfate (DHAS), whereas the circulating postmenopausal levels of androstenedione, testosterone, and estrogen remain relatively constant.

26. A
p.591

The symptoms frequently seen and related to decreasing ovarian follicular competence and then estrogen loss in this protracted climacteric are:

1. Disturbances in menstrual pattern, including anovulation and reduced fertility, decreased flow or hypermenorrhea, and irregular frequency of menses.
2. Vasomotor instability (hot flushes and sweats).
3. Psychological symptoms, including anxiety, increased tension, mood depression, and irritability, although a direct cause and effect relationship between these symptoms and estrogen is hard to

establish.
4. Atrophic conditions: atrophy of vaginal epithelium, formation of urethral caruncles, dyspareunia and pruritus due to vulvar, introital, and vaginal atrophy, general skin atrophy, urinary difficulties such as urgency and abacterial urethritis and cystitis.
5. Health problems secondary to long-term deprivation of estrogen: the consequences of osteoporosis and cardiovascular disease.

27. E   p.593

If vulva, vagina, and cervix appear normal on inspection, perimenopausal bleeding can be assumed to be intrauterine in origin. Confirmation requires the absence of abnormal cytology on the Pap smear. The principal symptom of endometrial cancer is abnormal vaginal bleeding, but carcinoma will be encountered in only about 2% of postmenopausal endometrial biopsies. Normal endometrium is found over half the time, polyps in about 3%, and endometrial hyperplasia about 15% of the time. Postmenopausal bleeding should always be taken seriously.

28. B   p.594,595

The vasomotor flush is viewed as the hallmark of the female climacteric, experienced to some degree by most postmenopausal women. The term "hot flush" is descriptive of a sudden onset of reddening of the skin over the head, neck, and chest, accompanied by a feeling of intense body heat and concluded by sometimes profuse perspiration. The duration varies from a few seconds to several minutes and rarely for an hour. The frequency may be rare to recurrent every few minutes. Flushes are more frequent and severe at night (when a woman is often awakened from sleep) or during times of stress. In a cool environment, hot flushes are fewer, less intense, and shorter in duration compared to a warm environment. Although the hot flush is the most common problem of the postmenopause, it presents no inherent health hazard.

29. C   p.597,598

Beyond age 40 resorption begins to exceed formation by about 0.5% per year. This adverse relationship accelerates after menopause and up to 5% of trabecular bone and 1–1.5% of total bone mass loss will occur per year after menopause. This accelerated loss will continue for 10–15 years, after which bone loss is considerably diminished but continues as the aging-related loss. For the first 20 years following cessation of menses, menopause-related bone loss results in a 50% reduction in trabecular bone and a 30% reduction in cortical bone. The process is slower in blacks.

The change in trabecular bone in postmenopausal women is attributed to estrogen deficiency; 75% or more of the bone loss that occurs in women during the first 15 years after menopause is attributable to estrogen deficiency rather than to aging itself. A study of the premenopausal daughters of women with osteoporosis revealed a reduction in bone mass, suggesting either a genetic influence or the sharing of a lifestyle which produces a relatively low peak bone mass.

30. C   p.598

Hip fractures begin to occur in the 10–15 years following menopause such that by age 90, 20% of all white women will have developed hip fractures, of which one-sixth will be fatal within three months. Hip fractures alone occur in about 250,000 women per year in the U.S. with a mortality of 40,000 annually and an associated cost of billions of dollars. In addition, the survivors are frequently severely disabled and may become permanent invalids.

Estrogen therapy will stabilize the process of osteoporosis or prevent it from occurring. With estrogen therapy one can expect a 50–60% decrease in fractures of the arm and hip, and when estrogen is supplemented with calcium, an 80% reduction in vertebral compression fractures can be observed. This reduction is seen primarily in patients who have taken estrogen for more than 5 years. If bone loss can be delayed with estrogen therapy for 8 years, fracture incidence can be reduced by 75%.

31. B   p.599

While progestational agents are considered antiestrogenic, they have been known to act independently, in a manner similar to estrogen, to reduce bone resorption. However, this effect may be limited to cortical bone. When added to estrogen, progestins actually lead to a synergistic increase in bone formation associated with a positive balance of calcium. The daily, continuous combination of estrogen-progestin is equally efficacious in maintaining bone density as the standard sequential regimens.

32. A   p.600

In order to remain in zero calcium balance, women on estrogen therapy require a total of 1,000 mg elemental calcium per day. Since the average woman receives only 500 mg of calcium in her diet, the minimal daily supplement equals an additional 500 mg. Women not on estrogen require a daily supplement of at least 1,000 mg calcium. Even with the commonly used therapeutic doses of calcium, nearly 40% of postmenopausal women will have inefficient absorption. Therefore estrogen improves calcium absorption and makes it possible to utilize supplemental calcium in effective doses without the side effects associated with higher doses (constipation and flatulence) that diminish compliance. Nevertheless, the calcium supplementation should be administered in divided doses with meals. We must emphasize that although calcium supplementation is important, it cannot provide the same degree of protection against osteoporosis as that achieved by hormonal therapy.

The addition of vitamin D or its active metabolite in some studies has no impact on the osteoporosis fracture rate and may cause hypercalcemia and renal stone formation. However, elderly people in nursing homes are usually deficient in vitamin D, and it is now recommended that individuals over age 70 should add 800 units of vitamin D to calcium supplementation. A large randomized trial in Finland has documented a reduced rate of fractures in elderly women receiving supplementation of vitamin D (by an annual intramuscular injection), and in France, supplementation of calcium and vitamin D reduced the number of hip fractures by 43%. Because adequate vitamin D depends upon cutaneous generation mediated by sun exposure, women who live in cloudy areas during the winter months are relatively vitamin D deficient and lose bone. Vitamin D supplementation is recommended for these women as well but at a lower level, 400 units daily. If uncertain regarding vitamin D supplementation, the serum level of the active metabolite, 1,25-dihydroxyvitamin D, can be measured; the normal range is 19–57 ng/L (45–137 pmol/L).

33. B   p.600,601

The addition of fluoride, a potent stimulator of bone formation, does offer some benefit but with a high rate of side effects (which may be greatly reduced with slow release preparations). A further concern is that this therapy may lead to more brittle bones subject to fracture.

Calcitonin will act to prevent bone resorption and eventually might be used in patients for whom hormone therapy is contraindicated. Given by injection in a dose of 100 IU daily to women early after menopause it has the same effectiveness as estrogen in conserving bone density. Studies with intranasal delivery of calcitonin (200 IU daily) suggest it may be similarly effective.

Etidronate disodium is an oral biphosphonate compound known to reduce bone resorption through the inhibition of osteoclastic activity. In postmenopausal women with osteoporosis randomized to intermittent cyclical etidronate (400 mg daily for 2 weeks followed by a 12-week drug free interval during which 1500 mg/day of calcium is administered) or placebo, a significant increase in vertebral bone mineral content and a significant decrease in fracture rate was observed in the treatment group. Newer biphosphates are more active than etidronate. Alendronate given in various doses to postmenopausal women for only 6 weeks increased bone density with a lack of side effects. Biphosphates may prove to be an effective addition to osteoporotic prevention because they are well tolerated and have no discernible side effects. However, unlike estrogens, biphosphates have no effect on cardiovascular disease, hot flushes, or the atrophic changes seen in menopause. At the present time further studies must be performed to evaluate the efficacy and value of biphosphates for prevention of osteoporosis.

Lifestyle can have a beneficial effect on bone density. Physical activity (weight bearing), as little as 30 minutes a day for 3 days a week, will increase the mineral content of bone in older women. The exercise need not be extreme. Walking 1.5 miles and ordinary calisthenics will suffice. The impact of exercise on bone is significantly less, however, than that achieved by hormone therapy. Women require the full combination of hormone therapy, calcium supplementation, and exercise in order to fully minimize the risk of fractures.

34. E   p.601

Adverse habits such as cigarette smoking or excessive alcohol consumption are associated with an increased risk of osteoporosis. The lower blood levels of estrogen in smokers have been correlated with an earlier menopause and a reduced bone density, and therefore estrogen therapy will not totally counteract the predisposition of smoking toward osteoporosis. The titration of estrogen dosage with circulating blood estradiol levels in smokers makes clinical sense, allowing the use of higher hormonal doses to mainain bone density. Clinicians should always remember that exposure to excessive thyroid and glucocorticoid hormones is associated with osteoporosis and an increased rate of fractures.

35. E   p.601

Patients with osteoporosis should be screened for other conditions that lead to osteoporosis:

1. Serum parathyroid hormone, calcium, phosphorus, and alkaline phosphatase: for primary hyperparathyroidism.
2. Renal function tests: for secondary hyperparathyroidism with chronic renal failure.
3. Blood count and smear, sedimentation rate, protein electrophoresis: for multiple myeloma, leukemia, or lymphoma.
4. Thyroid function tests: for hyperthyroidism.
5. Careful history and, when indicated, appropriate laboratory studies to rule out hypercortisolism, alcohol abuse, and metastatic cancer.

36. E   p.602

Standard x-rays do not provide an early assessment of fracture risk; 30–40% of bone must be lost before radiographic changes become apparent. Photon absorptiometry measures the transmission of photons through bone. Single photon absorptiometry uses an ^{125}I source of energy or, more recently, miniature x-ray tubes. This method measures bone density in the radius and the calcaneus. These measurements correlate with vertebral bone density but not very accurately. Dual energy absorptiometry employs photons from two energy sources. Dual energy x-ray absorptiometry (DEXA) provides good precision for all sites of osteoporotic fractures. Whole body scans by DEXA can measure total body calcium, lean body mass, and fat mass. Quantitative computed tomography for bone density measurements can be performed on most commercial computed tomography (CT) systems; however, radiation exposure is higher than with DEXA, and measurements of the femur are not available. The most accurate information is provided by the DEXA technique, measuring the three sites of greatest interest, the radius, the hip, and the spine. Serial measurements are usually at least one year apart.

37. E   p.602

Reasons to Measure Bone Mass
1. To help patients to make decisions regarding hormone therapy.
2. To assess response to therapy in selected patients, e.g., smokers.
3. To confirm the diagnosis and assess the severity of osteoporosis to aid in treatment decisions.

38. A   p.605

In cohort studies, only two produced conflicting data. The Walnut Creek Study, one initially with conflicting data, had, in its first report, only 26 women with infarctions, and only 9 were estrogen users. An update of the Walnut Creek data now documents a 50% reduction in death from diseases of the circulatory system when adjusted for all other factors.

The Framingham Heart Study presented data in 1978, and in 1985, which argued that there was a 50% increased risk for cardiovascular disease among estrogen users, although there was no difference in fatality rates between users and nonusers. Because of the respect the Framingham Heart Study carries, its impact was significant. There are, however, major criticisms of the Framingham report. First, the patient numbers were relatively small (302 postmenopausal women on estrogen) in comparison to the patient numbers in other studies on this particular issue. Furthermore, the effect of dose and duration of treatment could not be ascertained; they were not recorded. Finally and most conclusively, a subsequent reanalysis of the Framingham data (eliminating angina as a consideration) by the authors of the study reversed their conclusion. The early reports from the Framingham Heart Study, therefore, stand in lonely opposition to overwhelming evidence that appropriately low doses of estrogen protect postmenopausal women against cardiovascular disease.

The Leisure World Study (a prospective, longitudinal study in a large retirement community under relatively controlled and accurate conditions) has documented a reduced risk of death due to myocardial infarction in current and past users of estrogen.

The Nurses' Health Study has reached 10 years of follow-up; 48,470 postmenopausal women were free of coronary heart disease when initially evaluated, and subsequently 629 had either nonfatal or fatal disease. The age-adjusted relative risk of coronary disease in current users showed approximately a 50% reduction. No association between use and stroke was observed. It was suggested that higher doses might be harmful in that there was an apparent increase in the risk of coronary disease among women taking more than 1.25 mg conjugated estrogens per day.

The Lipid Research Clinics Follow-up Study (a prospective 8.5-year follow-up of 2,270 women) has demonstrated a 63% reduction in the relative risk of fatal cardiovascular disease in current estrogen users, including a protective effect in current and exsmokers.

39. E p.608

The possible beneficial actions of estrogens on cardiovascular disease include all of the following:

1. A favorable impact on the circulating lipid and lipoprotein profile, specifically a decrease in total cholesterol and LDL-cholesterol and an increase in HDL-cholesterol.
2. A direct antiatherosclerotic effect in arteries.
3. Augmentation of vasodilating and antiplatelet aggregation factors, especially nitric oxide and prostacyclin (endothelium-dependent mechanisms).
4. Vasodilatation by means of endothelium-independent mechanisms.
5. Direct inotropic actions on the heart.
6. Improvement of peripheral glucose metabolism with a subsequent decrease in circulating insulin levels.
7. Inhibition of lipoprotein oxidation.
8. Favorable impact on the clotting mechanism.

40. C p.611

Estrogen normally promotes mitotic growth of the endometrium. Abnormal progression of growth through simple hyperplasia, complex hyperplasia, atypia, and early carcinoma has been associated with unopposed estrogen activity, administered either continuously or in cyclic fashion. Only one year of treatment with unopposed estrogen (0.625 mg conjugated estrogens or the equivalent) will produce a 20% incidence of hyperplasia. Some 10% of women with complex hyperplasia progress to frank cancer, and complex hyperplasia is observed to antedate adenocarcinoma in 25–30% of cases. If atypia is present, 20–25% of cases will progress to carcinoma within a year. The average time required for progression from hyperplasia to carcinoma is approximately 5 years, and atypia is expected to appear prior to the malignant change. Retrospective studies have estimated that the risk of endometrial cancer in women on estrogen therapy (unopposed by a progestational agent) is increased by a factor of somewhere from 2 to 10 times the normal incidence of 1 per 1,000 postmenopausal women per year. The risk increases with duration of exposure and dose of estrogen, lingers for up to 10 years after estrogen is discontinued, and the risk of cancer that has already spread beyond the uterus is increased 3-fold in women who have used estrogen a year or longer.

41. A p.619

Relative Estrogen Potencies

Estrogen	FSH levels	Liver proteins	Bone density
Piperazine estrone sulfate	1.0 mg	2.0 mg	0.625 mg
Micronized estradiol	1.0 mg	1.0 mg	1.0 mg
Conjugated estrogens	1.0 mg	0.625 mg	0.625 mg
Ethinyl estradiol	5.0 µg	2–10 µg	5–10 µg
Transdermal estradiol	—	—	50 µg

42. C p.620

Daily estrogen:	0.625 mg conjugated estrogens, or 0.625 mg estrone sulfate, or 1.0 mg micronized estradiol
Daily progestin:	2.5 mg medroxyprogesterone acetate, or 0.35 mg norethindrone

Combined with calcium supplementation (250 mg bid with meals), and Vitamin D (400 IU in cloudy winter months and 800 IU for elderly women).

43. C p.621

Compliance with hormone therapy programs is notoriously poor. The two most common reasons why women discontinue or do not start hormone treatment are fear of cancer and vaginal bleeding. The current data on breast cancer are reassuring, and the addition of a progestational agent has effectively prevented endometrial cancer. But the persistence of bleeding with the traditional sequential regimen continues to be a barrier to good compliance. To go from 80–90% withdrawal bleeding to 80% no bleeding represents a major accomplishment, and thus, the continuous approach has a significant advantage.

44. A p.621

The single most aggravating and worrisome problem with daily, continuous therapy is breakthrough bleeding. One can expect 40–60% of patients to experience breakthrough bleeding during the first 6 months of treatment; however, this percentage decreases to approximately 20% after one year. While this percentage of amenorrhea is a gratifying accomplishment, the number of women who experience breakthrough bleeding is considerable and it is a difficult management problem.

This breakthrough bleeding is similar to that seen with oral contraceptives. It originates from an endometrium dominated by progestational influence; hence the endometrium is usually atrophic and yields little, if anything, to the exploring biopsy instrument. It takes confidence and experience with this method to withstand the urge to biopsy. The endometrial biopsy in this circumstance, no matter what the instrument or method, is not cost-effective. Patients require constant support through the early months of continuous therapy. If bleeding persists for 6 months, consider an office hysteroscopy; an impressive number of polyps and intrauterine fibroids will be discovered.

There is no effective method of drug alteration or substitution to manage this breakthrough bleeding. The breakthrough bleeding rate is not much better with a higher dose of progestin (5.0 mg medroxyprogesterone acetate) compared to the lower dose (2.5 mg). Therefore, there is no reason to use the higher dose, thus minimizing side effects. The best approach is to gain time, as most patients will cease bleeding. This means good educational preparation of the patient beforehand and frequent telephone contact to allay anxiety and encourage persistence.

45. C p.622

It is not essential to perform endometrial biopsies prior to treatment. Endometrial abnormalities in asymptomatic postmenopausal women are very rare. A reasonable economic moderation would be to limit pretreatment biopsies (using the plastic endometrial suction device in the office) to patients at higher risk for endometrial changes: those women with conditions associated with chronic estrogen exposure (obesity, dysfunctional uterine bleeding, anovulation and infertility, hirsutism, high alcohol intake, hepatic disease, metabolic problems such as diabetes mellitus and hypothyroidism) and those women in whom irregular bleeding occurs while on estrogen-progestin therapy. In the absence of abnormal bleeding, a certain amount of trust in the protective effects of the progestin is justified, and routine, periodic biopsies are not necessary. *Abnormal endometrium is more frequently encountered in patients on combination estrogen-progestin when the patients have previously been treated for a period of time with unopposed estrogen. Breakthrough bleeding in these patients requires endometrial sampling because an increased risk for endometrial cancer persists beyond the period of exposure to unopposed estrogen, and it is unknown how effective the subsequent protective exposure to a progestin will be.*

The timing of withdrawal bleeding in women on a sequential estrogen-progestin program has been suggested as a screening method for biopsy decision-making. In women taking a variety of progestins for 12 days each month, bleeding on or before day 10 after the addition of the progestin was associated with proliferative endometrium.

Bleeding beginning on day 11 or later was associated with secretory endometrium, presumably indicating less need for biopsy. Whether this truly correlates with the risk of hyperplasia and cancer is not known.

Women who elect to be treated with unopposed estrogen require endometrial surveillance at least once a year.

46. A   p.623

Many women do not tolerate treatment with progestational hormones. Typical side effects include breast tenderness, bloating, and depression. These reactions are significant detrimental factors with compliance.

47. B   p.623

The potential benefits of androgen treatment include improvement in psychological well-being and an increase in sexually motivated behavior. These effects, however, follow the administration of relatively large doses of androgen. In a well-designed, placebo-controlled study, lower doses of androgen contributed little to actual sexual behavior, although an increase in sexual fantasies and masturbation could be documented.

Any benefit must be balanced by the unwanted effects, in particular, a negative impact on the cholesterol-lipoprotein profile. Unfortunately, data are scanty on this issue. In a short-term study comparing a product with estrogen and a relatively low dose of testosterone (1.25 mg methyltestosterone) to estrogen alone, a negative impact on the lipid profile was apparent within 3 months. It should also be remembered that the addition of androgen does not protect the endometrium, and the addition of a progestin is still necessary. It is uncertain (and unstudied) how much aromatization of the administered testosterone increases the estrogen impact and whether this might further increase the risk of endometrial and/or breast cancer. The addition of testosterone to an estrogen therapy program provides no additional beneficial impact on bone.

There is no doubt that pharmacologic amounts of androgen can increase libido, but these same doses produce unwanted effects. In addition, patients on high doses of androgens often are somewhat addicted to this therapy. Small amounts of androgen supplementation can be provided in situations where the patient and clinician are convinced a depressed libido cannot be explained by psychosocial circumstances. In these cases, the lipid profile should be carefully monitored. Any positive clinical response may well be a placebo effect. After some months or a few years, conversion to a standard program is recommended.

48. E   p.627

Pregnancy and Breast Cancer. At one point in time, it was believed that pregnancy (and its impressive levels of estrogens and progesterone) had an adverse impact on the prognosis of breast cancer diagnosed during the pregnancy. It is now apparent that there is no difference in survival when pregnant women with breast cancer are matched to nonpregnant women by age and stage of disease, and termination of pregnancy is not associated with improved survival. Pregnant women do have a 2.5-fold higher risk of metastatic disease, but the reason is later diagnosis because the breast changes associated with pregnancy make diagnosis difficult. Because of diagnosis at a more advanced stage of disease, pregnant women with breast cancer usually have less well-differentiated (receptor negative) tumors. Thus, it can be argued, the intense hormonal stimulation of pregnancy (both estrogen and progesterone) has no adverse impact on the course of breast cancer.

Breast Cancer and Subsequent Pregnancy. As with breast cancer diagnosed in already pregnant women, subsequent pregnancy, after diagnosis and treatment, has no negative impact on prognosis. This, too, would argue against an impact of hormonal stimulation on the risk of recurrent or new disease.

Oral Contraception and the Risk of Breast Cancer. The experience with oral contraceptives over the last 30 years has provided neither definitive evidence that exogenous estrogen and progestin increase the risk of breast cancer, nor evidence that exposure to these exogenous hormones offers major protection against breast cancer. The lack of a major detrimental effect is an effective argument against a major link between breast cancer and exogenous hormone treatment.

Depo-Provera and the Risk of Breast Cancer. Medroxyprogesterone acetate, in large continuous doses, produced breast tumors in beagle dogs. This is an effect unique to the beagle dog and has not appeared in other animals or in women after years of use. A very large, hospital-based case-control World Health Organization study conducted over 9 years in 3 developing countries has indicated that exposure to Depo-Provera very slightly increased the risk of breast cancer in the first 4 years of use, but there was no evidence for an increase in risk with increased duration of use. The results were interpreted to suggest that growth of already existing tumors is enhanced. The number of cases was not large, and the confidence intervals reflected this. For example, the relative risk for recent users (based on a total of 19 cases) was 1.21, but the confidence interval included 1.0 and thus was not statistically significant.

Two earlier population-based case-control studies indicated a possible association between breast cancer and Depo-Provera. One, from Costa Rica, was subject to several biases. The other, from New Zealand, did not find an increased relative risk in ever users but did find an indication of increased risk shortly after initiating use in early age. These studies have been all limited by very small numbers and thus have been inconclusive.

Certainly the risk, if real, is very slight, and it is equally possible that the suggestions of increased risk have not been free of confounding variables. It is more appropriate to emphasize that these studies did not find evidence for an increased risk of breast cancer with long durations of use. Thus, experience with exposure to a pure progestational agent does not support the argument that progestational influence will increase the risk of breast cancer.

49. A   p.629

Tamoxifen, it has been argued, is a better choice for women who have had breast cancer. This argument stresses that the agonistic, estrogenic actions of tamoxifen on bone and lipids will offer protection against osteoporosis and cardiovascular disease, while tamoxifen's antagonism of estrogen at the breast will prevent recurrence and contralateral disease. An important assumption is that tamoxifen and estrogen provide equal protection against osteoporosis and cardiovascular disease.

In general, thus far, the studies indicate that the estrogenic, agonistic actions of tamoxifen do prevail upon the cholesterol profile and bone density. Bone density studies demonstrate no loss of bone, indicating an estrogen agonistic action of tamoxifen to maintain bone in comparison to the loss usually encountered after menopause. In a two-year randomized study tamoxifen had a positive impact on trabecular bone in the lumbar spine. At the end of two years, the difference between tamoxifen and the placebo group was 3%, identical to the difference observed with the use of etidronate. This difference is less than the usual 5–10% difference comparing women who use calcitonin or estrogen to placebo. Thus, the bone density data (still limited) suggest that the degree of protection is not equivalent to that of estrogen. Furthermore, in premenopausal women, tamoxifen may, in the presence of higher levels of estrogen, exert an antagonistic action on the bone, resulting in bone loss (clinical data in premenopausal women are not yet available).

Tamoxifen is associated with an estrogen-like decrease in total cholesterol and LDL-cholesterol, with an increase in triglycerides and HDL-cholesterol (although some studies do not find a significant impact on HDL). In a report from the Scottish cancer trial, 10 myocardial infarctions were observed in the tamoxifen arm and 25 in the placebo group, a statistically significant difference.

Postmenopausal patients can be reassured that the antagonistic actions of tamoxifen do not prevail in regard to osteoporosis and cardiovascular disease; however, to what extent the agonistic effect protects against clinical events and how it compares to the benefits of a hormone treatment program will require future epidemiologic studies. At this point in time, one cannot assume that tamoxifen protects against cardiovascular disease and osteoporosis with an impact equal to that of hormone treatment.

50. A   p.630

While it is known that the doses of estrogen used for postmenopausal treatment have no significant impact on the clotting mechanism and no increased risks for thrombotic clinical events have been demonstrated, these findings are derived from women without previous events. Does the woman with a previous event represent a different risk? On the other hand, the woman with a previous event may be the very woman who needs the protection of estrogen against cardiovascular disease. There is evidence to support this contention. In the Leisure World study, estrogen users with previous myocardial infarctions, strokes, or hypertension had a 50% reduction in risk for death from a subsequent stroke or myocardial infarction. In the Lipid Research Clinics study, the cardiovascular mortality in women with previous cardiovascular disease was reduced 85%. And finally, and most impressively, in women with severe coronary disease (documented by arteriography), estrogen users had a 97% survival rate at 5 years compared to a significantly different 81% rate in nonusers. In women with mild to moderate disease, there was no difference at 5 years, but at 10 years, estrogen users had a 96% survival rate compared to 85% in nonusers. In our opinion, estrogen treatment is indicated for these patients.

Metabolic contraindications to estrogen include impaired liver function and acute vascular disease (including embolus and thrombosis). Close surveillance is indicated for some patients with seizure disorders, familial hyperlipidemias (elevated triglycerides), and migraine headaches. Patients with migraine headaches often improve if a daily, continuous method of treatment is used, eliminating a cyclic change in hormone levels that can serve to trigger headaches.

Conditions that do not represent contraindications include controlled hypertension, diabetes mellitus, and varicose veins. The belief that estrogen is potentially harmful with each of these clinical situations is derived from old studies of high dose birth control pills. Estrogen in appropriate doses is acceptable in the presence of these conditions.

Fibroid tumors of the uterus almost always are not stimulated to grow by postmenopausal doses of estrogen. Nevertheless, pelvic examination surveillance is a wise course. No other cancers (besides those mentioned above) are known to be adversely affected by hormone therapy. Postmenopausal hormone therapy can be administered to all patients with cervical, ovarian, or vulvar malignancies. Interestingly, the Nurses' Health Study reported a marginally significant reduced risk of colorectal cancer in past users of postmenopausal estrogen.

51. D p.632

Clonidine, bromocriptine, and naloxone given orally are only partially effective for the relief of hot flushes and require high doses with a high rate of side effects. Bellergal treatment is better than a placebo, but it is also a potent sedative. Veralipride, a dopamine antagonist that is active in the hypothalamus, is relatively effective in inhibiting flushing at a dose of 100 mg daily. Mastodynia and galactorrhea are the major side effects. Medroxyprogesterone acetate (10–20 mg daily) and megestrol acetate (20 mg bid) are also effective, but concerns regarding exogenous steroids (especially in patients who have had breast cancer) would apply to progestins as well. Methyldopa, in doses of 250–500 mg/day, is said to be effective, but there have been no properly controlled studies with this agent. Propranolol and similar agents are ineffective as is Vitamin E.

We recommend transdermal clonidine, applied with the 100 mg dose once weekly. Side effects are minimal, and the treatment is twice as effective as a placebo.

Patients should be questioned regarding the use of "natural" therapies. The herbs that contain estrogen-like compounds include ginseng, agnus castus, red sage, black cohosh, and beth root. The dosage and purity of herbal preprations is unknown, and most importantly, there are no substantial studies documenting either harmful or beneficial effects. Herbs are often contanimated with heavy metals. In our view, the use of products without scientific study should be discouraged.

19 Obesity

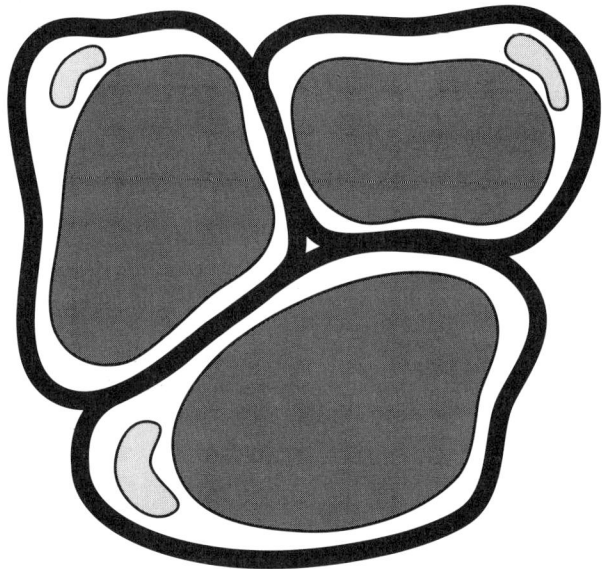

Learning Objectives

Be able to:

1. Describe methods of determining ideal body weight and defining obesity.

2. Understand the physiology of adipose tissue.

3. Detail the different types of anatomic obesity and the physiologic significance of each.

4. Discuss what is known regarding diet management of obesity and its long-term effects upon cardiovascular disease.

Pre-Test

A. Instructions: Fill in the blanks

1. The most important endocrine change in obesity is elevation of the basal blood _____ level.

2. To lose a pound of fat, the equivalent of a _____ calorie intake must be expended.

B. Instructions: True or False

3. A body mass index of greater than 40 is comparable with respect to risk of morbidity to that associated with hypertension and heavy smoking.

4. The simplest way to assess insulin resistance is to measure the ratio of fasting glucose to fasting insulin.

C. Instructions: For the following question choose:

A. if only 1, 2 and 3 are correct
B. if only 1 and 3 are correct
C. if only 2 and 4 are correct
D. if only 4 is correct
E. if all are correct

5. Women with android obesity
   1. should be tested for hyperinsulinemia
   2. have a waist:hip ratio less than 0.75
   3. are at greater risk of developing cardiovascular disease than women with gynoid obesity
   4. have less adrenal activity with decreases in ACTH and cortisol secretion

Post-Test

A. Instructions: Fill in the blanks

1. Obesity is an excess storage of _____ in adipose cells.

2. The formula for the ideal weight in pounds for women is _____ + (4 x (height in inches minus _____)).

3. The body mass index is the ratio of the _____ in _____ divided by the _____ squared in _____.

4. _____ obesity (the pear shape) refers to fat distribution in the lower body (femoral and gluteal regions), while _____ obesity (the apple shape) refers to central body distribution.

5. _____ obesity is associated with hyperinsulinemia, impaired glucose tolerance, diabetes mellitus, decreased levels of sex hormone binding, globulin and increased levels of free testosterone and estradiol.

6. The _____ to _____ ratio is the variable most strongly and inversely associated with the level of _____, the fraction of HDL-cholesterol most consistently linked with protection from cardiovascular disease.

7. After adjusting for age and smoking, the Nurses' Health Study documented a 3-fold increase in risk for coronary disease among women with a body mass index of _____ or greater.

8. The best diet is limitation of calories to between _____ and _____ calories per day. The ideal diet consists of _____% carbohydrates, _____% protein and less than _____% fat.

9. Phenylpropanolamine taken in combination with _____ can precipitate a hypertensive crisis.

10. Both weight loss and increased physical activity lower the level of _____-cholesterol and increase the level of _____-cholesterol.

B. Instructions: True or False

11. Being overweight in adolescence is a more powerful predictor of cardiovascular adverse health effects than being overweight as an adult.

12. The incidence of heart disease, gout, colorectal cancer and arthritis is elevated in overweight people.

13. Men have a greater prevalence of obesity compared to women.

14. The prevalence of obesity is inversely related to the level of physical activity and education and directly related to parity.

15. Hypothyroidism can cause obesity.

16. Women with android obesity are less likely than women with gynoid obesity to develop diabetes mellitus and coronary heart disease.

17. Weight loss in women with lower body obesity is mainly cosmetic, whereas loss of central body weight is more important for general health.

18. The waist measurement is measured as the smallest circumference between the rib cage and iliac crests while the hip measurement is the largest circumference between the waist and thighs.

19. A regular pattern of physical exercise reduces the risk of myocardial infarction in all people.

C. Match each activity with the appropriate calories per hour

A. 90
B. 240
C. 300
D. 360
E. greater than 750

20. swimming
21. housework
22. sleeping
23. golf
24. bicycling
25. cross country skiing
26. running

D. Instructions: For each of the following questions choose:

    A. if only 1, 2 and 3 are correct
    B. if only 1 and 3 are correct
    C. if only 2 and 4 are correct
    D. if only 4 is correct
    E. if all are correct

27. Obesity is associated with increased morbidity associated with the following diseases
    1. diabetes mellitus
    2. gallbladder disease
    3. renal disease
    4. cirrhosis of the liver

28. Obesity is associated with major risk factors for atherosclerosis which include
    1. hypertension
    2. diabetes
    3. hypercholesterolemia
    4. hypertriglycerides

29. Hyperinsulinemia
    1. affects the metabolism of carbohydrate, fat and protein
    2. leads to a decrease in HDL-cholesterol and an increase in LDL-cholesterol
    3. is directly associated with hypertension
    4. associated with obesity and is not reversible with weight loss

30. The effectiveness of diets
    1. are more successful when managed by commercial organizations rather than nonprofit self-help groups
    2. is disappointing in that only 30% lose 20 pounds or more
    3. has little to do with changes in lifestyle
    4. is disappointing in that only 4% lose 40 pounds or more

---

Answers for Chapter 19 — Pre-Test Questions

1. insulin   p.658

The most important endocrine change in obesity is elevation of the basal blood insulin level. Increases in body fat change the body's secretion and sensitivity to insulin. There is a decrease in the number of insulin receptor sites at a cellular level, most significantly in fat, liver, and muscle tissue. The key factors which affect insulin resistance are the amount of fat tissue in the body, the caloric intake per day, the amount of carbohydrates in the diet, and the amount of daily exercise. At least one mechanism for the increased resistance to insulin observed with increasing weight is down-regulation of insulin receptors brought about by the increase in insulin secretion.

2. 3500   p.660

The discouraging aspect is that to lose a pound of fat, the equivalent to a 3,500 calorie intake must be expended. Dieting has to be slow and steady to be effective. Successful programs include behavior modification, frequent visits to the physician, and involvement of family members. Behavior modification starts with daily recording of activity and behavior related to food intake, followed by the elimination of inappropriate cues (other than hunger) that lead to eating.

3. true   p.652

The average adult has a body mass index of 25. A body mass index of 28 or more warrants treatment. A body mass index of about 30 is roughly equivalent to 30% excess body weight, the point at which excess mortality begins (approximately

10–12% of people in the U.S. have a body mass index of 30 or greater). Above 40, the risk from obesity itself is comparable to that associated with major health problems such as hypertension and heavy smoking.

4. true   p.658

The simplest way to assess insulin resistance is to measure the ratio of fasting glucose to fasting insulin. A ratio lower than 3 is characteristic of obesity. This method has limitations, the most notable being the variation due to assay precision and pulsatile secretion of insulin. It is more reliable to measure the insulin response to 1 g/kg glucose; the maximal response should not be greater than 150 mU/mL (1,076 pmol/L). However, if a patient is obese, one can assume the patient is insulin resistant.

5. B   p.659,660

Android obesity refers to fat located in the abdominal wall and visceral-mesenteric locations. This fat is more sensitive to catecholamines and less sensitive to insulin and thus more active metabolically. It more easily delivers triglyceride to other tissues to meet energy requirements. This fat distribution is associated with hyperinsulinemia, impaired glucose tolerance, diabetes mellitus, an increase in androgen production rates, decreased levels of sex hormone binding globulin, and increased levels of free testosterone and estradiol. In addition, women with central obesity have greater adrenal activity with increases in ACTH and cortisol secretion.

It is central body obesity that is associated with cardiovascular risk factors, including hypertension and adverse cholesterol-lipoprotein profiles. The adverse impact of excess weight in adolescence can be explained by the fact that deposition of fat in adolescence is largely central in location.

The waist:hip ratio is a means of estimating the degree of upper to lower body obesity; the ratio accurately predicts the amount of intra-abdominal fat (which is greater with android obesity). The waist measurement is measured as the smallest circumference (girth) between the rib cage and iliac crests. The hip measurement is the largest circumference between the waist and thighs. Interpretation is as follows:

Greater than 0.85 — Android Obesity
Less than 0.75 — Gynoid Obesity

Answers for Chapter 19 — Post-Test Questions

1. triglycerides   p.652,653

Obesity is an excess storage of triglycerides in adipose cells. There is a difference between obesity and overweight. Obesity is an excess of body fat. Overweight is a body weight in excess of some standard or ideal weight. The ideal weight for any adult is believed to correspond to his or her ideal weight from age 20 to 30.

2. 100; 60   p.652

Women: 100 + (4 x (height in inches minus 60))
Men: 120 + (4 x (height in inches minus 60))

3. weight; kilograms; height; meters   p.652

The body mass index (the Quetelet index) is the ratio of weight divided by the height squared (in metric units):

Quetelet Index = $kilograms/meters^2$

4. Gynoid; android   p.659

Gynoid obesity (the pear shape) refers to fat distribution in the lower body (femoral and gluteal regions), while android obesity (the apple shape) refers to central body distribution. Gynoid fat is more resistant to catecholamines and more sensitive to insulin than abdominal fat; thus extraction and storage of fatty acids easily occur, and fat is accumulated more readily in the thighs and buttocks. This fat is associated with minimal fatty acid flux, and therefore the negative consequences of fatty acid metabolism are less.

5. Android
p.659

Android obesity refers to fat located in the abdominal wall and visceral-mesenteric locations. This fat is more sensitive to catecholamines and less sensitive to insulin and thus more active metabolically. It more easily delivers triglyceride to other tissues to meet energy requirements. This fat distribution is associated with hyperinsulinemia, impaired glucose tolerance, diabetes mellitus, an increase in androgen production rates, decreased levels of sex hormone binding globulin, and increased levels of free testosterone and estradiol. In addition, women with central obesity have greater adrenal activity with increases in ACTH and cortisol secretion.

6. waist; hip; HDL_2
p.659

The waist:hip ratio is the variable most strongly and inversely associated with the level of HDL_2, the fraction of HDL-cholesterol most consistently linked with protection from cardiovascular disease.

7. 29
p.660

Aside from not smoking cigarettes, weight reduction is the most important health measure available for reducing the risk of cardiovascular disease. After adjusting for age and smoking, the Nurses' Health Study documented a 3-fold increase in risk for coronary disease among women with a body mass index of 29 or greater. Even women who are mildly or moderately overweight have a substantial increase in coronary risk. In the Nurses' Health Study, 40% of coronary events could be attributed to excessive body weight, and in the heaviest women, 70%.

8. 900; 1200; 50; 15–20; 30
p.660

Despite various fads and diet books, the best diet continues to be a limitation of calories to between 900 and 1200 calories per day, the actual amount depending on what the individual patient will accept and pursue. When energy intake is less than this, it is very difficult to obtain the recommended levels of vitamins and minerals.

Ideal Diet: Carbohydrates — 50%
               Protein   — 15–20%
               Fat   — <30%

9. bromocriptine or monoamine oxidase inhibitor
p.661

Over-the-counter products contain phenylpropanolamine as the active ingredient. This drug is a sympathomimetic derived from ephedrine and can act synergistically with caffeine to produce amphetamine-like reactions. ***It should be noted that phenylpropanolamine taken in combination with bromocriptine or a monoamine oxidase inhibitor can precipitate a hypertensive crisis.***

10. LDL; HDL
p.662

A regular pattern of physical exercise reduces the risk of myocardial infarction in all people. Both weight loss and increased physical activity, through an unknown mechanism, lower the level of low density lipoprotein (LDL), and increase the level of high density lipoprotein (HDL). A further benefit of strenuous or prolonged exercise is an inhibition of appetite that lasts many hours and that is associated with an increase in the resting metabolic rate for 24–48 hours. There is one study, however, that indicates a rebound increase in appetite 1–2 days after exercise. The optimal program includes, therefore, a *daily* period of exercise. The best time for exercise is before meals or about 2 hours after eating. It is probably wise to take a day off at least once a week to give muscles and joints a rest.

11. true
p.651

Being overweight in adolescence is a more powerful predictor of cardiovascular adverse health effects than being overweight as an adult.

12. true
p.651

The incidence of heart disease, noninsulin dependent diabetes mellitus, gout, colorectal cancer, and arthritis is elevated in overweight people. When the personal and social problems encountered by obese persons are also considered, it is no wonder that a physician without a weight problem cannot comprehend why fat individuals remain overweight.

13. false
p.652

It is well recognized that women have a greater prevalence of obesity compared to men. One reason may be the fact that women have a lower metabolic rate than men, even when adjusted for differences in body composition and level of activity. Another reason that more women gain weight with age is the postmenopausal loss of the increase in metabolic rate that is associated with the luteal phase of the menstrual cycle. The difference between men and women is even greater in older age. Unfortunately the basal metabolic rate decreases with age. After age 18, the resting metabolic rate declines about 2% per decade. A 30-year-old individual will inevitably gain weight if there is no change in caloric intake or exercise level over the years. The middle-age spread is both a biologic and a psychosociologic phenomenon. It is therefore important for both our patients and ourselves to understand adipose tissue and the problem of obesity.

14. true p.658

Genetics and biochemistry are against many obese people. It is best to recognize that an obese individual who has suffered with the problem lifelong does have a disorder, a disorder which is not well understood. However, for each individual, the extent to which the genetic predisposition is expressed depends upon environmental influences. The prevalence of obesity is inversely related to the level of physical activity and education and directly related to parity. Thus, socioeconomic and behavioral factors are important determinants of body weight, and surely each individual will reflect varying impacts of genetics and environment.

15. false p.659

Contrary to popular misconception, hypothyroidism does not cause obesity. Weight gain due to hypothyroidism is confined to the fluid accumulation of myxedema. There is no place, therefore, for thyroid hormone administration in the treatment of obesity when the patient is euthyroid.

16. false p.659

Gynoid fat is principally stored fat. The clinical meaning of this is that women with gynoid obesity are less likely than women with android obesity to develop diabetes mellitus and coronary heart disease.

17. true p.660

Weight loss in women with lower body obesity is mainly cosmetic, whereas loss of central body weight is more important for general health in that an improvement in cardiovascular risk is associated with loss of central body fat.

18. true p.660

The waist:hip ratio is a means of estimating the degree of upper to lower body obesity; the ratio accurately predicts the amount of intra-abdominal fat (which is greater with android obesity). The waist measurement is measured as the smallest circumference (girth) between the rib cage and iliac crests.

19. true p.662

20. D

21. C

22. A

23. C

24. D

25. E

26. E
(See table on page 274 in this Study Guide)

27. E p.651
The lack of success in treating obesity is not due to an unawareness of the implications of obesity; there is a clear-cut

Activity	Calories per Hour
Sleeping	90
Office work	240
Walking	240
Golf	300
Housework	300
Bicycling	360
Swimming	360
Tennis	480
Bowling	510
Running slowly	750 (ca. 120/mile)
Cross country skiing	840
Running fast	960 (ca. 160/mile)

relationship between mortality and weight. The death rate from diabetes mellitus, for example, is approximately 4 times higher among obese diabetics than among those who control their weight. Also higher among obese individuals is the incidence of gallbladder disease, cardiovascular disease, renal disease, and cirrhosis of the liver. The death rate from appendicitis is double, presumably from anesthetic and surgical complications. Even the rate of accidents is higher, perhaps because fat people are awkward or because their view of the ground or floor is obstructed.

28. E p.652

A person is obese when the amount of adipose tissue is sufficiently high (20% or more over ideal weight) to detrimentally alter biochemical and physiologic functions and to shorten life expectancy. Obesity is associated with four major risk factors for atherosclerosis: hypertension, diabetes, hypercholesterolemia, and hypertriglyceridemia. Overweight individuals have a higher prevalence of hypertension at every age, and the risk of developing hypertension is related to the amount of weight gain after age 25. The two in combination (hypertension and obesity) increase the risk of heart disease, cerebrovascular disease, and death.

29. A p.658

The increase in insulin resistance affects the metabolism of carbohydrate, fat and protein. Circulating levels of free fatty acids increase as a result of inadequate insulin suppression of the fat cell. Insulin resistance results in decreased catabolism of triglycerides, yielding a decrease in HDL-cholesterol and an increase in LDL-cholesterol. This, of course, is a major mechanism for the development of atherosclerosis. Hyperinsulinemia is also directly associated with hypertension. The hyperinsulinemia associated with obesity is reversible with weight loss.

30. C p.661

As an index of the general lack of success with diets, a summary of 10 studies (approximately 1200 patients) revealed that only 30% lose 20 pounds or more, and only 4% lose 40 pounds or more. Commercial organizations are no more successful than physician-directed programs or nonprofit self-help groups. Thus, it is obvious why gimmicks abound in this area of patient management.

It is not unusual to encounter patients who claim to be unable to lose weight despite following a diet with less than 1200 calories per day. In a study of such patients, it was discovered that underreporting of actual food intake and overreporting of physical activity are both common. While it may not be true for all patients, certainly some individuals do eat more than they think and exercise less than they report to their physicians. This is not a deliberate conscious attempt to deceive the physician. These patients truly believe their resistance to weight loss is genetic and not due to their own personal behavior. They are astonished and distressed to learn the results of accurate recording of dietary intake and physical exercise. The use of a dietitian to record a typical week's worth of eating and exercise is worthwhile. This kind of knowledge proves to be a powerful lever in providing the motivation to make the changes in lifestyle that can yield loss of weight.

20 Reproduction and the Thyroid

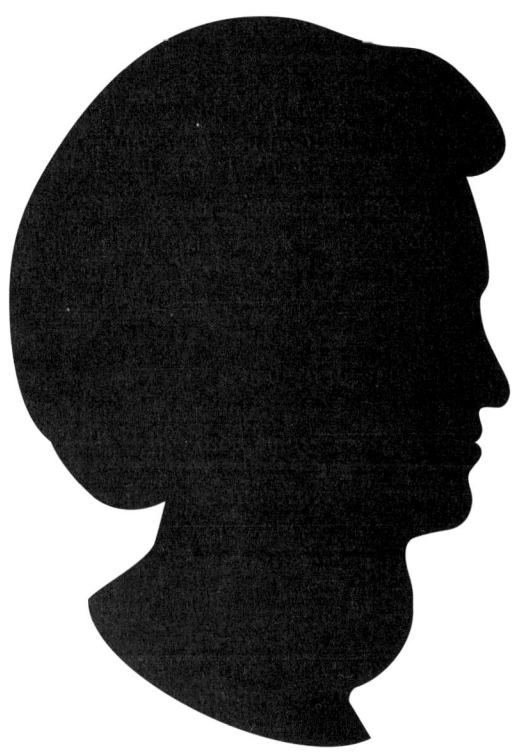

Learning Objectives

Be able to:

1. Describe the functional changes of the thyroid with aging.

2. Detail the screening and workup for nonpregnant and pregnant women with hypo-and hyperthyroidism.

3. Discuss the treatment of hypothyroidism and hyperthyroidism in both nonpregnant and pregnant women.

4. Explain the association between osteoporosis and thyroid dysfunction.

5. Discuss the natural history of postpartum thyroiditis.

Pre-Test

A. Instructions: True or False

1. The most common cause of hypothyroidism in areas with normal iodine intake is _____.

2. The full response of TSH to changes in T_4 is relatively slow; a minimum of _____ weeks is necessary between changes in dosage and assessment of TSH.

B. Instructions: True or False

3. TRH inhibits prolactin secretion by the pituitary.

4. Women receiving TSH suppressive doses of thyroxine must be considered at increased risk for osteoporosis.

C. Instructions: For each of the following questions choose:

A. if only 1, 2 and 3 are correct
B. if only 1 and 3 are correct
C. if only 2 and 4 are correct
D. if only 4 is correct
E. if all are correct

5. Functional changes which occur in thyroid physiology with aging include
   1. a decrease in TSH levels
   2. a decrease in conversion of T_4 to T_3
   3. a dramatic decrease in TBG concentrations
   4. a normal TSH response to TRH

6. Treatment of hypothyroidism
   1. involves synthetic thyroxine T_4 given daily
   2. requires standard replacement amounts of synthetic T_4 regardless of a woman's age
   3. should not exceed 25–50 µg per day for 5 weeks in older women
   4. requires a minimum of 4 weeks between changes in dosage and assessment of TSH

Post-Test

A. Instructions: Fill in the blanks

1. Removal of one iodine from the phenolic ring of T_4 yields _____, while removal of an iodine from the nonphenolic ring yields _____ which is biologically inactive.

2. Hypothyroidism accompanied by goiter formation and the presence of antithyroid antibodies is consistent with a diagnosis of _____ thyroiditis.

3. Women who have subclinical hypothyroidism and abnormal cholesterol-lipoprotein profile may show improvement with _____ treatment.

4. The two primary causes of hyperthyroidism are _____ disease and _____ disease.

5. The drug of choice for treatment of hyperthyroidism in most circumstances will be _____ because it has fewer adverse effects.

6. All patients definitively treated for hyperthyroidism must be monitored for the onset of _____.

7. Mild chronic excess thyroid hormone replacement might increase the risk of _____.

8. The most common cause of thyrotoxicosis in pregnancy is _____.

B. Instructions: True or False

9. T_4 is 3–5 times more potent than T_3.

10. Carbohydrate calories appear to be the primary determinant of T_3 levels in adults.

11. The free thyroxine (FT_4) assay has virtually replaced the total thyroxine (TT_4) and the free thyroxine index (FTI or T7) assays.

12. A normal sensitive TSH assay essentially excludes hypothyroidism or hyperthyroidism.

13. In most cases of hypothyroidism, a specific cause is apparent.

14. Thyroid hormone treatment does not help infertility in euthyroid women.

15. Patients with elevated TSH and normal free T_4 should be tested for antithyroid antibodies.

16. When abnormal thyroid function is present, a single thyroid nodule is almost always benign.

17. Maternal TSH levels reach a nadir at the same time HCG reaches a peak at 10 weeks of pregnancy.

C. Match each phrase with the appropriate medication

    A. methimazole
    B. thyroxine
    C. propranolol

18. the half-life is about one week with the maximum effect of this medication occurring at 4 to 8 weeks
19. inhibits organification of iodide and decreases production of T_4 and T_3
20. controls effects of thyroid hormone on peripheral tissues
21. major side effects are rash, gastrointestinal symptoms and granulocytopenia
22. side effects may be bronchospasm, worsening of congestive heart failure, fatigue, depression

D. Instructions: For each of the following questions choose:

A. if only 1, 2 and 3 are correct
B. if only 1 and 3 are correct
C. if only 2 and 4 are correct
D. if only 4 is correct
E. if all are correct

23. Normal thyroid physiology states that
    1. although T_4 is secreted at 20 times the rate of T_3, it is T_3 which is responsible for most of the thyroid action in the body
    2. during periods of stress, the body produces more reverse T_3 and less T_3
    3. binding proteins have a greater affinity for T_4 and thus allows T_3 to have greater entry into cells
    4. the thyroid axis is stimulated by TRH and inhibited by somatostatin and dopamine

24. To screen for thyroid disease
    1. a sensitive TSH assay is the initial screening assay
    2. if the TSH is low or high a free T_4 should be obtained
    3. if the TSH is low and the free T_4 is normal, a normal free T_3 would confirm subclinical hyperthyroidism
    4. if the TSH is low and the free T_4 is normal, a high free T_3 would confirm hyperthyroidism

25. With aging of women
    1. there is an increase in hypothyroidism
    2. the incidence of antithyroglobulin antibodies decreases
    3. screening with the highly sensitive TSH should begin at age 45
    4. there is a decrease in thyroiditis

26. Hypothyroidism may present as
    1. menstrual irregularities
    2. carpal tunnel syndrome
    3. bradycardia
    4. decreased cholesterol and LDL-cholesterol

27. Graves' disease is
    1. characterized by pretibial myxedema
    2. associated with unpredictable menstrual changes
    3. characterized by a low TSH and high T_4 or high T_3
    4. a risk factor for osteoporosis if untreated

28. Thyroid nodules
    1. are less likely to be cancerous in women than men
    2. if single, are 4 times more common in women than men
    3. do not require medical attention
    4. if single, are malignant in 12% of the cases with the vast majority being benign

29. Major risk factors for thyroid cancer are
    1. family history of thyroid cancer
    2. history of having taken Lugol's solution
    3. history of irradiation to the head or neck
    4. history of thyroiditis

30. The thyroid gland in pregnancy
    1. secretes more free T_4 than in the nonpregnant state
    2. is more sensitive to TSH than in the nonpregnant state
    3. is unaffected by levels of HCG
    4. increases in size

31. Fetal and newborn thyroid changes are characterized by
    1. reverse T_3 exceeding normal adult levels
    2. T_3 levels rising, but concentrations are relatively low, similar to hypothyroid adults
    3. TSH and T_4 appearing in the fetus at 10–13 weeks
    4. T_4 rises slowly and does not exceed maternal values at term

32. Congenital hypothyroidism
    1. is not apparent clinically at birth
    2. is accompanied by low TSH and low T_4
    3. has the best prognosis for normal mental development if treated prior to 3 months of age
    4. can not result from women treated with antithyroid drugs for hyperthyroidism during pregnancy

33. Hyperthyroidism in pregnancy
    1. if untreated, is associated with a higher risk of preeclampsia, intrauterine growth retardation and stillbirth
    2. is most commonly caused by Graves' disease
    3. may present as hyperemesis gravidarum
    4. is preferably treated with methimazole instead of propylthiouracil

34. Hypothyroidism is pregnancy
    1. is not infrequent during pregnancy
    2. if untreated, is associated with preeclampsia and intrauterine growth retardation
    3. is not associated with an increased incidence of SAB
    4. when treated, requires monthly TSH levels in the first trimester in order to keep it in the normal range

35. Postpartum thyroiditis
    1. becomes apparent 3–6 months after delivery
    2. is manifested by transient hypothyroidism followed by hyperthyroidism
    3. results in symptoms lasting 1–3 months and then usually spontaneous remission
    4. is responsive to antithyroid medications

Answers for Chapter 20 — Pre-Test Questions

1. autoimmune   p.672
Hypothyroidism can occur due to pituitary failure in which case the TSH will be inappropriately low for the T_4. The most common cause will be autoimmune thyroid disease (elevated titers of antithyroid antibodies) in areas with normal iodine intake. However, making an etiologic diagnosis in women adds little to the clinical management.

2. 8   p.673
When the patient appears clinically euthyroid, evaluation of TSH levels will provide the most accurate assessment of the adequacy of thyroid hormone replacement. A patient being treated with thyroid hormone should be evaluated once every year with the sensitive TSH assay. Thyroid hormone requirements tend to decrease with age. If the sensitive TSH assay is low, then the free T_4 should be measured to help adjust the thyroxine dose. ***The full response of TSH to changes in T_4 is relatively slow; a minimum of 8 weeks is necessary between changes in dosage and assessment of TSH.***

3. false p.669

TRH also stimulates prolactin secretion by the pituitary. The smallest doses of TRH that are capable of producing an increase in TSH, also increase prolactin levels, indicating a physiologic role for TRH in the control of prolactin secretion. However, except in hypothyroidism, normal physiologic changes as well as abnormal prolactin secretion can be understood in terms of dopaminergic inhibitory control, and TRH need not be considered.

4. true p.675

Some patients who require TSH suppressive doses of thyroxine, such as patients with nodules, goiters, and cancer, must be considered at increased risk of osteoporosis. The use of hormone therapy, exercise programs, and possibly biphosphate treatment must be seriously considered for these patients. Thus, hyperthyroidism must be added to the risk factors for osteoporosis.

5. C p.669

Thyroxine metabolism and clearance decrease in older people, and thyroxine secretion decreases in compensation to maintain normal serum thyroxine concentrations. With aging, conversion of T_4 to T_3 decreases, and TSH levels increase. The TSH response to TRH is normal in older women. TBG concentrations decrease slightly in postmenopausal women but not enough to alter measurements in serum.

6. B p.673

Initial therapy is straightforward with synthetic thyroxine, T_4, given daily. Mixtures of T_4 and T_3, such as desiccated thyroid, provide T_3 in excess of normal thyroid secretion. It is better to provide T_4 and allow the peripheral conversion process to provide the T_3. "Natural" thyroid preparations are not better, and in fact are potentially detrimental. Patients taking biological preparations should be switched to synthetic thyroxine. Because of a risk of coronary heart disease in older women, the initial dose should be 25–50 mg per day for about 5 weeks, at which time the dose is adjusted according to the clinical and biochemical assessment. Usually the dose required will be close to 1.5 mg/lb body weight, but it may be less in very old women. The average final dose required in the elderly is approximately 70% of that in younger patients. *Patients who have been on thyroid hormone for a long time may have their medication discontinued. Recovery of the hypothalamic-pituitary axis usually requires 8 weeks at which time the TSH and free T_4 levels can be measured.*

Answers for Chapter 20 — Post-Test Questions

1. T_3; reverse T_3 p.668

Removal of one iodine from the phenolic ring of T_4 yields T_3, while removal of an iodine from the nonphenolic ring yields reverse T_3 (RT_3) which is biologically inactive. In a normal adult, about one-third of the T_4 secreted each day is converted in peripheral tissues, largely liver and kidney, to T_3, and about 40% is converted to the inactive, reverse T_3 (RT_3). About 80% of the T_3 generated is derived outside the thyroid gland, chiefly in the liver and kidney. While T_4 may have some intrinsic activity of its own, it serves mainly as a prohormone of T_3. It is hard to think of a body process or function that doesn't require thyroid hormone for its normal operation, not only metabolism but also development, steroidogenesis, and most specific tissue activities.

2. Hashimoto's p.670

It is believed that the hypothyroidism is secondary to an autoimmune reaction, and when goiter formation is present, it is called Hashimoto's thyroiditis.

3. thyroxine p.672

In early hypothyroidism, with undetectable symptoms or signs, a compensated state can be detected by an elevated TSH and normal T_4 (called subclinical hypothyroidism). Many of these patients (but not all) will eventually become clinically hypothyroid with low T_4 concentrations. A good reason to treat subclinical hypothyroidism is to avoid the appearance of a goiter. Furthermore, some patients in retrospect (after treatment) recognize improved physical and mental well-being. With only very slight elevations of TSH, it is reasonable not to treat and to check thyroid function every year to detect further deterioration. Patients with an abnormal cholesterol-lipoprotein profile may show improvement with thyroxine treatment.

4. Graves'; Plummer's   p.673

The two primary causes of hyperthyroidism are Graves' disease (toxic diffuse goiter) and Plummer's disease (toxic nodular goiter). Plummer's disease is usually encountered in postmenopausal women who have had a long history of goiter. Twenty percent of hyperthyroid patients are over 60, and 25% of older women with hyperthyroidism present with an apathetic or atypical syndrome.

5. methimazole   p.674

The drug of choice in most circumstances will be methimazole because it has fewer adverse effects. The onset of effect takes 2–4 weeks. The dose can be titrated down once the disease is controlled. Rarely inorganic iodine will be needed to block release of hormone from the gland. Lugol's solution, 2 drops in water daily, is sufficient. The onset of effect is 1–2 days, with maximal effect in 3–7 days. There may be an escape from protection in 2–6 weeks, and the drug can cause rash, fever, and parotitis.

6. hypothyroidism   p.674

After the symptoms are controlled, and the patient is euthyroid, a dose of radioactive iodine can be selected, the thiouracil withheld temporarily, and definitive therapy accomplished. Patients with solitary nodules will be treated in the same fashion. Some patients with hot nodules in multinodular glands will require surgery because of the size of the gland and because the hyperthyroidism tends to recur in new nodules after the ablation of the original hot nodule. This can result in repetitive treatments with substantial doses of radioactive iodine, and surgery may be preferable. All patients definitively treated for hyperthyroidism must be monitored for the onset of hypothyroidism.

7. osteoporosis   p.675

Bone density has been found to be reduced (9%) in premenopausal women receiving enough thyroxine to suppress TSH for 10 years or more. In another study with lower bone densities in women being treated with levothyroxine, the hormone levels indicated that many were being overtreated for their hypothyroidism. On the other hand, a careful comparison of treated patients to controls matched for age and menopausal status failed to detect a difference in bone density. Perhaps this was because the increases in circulating thyroid hormone were relatively mild. It still makes sense to monitor patients receiving thyroxine with the sensitive TSH assay to ensure that levothyroxine doses are "physiologic."

8. Graves'   p.680

The most common cause of thyrotoxicosis in pregnancy is Graves' disease. However, the clinican should always keep in mind that trophoblastic disease can cause hyperthyroidism due to the TSH property inherent in human chorionic gonadotropin. The maternal changes with pregnancy can make diagnosis difficult. Tachycardia upon awakening from sleep and a failure to gain weight should make a clinician suspicious. Hyperemesis gravidarum is a common presentation of hyperthyroidism in pregnancy.

9. false   p.668

T_3 is 3–5 times more potent than T_4, and virtually all the biologic activity of T_4 can be attributed to the T_3 generated from it. Although T_4 is secreted at 20 times the rate of T_3, it is T_3 which is responsible for most if not all the thyroid action in the body. T_3 is more potent than T_4 because the nuclear thyroid receptor has a ten-fold greater affinity for T_3 compared to T_4.

10. true   p.668

Carbohydrate calories appear to be the primary determinant of T_3 levels in adults. A reciprocal relationship exists between T_3 and RT_3. Low T_3 and elevated RT_3 are seen in a variety of illnesses such as febrile diseases, burn injuries, malnutrition, and anorexia nervosa. The metabolic rate is determined to a large degree by the relative production of T_3 and RT_3.

11. true   p.669,670

Free Thyroxine (FT_4). Assays are now available to measure free T_4. These are usually displacement assays using an antibody to T_4. The result is not affected by changes in TBG and binding. The free T_4 level has a different range of normal values from laboratory to laboratory.

Total Thyroxine (TT_4). The total thyroxine, both the bound portion to TBG and the free unbound portion, is measured by displacement assays, and in the absence of hormone therapy or other illnesses, estimates the thyroxine concentration in the blood. However, the free thyroxine assay is now available and preferred.

Free Thyroxine Index (FTI or T7). The free thyroxine index is calculated from the TT_4 and the T_3 resin uptake measurements. This test too has been replaced by the free T_4 assay.

12. true p.670,671
(See figure on page 285 in this Study Guide)

13. false p.670
In most cases of hypothyroidism, a specific cause is not apparent. Unless abnormal thyroid function can be documented by specific laboratory assessment, empiric treatment with thyroid hormone is not indicated

14. true p.670
It is especially worth emphasizing that thyroid hormone treatment does not help infertility in euthyroid women. It is uncertain whether hypothyroidism can be a cause of recurrent abortions, but an assessment of thyroid function is worthwhile in these patients.

15. true p.672
In those patients who are asymptomatic, it is worth measuring antithyroid antibodies. A positive test identifies those who are likely to become clinically hypothyroid.

16. true p.676
In patients with a thyroid nodule, laboratory assessment of thyroid function is essential. When abnormal thyroid function is present, the nodule is almost always benign. Detection of a thyroid nodule is followed by clinical characterization of the nodule, examination of the lymph nodes, and inquiry regarding rapid growth, family history, and history of thyroid irradiation. In the presence of any of these findings, surgery is recommended for excision of the nodule. If none of these is present, proceed directly to fine needle aspiration biopsy.

17. true p.677
(See figure on page 286 in this Study Guide)

18. B p.674
Remember that the half-life of thyroxine is about one week, and the gland usually has large stores of T_4. Maximal effect occurs at 4–8 weeks.

19. A p.674
Methimazole inhibits organification of iodide and decreases production of T_4 and T_3. The dose is 10–15 mg, every 8 hours, orally.

20. C p.674
Propranolol and other beta-blockers are effective in rapidly controlling the effects of thyroid hormone on peripheral tissues. The dose is usually 20–40 mg, every 6 hours, orally, and the dose is titrated to maintain a heart rate of about 100 beats/minute.

21. A p.674
The major side effects are rash, gastrointestinal symptoms, and granulocytopenia.

22. C p.674
The drug may cause bronchospasm, worsening congestive heart failure, fatigue, and depression.

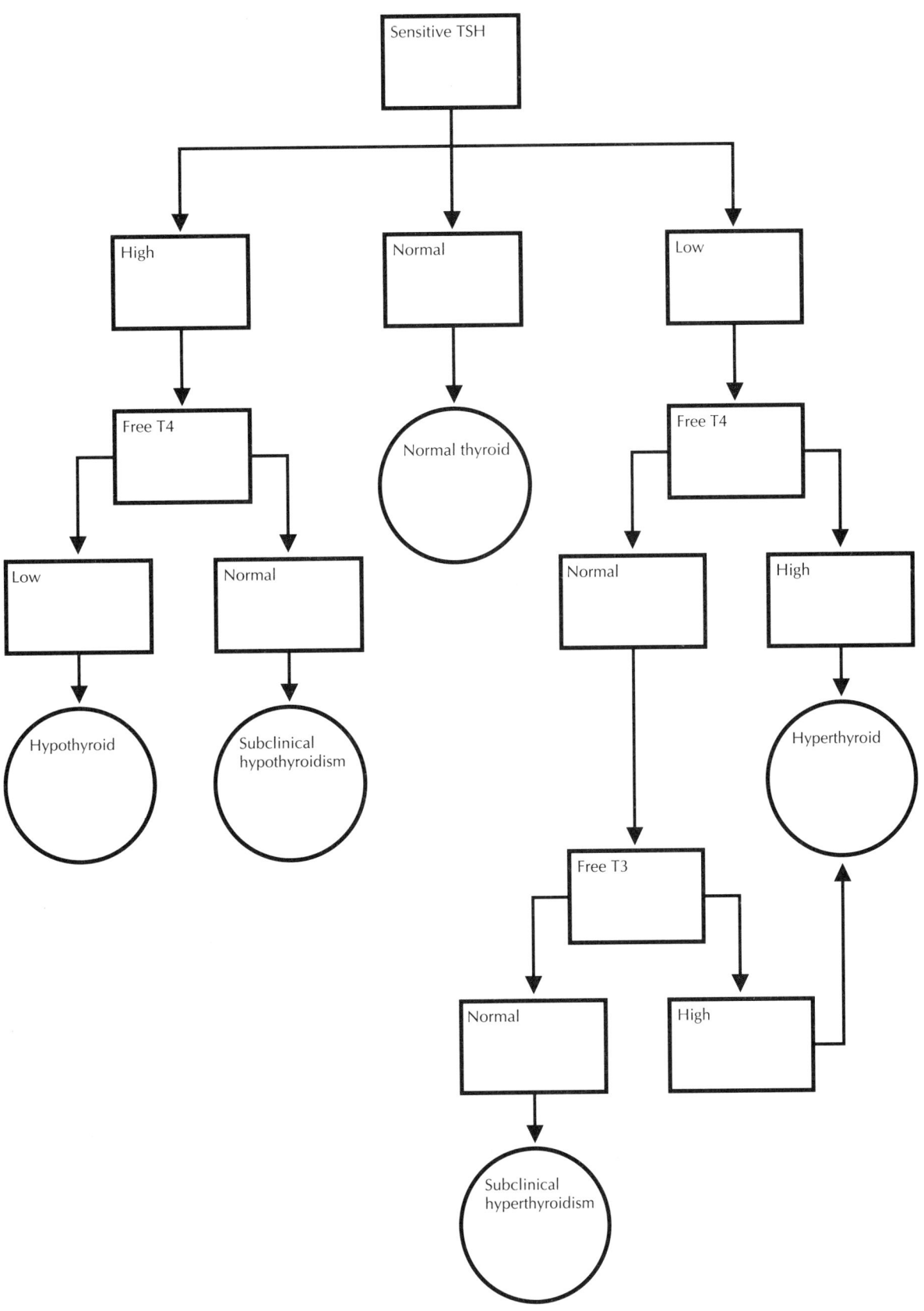

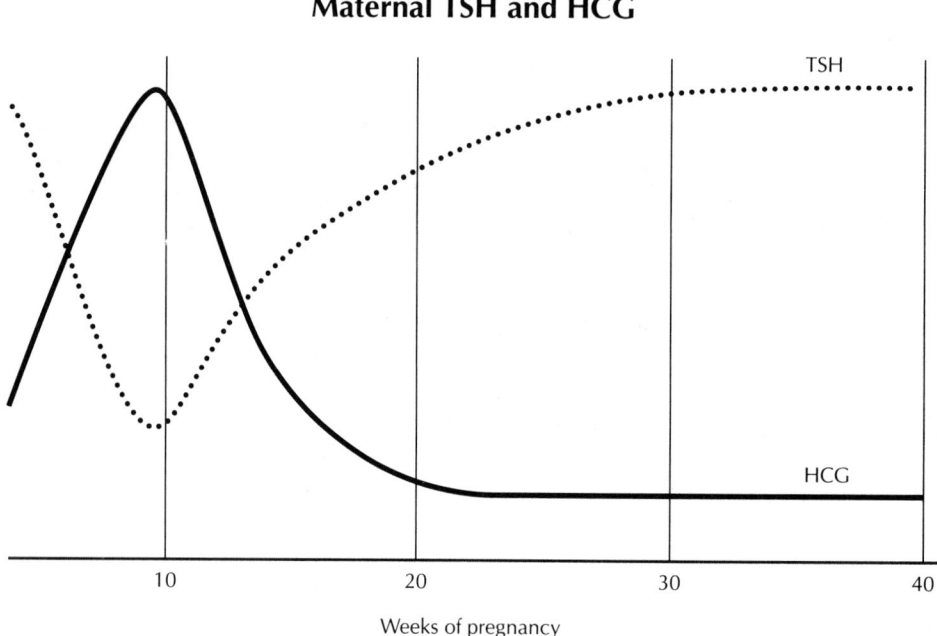

Maternal TSH and HCG

23. E p.668,669

Although T_4 is secreted at 20 times the rate of T_3, it is T_3 which is responsible for most if not all the thyroid action in the body. During periods of stress, when a decrease in metabolic rate would conserve energy, the body produces more RT_3 and less T_3, and metabolism slows. Upon recovery, this process reverses and metabolic rate increases. Circulating thyroid hormones are present in the circulation mainly bound to proteins. Approximately 75–80% of thyroid hormones are bound to thyroxine-binding globulin (TBG), which therefore, is the major determining factor in the total thyroid hormone concentration in the circulation. The remaining 20–25% is bound to thyroxine-binding prealbumin and albumin. The binding proteins have a greater affinity for T_4 and thus allow T_3 to have greater entry into cells. TBG is synthesized in the liver, and this synthesis is increased by estrogens.

The thyroid axis is stimulated by the hypothalamic factor, thyrotropin releasing hormone (TRH) and inhibited by somatostatin and dopamine. Thyroid hormones regulate TSH by suppressing TRH secretion, but primarily affecting the pituitary sensitivity to TRH (by reducing the number of TRH receptors). Pituitary secretion of TSH is very sensitive to changes in the circulating levels of thyroid hormone; a slight change in the circulating level of T_4 will produce a many-fold greater response in TSH. TSH-secreting cells are regulated by T_4, but only after the T_4 is converted to T_3 in the pituitary cells. Although modulation of thyroid hormone occurs at the pituitary level, this function is permitted by the hypothalamic releasing hormone, TRH. Although some tissues depend mainly on the blood T_3 for their intracellular T_3, the brain and the pituitary depend on their own intracellular conversion of T_4. The measurement of T_4 and TSH, therefore, provides the most accurate assessment of thyroid function.

24. E p.670

For screening purposes, or when there is a relatively low clinical suspicion of thyroid disease, the initial step is to measure the TSH by a sensitive assay. A normal TSH essentially excludes hypothyroidism or hyperthyroidism. A high TSH requires the measurement of free T_4 to confirm the diagnosis of hypothyroidism.

If the initial TSH is low, especially less than 0.08 mU/mL, then measurement of a high T_4 will confirm the diagnosis of hyperthyroidism. If the T_4 is normal, the T_3 level is measured, since some patients with hyperthyroidism will have predominantly T_3 toxicosis. If the T_3 is normal, it implies that thyroxine secretion is autonomous from TSH, and this is called subclinical hyperthyroidism. Some of these patients will eventually have increased T_4 or T_3 levels with true hyperthyroidism.

25. B   p.672

Hypothyroidism increases with aging and is more common in women. Up to 45% of thyroid glands from women over age 60 show evidence of thyroiditis. The incidence of antithyroglobulin antibodies is 7.4% in women over age 75 years, while 16.9% of women age 60 and 17.4% of women over age 75 have elevated TSH levels. In women admitted to geriatric wards, 2–4% have clinically apparent hypothyroidism. ***Therefore, hypothyroidism is frequent enough to warrant consideration in most older women, justifying screening even in asymptomatic older women. We recommend that older women be screened with the highly sensitive TSH assay at age 45, then every 2 years beginning at age 60, or with the appearance of any symptoms suggesting hypothyroidism.***

26. A   p.672

Menstrual irregularites and bleeding problems are common in hypothyroid women. Amenorrhea can be a consequence of hypothyroidism, either with TRH-induced increases in prolactin or with normal prolactin levels. Other clinical manifestations of hypothyroidism include constipation, cold intolerance, psychomotor retardation, carpal tunnel syndrome, and decreased exercise tolerance. However, patients often appear asymptomatic. Close evaluation can reveal mental slowness, decreased energy, fatigue, poor memory, somnolence, slow speech, a low pitched voice, water retention, periorbital edema, delayed reflexes, or a low body temperature and bradycardia. Hypothyroidism can cause hypertension, cognitive abnormalities, pericardial effusion, asymmetric septal myocardial hypertrophy, myopathy, neuropathy, ataxia, anemia, elevated cholesterol and LDL-cholesterol, or hyponatremia. The increase in cholesterol is due to impaired LDL-cholesterol clearance secondary to a decrease in cell membrane LDL receptors. The mechanism for this LDL effect is attributed to a thyroid response element in the LDL receptor gene.

27. E   p.674,675

Graves' disease is characterized by the triad of hyperthyroidism, exophthalmos, and pretibial myxedema and is believed to be caused by autoantibodies that have TSH properties and therefore bind to and activate the TSH receptor. Menstrual changes associated with hyperthyroidism are unpredictable, ranging from amenorrhea to oligomenorrhea to normal cycles (hence, the amenorrhea in a thyrotoxoic woman can be due to pregnancy).

28. C   p.675

The major concern with thyroid nodules is the potential for thyroid cancer. Single nodules are 4 times more common in women, and carcinoma of the thyroid is nearly 3 times more common in women than in men. The incidence rises steadily from the age of 55. Mortality from thyroid cancer occurs predominantly in the middle-aged and the elderly. There are 4 major types of primary thyroid carcinoma: papillary, follicular, anaplastic, and medullary. In solitary nodules that are "cold" (those that do not take up radioactive iodine or pertechnetate on thyroid scan), 12% prove to be malignant. This also means that the majority are benign. Surgical excision of nodules can result in vocal cord paralysis, hypoparathyroidism, and other complications. Therefore, the goal is to select patients for curative surgery who have the greatest likelihood of having cancer in the nodule.

29. B   p.675

The major risk factors for thyroid cancer are family history of this disease and a history of irradiation to head or neck. In those who have received thyroid irradiation, about one-third will have thyroid abnormalities, and about one-third of those with abnormalities will have thyroid cancer (about 10% overall). The carcinogenic risk has been estimated to be 1% per 100 rads in 20 years. A rapidly growing nodule, a hard nodule, the presence of palpable regional lymph nodes, or vocal cord paralysis greatly increase the probability of thyroid cancer.

Thyroid nodules in multinodular thyroid glands, not previously exposed to thyroid irradiation, have no greater risk of thyroid carcinoma than normal glands. Therefore, predominant thyroid nodules in multinodular glands should be followed and, if a nodule grows, then biopsy or surgery considered.

30. D   p.676, 677

The increase in thyroid activity during pregnancy is attributed to the thyrotropic substances secreted by the placenta: a chorionic thyrotropin and the thyrotropic activity in human chorionic gonadotropin (HCG). The increase in thyroid activity in pregnancy is compensated by an marked increase in the circulating levels of TBG in response to estrogen; therefore, a new equilibrium is reached with an increase in the bound portion of the thyroid hormone. The mechanism for the estrogen effect on TBG is an increase in hepatic synthesis and an increase in glycosylation of the TBG molecule that leads to decreased clearance.

TBG levels reach a peak (twice nonpregnant levels) at about 20 weeks, which is maintained throughout the rest of pregnancy. T_4 undergoes a simlar change, but T_3 increases more markedly. Because of the increase in TBG, free T_4 and T_3 levels actually decrease, although they remain within the normal range. There is an inverse relationship between maternal circulation levels of TSH and HCG. TSH reaches a nadir at the same time that HCG reaches a peak at 10 weeks of pregnancy. TSH levels then increase as HCG levels drop to their stable levels throughout the rest of pregnancy. These changes support a role for HCG stimulation of the maternal thyroid gland during early pregnancy.

31. A p.680

Summary of Fetal and Newborn Thyroid Changes
1. TSH and T_4 appear in the fetus at 10–13 weeks. Levels are low until an abrupt rise at 20 weeks.
2. T_4 rises rapidly and exceeds maternal values at term.
3. T_3 levels rise, but concentrations are relatively low, similar to hypothyroid adults.
4. RT_3 levels exceed normal adult levels.
5. The fetal pattern of low T_3 and high RT_3 is similar to that seen with calorie malnutrition.
6. After delivery, TSH peaks at 30 minutes of age, followed by a T_3 peak at 24 hours and a T_4 peak at 24–48 hours. The T_3 increase is independent of the TSH change.
7. High RT_3 levels persist for 3–5 days after delivery, then reach normal values by 2 weeks.

32. B p.680

The incidence of neonatal hypothyroidism is about one in 4,000 live births. The problem is that congenital hypothyroidism is not apparent clinically at birth. Fortunately, infants with congenital hypothyroidism have low T_4 and high TSH concentrations easily detected in blood, and early treatment before 3 months of age is usually associated with normal mental development. Less than normal development can be a consequence of a delay in treatment or extremely low thyroid hormone production in the fetus.

There is a familial tendency for hypothyroidism, and if the diagnosis is made in the antepartum period, intraamniotic injections of thyroxine can raise fetal levels of thyroid hormone. Ultrasonographic examination of patients with polyhydramnios should include a search for a fetal goiter. In addition, the fetus should be monitored for goiter formation in women treated with antithyroid drugs for hyperthyroidism during pregnancy. Amniotic fluid iodothyronines and TSH reflect fetal plasma levels, and abnormal values may allow prenatal diagnosis of fetal hypothyroidism by amniocentesis. However, cord blood sampling is advocated for accurate diagnosis. Treatment of fetal hypothyroidism is important because there is a concern that prenatal hypothyroidism can affect some aspects of development, e.g., the full function of physical skills.

33. A p.680,681

Untreated thyrotoxicosis in pregnancy is associated with a higher risk of preeclampsia, heart failure, intrauterine growth retardation, and stillbirth. Heart failure is a consequence of the demands of pregnancy superimposed upon the hyperdynamic cardiovascular state induced by the increased thyroid hormone.

The most common cause of thyrotoxicosis in pregnancy is Graves' disease. However, the clinican should always keep in mind that trophoblastic disease can cause hyperthyroidism due to the TSH property inherent in human chorionic gonadotropin. The maternal changes with pregnancy can make diagnosis difficult. Tachycardia upon awakening from sleep and a failure to gain weight should make a clinician suspicious. Hyperemesis gravidarum is a common presentation of hyperthyroidism in pregnancy. Laboratory assessment is unaffected by pregnancy and should follow our algorithm.

The choice of treatment is between surgery and antithyroid drugs. However prior to surgery, the thyroid gland has to be controlled with medical therapy. Most women can be successfully treated with thioamide drugs. Propylthiouracil is preferred for pregnant women because methimazole crosses the placenta more readily.

34. C p.681

Serious hypothyroidism is rarely encountered during pregnancy. Patients with this degree of illness probably do not get pregnant. Patients with mild hypothyroidism probably never have a laboratory assessment for thyroid function during pregnancy and go undetected. Preeclampsia and intrauterine growth retardation are more frequent in women with significant hypothyroidism. There is also reason to believe that patients with hypothyroidism have an increased rate of spontaneous abortion. The mechanism may be impaired ability of important organs such as the endometrium and the corpus luteum. Women being treated for hypothyroidism require a small increase in thyroxine during pregnancy. TSH should be monitored monthly in the first trimester and again in the postpartum period, and dosage should be adjusted to keep the TSH level in the normal range.

35. B p.681,682

Autoimmune thyroid disease is suppressed to some degree by the immunologic changes of pregnancy. Thus, there is a relatively high incidence of postpartum thyroiditis (5–10%), usually 3–6 months after delivery, manifested by either hyperthyroidism or hypothyroidism, although commonly transient hyperthyroidism is followed by hypothyroidism. This condition is due to a destructive thyroiditis associated with thyroid microsomal autoantibodies. Women at high risk for postpartum thyroiditis are those with a personal or family history of autoimmune disease, and those with a previous postpartum episode.

Most importantly, the symptoms in these women are often attributed to anxiety or depression, and the obstetrician must have a high index of suspicion for hypothyroidism. The symptoms usually last 1–3 months and almost all women return to normal thyroid function. Postpartum thyroiditis tends to recur with subsequent pregnancies, and eventually hypothyroidism remains. The symptoms of hyperthyroidism in this condition are not responsive to antithyroid medication, and patients are usually not treated or given beta-adrenergic blocking agents (e.g., propranolol in a dose sufficient to reduce the resting pulse to less than 100 per minute). Because spontaneous remission is common, patients who are treated with hypothyroidism should be reassessed one year after gradual withdrawal of thyroxine. Patients who return to normal should undergo periodic laboratory surveillance of their thyroid status.

21 Use of Contraception, Sterilization, and Abortion

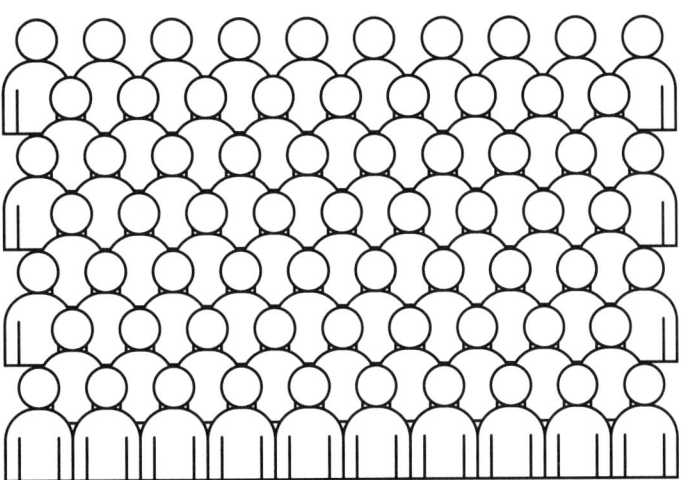

Learning Objectives

Be able to:

1. Define methods presently used to measure contraceptive efficacy.

2. Describe the current available reversible and irreversible contraceptive methods. Discuss their unique advantages, disadvantages and typical failure rates during the first year of use.

3. Explain the characteristic patient concerns which need to be addressed when counseling couples for sterilization.

4. Discuss the preoperative care, counseling, methods and complications of first and second trimester abortions.

Pre-Test

A. Instructions: Fill in the blanks

1. Vasectomy reversal is associated with pregnancy rates greater than ____%. The best results are achieved when reversal is performed within _____ years after vasectomy.

B. Instructions: True or False

2. After several years of use, efficacy with the IUD remains less than the efficacy of the oral contraceptives.

C. Instructions: For the following question choose:

A. if only 1, 2 and 3 are correct
B. if only 1 and 3 are correct
C. if only 2 and 4 are correct
D. if only 4 is correct
E. if all are correct

3. Sterilization techniques
   1. that involve more complicated techniques of tubal occlusion have higher technical failure rates
   2. resulting in failures are due to technical errors in 50% of these cases
   3. involving bipolar tubal coagulation are more likely to result in an ectopic pregnancy than is mechanical occlusion
   4. performed vaginally has a greater chance of failure than does a tubal procedure performed by laparoscopy

Post-Test

A. Instructions: Fill in the blanks

1. The two methods that have been used to measure contraceptive efficacy are the _____ and _____.

2. The world population is expected to stabilize at approximately _____ billion by the year 2100.

3. Contraceptive failures account for about ____% of the 1.6 million annual abortions in the U.S.

4. A patient visit for contraception is an excellent time for _____ screening.

5. The highest number of births in the U.S. occurred between _____ and _____ known as the post-World War II baby boom.

B. Instructions: True or False

6. With most methods of contraception, failure rates increase with duration of use.

7. During the years of maximal fertility, oral contraceptives are the most common method peaking at age 20–24.

8. As more and more couples defer pregnancy until later in life, the use of sterilization under age 35 will decline and the need for reversible contraception will increase.

9. Deaths specifically attributed to sterilization now account for a fatality rate lower than that for childbearing in the U.S.

10. When the risk of pregnancy from contraceptive method failure is taken into account, sterilization is the safest of all contraceptive methods.

11. Vasectomy is highly effective once the supply of remaining sperm in the vas deferens is exhausted. After 6 weeks or 15 ejaculations essentially all men are sterile.

12. Vasectomy is safer, easier and less expensive than female sterilization.

C. Instructions: Match each failure rate during the first year of use for contraceptive methods used in the U.S.

A. less than 1%
B. less than 5%
C. less than 10%
D. less than 20%
E. less than 30%

13. norplant
14. sponge
15. diaphragm and spermicides
16. condoms
17. withdrawal
18. combination OC
19. female sterilization
20. male sterilization

D. Instructions: Match each sterilization technique with each illustration

A. Uchida
B. Irving
C. Pomeroy

21.

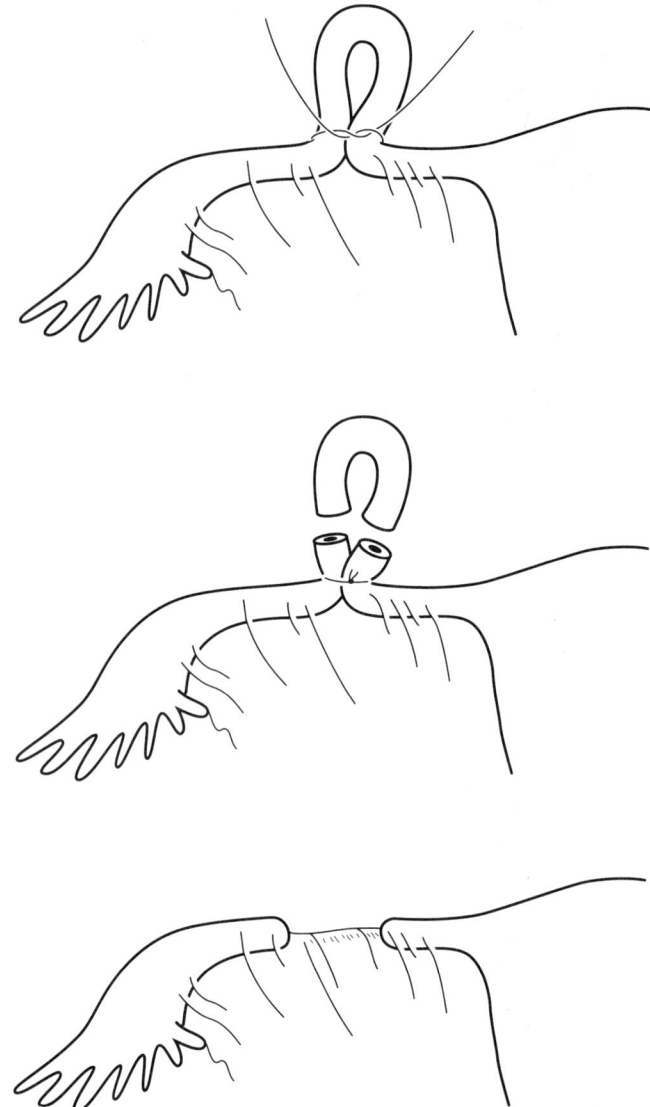

22.

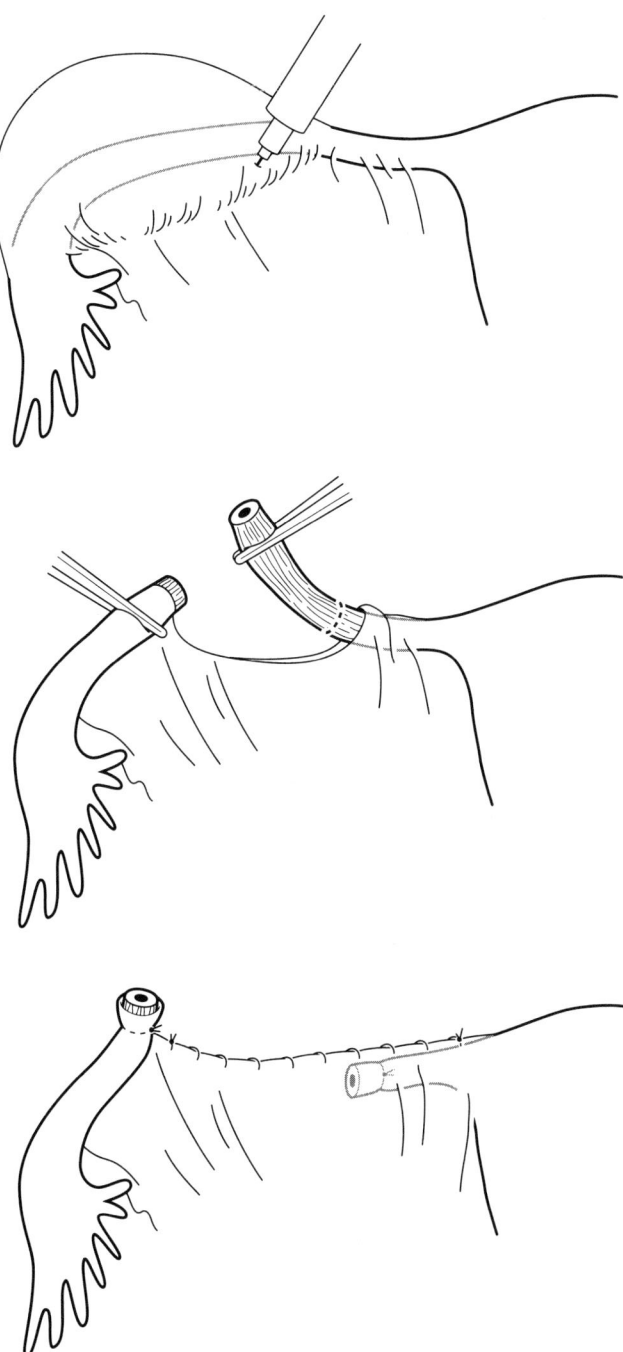

23.

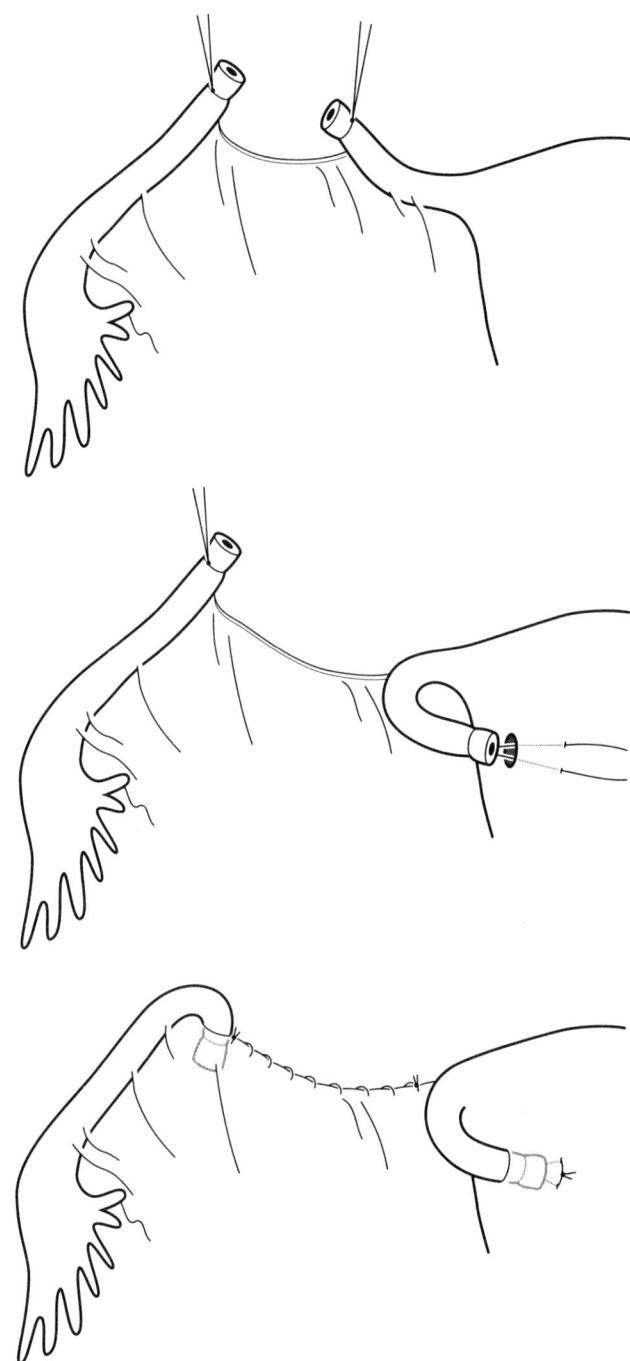

E. Instructions: For each of the following questions choose:

A. if only 1, 2 and 3 are correct
B. if only 1 and 3 are correct
C. if only 2 and 4 are correct
D. if only 4 is correct
E. if all are correct

24. The Pearl Index
    1. is defined as the number of failures per 100 woman-years of exposure
    2. fails to accurately compare methods at various durations of exposure
    3. is usually based on 1 year of exposure
    4. may be the most precise method of assessing efficacy of contraception

25. Life Table Analysis
    1. calculates a failure rate for each month of use
    2. does not provide a cumulative failure rate
    3. removes women from the analysis who leave the study prior to its completion
    4. does not add additional information to that already provided by the Pearl Index

26. Reasons for a predicted increase in demand for reversible contraception include
    1. deferment of marriage
    2. fewer numbers of women between the ages of 35 and 49
    3. postponement of pregnancy in marriage
    4. an increasing rate of failure among irreversible methods of contraception

27. Vasectomy
    1. is more popular in the U.S. than anywhere else in the world
    2. is associated with an increase incidence of atherosclerosis and prostate cancer
    3. is less expensive than tubal sterilization
    4. is associated with a higher morbidity and mortality than tubal sterilization

28. Tubal occlusion by bipolar cautery
    1. is safer than by unipolar cautery
    2. has higher failure rates compared to unipolar cautery
    3. can be performed with either a single incision operating laparoscope or with dual incision instruments
    4. may fail if incomplete electrocoagulation occurs due to damaged instruments

29. In counseling patients for sterilization you should state that
    1. there is evidence that there is a detrimental effect on sexuality
    2. some women experience menstrual changes but most do not
    3. up to 10% of U.S. women have been reported to express regret up to 2 years following the procedure
    4. it is important to involve both partners in the counseling session

30. Tubal anastomosis pregnancy rates depend upon
    1. segment length of damaged tube
    2. length of remaining tube
    3. type of sterilization procedure initially performed
    4. presence of pelvic adhesions

31. First trimester therapeutic abortion by suction aspiration is not associated with an increase incidence of future
    1. ectopic pregnancies
    2. infertility
    3. spontaneous abortions
    4. uterine infections

32. Possible complications following a therapeutic abortion include
    1. infection
    2. incomplete abortion
    3. uterine perforation
    4. Asherman's syndrome

33. RU486
    1. in combination with a prostaglandin analogue is an effective method of abortion up to 9 weeks of gestation
    2. opens and softens the cervix
    3. blocks progesterone receptors in the endometrium
    4. is an effective treatment for ectopic pregnancy

34. Abortion in the second trimester
    1. does not require preoperative cervical dilatation
    2. performed by dilatation and evacuation is safer and less expensive than by medical methods
    3. is not accompanied by an increase risk of complications compared to first trimester abortion
    4. includes medical treatment options of prostaglandins and intra-amniotic injection of hypertonic saline or urea

Answers for Chapter 21 — Pre-Test Questions

1. 50; 3   p.706

Vasectomy reversal is associated with pregnancy rates greater than 50%. The prospect for pregnancy diminishes with time elapsed from vasectomy, decreasing significantly to 30% after 10 years; the best results are achieved when reversal is performed within 3 years after vasectomy.

2. false   p.693

The growing need for reversible contraception would also be served by increased utilization of the IUD. After several years of use, efficacy with the IUD is similar to that of oral contraceptives. The decline in IUD use in the U.S. is in direct contrast to the experience in the rest of the world, a complicated response to publicity and litigation. An increased risk of pelvic infection with contemporary IUDs in use is limited to the act of insertion and the transportation of pathogens to the upper genital tract. This risk is effectively minimized by careful screening with preinsertion cultures and the use of good technique. A return to IUD use by American couples is both warranted and desirable.

3. E   p.698,699

Besides the specific operation employed, the skill of the operator and characteristics of the patient make important contributions to the efficacy of female sterilization. Up to 50% of failures are due to technical errors. The methods employing complicated equipment, such as spring-loaded clips and silastic rings, fail for technical reasons more commonly than do simpler procedures such as the Pomeroy tubal ligation. Minilaparotomy failures, therefore, occur much less frequently from technical errors.

Ectopic pregnancies can occur following tubal occlusion, and the incidence is much higher with some types of tubal occlusion. Bipolar tubal coagulation is more likely to result in ectopic pregnancy than is mechanical occlusion. The probable explanation is that microscopic fistulae in the coagulated segment connecting to the peritoneal cavity permit sperm to reach the ovum. Ectopic pregnancies following tubal ligation are more likely to occur 2 or more years after sterilization, rather than immediately after. In the first year after sterilization, about 6% of pregnancies will be ectopic, but the majority of pregnancies that occur 2–3 years after occlusion will be ectopic. The rate of intrauterine pregnancies decreases with time, but ectopic rates remain constant. Overall, however, the risk of an ectopic pregnancy in sterilized women is lower than if they had not been sterilized.

Vaginal procedures have higher failure rates than laparoscopy or minilaparotomy, but the principal disadvantage is a higher rate of infection. Intraperitoneal infection is a rare complication of minilap or laparoscopic techniques, but in vaginal procedures, abscess formation approaches 1%. This risk can be reduced by the use of prophylactic antibiotics administered intraoperatively, but open laparoscopy is usually easier and safer than vaginal sterilization even in obese women.

Answers for Chapter 21 — Post-Test Questions

1. Pearl index; Life Table Analysis p.688
Contraceptive efficacy is generally assessed by measuring the number of unplanned pregnancies that occur during a specified period of exposure and use of a contraceptive method. The two methods that have been used to measure contraceptive efficacy are the Pearl index and life table analysis.

2. 10–11 p.691
The world population is expected to stabilize at between 10 and 11 billion by the year 2100. Approximately 95% of the growth will occur in developing countries, so that by 2100, 13% of the population will live in developed countries, a decrease from the current 25%.

3. 50 p.691, 692
Inadequate access to contraception is associated with a high abortion rate. Effective contraceptive use largely, although not totally, replaces the resort to abortion. The combination of restrictive abortion laws and the lack of safe abortion services continues to make unsafe abortion a major cause of morbidity and mortality throughout the world. Both safe and unsafe abortions can be minimized by maximizing contraceptive services. However, the need for safe abortion services will persist. Contraceptive failures account for about half of the 1.6 million annual induced abortions in the U.S.

4. STD p.692
The interaction between clinician and patient for the purpose of contraception provides an opportunity to control sexually transmitted diseases (STDs). The modification of unsafe sexual practices reduces the risk of unplanned pregnancy and the risk of infections of the reproductive tract. A patient visit for contraception is an excellent time for STD screening; if an infection is symptomatic, it should be diagnosed and treated during the same visit in which contraception is requested. A positive history for STDs should trigger both screening for asymptomatic infections and counseling for safer sexual practices. Attention should be given to the contraceptive methods that have the greatest influence on the risk of STDs.

5. 1947; 1965 p.692
The need for reversible contraception in women over the age of 30 is growing, not diminishing. The highest number of births in the U.S. occurred between 1947 and 1965 — the post-World War II baby boom. Women born in this period won't be through reaching their 45th birthday until around 2010. For approximately a 20-year period, therefore, there will be an unprecedented number of women in the later childbearing years.

6. false p.688
With most methods of contraception, failure rates decline with duration of use. The Pearl index is usually based on a lengthy exposure (usually one year) and therefore fails to accurately compare methods at various durations of exposure. This limitation is overcome by using the method of life table analysis.

7. true
                                                                                                     p.691

U.S. couples have made up for the lack of contraceptive choices by greater reliance on voluntary sterilization. Although the use of sterilization has remained steady for the last several years, approximately one-half of American couples choose sterilization within 15 to 20 years of their last wanted birth. During the years of maximal fertility, oral contraceptives are the most common method peaking at age 20–24. The use of condoms is the second most widely used method of reversible contraception, rising from about 9% in the mid 1980s to approximately 15% of couples in 1991. Most IUD users are concentrated between ages 25 and 40.

8. true
                                                                                                     p.692

From 1970 to 1986, the number of births in women over 30 quadrupled. As more and more couples defer pregnancy until later in life, the use of sterilization under age 35 will decline, and the need for reversible contraception will increase. In 1988, 75% of pill users were under age 30. Only 5% of women aged 35–44 used oral contraception, compared to 38% under age 25. These numbers will change only if clinicians and patients understand and accept that low dose oral contraception is safe for healthy, nonsmoking older women.

9. true
                                                                                                     p.696

The great majority of sterilization procedures are accomplished in hospitals by physicians in private practice, but a rapidly increasing proportion are performed outside of hospitals in ambulatory surgical settings, including physician's offices. In either hospital or outpatient settings, female sterilization is a very safe operation. Deaths specifically attributed to sterilization now account for a fatality rate of only 1.5 per 100,000 procedures, a mortality rate that is lower than that for childbearing (about 10 per 100,000 births in the U.S.).

10. true
                                                                                                     p.696

When the risk of pregnancy from contraceptive method failure is taken into account, sterilization is the safest of all contraceptive methods.

11. true
                                                                                                     p.698

Laparoscopic and minilaparotomy sterilization are not only convenient, they are almost as effective at preventing pregnancy as were the older, more complex operations. Vasectomy is also highly effective once the supply of remaining sperm in the vas deferens is exhausted. After 6 weeks or 15 ejaculations, essentially all men are sterile.

12. true
                                                                                                     p.706

Vasectomy is safer, easier, and less expensive than female sterilization. Hematomas and infection occur rarely and are easily treated with heat, scrotal support, and antibiotics. Most men will develop sperm antibodies following vasectomy, but no long-term sequelae have been observed, including no increased risk of cardiovascular disease. Adverse psychological and sexual effects have not been reported. Since the other constituents of semen are made downstream from the testes, men do not notice a decreased volume or velocity of ejaculate.

13. A   p.689

14. E   p.689

15. D   p.689

16. D   p.689

17. D   p.689

18. B   p.689

19. A   p.689

20. A   p.689

Failure Rates During the First Year of Use, United States

Method	Percent of Women with Pregnancy	
	Lowest Expected	Typical
No method	85.0%	85.0%
Combination Pill	0.1	3.0
Progestin only	0.5	3.0
IUDs		3.0
Progesterone IUD	2.0	<2.0
Copper T 380A	0.8	<1.0
Norplant	0.2	0.2
Female sterilization	0.2	0.4
Male sterilization	0.1	0.15
Depo-Provera	0.3	0.3
Spermicides	3.0	21.0
Periodic abstinence		20.0
Calendar	9.0	
Ovulation method	3.0	
Symptothermal	2.0	
Post–ovulation	1.0	
Withdrawal	4.0	18.0
Cervical cap	6.0	18.0
Sponge		
Parous women	9.0	28.0
Nulliparous women	6.0	18.0
Diaphragm and spermicides	6.0	18.0
Condom	2.0	12.0

21. C

The Pomeroy

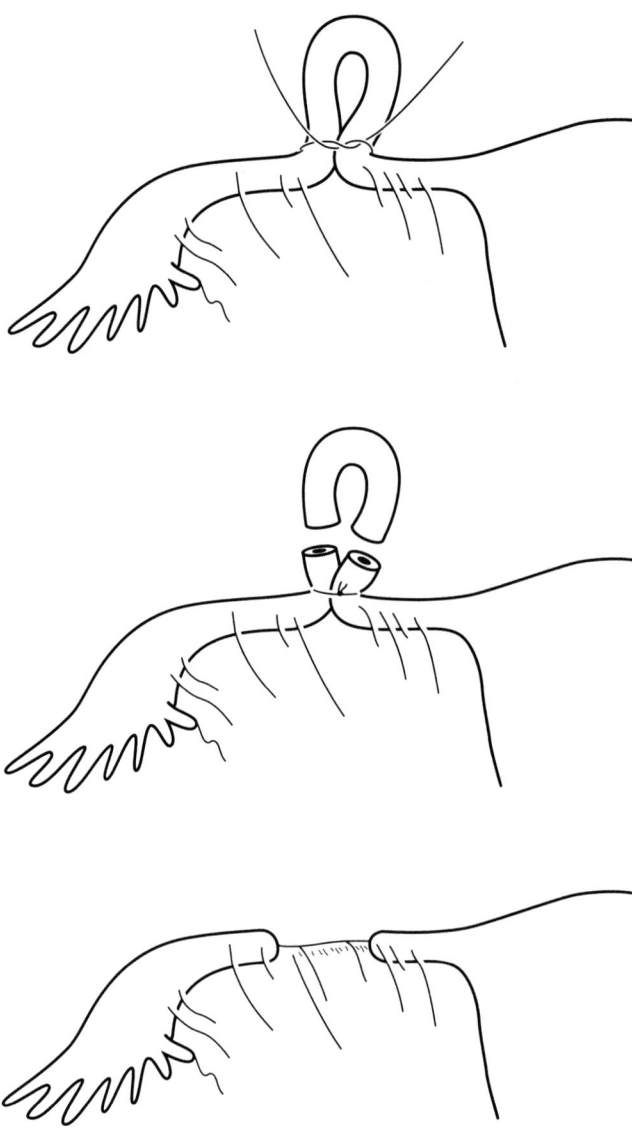

22. A

The Uchida

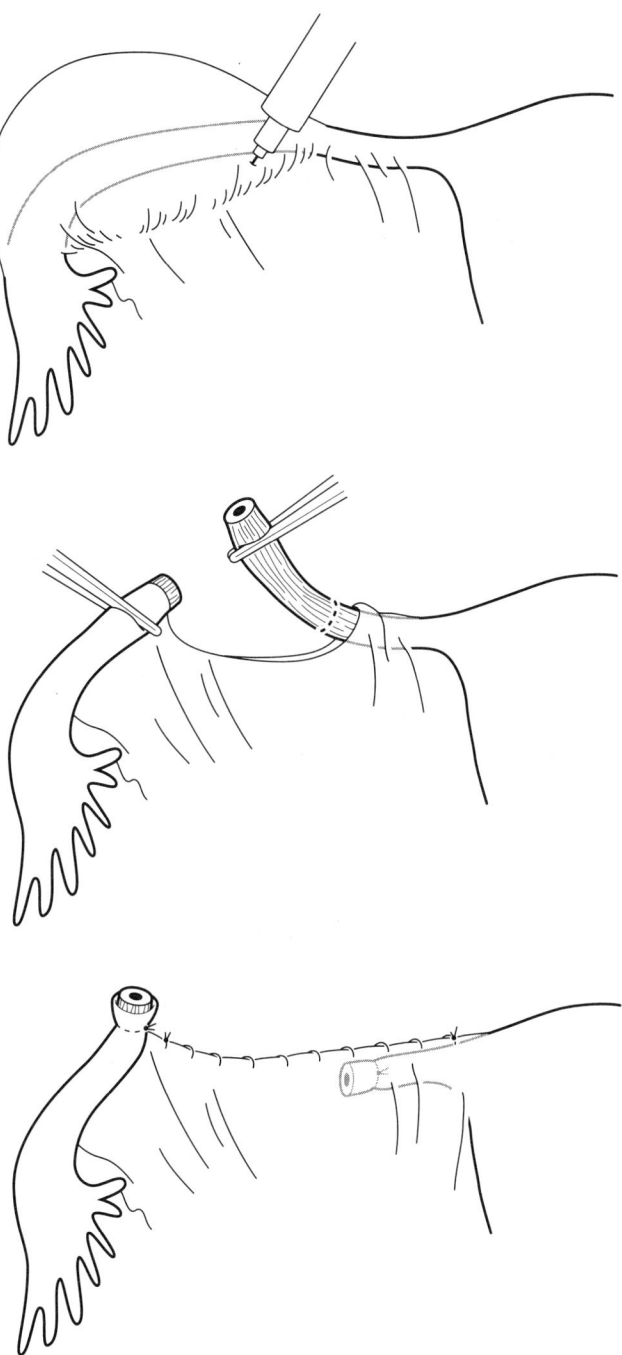

23. B

The Irving

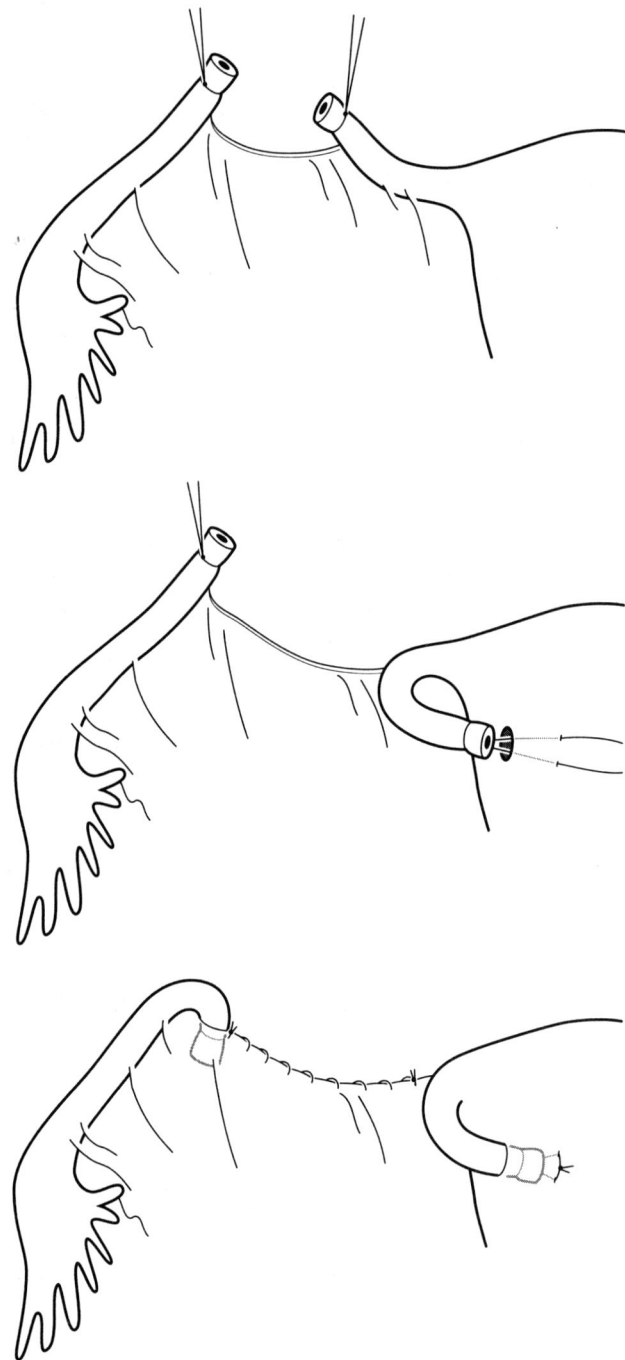

Chapter 21 Use of Contraception, Sterilization and Abortion

24. A   p.688

The Pearl index is defined as the number of failures per 100 woman-years of exposure. The denominator is the total months or cycles of exposure from the onset of a method until completion of the study, an unintended pregnancy, or discontinuation of the method. The quotient is multiplied by 1,200 if the denominator consists of months or by 1,300 if the denominator consists of cycles.

25. B   p.688

Life table analysis calculates a failure rate for each month of use. A cumulative failure rate can then compare methods for any specific length of exposure. Women who leave a study for any reason other than unintended pregnancy are removed from the analysis, contributing their exposure until the time of the exit.

26. B   p.692,693

It is estimated that the number of women aged 35–49 will increase 61% between 1982 and 1995. The proportion of births accounted for by this group of women will increase by about 72%, from 5% in 1982 to 8.6% in 2000. This group of women is not only increasing in number, but it is changing its fertility pattern.

The deferment of marriage is a significant change in our society. In 1960, 28% of women aged 20–24 were single; in 1985, 58.5%. In 1960, 10% of women 25–29 were single; in 1985, 26%. But only 16% of the decline in the total fertility rate is accounted for by the increase in the average age at first marriage. Eighty-three percent of the decline in total fertility rate is accounted for by changes in marital fertility rates. In other words postponement of pregnancy in marriage is the more significant change. This combination of increasing numbers, deferment of marriage, and postponement of pregnancy in marriage is responsible for the fact that we will be seeing more and more older women who will need reversible contraception. In short, there will continue to be longer duration of use in younger women and greater use in older women, the pattern of use which was being observed by 1990.

27. B   p.697,706

Vasectomy has long been more popular in the U.S. than anywhere else in the world, but why don't more men use it? One explanation is that women have chosen laparoscopic sterilization in increasing numbers. Another is that men have been frightened by reports, often from animal data, of associations with autoimmune diseases, atherosclerosis, and most recently, prostatic cancer. Large epidemiologic studies have failed to confirm any definite adverse consequences. In addition, vasectomy is less expensive than tubal sterilization, morbidity is less, and mortality is essentially zero.

28. E   p.701

The bipolar method can be used with either a single incision operating laparoscope or with dual incision instruments. The forceps are, however, more delicate than unipolar equipment and must be kept meticulously clean. Damage to the instruments can alter the ability to coagulate, and inadequate or incomplete electrocoagulation is the main cause of failure.

Bipolar cautery is safer than unipolar cautery with regard to burns of abdominal organs, but most studies indicate higher failure rates. Although the bipolar forceps will not burn tissues that are not actually grasped, care must be taken to avoid coagulating structures adherent to the tubes. For example, the ureter can be damaged when the tube is adherent to the pelvic side wall.

29. C   p.704, 705

All patients undergoing a surgical procedure for permanent contraception should be aware of the nature of the operation, its alternatives, efficacy, safety, and complications. The operation can be described using drawings or pelvic models, as well as films, slides, or video tapes. The description of the operation should emphasize its similarities to and differences from laparoscopy and pelvic surgery, especially hysterectomy or ovariectomy which may be confused with simple tubal ligation. Alternatives, including vasectomy, oral contraception, long-acting hormone methods, barrier methods, and IUDs, should be reviewed. It should be emphasized to the patient that tubal ligation is not intended to be reversible, and that it cannot be guaranteed to prevent intrauterine or ectopic pregnancy. Informed consent is best obtained at a time when a patient is not distracted or distraught, e.g., not immediately before or after a therapeutic abortion.

30. A p.706

Microsurgery for tubal reanastomosis is associated with excellent results if only a small segment of the tube has been damaged. Pregnancy rates correlate with the length of remaining tube, a length of 4 cm or more is optimal. Thus, the pregnancy rates are lowest with electrocoagulation, and reach 70–80% with clips, rings, and surgical methods such as the Pomeroy. About 2 per 1,000 sterilized women will eventually undergo tubal reanastomosis.

31. E p.707

The most important determinants of abortion mortality are duration of gestation and type of anesthesia: later abortions and general anesthesia are more hazardous. As with mortality, morbidity rates vary primarily with duration of pregnancy, but other factors are important as well, including type of operation, age of patient, type of anesthesia, operator's skill, and method of cervical dilatation.

The possibility that abortion can result in longer-term complications has been examined in over 150 studies. First trimester abortion by vacuum aspiration is not associated with any adverse consequences on the following: subsequent fertility, subsequent pregnancies, or the risk of ectopic pregnancy. It is not yet certain if second trimester abortions or multiple first trimester abortions can affect the outcome of later pregnancies.

32. E p.708

Postoperative complications of elective abortions are classified as either immediate or delayed. Uterine perforation and uterine atony are examples of immediate complications. Delayed complications can occur several hours to several weeks after the operation. These usually present according to the major complaint: bleeding, pain, and continuing symptoms of pregnancy.

33. A p.708

Since September, 1988, RU486 has been available as a medical abortifacient in France and China, and more recently it has become available in other countries. RU486 (the trade name is Mifepristone) is a synthetic relative of the progestational agents in birth control pills. It acts primarily, but not totally, as an antiprogestational agent. RU486 is administered together with a prostaglandin analogue. The combination allows a reduction in dosage of both agents. When administered early in pregnancy, this medical treatment carries with it a success and complication rate similar to that achieved with vacuum curettage. Misoprostol is a stable, orally active synthetic analogue of prostaglandin E_1, available commercially for the treatment of peptic ulcer. By itself it is very ineffective for therapeutic abortion, but combined with RU486 it provides an effective, simple, inexpensive, completely oral method.

It is likely that abortion with RU486 is the result of multiple actions. Although RU486 does not induce labor, it does open and soften the cervix (this may be an action secondary to endogenous prostaglandins). Its major action is its blockade of progesterone receptors in the endometrium. This leads to a disruption of the embryo and the production of prostaglandins. The disruption of the embryo and perhaps a direct action on the trophoblast lead to a decrease in human chorionic gonadotropin (HCG) and a withdrawal of support from the corpus luteum. The success rate is dependent upon the length of pregnancy — the more dependent the pregnancy is upon progesterone from the corpus luteum, the more likely the progesterone antagonist, RU486, will result in abortion. The combined RU486-prostaglandin analogue method is usually restricted to pregnancies that are not beyond 9 weeks gestation.

34. C p.710

Second trimester abortions can be accomplished surgically or medically. The surgical procedure is termed dilatation and evacuation (D and E). Several approaches have been utilized for the medical termination of pregnancy. These include the vaginal, intramuscular, or intra-amniotic administration of prostaglandins and the intra-amniotic injection of hypertonic saline or urea. The D and E procedure is safer and less expensive than the medical methods and is better tolerated (and thus preferred) by patients.

The training, experience, and skills of the surgeon are the primary factors which limit the gestational age at which abortion can be safely performed. Advanced gestational age by itself incurs increased risks for all types of complications. These are multiplied when the duration of pregnancy is discovered, after beginning uterine evacuation, to be beyond the experience and skill of the surgeon or capacity of the equipment. Uterine perforation, infection, bleeding, amniotic fluid embolism, and anesthetic reactions are increased as gestational age increases.

Preoperative cervical dilatation with osmotic dilators makes first trimester abortion safer and easier and is essential for second trimester abortion. Local anesthesia instead of general anesthesia also makes abortion safer. Some patients are not good candidates for surgical procedures of any kind under local anesthesia, and others may have special reasons to prefer that an abortion be performed under general anesthesia. Patient requests should be seriously considered, but the clinician also has a responsibility to inform the patient of the risks and benefits of local versus general anesthesia.

In the United Kingdom, prostaglandin analogues are favored for a noninvasive method of second trimester abortion. A combination of the progesterone antagonist, RU486, (a single oral 200 mg dose of mifepristone administered 36 hours before prostaglandin treatment) and an E prostaglandin analogue (gemeprost) placed vaginally is highly effective, and the combination allows a lesser dose of both agents which results in fewer side effects. In addition this combination does not require the use of cervical laminaria for dilatation.

22 Oral Contraception

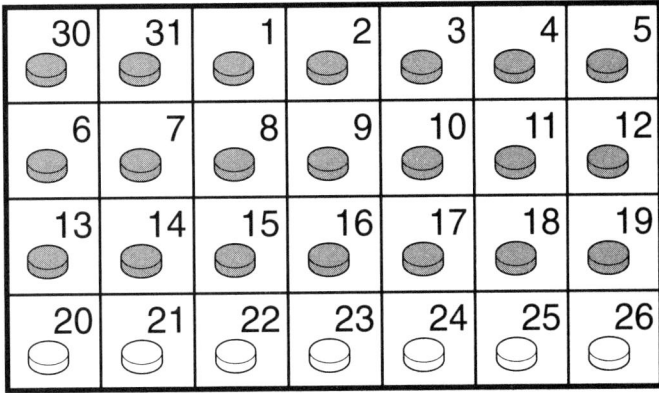

Learning Objectives:

Be able to:

1. Describe the estrogenic and progestational components of traditional oral contraceptives.

2. Discuss the mechanisms of action in oral contraceptives in preventing pregnancy.

3. Detail the non-contraceptive benefits of oral contraceptives.

4. Explain the absolute and relative contraindications for the use of oral contraceptives.

5. Discuss the advantages of the new progestins and how they differ from traditional progestins.

6. Detail possible options for emergency postcoital contraception.

Pre-Test

A. Instructions: Fill in the blanks

1. Cardiovascular side effects are now known to be due to a dose-related stimulation of _____ by estrogen.

2. The _____ androgenicity of the new progestins is reflected in _____ sex hormone binding globulin and _____ free testosterone concentrations to a greater degree than the older established oral contraceptives.

B. Instructions: True or False

3. Oral contraceptive progestin potency is no longer a consideration when it comes to prescribing oral contraception, because the potency of various progestins has been accounted for by appropriate adjustments of dose.

4. Cirrhosis and previous hepatitis are absolute contraindications to oral contraceptive use.

C. Instructions: For each of the following questions choose:

A. if only 1, 2 and 3 are correct
B. if only 1 and 3 are correct
C. if only 2 and 4 are correct
D. if only 4 is correct
E. if all are correct

5. The norethindrone family contains the following 19-nortestosterone progestins
   1. ethynodiol diacetate
   2. norethindrone
   3. norgestrel
   4. gestodene

6. The use of oral contraceptives during pregnancy
   1. is of concern because of the VACTERL complex
   2. is of concern because of the increased risk of virilization
   3. is of concern because of the increased risk of hypospadias
   4. does not increase the risk for major malformations, congenital heart defects or limb reduction defects

Post-Test

A. Instructions: Fill in the blanks

1. The plant from which progesterone was originally derived from was the _____.

2. The first human trials of the oral contraceptive took place in _____.

3. The first oral contraceptive was marketed for commercial use in _____.

4. It was not until the late _____ that a dose-response relationship between problems and the amount of steroids in the pill was appreciated.

5. _____ is the most potent natural estrogen and the major estrogen secreted by the ovaries.

6. _____ is the active isomer of norgestrel.

7. Estrogen-induced thrombosis is a _____-related event.

8. The best estimate of subsequent tubal infertility is approximately ____% after one episode of PID, _____% after 2 episodes and _____% after 3 episodes.

9. The incidence of amenorrhea in the first year of use with low dose oral contraception is approximately _____%. This incidence increases with duration, reaching _____% after several years of use.

10. A simple test for pregnancy is to assess the basal body temperature during the end of the pill-free week; a basal body temperature of less than _____°F (____°C) is inconsistent with pregnancy.

B. Instructions: True or False

11. The addition of an ethinyl group at the 17 position makes estradiol orally active.

12. Mestranol is weaker than ethinyl estradiol, because mestranol must first be converted to ethinyl estradiol in the body.

13. All low dose oral contraceptives contain ethinyl estradiol.

14. From a clinical point of view, there are distinct advantages of multiphasic formulations to low dose monophasic products.

15. The minimal risk of thrombosis associated with oral contraceptive use does not justify the cost of routine screening for deficiencies in the coagulation system.

16. There is evidence from studies in monkeys that estrogen may have protective action against atherosclerosis by a mechanism independent of the cholesterol-lipoprotein profile.

17. Carbohydrate metabolism is affected mainly by the estrogenic component of the oral contraceptive.

18. Long-term use of oral contraception during the reproductive years is not associated with a significant increase in risk of breast cancer after age 45.

19. The inadvertent use of medroxyprogesterone acetate during pregnancy does not increase the risk of a significant congenital anomaly greater than the general rate of 2–3%.

20. Oral contraception should not be started immediately after a second trimester abortion or a premature delivery.

21. The approximate incidence of "postpill amenorrhea" is less than 1%, which is equal to the incidence of spontaneous secondary amenorrhea.

22. Oral contraceptives offer protection against pelvic inflammatory disease.

23. If a woman misses 2 pills in the first two weeks, she should take 2 pills on each of the next two days and use a means of backup contraception for the next week.

C. Match each structure with the appropriate name

A.

B.

C.

D.

E.

F.

G.

24. a type of new progestin
25. a synthetic progestin given to induce withdrawal bleeding
26. the active isomer of norgestrel
27. the estrogen component of all low dose oral contraceptives
28. the activity of ethynodiol diacetate is due to its rapid conversion to this parent compound

D. Instructions: *For each of the following questions choose:*

A. if only 1, 2 and 3 are correct
B. if only 1 and 3 are correct
C. if only 2 and 4 are correct
D. if only 4 is correct
E. if all are correct

29. The new progestins
    1. include desogestrel, gestodene and norgestimate
    2. cause an increase in coagulation disorders
    3. have reduced androgenicity
    4. cause greater breakthrough bleeding than existing low dose oral contraceptives

30. The mechanisms of action of combination oral contraceptives includes
    1. the progestational agent suppresses FSH
    2. the cervical mucus becoming thick and impervious to sperm transport
    3. the estrogenic agent suppress LH
    4. the progestin produces an endometrium which is not receptive to implantation

31. Deleterious metabolic effects of oral contraception include
    1. an increased incidence of cardiovascular disease
    2. an increased incidence of hypertension
    3. a derangement of carbohydrate metabolism
    4. an accelerated incidence of gallbladder disease during the first years of use

32. The use of oral contraceptives
    1. protects against endometrial cancer
    2. protects against ovarian cancer
    3. is associated with an increased incidence for cervical dysplasia
    4. protects against benign breast disease

33. Oral contraceptives
    1. increase cortisol levels
    2. increase thyroxine-binding globulin
    3. do not interfere with accurate assessment of the thyroid function if TSH and free T_4 are measured
    4. increase risk of colon and kidney cancer

34. Absolute contraindications to the use of oral contraception include
    1. a past history of cerebral vascular disease
    2. smokers over the age of 35
    3. suspected breast cancer
    4. gallbladder disease

35. The noncontraceptive benefits of oral contraception include
    1. fewer ectopic pregnancies
    2. increased bone density
    3. less rheumatoid arthritis
    4. less anemia

36. The progestin-only minipill
    1. consistently suppresses gonadotropins
    2. causes the endometrium to involute
    3. has a delay of months before returning of fertility after its discontinuation
    4. will allow up to 40% of patients to ovulate normally

37. The progestin-only minipill may be useful for
    1. lactating women
    2. women for whom estrogen is contraindicated
    3. women over 40 years old
    4. women who report diminished libido on combination oral contraceptives

38. Emergency postcoital contraception
    1. ethinyl estradiol 2.5 mg bid for 5 days
    2. Ovral 4 tablets (2 given 12 hours apart)
    3. LoOvral or Levelen 8 tablets (4 given 12 hours apart)
    4. Ortho Novum 4 tablets (2 given 12 hours apart)

Answers for Chapter 22 — Pre-Test Questions

1. thrombosis   p.718
The estrogen content (dosage) of the pill is of major clinical importance. Thrombosis is one of the most serious side effects of the pill, playing a key role in the increased risk of death from a variety of circulatory problems. This side effect is related to estrogen, and it is dose related. Therefore, the dose of estrogen is a critical issue in selecting an oral contraceptive.

2. decreased; increased; decreased   p.722
The decreased androgenicity of the progestins in the new products is reflected in increased sex hormone binding globulin and decreased free testosterone concentrations to a greater degree than the older established oral contraceptives. This difference may be of greater clinical value in the treatment of acne and hirsutism, but whether a better clinical response is possible is yet to be documented in clinical studies.

3. true   p.722
Oral contraceptive progestin potency is no longer a consideration when it comes to prescribing oral contraception, because the potency of the various progestins has been accounted for by appropriate adjustments of dose. In other words, the biologic effect (in this case the clinical effect) of the various progestational components in current low dose oral contraceptives is approximately the same. The potency of a drug does not determine its efficacy or safety, only the amount of a drug required to achieve an effect.

Clinical advice based on potency ranking is an artificial exercise that has not stood the test of time. There is no clinical evidence that a particular progestin is better or worse in terms of particular side effects or clinical responses. Thus oral contraceptives should be judged by their clinical characteristics: efficacy, side effects, risks, and benefits. Our progress in lowering the doses of the steroids contained in oral contraceptives has yielded products with little serious differences. Potency is no longer an important clinical issue.

4. false   p.727

The only absolute hepatic contraindication to oral contraceptive use is acute or chronic cholestatic liver disease. Cirrhosis and previous hepatitis are not aggravated. Once recovered from the acute phase of liver disease, a woman can use oral contraception.

5. E   p.719

The norethindrone family contains the following 19-nortestosterone progestins: norethindrone, norethynodrel, norethindrone acetate, ethynodiol diacetate, lynestrenol, norgestrel, norgestimate, desogestrel, and gestodene.

6. D   p.732

One of the reasons, if not the major reason, why a lack of withdrawal bleeding while using oral contraceptives is such a problem is the anxiety produced in both patient and clinician. The patient is anxious because of the uncertainty regarding pregnancy, and the clinician is anxious because of the concerns stemming from early retrospective studies which indicated an increased risk of congenital malformations among the offspring of women who were pregnant and using oral contraception. The initial positive reports linking the use of contraceptive steroids to congenital malformations have not been substantiated. Many suspect a strong component of recall bias in the few positive studies due to a tendency of patients with malformed infants to recall details better than those with normal children. Other confounding problems have included a failure to consider the reasons for the administration of hormones (e.g., bleeding in an already abnormal pregnancy), and a failure to delineate the exact timing of the treatment (e.g., treatment was sometimes confined to a period of time during which the heart could not have been affected).

There is no relationship between oral contraception and the following problems: hypospadias, limb reduction anomalies, neural tube defects, and mutagenic effects which would be responsible for chromosomally abnormal fetuses. Even virilization is not a practical consideration because the doses required (e.g., 20–40 mg norethindrone per day) are in excess of anything currently used. These conclusions reflect use of combined oral contraceptives as well as progestins alone.

In the past there was a concern regarding the VACTERL complex. VACTERL refers to a complex of vertebral, anal, cardiac, tracheoesophageal, renal, and limb anomalies. While case-control studies indicated a relationship with oral contraception, prospective studies have failed to observe any connection between sex steroids and the VACTERL complex. A meta-analysis of 26 prospective studies of the risk of birth defects with oral contraceptive ingestion during pregnancy concluded that there was no increase in risk for major malformations, congenital heart defects, or limb reduction defects.

Answers for Chapter 22 — Post-Test Questions

1. yam   p.716

Marker organized extensive botanical expeditions in the Southwest and Mexico, sending home more than 100,000 pounds of material. In 1942, he collected the roots of the Mexican yam, and back in Pennsylvania, he worked out the degradation of diosgenin to progesterone. United States pharmaceutical companies refused to back Marker, and even the university refused, despite Marker's urging, to patent the process.

In 1943, Marker resigned from Pennsylvania State University and went to Mexico where he collected the roots of *Dioscorea mexicana,* 10 tons worth! In an old pottery shed in Mexico City, he prepared several pounds of progesterone (worth $600,000) in two months. This progesterone gained him entry to Hormone Laboratories in Mexico City. The two partners in Hormone Laboratories and Marker formed a company that they called Syntex. The price of progesterone fell from $200 to $2 a gram.

2. 1956   p.716

Both the Syntex and Searle compounds (norethindrone and norethynodrel) were tested in animals in 1953–1954 by Gregory Pincus, John Rock, and colleagues, and in the first human trial, in 1956, with the help of Edris Rice-Wray, a pioneer in family planning who was working at the time in Puerto Rico. The initial progestin products were contaminated with about 1% mestranol. In the amounts being used, this added up to 50–500 micrograms of mestranol, a sufficient amount of estrogen to inhibit ovulation by itself. When efforts to lower the estrogen content yielded breakthrough bleeding, it was decided to retain the estrogen for cycle control, thus establishing the principle of the combined estrogen-progestin oral contraceptive.

3. 1960 p.717

Pincus, a long-time consultant to Searle, picked the Searle compound for extended use. Syntex, a wholesale drug supplier, was without marketing experience or organization. Pincus with great effort convinced Searle that the commercial potential of an oral contraceptive warranted the risk of possible negative public reaction. By the time Syntex had secured arrangements with Ortho for a sales outlet, Searle marketed Enovid in 1960 (150 ug mestranol and 9.85 mg norethynodrel). Ortho-Novum using norethindrone from Syntex appeared in 1962.

4. 1970s p.717

Wyeth Laboratories introduced norgestrel in 1968, the same year in which the first reliable prospective studies were initiated. It was not until the late 1970s that a dose-response relationship between problems and the amount of steroids in the pill was appreciated. As a result, health care providers and patients, over the years, have been confronted by a bewildering array of different products and formulations. The solution to this clinical dilemma is relatively straightforward: use the lowest doses that provide effective contraception.

5. Estradiol p.717

Estradiol is the most potent natural estrogen and the major estrogen secreted by the ovaries. The major obstacle to the use of sex steroids for contraception was inactivity of the compounds when given orally.

6. Levonorgestrel p.720

Norgestrel is a racemic equal mixture of the dextrorotatory enantiomer and the levorotatory enantiomer. These enantiomers are mirror images of each other and rotate the plane of polarized light in opposite directions. The dextrorotatory form is known as *d*-norgestrel, and the levorotatory form is *l*-norgestrel (known as levonorgestrel). Levonorgestrel is the active isomer of norgestrel.

7. dose p.724

There is no evidence of an increase in risk of cardiovascular disease among past users of oral contraception. Part of the concern for a possible lingering effect of oral contraceptive use was based upon a presumed adverse impact on the atherosclerotic process which would then be added to the effect of aging and thus would be manifested later in life. Instead, the findings are consistent with the contention that cardiovascular disease due to oral contraception is secondary to acute effects, specifically estrogen-induced thrombosis, a dose-related event.

8. 12; 23; 54 p.735

Sexually transmitted diseases (STDs) are one of the most common public health problems in the United States. Pelvic inflammatory disease (PID) is usually a consequence of STDs. The best estimate of subsequent tubal infertility is approximately 12% after one episode of PID, 23% after 2 episodes, and 54% after 3 episodes. Because pelvic infection is the single greatest threat to the reproductive future of a young woman, the now recognized protection offered by oral contraception against pelvic inflammatory disease is very important.

9. 1; 5 p.741

The incidence of amenorrhea in the first year of use with low dose oral contraception is approximately 1%. This incidence increases with duration, reaching perhaps 5% after several years of use. It is important to alert patients upon starting oral contraception that diminished bleeding and possibly no bleeding may ensue.

10. 98; 36.8 p.741

Amenorrhea is a difficult management problem. A pregnancy test will allow reliable assessment for the presence of pregnancy even at this early stage. However, routine, repeated use of such testing is expensive and annoying, and may lead to discontinuation of oral contraception. ***A simple test for pregnancy is to assess the basal body temperature*** *during the END of the pill-free week; a basal body temperature of less than 98°F (36.8°C) is consistent with pregnancy, and oral contraception can be continued.*

11. true   p.717

A major breakthrough occurred in 1938 when it was discovered that the addition of an ethinyl group at the 17 position made estradiol orally active. Ethinyl estradiol is a very potent oral estrogen and is one of the two forms of estrogen in every oral contraceptive. The other estrogen is the 3-methyl ether of ethinyl estradiol, mestranol.

12. true   p.717

Mestranol and ethinyl estradiol are different from natural estradiol and must be regarded as pharmacologic drugs. Animal studies have suggested that mestranol is weaker than ethinyl estradiol, because mestranol must first be converted to ethinyl estradiol in the body. Indeed, mestranol will not bind to the estrogen receptor. Therefore, unconjugated ethinyl estradiol is the active estrogen in the blood for both mestranol and ethinyl estradiol.

13. true   p.717

In the human body, differences in potency between ethinyl estradiol and mestranol do not appear to be significant, certainly not as great as indicated by assays in rodents. This is now a minor point since all of the low dose oral contraceptives contain ethinyl estradiol.

14. false   p.722

The multiphasic preparations alter the dosage of both the estrogen and progestin components periodically throughout the pill-taking schedule. The aim of these formulations is to alter steroid levels in an effort to achieve fewer metabolic effects and minimize the occurrence of breakthrough bleeding and amenorrhea, while maintaining efficacy. We are probably at or very near the lowest dose levels which can be achieved without sacrificing efficacy. Metabolic studies with the multiphasic preparations indicate no differences or slight improvements over the metabolic effects of low dose monophasic products. From a clinical point of view, there are no outstanding advantages or disadvantages comparing multiphasic formulations to low dose monophasic products.

15. true   p.724

Today, the rare young woman on oral contraception who has a thrombotic episode probably represents someone with an underlying clotting problem, an individual who shows an extreme response to oral contraceptives, or an individual with an unknown lesion of a vessel wall or an unknown local disturbance of circulation. The minimal risk of thrombosis associated with oral contraceptive use does not justify the cost of routine screening for deficiencies in the coagulation system. If a patient develops a thrombotic complication while taking oral contraceptives, an evaluation to search for an underlying abnormality in the coagulation system is warranted (measurement of antithrombin III, protein C, protein S, activated partial thromboplastin time, fibrinogen, and plasminogen).

16. true   p.725

An important study in monkeys has indicated a protective action of estrogen against atherosclerosis, but by a mechanism independent of the cholesterol-lipoprotein profile. Oral administration of a combination of estrogen and progestin to monkeys fed a high cholesterol, atherogenic diet decreased the extent of coronary atherosclerosis despite a reduction in HDL-cholesterol levels. In considering the impact of progestational agents, lowering of HDL is not necessarily atherogenic if accompanied by other significant estrogen effects. These animal studies help explain why older, higher dose combinations which had an adverse impact on the lipoprotein profile did not increase subsequent cardiovascular disease. The estrogen component provided protection through a direct effect on vessel walls. Perhaps the low dose combinations will even be associated with a favorable impact on the risk of cardiovascular disease.

17. false   p.726

Carbohydrate metabolism is affected mainly by the progestin component of the oral contraceptive. The derangement of carbohydrate metabolism may also be affected by estrogen influences on lipid metabolism, hepatic enzymes, and elevation of unbound cortisol. The glucose intolerance is dose-related, and once again effects are less with the low dose formulations. Insulin and glucose changes with low dose monophasic and multiphasic oral contraceptives are so minimal, that it is now believed that they are of no clinical significance. This includes long-term evaluation with hemoglobin A1c. The one exception is the claim that the levonorgestrel monophasic has an excessively negative impact.

18. true   p.730

The crucial question is this: as studies gain more statistical power, will they confirm a slightly increased risk for premenopausal breast cancer or will the present suggestion of an increased risk disappear? For some time to come, probably a decade or more, clinical advice will have to be based on the current conflicting findings. With considerable confidence, it can be stated that long-term use of oral contraception during the reproductive years is **NOT** associated with a significant increase in the risk of breast cancer after age 45. There is the possibility that a subgroup of young women who use contraception early and for a long time (greater than 4 years) has a slightly increased risk of breast cancer before the age of 45, a relative risk of less than 1.5. It is not cost-effective to promote mammographic surveillance of this group of patients, but it should not be denied to any woman of this group who makes the request. There is also the possibility that previous users of oral contraception are provided some protection against postmenopausal breast cancer. Keep in mind that these conclusions depend upon data derived from use of higher dose oral contraception. It is important to be aware that there has been consistent failure to demonstrate an increased risk with oral contraceptive use in women with positive family histories of breast cancer or in women with proven benign breast disease.

19. true   p.732

Women who become pregnant while taking oral contraceptives or women who inadvertently take birth control pills early in pregnancy should be advised that the risk of a significant congenital anomaly is no greater than the general rate of 2–3%. This recommendation can be extended to those pregnant woman who have been exposed to a progestational agent such as medroxyprogesterone acetate or 17-hydroxyprogesterone caproate.

20. false   p.735

After the termination of a pregnancy of less than 12 weeks, oral contraception can be started immediately. After a pregnancy of 12 or more weeks, oral contraception has traditionally been started 2 weeks after delivery to avoid an increased risk of thrombosis during the initial postpartum period. This practice has been based on a theoretical concern that is probably no longer an issue with low dose oral contraception. Oral contraception can be started immediately after a second trimester abortion or premature delivery.

21. true   p.735

The approximate incidence of "postpill amenorrhea" is 0.7–0.8%, which is equal to the incidence of spontaneous secondary amenorrhea, and there is no evidence to support the idea that oral contraception causes secondary amenorrhea. If a cause and effect relationship exists between oral contraception and subsequent amenorrhea, one would expect the incidence of infertility to be increased after a given population discontinues use of oral contraception. In those women who discontinue oral contraception in order to get pregnant, 50% conceive by 3 months, and after 2 years, a maximum of 15% of nulliparous women and 7% of parous women fail to conceive, figures comparable to those quoted for the prevalence of spontaneous infertility. While patients with this problem come more quickly to our attention because of previous oral contraceptive use and follow-up, there is no cause and effect relationship. Women who have not resumed menstrual function within 12 months should be evaluated as any other patient with secondary amenorrhea.

22. true   p.735,736

The risk of hospitalization for PID is reduced by approximately 50–60%, but at least 12 months of use is necessary, and the protection is limited to current users. If a woman does get a pelvic infection, the severity of the salpingitis found at laparoscopy is decreased. The mechanism of this protection remains unknown. Speculation includes thickening of the cervical mucus to prevent movement of pathogens and bacteria-laden sperm into the uterus and tubes, and decreased menstrual bleeding which reduces movement of pathogens into the tubes as well as a reduction in "culture medium."

23. true   p.739

If a woman misses 2 pills in the first two weeks, she should take two pills on each of the next two days; it is unlikely that a back-up method is needed, but the official consensus is to recommend back-up for the next 7 days.

24. F

Gestodene

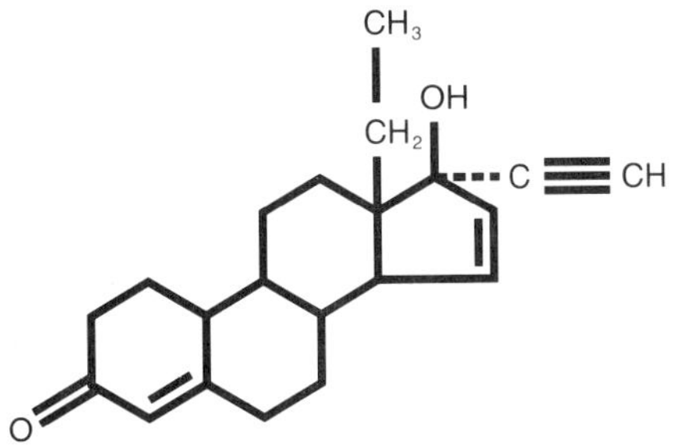

p.720

25. G

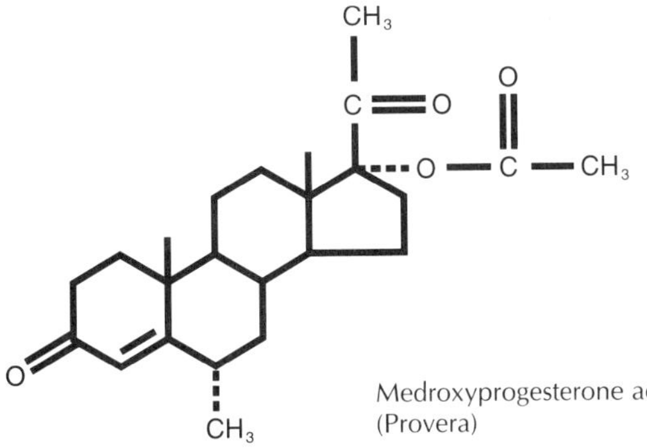

Medroxyprogesterone acetate (Provera)

p.721

26. B

Levonorgestrel

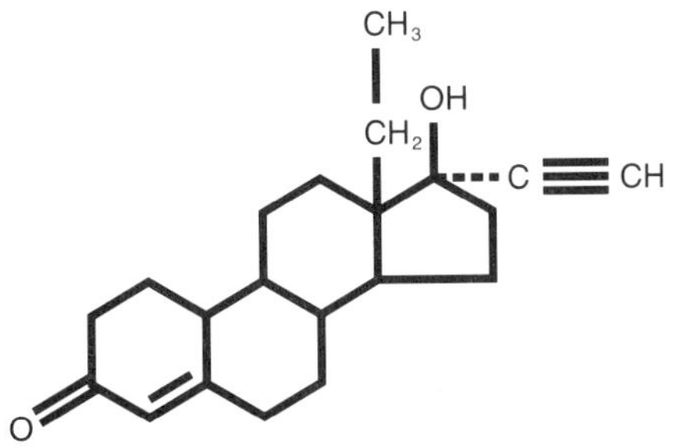

P.719

27. D

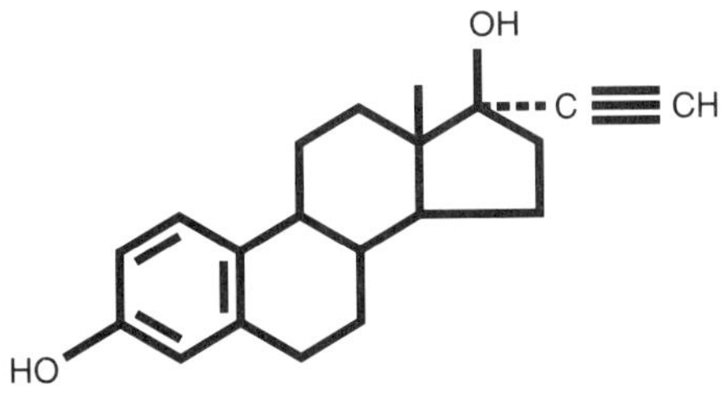

Ethinyl estradiol

P.717

28. A   P.719

Norethindrone

29. B   p.721,722
The new progestins include desogestrel, gestodene, and norgestimate. With the combined products containing the new progestins, the changes in the coagulation system are very similar to those with the current low dose formulations. A slight prothrombotic effect is characterized by increased levels of fibrinopeptide A that is balanced by antithrombin III and protein C. Thus any coagulation tendency is counteracted. The protime and the activated partial thromboplastin time measure the overall activity of the coagulation pathways — there is no significant increase in these measurements with the new formulations. In a controversial issue, it has been argued that gestodene affects the pharmocokinetics of ethinyl estradiol differently, causing higher circulating levels of the estrogen component. Intense evaluation of this issue, however, has failed to reveal any effects unique to gestodene.

In regard to cycle control (breakthrough bleeding and amenorrhea), the new formulations are comparable to existing low dose products.

All progestins derived from 19-nortestosterone have the potential to decrease glucose tolerance and increase insulin resistance. The impact of the current low dose formulations is very minimal, and the impact of the new progestins is negligible. Most changes are not statistically significant, and when they are, they are so subtle as to be of no clinical significance. For example, there are no changes in hemoglobin A1c.

The decreased androgenicity of the progestins in the new products is reflected in increased sex hormone binding globulin and decreased free testosterone concentrations to a greater degree than the older established oral contraceptives. This difference may be of greater clinical value in the treatment of acne and hirsutism, but whether a better clinical response is possible is yet to be documented in clinical studies.

The new progestins, because of their reduced androgenicity, predictably do not adversely affect the cholesterol-lipoprotein profile. Indeed, the estrogen-progestin balance of combined oral contraceptives containing one of the new progestins may even promote favorable lipid changes. Thus, the new formulations have the potential to offer protection against cardiovascular disease, an important consideration as we enter an era of women using oral contraceptives for longer durations and later in life. But one must be cautious regarding the clinical significance of subtle changes, and it will be a long time before epidemiologic data on this issue are available.

30. C   p.723
The combination oral contraceptive, consisting of the estrogen and progestin components, is given daily for 3 out of every 4 weeks. The combination oral contraceptive prevents ovulation by inhibiting gonadotropin secretion via an effect on both pituitary and hypothalamic centers. The progestational agent primarily suppresses luteinizing hormone (LH) secretion (and thus prevents ovulation), while the estrogenic agent suppresses follicle-stimulating hormone (FSH) secretion (and thus prevents the selection and emergence of a dominant follicle). Therefore, the estrogenic component significantly contributes to the contraceptive efficacy. However, even if follicular growth and development were not sufficiently inhibited, the progestational component would prevent the surge-like release of LH necessary for ovulation.

The estrogen in the oral contraceptive serves two other purposes. It provides stability to the endometrium so that irregular shedding and unwanted breakthrough bleeding can be minimized, and the presence of estrogen is required to potentiate the action of the progestational agents. The latter function of estrogen has allowed reduction of the progestational dose in the oral contraceptive. The mechanism for this action is probably estrogen's effect in increasing the concentration of intracellular progestational receptors. Therefore, a certain pharmacologic level of estrogen is necessary to maintain the potency of the combination oral contraceptive.

Since the effect of a progestational agent will always take precedence over estrogen (unless the dose of estrogen is increased many, many fold), the endometrium, cervical mucus, and perhaps tubal function reflect progestational stimulation. The progestin in the combination pill produces an endometrium which is not receptive to ovum implantation, a decidualized bed with exhausted and atrophied glands. The cervical mucus becomes thick and impervious to sperm transport. It is possible that progestational influences on secretion and peristalsis within the fallopian tubes provide additional contraceptive effects.

31. D   p.724–727

A review of the massive Medicaid data in the state of Michigan confirms the fact that the risk of venous thrombosis is increased at the 50 mg dose. It is still unknown whether a risk of thrombosis persists at the lower doses. A case-control study of all 794 women in Denmark who suffered a cerebral thromboembolic attack during 1985–1989 concluded that there was an increased relative risk (1.8) associated with oral contraceptives containing 30–40 µg estrogen. Whether the conclusion of this retrospective case-control study (which relied upon questionnaires) is real or not must be verified by the ongoing cohort studies. An analysis of fatal venous thromboembolism in England and Wales between 1986 and 1988 failed to find a statistically significant increase in the relative risk for current users of oral contraceptives.

Evidence indicates that small increases in blood pressure can be observed even with 30 mg estrogen, monophasic pills, including those containing the new progestins. However, an increased incidence of clinically significant hypertension has not been reported.

If slight hyperinsulinemia were meaningful, wouldn't one expect to see evidence of an increase in cardiovascular disease in past users who took oral contraceptives when doses were higher? Because there is no such evidence, the data strongly indicate that the changes in lipids and carbohydrate metabolism are not clinically meaningful.

Data from the RCGP prospective study indicated that an increase in the incidence of gallstones occurred in the first years of oral contraceptive use, apparently due to an acceleration of gallbladder disease in women already susceptible. In other words, the overall risk of gallbladder disease was not increased, but in the first years of use disease was activated or accelerated in women who were vulnerable because of asymptomatic disease or a tendency toward gallbladder disease. The Nurses' Health Study reported no significant increase in the risk of symptomatic gallstones among ever-users, but slightly elevated risks among current and long-term users. Although oral contraceptive use has been linked to an increased risk of gallbladder disease, the epidemiologic evidence has been inconsistent. It has been suggested that the mechanism is due to induced alterations in the composition of gallbladder bile, specifically a rise in cholesterol saturation that is presumably an estrogen effect. If this is the case, we would anticipate an even lesser effect in the forthcoming reports describing the impact of low dose oral contraceptives. Keep in mind that while some studies have found a statistically significant modest increase in the relative risk of gallbladder disease, because the actual incidence of this problem is low, the effect is of minimal clinical importance.

32. E   p.728,729

The use of oral contraception protects against endometrial cancer. Use for at least 12 months reduces the risk of developing endometrial cancer by **50%**, with the greatest protective effect gained by use for more than 3 years. The risk of developing epithelial ovarian cancer in users of oral contraception is reduced by **40%** compared to that of nonusers. This protective effect increases with duration of use (taking 5–10 years to become apparent) and continues for at least 10–15 years after stopping the medication. This protection is seen in women who use oral contraception for as little as 3 to 6 months, reaches an 80% reduction in risk with more than 10 years of use, and is a benefit associated with all monophasic formulations, including the low dose formulations. Studies have indicated that the risk for dysplasia and carcinoma-in-situ of the uterine cervix increases with the use of oral contraception for more than one year. After 2 years there is a progressive reduction (about 40%) in the incidence of fibrocystic disease of the breast. Women who used oral contraception were one-fourth as likely to develop benign breast disease as nonusers, but this protection was limited to current and recent users. It is still unknown whether this same protection is provided by the lower dose products.

33. A p.731

The Walnut Creek study suggested that melanoma was linked to oral contraception; however, the major risk factor for melanoma is exposure to sunlight. More recent and accurate evaluation utilizing both of the RCGP and OFPA prospective cohorts and accounting for exposure to sunlight has not indicated a significant difference in the risk of melanoma comparing users to nonusers. There is no evidence linking oral contraceptive use to kidney cancer, colon cancer, gallbladder cancer, or pituitary tumors.

For some time it has been known that estrogen increases the cortisol-binding globulin, transcortin. It had been thought that the increase in plasma cortisol while on oral contraception was due to increased binding by this globulin and not an increase in free active cortisol. Now it is apparent that free and active cortisol levels are also elevated. Estrogen decreases the ability of the liver to metabolize cortisol, and in addition, progesterone and related compounds can displace cortisol from transcortin and thus contribute to the elevation of unbound cortisol. The effects of these elevated levels over prolonged periods of time are unknown. To put this into perspective, the increase is not as great as that which occurs in pregnancy, and, in fact it is within the normal range for nonpregnant women.

As with transcortin, estrogen increases thyroxine-binding globulin. Prior to the introduction of new methods for measuring free thyroxine levels, evaluation of thyroid function was a problem. Measurement of TSH (thyroid-stimulating hormone) and the free thyroxine level in a woman on oral contraception provides an accurate assessment of a patient's thyroid state. Oral contraception affects the total thyroxine level in the blood as well as the amount of binding globulin, but the free thyroxine level is unchanged.

34. A p.737,743-745

Absolute contraindications to the use of oral contraception
1. Thrombophlebitis, thromboembolic disorders, cerebral vascular disease, coronary occlusion, a past history of these conditions, or conditions predisposing to these problems.
2. Markedly impaired liver function. Steroid hormones are contraindicated in patients with hepatitis until liver function tests return to normal.
3. Known or suspected breast cancer.
4. Undiagnosed abnormal vaginal bleeding.
5. Known or suspected pregnancy.
6. Smokers over the age of 35.

35. E p.745

The noncontraceptive incidental benefits can be listed as follows:

Effective contraception.
 -less need for therapeutic abortion.
 -less need for surgical sterilization.
Less endometrial cancer.
Less ovarian cancer.
Less benign breast disease.
Fewer ectopic pregnancies.
More regular menses.
 -less flow.
 -less dysmenorrhea.
 -less anemia.
Less salpingitis.
Less rheumatoid arthritis.
Increased bone density.
Probably less endometriosis.
Possibly protection against atherosclerosis.
Possibly fewer fibroids.
Possibly fewer ovarian cysts.

36. C   p.749

The small amount of progestin in the circulation will have a significant impact only on those tissues very sensitive to the female sex steroids, estrogen and progesterone. The contraceptive effect is more dependent upon endometrial and cervical mucus effects, since gonadotropins are not consistently suppressed. The endometrium involutes and becomes hostile to implantation, and the cervical mucus becomes thick and impermeable. Approximately 40% of patients will ovulate normally. Tubal physiology may also be affected, but this is speculative.

Ectopic pregnancy is not prevented as effectively as intrauterine pregnancy. Although the overall incidence of ectopic pregnancy is not increased, when pregnancy occurs, the clinician must suspect that it is more likely to be ectopic. There are no significant metabolic effects, and there is an immediate return to fertility upon discontinuation (unlike the delay seen with the combination oral contraceptive).

37. E   p.750,751

There are two situations where excellent efficacy, probably near total effectiveness, is achieved: lactating women and women over age 40. In lactating women, the contribution of the minipill is combined with prolactin-induced suppression of ovulation, adding up to very effective protection. In women over age 40, reduced fecundity adds to the minipill's effects. The minipill is a good choice in situations where estrogen is contraindicated, such as patients with serious medical conditions (diabetes with vascular disease, severe systemic lupus erythematosus, cardiovascular disease). It should be noted that the freedom from estrogen effects, although likely, is presumptive. Substantial data, e.g., on associations with vascular disease, blood pressure, and cancer, are not available because relatively small numbers have chosen to use this method of contraception. On the other hand, it is very logical to conclude that any of the progestin effects associated with the combination oral contraceptives can be related to the minipill according to a dose-response curve; all effects should be reduced.

The minipill is a good alternative for the occasional woman who reports diminished libido on combination oral contraceptives, presumably due to decreased androgen levels. The minipill should also be considered for the few patients who report minor side effects (gastrointestinal upset, breast tenderness, headaches) of such a degree that the combination oral contraceptive is not acceptable.

38. A   p.751,752

The following treatment regimens have been documented to be effective:

> Conjugated estrogens 15 mg bid for 5 days or 50 mg iv on each of 2 consecutive days.
> Ethinyl estradiol, 2.5 mg bid for 5 days.
> Ovral, 4 tablets (2 given 12 hours apart).
> LoOvral or Levelen, 8 tablets (4 given 12 hours apart).

Could other combination oral contraceptive products be used? Since other doses and other formulations have never been tested, the efficacy is unknown. It would not be appropriate to expose patients to an unknown failure rate. Levonorgestrel in a dose of 0.75 mg given twice, 12 hours apart, is as successful as the combination oral contraceptive method, but this dose is equivalent to 25 pills of the levonorgestrel progestin-only minipill. The use of danazol for this purpose is relatively untested, but RU486, the progesterone antagonist, has been without failures and with lower side effects in preliminary trials.

23 Long-Acting Methods of Contraception

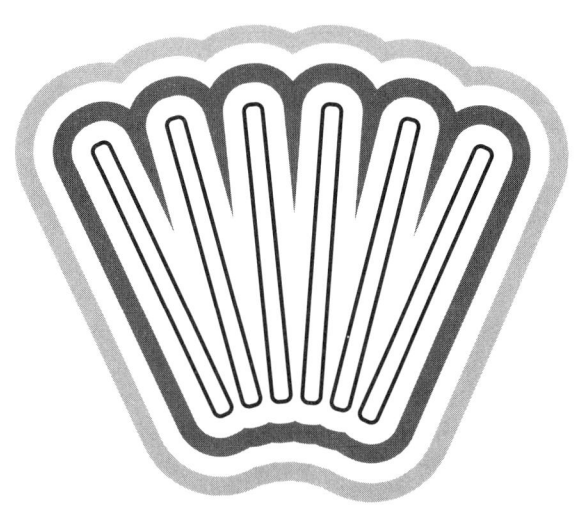

Learning Objectives

Be able to:

1. Name and describe the mechanisms of action of two currently available long-acting reversible methods of medical contraception.

2. Discuss the indications and absolute contraindications for using both methods.

3. Describe the advantages and disadvantages of each long-acting method.

Pre-Test

A. Instructions: Fill in the blank

1. The freedom from the side effects of estrogen allows _____ to be considered for patients with congenital heart disease, sickle cell anemia and patients with a previous history of thromboembolism.

B. Instructions: True or False

2. Return of fertility after Norplant removal is delayed up to 6 months.

C. Instructions: For the following question choose:

A. if only 1, 2 and 3 are correct
B. if only 1 and 3 are correct
C. if only 2 and 4 are correct
D. if only 4 is correct
E. if all are correct

3. Norplant capsule release
   1. is approximately 80 mg of levonorgestrel per 24 hours during the first 6–12 months of use
   2. is 30–35 mg of levonorgestrel per 24 hours after the first 12 months of use
   3. maintains mean plasma concentrations of levonorgestrel greater than 0.25 ng/ml for up to 5 years
   4. is subject to a large first pass effect through the liver

Post-Test

A. Instructions: Fill in the blanks

1. There are two effective and popular methods currently available as long-acting contraceptive methods. They are _____ and _____.

2. _____ utilizes silastic tubing permeable to _____ to provide stable circulating levels over _____ months.

3. Injectable _____ is a long-acting (_____ months) agent which has been part of the contraceptive program of many countries for more than 20 years.

4. The most common side effect of Norplant is _____.

5. The dose of medroxyprogesterone acetate given for contraceptive purposes is _____ mg intramuscularly every _____ months.

B. Instructions: True or False

6. The progestins release by Norplant circulate at levels of one-fourth to one-tenth of those obtained with combined oral contraceptives.

7. Current long-acting contraceptive methods are not associated with many of the side effects associated with more short-acting progestin-containing contraceptive methods.

8. Norplant is a more effective method of birth control than any of the other reversible methods.

9. Norplant's efficacy may be longer in duration for women greater than 70 kg than for slender women.

10. When pregnancy occurs in a patient who has Norplant in place, an ectopic pregnancy must be ruled out.

11. Ectopic pregnancy rates are higher in women using Norplant than in women not using contraception.

12. Exposure to the sustained, low dose of levonorgestrel delivered by implants is not associated with significant metabolic changes.

13. Norplant and Depo-Provera deserve consideration in those situations where combination estrogen-progestin is unacceptable.

C. Instructions: For each of the following questions choose:

A. if only 1, 2 and 3 are correct
B. if only 1 and 3 are correct
C. if only 2 and 4 are correct
D. if only 4 is correct
E. if all are correct

14. Norplant
    1. capsules contain 36 mg of dry crystalline levonorgestrel for a total of 216 mg in the 6 capsules
    2. contains levonorgestrel which is stable in capsule form for more than 7 years
    3. has a release rate which is determined by its total surface area and thickness of the capsule wall
    4. releases enough levonorgestrel within 24 hours to prevent conception

15. Norplant may prevent contraception through several mechanisms which
    1. are similar to those attributed to the contraceptive effect of the progestin-only minipill
    2. includes thickening of the cervical mucus
    3. includes suppression of the LH surge
    4. includes eventual atrophy of the endometrium

16. Advantages of Norplant include
    1. freedom from compliance issues
    2. its use-effectiveness does not closely approximate its theoretical effectiveness
    3. may be used by women who have contraindications for the use of estrogen-containing oral contraceptives
    4. that it is less expensive compared to oral contraceptives

17. Disadvantages of Norplant include
    1. protection against STDs
    2. disruption of bleeding patterns in up to 80% of users
    3. the inability to see the capsules under the skin
    4. requirement of minor surgical procedures for placement and removal

18. Norplant is absolutely contraindicated in women who
    1. smoke heavily
    2. have active thrombophlebitis
    3. have hypercholesterolemia
    4. have acute liver disease

19. In addition to the menstrual changes the following side effects have been reported
    1. headache
    2. acne
    3. weight change
    4. depression

20. Depo-Provera administered for contraception
    1. should be given within 2 weeks of the current menstrual cycle otherwise a backup method is necessary
    2. can provide effective contraceptive levels for 4 months
    3. has a different mechanism of action than progestin-only methods
    4. will not result in symptoms of estrogen deficiency

21. Problems with Depo-Provera include
    1. irregular menstrual bleeding
    2. breast tenderness
    3. weight gain
    4. higher incidence of ectopic pregnancy

22. Metabolic changes which occur with Depo-Provera
    1. a possible change in lipoprotein profile
    2. a clinical change in carbohydrate metabolism
    3. a possible loss of bone density
    4. a clinical change in coagulation

23. After Depo-Provera is discontinued
    1. the pregnancy rate in women who desire pregnancy is decreased
    2. the delay to conception is about 9 months after the last injection
    3. the delay to conception increases with increasing duration of use
    4. if suppressed menstrual function persists beyond 1 year it deserves evaluation

24. Advantages of Depo-Provera include
    1. avoidance of compliance issues
    2. increasing amount of lactation in nursing mothers
    3. an improvement in seizure disorders
    4. a decreased risk of pelvic inflammatory disease and endometrial cancer

Answers for Chapter 23 — Pre-Test Questions

1. Depo-Provera p.772
Like other sustained release forms of contraception, this method is not associated with compliance problems and is not related to the coital event. The freedom from the side effects of estrogen allows Depo-Provera to be considered for patients with congenital heart disease, sickle cell anemia, patients with a previous history of thromboembolism, and women over 30 who smoke or have other risk factors. The absolute safety in regard to thrombosis is mainly theoretical; it has not been proven in a controlled study. However, an increased rate of thrombosis has not been observed in epidemiologic evaluation of Depo-Provera users.

2. false p.770
Circulating levels of levonorgestrel become too low to measure within 48 hours after removal of Norplant. Most women resume normal ovulatory cycles during the first month after removal. The pregnancy rates during the first year after removal are comparable to those of women not using contraceptive methods and trying to become pregnant. There are no long-term effects on future fertility, nor are there any effects on sex ratios, rates of ectopic pregnancy, spontaneous abortion, stillbirth, or congenital malformations.

3. A p.766
The release rate of the capsule is determined by its total surface area and the thickness of the capsule wall. The levonorgestrel diffuses through the wall of the tubing into the surrounding tissues where it is absorbed by the circulatory system and distributed systemically, avoiding an initial high level in the hepatic circulation. Within 24 hours after insertion, plasma concentrations of levonorgestrel range from 0.4 to 0.5 ng/mL, high enough to prevent conception. This level corresponds to the level reached 12 hours after taking the levonorgestrel progestin-only oral minipill. The capsules release approximately 80 mg levonorgestrel per 24 hours during the first 6–12 months of use. This rate declines gradually to 30–35 mg per day for the remaining duration of use. After 5 years, the implants release about 25 mg per day. The 80 mg per day of hormone released by the implants during the first 2–6 months of use is about the same as the daily dose of levonorgestrel delivered by the progestin-only, minipill oral contraceptive, and 25–50% of the dose delivered by low dose combined oral contraceptives. Mean plasma concentrations below 0.20 ng/mL are associated with increased pregnancy rates. After 6 months of use, daily levonorgestrel concentrations are about 0.35 ng/mL; at 2.5 years, the levels decrease to 0.25–0.35 ng/mL. Until the 5-year mark, mean levels remain above 0.25 ng/mL.

Answers for Chapter 23 — Post-Test Questions

1. Norplant; depot-medroxyprogesterone acetate (Depo-Provera) p.765
The high rate of unintended pregnancies and the relatively high failure rates with the typical use of reversible methods of contraception are strong indications of a need for long-acting contraceptive methods that simplify compliance. Two effective and popular methods are available, the Norplant system and depot-medroxyprogesterone acetate (Depo-Provera). Other products are in development.

2. Norplant; steroids p.765
Norplant employs silastic tubing permeable to steroid molecules to provide stable circulating levels of synthetic progestins over months and years.

3. medroxyprogesterone acetate; 3–6 p.765
Injectable medroxyprogesterone acetate is a long-acting (3–6 months) agent which has been part of the contraceptive programs of many countries for more than 20 years. This experience has demonstrated it to be safe, effective, and acceptable. It is not a "sustained release" system, but its action is the same.

4. irregular bleeding p.769
Menstrual bleeding patterns are highly variable among users of Norplant. Some alteration of menstrual patterns will

occur during the first year of use in approximately 60% of users. The changes include alterations in the interval between bleeding, the duration and volume of menstrual flow, and spotting. Oligomenorrhea and amenorrhea also occur but are less common. Irregular and prolonged bleeding usually occurs during the first year. Although bleeding problems occur much less frequently after the second year, they can occur at any time. Despite an increase in the number of spotting and bleeding days over preinsertion menstrual patterns, hemoglobin concentrations rise in Norplant users because of a decrease in the average amount of menstrual blood loss.

5. 150; 3   p.771

Medroxyprogesterone acetate (Depo-Provera) for contraception is administered as microcrystals, suspended in an aqueous solution, which dissolve very slowly. The dose of medroxyprogesterone acetate for contraceptive purposes is 150 mg intramuscularly every 3 months. The injection should be given within the first 5 days of the current menstrual cycle, otherwise a back-up method is necessary for 2 weeks. The effective contraceptive level is maintained for 4 months, providing a safety margin for reliable contraception.

6. true   p.765

The progestins, circulating at levels one-fourth to one-tenth of those obtained with combined oral contraceptives, prevent conception by suppressing ovulation and thickening cervical mucus to inhibit sperm penetration so that fertilization rarely occurs.

7. false   p.765

Because serum levels of progestin remain low and because no estrogen is administered, these long-acting contraceptive methods have not caused any serious health effects. These methods do, however, cause many of the same minor, but bothersome, side effects associated with the progestin component of combined oral contraceptives. The continuous presence of low levels of progestin leads to irregular endometrial sloughing, a problem common to all of these methods, and one that is highly variable from one woman to another.

8. true   p.768

Norplant is a more effective method of birth control than any of the other reversible methods. In studies conducted in 11 countries, totaling 12,133 woman-years of use, the pregnancy rate was 0.2 pregnancies per 100 woman-years of use. All but one of the pregnancies that occurred during this evaluation were present at the time of implant insertion. If these luteal phase insertions are excluded from analysis, the first-year pregnancy rate was 0.01 per 100 woman-years.

9. false   p.768

The overall pregnancy rate after 2 years of use in 9 countries was 0.2 per 100 woman-years of use. The pregnancy rate achieved in the U.S. trials during the second year of use was higher (2.1 per 100 woman-years). Two factors may account for this difference. First, users in the U.S. weighed, on the average, more than study participants in other countries. Clinical trials have demonstrated a direct correlation between weight greater than 70 kg (154 pounds) and an increased risk of pregnancy, but even for heavy women, pregnancy rates are lower than with oral contraception. Second, two different types of silastic tubing were used in the manufacture of Norplant capsules. The first type contained a larger proportion of inert filler and was more dense, while the second type contained less filler and was less dense. Higher pregnancy rates have been observed among women using the more dense capsules, and in the U.S. trials, capsules were more often of the more dense variety. The less dense tubing is now the only one used in the manufacture of Norplant and has a 15% higher release rate than denser tubing.

Using the less dense tubing, there now are no weight restrictions for Norplant users, but heavier women (more than 70 kg) may experience slightly higher pregnancy rates in the fourth and fifth years of use compared to lighter women. Even in the later years, however, pregnancy rates for heavier women using Norplant are lower than with oral contraception. The differences in pregnancy rates by weight are probably due to the dilutional effect of larger body size on the low, sustained serum levels of levonorgestrel. Heavier women should not rely on Norplant beyond the 5-year limit. For slender women the duration of Norplant's efficacy may extend well into the fifth year of use.

10. true   p.769

The ectopic pregnancy rate during Norplant use has been 0.28 per 1,000 woman-years. This compares to the rate of 1.5 per 1,000 among U.S. women aged 15–44. Although the risk of developing an ectopic pregnancy during use of Norplant is low, when pregnancy does occur, ectopic pregnancy should be suspected, especially if the patient has additional risk factors.

11. false p.769

Ectopic Pregnancy Rates per 1,000 Woman-Years

All U.S. women	1.50
Non-contraceptive users	3.00
Copper T-380 IUD	0.20
Norplant	0.28

12. true p.769
Exposure to the sustained, low dose of levonorgestrel delivered by the implants is not associated with significant metabolic changes. Studies of carbohydrate metabolism, liver function, blood coagulation, immunoglobulin levels, serum cortisol levels, and blood chemistries have failed to detect changes outside of normal ranges.

13. true p.766
A progestin-only method may be utilized by women who have contraindications for the use of estrogen-containing oral contraceptives. The sustained release of low doses of progestin avoids the high initial dose delivered by injectables and the daily hormone surge associated with oral contraceptives. Norplant is not a coitus-related contraceptive method. The use-effectiveness closely approximates the theoretical effectiveness. Norplant is an excellent choice for a breastfeeding woman (there is no effect on breastfeeding) and can be inserted immediately postpartum.

14. A p.766
The Norplant system consists of 6 capsules, each measuring 34 mm in length with a 2.4 mm outer diameter and containing levonorgestrel. The capsule is made of flexible, medical grade silastic (polydimethylsiloxane) tubing which is sealed shut with silastic medical adhesive, silicone type A. The cavity of the capsule has an inner diameter of 1.57 mm, with an inner length of 30 mm. Each capsule contains 36 mg dry crystalline levonorgestrel for a total of 216 mg in the 6 capsules. The levonorgestrel is very stable and has remained unchanged in capsules examined after more than 7 years of use. Norplant II, which consists of two implants, is a system nearing completion of clinical trials.

The release rate of the capsule is determined by its total surface area and the thickness of the capsule wall. The levonorgestrel diffuses through the wall of the tubing into the surrounding tissues where it is absorbed by the circulatory system and distributed systemically, avoiding an initial high level in the hepatic circulation. Within 24 hours after insertion, plasma concentrations of levonorgestrel range from 0.4 to 0.5 ng/mL, high enough to prevent conception.

15. E p.766
The mechanism by which Norplant prevents conception is only partially explained. There are three probable modes of action, which are similar to those attributed to the contraceptive effect of the progestin-only minipills:

1. The levonorgestrel suppresses, at both the hypothalamus and the pituitary, the luteinizing hormone (LH) surge necessary for ovulation. As determined by progesterone levels in many users over several years, about one-third of all cycles are ovulatory.
2. The levonorgestrel has a marked effect on the cervical mucus. The mucus thickens and decreases in amount, forming a barrier to sperm penetration.
3. The constant level of levonorgestrel suppresses the estradiol-induced cyclic maturation of the endometrium and eventually causes atrophy. These changes could prevent implantation should fertilization occur; however, no evidence of fertilization can be detected in Norplant users.

16. B   p.766

Norplant is a safe, highly effective, continuous method of contraception that requires little user compliance or motivation and is rapidly reversible. Because this is a progestin-only method, it may be utilized by women who have contraindications for the use of estrogen-containing oral contraceptives. The sustained release of low doses of progestin avoids the high initial dose delivered by injectables and the daily hormone surge associated with oral contraceptives. Norplant is not a coitus-related contraceptive method. The use-effectiveness closely approximates the theoretical effectiveness. Norplant is an excellent choice for a breastfeeding woman (there is no effect on breastfeeding) and can be inserted immediately postpartum.

17. C   p.767

There are some disadvantages associated with the use of the Norplant system. Norplant frequently causes disruption of bleeding patterns in up to 80% of users, especially during the first year of use, and some women or their partners find these changes unacceptable. Endogenous estrogen is variably suppressed, and unlike the combined oral contraceptives, no exogenous estrogen is provided to maintain a stable endometrium. The absence of cyclic administration does not allow for regular withdrawal bleeding. Consequently, the relatively unstable endometrium sheds at unpredictable intervals. The implants must be inserted and removed in a surgical procedure performed by trained personnel. Women cannot initiate or discontinue the method without the assistance of a clinician. Because the insertion and removal of Norplant require a minor surgical procedure, initiation and discontinuation costs will be higher than with oral contraceptives or barrier methods. The implants can be visible under the skin. This sign of the use of contraception may be unacceptable for some women, and for some partners. Norplant is not known to provide protection against sexually transmitted diseases (STDs) such as herpes, human papillomavirus, human immunodeficiency virus (HIV), gonorrhea, or chlamydia. Users at risk for STDs must consider adding a barrier method to prevent infection.

18. C   p.767

Absolute Contraindications for Norplant Use
Norplant use is contraindicated in women who have:
1. Active thrombophlebitis or thromboembolic disease.
2. Undiagnosed genital bleeding.
3. Acute liver disease.
4. Benign or malignant liver tumors.
5. Known or suspected breast cancer.

19. E   p.770

In addition to the menstrual changes, the following side effects have been reported: headache, acne, weight change, mastalgia, hyperpigmentation over the implants, hirsutism, depression, mood changes, anxiety, nervousness, ovarian cyst formation, and galactorrhea. It is difficult, of course, to be certain which of these effects were actually caused by the levonorgestrel. Although these side effects are minor in nature, they can cause patients to discontinue the method. Patients often find common side effects tolerable after assurance that they do not represent a health hazard. Many complaints respond to reassurance; others can be treated with simple therapies. The most common side effect experienced by users is headache; about 20% of women who discontinue use do so because of headache.

20. C   p.771

The injection should be given within the first 5 days of the current menstrual cycle, otherwise a back-up method is necessary for 2 weeks. The effective contraceptive level is maintained for 4 months, providing a safety margin for reliable contraception. The efficacy of this method is equal to that of sterilization. The mechanism of action is the same as with all progestin-only methods, except the circulating level of the progestin is high enough to effectively block the LH surge, and therefore it is unlikely that any patient will ovulate with this method. Depo-Provera also affects the endometrium and cervical mucus, producing barriers to implantation and sperm penetration, as with Norplant. Suppression of FSH is not as intense as with the combination oral contraceptive, therefore follicular growth is maintained sufficiently to produce estrogen levels comparable to those in the early folllicular phase of a normal menstrual cycle. Symptoms of estrogen deficiency, such as vaginal atrophy or a decrease in breast size, do not occur.

21. A   p.771

Major problems with Depo-Provera are irregular menstrual bleeding, breast tenderness, weight gain, and depression.

The incidence of irregular bleeding is 30% in the first year, and 10% thereafter. After several injections, the majority of women become totally amenorrheic. If necessary, the bleeding can be treated with exogenous estrogen, 1.25 mg conjugated estrogens, or 2 mg estradiol, given daily for 7 days. Serious weight gain and depression (less than 5% incidence) are not relieved until the drug clears the body 6–8 months after the last injection.

22. B   p.772

The impact of Depo-Provera on the lipoprotein profile is uncertain. While some fail to detect an adverse impact, and claim that this is due to the avoidance of a first pass through effect in the liver, others have demonstrated a decrease in HDL-cholesterol and increases in total cholesterol and LDL-cholesterol. In a multicenter clinical trial by the World Health Organization, a transient adverse impact was present only in the few weeks after injection when blood levels were high. The clinical impact of these changes, if any, have yet to be reported. It seems prudent to monitor the lipid profile annually in women using Depo-Provera for long durations. The emergence of significant adverse changes in LDL-cholesterol and HDL-cholesterol warrant reconsideration of contraceptive choice. There are no clinically significant changes in carbohydrate metabolism or in coagulation factors.

There is some concern that the blood levels of estrogen with this method of contraception are relatively lower over a period of time compared to a normal menstrual cycle, and therefore patients can lose bone to some degree. Another possible mechanism is displacement of cortisol by the progestin from its binding globulin in the circulation, resulting in elevated levels of free cortisol. It is unlikely that this bone loss is sufficient to raise the risk of osteoporosis later in life. Furthermore, it is probable that any loss is regained with discontinuation of the method. This concern will require on-going surveillance, especially of past users, but at the present time, this should not be a reason to avoid this method of contraception.

23. C   p.772

The concern that infertility with suppressed menstrual function may be caused by Depo-Provera has not been supported by epidemiologic data. The pregnancy rate in women discontinuing the injections because of a desire to become pregnant is normal. The delay to conception is about 9 months after the last injection, and the delay does not increase with increasing duration of use. Suppressed menstrual function persisting beyond 12 months after the last injection is not due to the drug and deserves evaluation.

24. E   p.772,773

Like other sustained release forms of contraception, this method is not associated with compliance problems and is not related to the coital event. The freedom from the side effects of estrogen allows Depo-Provera to be considered for patients with congenital heart disease, sickle cell anemia, patients with a previous history of thromboembolism, and women over 30 who smoke or have other risk factors. The absolute safety in regard to thrombosis is mainly theoretical; it has not been proven in a controlled study. However, an increased rate of thrombosis has not been observed in epidemiologic evaluation of Depo-Provera users.

A further advantage in patients with sickle-cell disease is evidence indicating an inhibition of in vivo sickling with hematologic improvement during treatment. Depo-Provera is useful for cases where compliance is a problem, e.g., mentally retarded young women. Another advantage is the finding that Depo-Provera increases the quantity of milk in nursing mothers, a direct contrast to the effect seen with combination oral contraception. The concentration of the drug in the breast milk is very small, and no effects of the drug on infant growth and development have been observed. Depo-Provera should be considered in patients with seizure disorders; an improvement in seizure control can be achieved probably because of the sedative properties of progestins.

Other benefits associated with Depo-Provera use include a decreased risk of endometrial cancer and probably the same benefits associated with the progestin impact of oral contraceptives: reduced menstrual flow and anemia, less pelvic inflammatory disease, less endometriosis, and fewer ectopic pregnancies. A failure to document a reduced risk of ovarian cancer by the World Health Organization probably reflects the study's low statistical power and the high parity in the Depo-Provera users. A large case-control study could detect no increase in risk of invasive cervical cancer even after over 12 years since exposure. However, women at higher risk because of their sexual behavior (multiple partners, history of STDs) should have Pap smears every 6 months.

24 The Intrauterine Device (IUD)

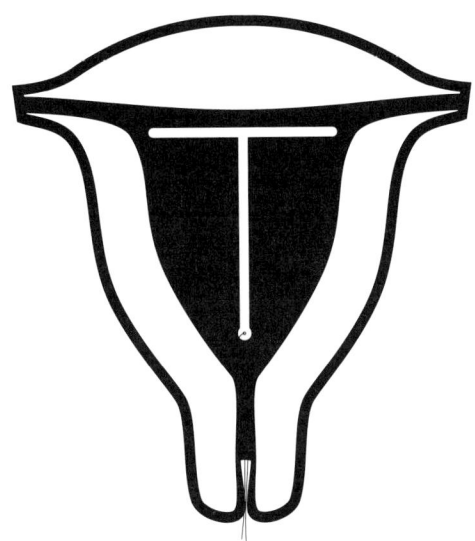

Learning Objectives

Be able to:

1. Describe the different broad categories of IUDs and their mechanisms of action.

2. Detail the efficacy of different types of IUDs.

3. Discuss who and who is not appropriate to have placement of an IUD.

4. Explain the management plan for finding a displaced IUD or an IUD in situ during pregnancy.

Pre-Test

A. Instructions: Fill in the blanks

1. By adding _____ to the IUD it can reduce cramping and blood loss.

2. The progesterone-releasing IUD must be replaced every _____ because the reservoir of progesterone is depleted in _____ months.

B. Instructions: True or False

3. IUDs do not provide protection against ectopic pregnancy.

4. Nonmedicated IUDs never have to be replaced.

C. Instructions: For each of the following questions choose:

A. if only 1, 2 and 3 are correct
B. if only 1 and 3 are correct
C. if only 2 and 4 are correct
D. if only 4 is correct
E. if all are correct

5. After the first year of use for all IUDs
   1. the failure rate is 9%
   2. the expulsion rate is 10%
   3. with increasing duration of use, the failure rate increases
   4. 15% are removed for bleeding and pain

6. The IUD is not recommended for women
   1. at increased risk of bacterial endocarditis
   2. who have prosthetic heart valves
   3. who have rheumatic heart disease
   4. who have mitral valve prolapse

Post-Test

A. Instructions: Fill in the blanks

1. The Dalkon Shield was introduced in _____.

2. A call for removal of all Dalkon Shields was in the early _____.

3. The metal _____ was added to IUDs and was noted to act upon the endometrium locally.

4. The Lippes-Loop is made of plastic (polyethylene) and impregnated with _____.

Chapter 24 The Intrauterine Device (IUD)

5. The more modern _____ IUDs contain more _____ and part of this is in the form of solid tubular sleeves, rather than wire, increasing efficacy and extending lifespan.

6. The only hormone-releasing device marketed in the U.S. since 1976 is the _____.

7. The symptoms most responsible for IUD discontinuation are increased _____ and increased _____.

8. IUDs should be removed immediately when an intrauterine pregnancy is diagnosed in order to avoid a _____ abortion.

9. High _____ placement is a key to minimizing IUD expulsion rates.

10. IUD perforations usually occur at the time of _____.

11. The IUD is a good reversible contraceptive choice for _____ women.

B. Instructions: True or False

12. The number of women using the IUD in the U.S. decreased by two-thirds from 1981 to 1988.

13. Worldwide, the IUD is the most popular method of reversible contraception.

14. The contraceptive action of all IUDs is mainly in the uterine cavity.

15. Progestin IUDs do not decrease menstrual blood loss and dysmenorrhea.

16. Following removal of IUDs, there is no delay in achieving pregnancy.

17. The levonorgestrel IUD that releases 20 µg levonorgestrel per day is less effective than the new copper IUDs.

18. Women use IUDs longer than other reversible methods of contraception.

19. IUDs increase the risk of ectopic pregnancy.

20. When an IUD user becomes pregnant, the pregnancy is more likely to be ectopic.

21. IUDs commonly cause intermenstrual bleeding and thus such bleeding does not require evaluation.

22. IUD-related infections are due to contamination of the endometrial cavity at the time of insertion.

23. Asymptomatic IUD users whose cervical cultures show gonorrheal or chlamydia infection should be treated with the recommended antibiotics without removal of the IUD.

24. If tubal infection is present, parenteral treatment with antibiotics is indicated without removal of the IUD.

25. Fertility returns promptly and pregnancies after removal of an IUD occur sooner than after oral contraception or those using the diaphragm.

26. All IUDs are radiopaque.

C. Instructions: For each of the following questions choose:

A. if only 1, 2 and 3 are correct
B. if only 1 and 3 are correct
C. if only 2 and 4 are correct
D. if only 4 is correct
E. if all are correct

27. IUDs may contain
    1. copper
    2. progestins
    3. no hormones or metals (nonmedicated)
    4. testosterone

29. IUDs
    1. if containing copper can enhance prostaglandin production and inhibit endometrial enzymes
    2. if made of copper can raise serum copper levels of those using it
    3. if containing progestin can result in decidualized endometrium with atrophic glands
    4. all have non-contraceptive benefits

29. Which of the following IUDs can not be left in place for 5 years or more due to the loss of their effectiveness
    1. TCu-380A
    2. Multiload-375
    3. Nova-T
    4. Progestasert

30. Failure rates with IUDs
    1. is less than with oral contraception
    2. is slightly higher in younger (less than age 25) more fertile women
    3. is approximately 3% after one year of experience
    4. are similar if made of copper or levonorgestrel

31. Ectopic pregnancy rates
    1. are lowest using the most effective IUDs
    2. are highest among progesterone-containing IUDs
    3. are among the lowest using levonorgestrel-containing IUD
    4. are higher among non-contraceptive users than among IUD users with the exception of the progesterone IUD

32. Side effects of IUDs include
    1. increased uterine bleeding
    2. increased uterine pain
    3. amenorrhea with the progestin-containing IUDs
    4. increased incidence of vaginitis

33. Pregnancy with an IUD in situ
    1. is accompanied by a spontaneous abortion rate of 50%
    2. requires that the IUD be removed immediately if the string is visible
    3. results in spontaneous abortion in 30% of cases after removal of an IUD with a visible string
    4. should initiate discussion regarding termination if the IUD can not be easily removed

34. IUDs are not recommended for women
    1. with uterine anomalies
    2. with allergies to copper
    3. with immunosuppression
    4. with diabetes

Answers for Chapter 24 — Pre-Test Questions

1. progesterone   p.780
The Progestasert was developed by the Alza Corporation at the same time that the copper IUDs were developed. This T-shaped device releases 65 mg progesterone per day for at least one year. The progesterone diminishes the amount of cramping and the amount of blood loss; thus, it is especially useful for women who have heavy periods and cramping. The short lifespan can be and has been solved by using a more potent progestin, such as levonorgestrel.

2. year; 12–18   p.783
The progesterone-releasing IUD must be replaced every year because the reservoir of progesterone is depleted in 12–18 months. The levonorgestrel IUD can be used for at least 7 years, and probably 10.

3. false   p.784
IUDs do not increase the risk of ectopic pregnancy, and they offer some protection. The largest study, a World Health Organization multicenter study, concluded that IUD users were 50% less likely to have an ectopic pregnancy when compared to women using no contraception.

4. true   p.783
The nonmedicated IUDs never have to be replaced. The deposition of calcium salts on the IUD can produce a structure that is irritating to the endometrium. If bleeding increases after a nonmedicated IUD has been in place for some time, it is worth replacing.

5. C   p.783
The actual use failure rate in the first year of use for all IUDs is approximately 3%, with a 10% expulsion rate and a 15% rate of removal, mainly for bleeding and pain. With increasing duration of use and increasing age, the failure rate decreases, as do removals for pain and bleeding.

In careful studies, with attention to technique and participation by motivated patients, the failure rate with the TCu-380A and the other newer copper IUDs is less than one per 100 women per year. The cumulative net pregnancy rate after 7 years of use is 1.5 per 100 woman-years. In developing countries, the failure rate with IUDs is less than that with oral contraception. Failure rates are slightly higher in younger (less than age 25), more fertile women.

6. A   p.785
The IUD is not recommended for women who are at increased risk of bacterial endocarditis (previous endocarditis, rheumatic heart disease, or the presence of prosthetic heart valves). ***Women with mitral valve prolapse can use an IUD, but antibiotic prophylaxis (amoxicillin 2 g) should be provided one hour before insertion.***

Answers for Chapter 24 — Post-Test Questions

1. 1970   p.778
The Dalkon Shield was introduced in 1970. Within 3 years, a high incidence of pelvic infection was recognized. There is no doubt that the problems with the Dalkon Shield were due to defective construction, pointed out as early as 1975

by Tatum. The multifilamented tail (hundreds of fibers enclosed in a sheath) of the Dalkon Shield provided a pathway for bacteria to ascend protected from the barrier of cervical mucus.

2. 1980s p.778

Although sales were discontinued in 1975, a call for removal of all Dalkon Shields was not issued until the early 1980s. The large number of women with pelvic infections led to many lawsuits against the pharmaceutical company, ultimately causing its bankruptcy. Unfortunately, the Dalkon Shield problem tainted all IUDs, and ever since, media and the public have inappropriately regarded all IUDs in a single, generic fashion.

3. copper p.780

The addition of copper to the IUD was suggested by Jaime Zipper of Chile, whose experiments with metals indicated that copper acted locally on the endometrium. Howard Tatum combined Zipper's suggestion with the development of the T-shape to diminish the uterine reaction to the structural frame, and produced the copper-T. The first copper IUD had copper wire wound around the straight shaft of the T, the TCu-200 (200 mm^2 of exposed copper wire), also known as the Tatum-T. Tatum's reasoning was that the T-shape would conform to the shape of the uterus in contrast to the other IUDs which required the uterus to conform to their shape. Furthermore, the copper IUDs could be much smaller than those of simple, inert plastic devices and still provide effective contraception. Recent studies indicate that copper exerts its effect before implantation of a fertilized ovum; it may be spermicidal, or it may diminish sperm motility or fertilizing capacity. The addition of copper to the IUD and reduction in the size and structure of the frame improved tolerance, resulting in fewer removals for pain and bleeding.

4. barium sulfate p.781

The Lippes Loop, made of plastic (polyethylene) impregnated with barium sulfate, is still used throughout the world (except in the U.S.). Flexible stainless steel rings are widely used in China, but not elsewhere.

5. copper; copper p.781

The first copper IUDs were wound with 200 to 250 mm^2 of wire, and two of these are still available (except in the U.S.), the TCu-200 and the Multiload-250. The more modern copper IUDs contain more copper, and part of the copper is in the form of solid tubular sleeves, rather than wire, increasing efficacy and extending lifespan. This group of IUDs is represented in the U.S. by the TCu-380A (the ParaGard), and in the rest of the world by the TCu-220C, the Nova T, and the Multiload-375.

6. Progestasert p.781

The only hormone-releasing device marketed in the U.S. (since 1976) is the Progestasert. The Progestasert is a T-shaped IUD made of ethylene/vinyl acetate copolymer containing titanium dioxide. The vertical stem contains a reservoir of 38 mg progesterone together with barium sulfate dispersed in silicone fluid. The horizontal arms are solid and made of the same copolymer. Two blue-black, monofilament strings are attached at a hole in the base of the stem. Progesterone is released at a rate of 65 mg per day.

7. bleeding; menstrual pain p.784

The symptoms most often responsible for IUD discontinuation are increased uterine bleeding and increased menstrual pain. Within one year, 5–15% of women discontinue IUD use because of these problems. Smaller copper and progestin IUDs have reduced the incidence of pain and bleeding considerably, but a careful menstrual history is still important in helping a woman consider an IUD.

8. septic p.786

Spontaneous abortion occurs more frequently among women who become pregnant with IUDs in place, a rate of approximately 50%. Because of this high rate of spontaneous abortion and the hazard of septic abortion, IUDs should always be removed if pregnancy is diagnosed and the string is visible.

9. fundal p.787

An IUD can be safely inserted at any time after delivery, abortion, or during the menstrual cycle. Expulsion rates were higher when the older, large plastic IUDs were inserted sooner than 8 weeks postpartum; however, studies indicate that the copper IUDs can be inserted between 4 and 8 weeks postpartum without an increase in pregnancy rates, expulsion, or removals for bleeding and/or pain. Postpartum insertions immediately after expulsion of the placenta or during the first postpartum week can be safely accomplished; however, an expulsion rate of 7–15 per 100 users can be expected in the first 6 months. Expulsion rates are lower after placement at cesarean section. High fundal placement is a key to minimizing expulsion rates. Insertion is easier and tolerance is better with the TCu-380A in breastfeeding women.

10. insertion p.788

Copper in the abdominal cavity can lead to adhesion formation, making laparoscopic removal difficult. Although inert perforated devices without closed loops were previously allowed to remain in the abdominal cavity, current practice is to remove any perforated IUD. Because IUD perforations usually occur at the time of insertion, it is important to check for correct position by identifying the string within a few weeks after insertion. Uterine perforation itself is unlikely to cause more than transient pain and bleeding, and can go undetected at the time of IUD insertion. If you believe perforation has occurred, prompt sonography is indicated so that the device can be removed before adhesion formation can occur.

11. older p.789

The IUD is a good reversible contraceptive choice for older women. An older woman is more likely to be mutually monogamous and less likely to develop PID, and for those women who have already had their children, concern with fertility and problems with cramping and bleeding are both lesser issues. If protection from STDs is not a concern, insertion of a copper IUD can provide very effective contraception until the menopause without the need to do anything other than check the string occasionally. On the other hand, because alterations of bleeding patterns become more common in this age group, it may be necessary to remove an IUD.

12. true p.779

The 1980s saw the decline of IUD use in the United States as manufacturers discontinued marketing in response to the burden of litigation. Despite the fact that most of the lawsuits against the copper devices were won by the manufacturer, the cost of the defense combined with declining use affected the financial return. It should be emphasized that this action was the result of corporate business decisions related to concerns for profit and liability, not for medical or scientific reasons. The number of women using the IUD in the U.S. decreased by two-thirds from 1981 to 1988, from 2.2 million to 0.7 million (7.1% to 2% of married couples).

13. true p.780

Worldwide, the IUD is the most popular method of reversible contraception. Ironically, the IUD declined in the country that developed the modern IUD.

14. true p.782

The contraceptive action of all IUDs is mainly in the uterine cavity. Ovulation is not affected, nor is the IUD an abortifacient. It is currently believed that the major mechanism of action for IUDs is the production of an intrauterine environment that is spermicidal. The protection provided by IUDs against ectopic pregnancy (see below) argues that there exists an extrauterine action as well, perhaps a cytotoxic effect on ova or a disruption of tubal function.

15. false p.782

With the exception of the progestin-releasing IUDs, no major noncontraceptive benefits are associated with IUD use. The progestin IUDs decrease menstrual blood loss (about 40–50%) and dysmenorrhea. Average hemoglobin and iron levels increase over time compared to preinsertion values.

16. true p.782

Following removal of IUDs, the normal intrauterine environment is rapidly restored. In large studies, there is no delay in achieving pregnancy, which belies the assertion that IUD use is associated with infection leading to infertility.

17. false p.783

The progesterone IUD has a slightly higher failure rate, but the levonorgestrel device that releases 20 mg levonorgestrel per day is as effective as the new copper IUDs.

18. true p.783

Women use IUDs longer than other reversible methods of contraception. The IUD continuation rate is higher than that with oral contraception, condoms, or diaphragms. This may reflect the circumstances surrounding the choice of an IUD (older, parous women).

19. false p.784

Ectopic Pregnancy Rates per 1,000 Woman-Years

All U.S. women	1.50
Non-contraceptive users	3.00
Copper T-380A IUD	0.20
Copper T-200 IUD	0.60
Progesterone IUD	6.80
Levonorgestrel IUD	0.20

20. true p.784

Protection against ectopic pregnancy is not as great as that achieved by inhibition of ovulation with oral contraception. Therefore, when an IUD user becomes pregnant, the pregnancy is more likely to be ectopic. About 3–4% of IUD pregnancies have been ectopic, making the actual occurrence a rare event.

21. false p.784

IUDs rarely cause intermenstrual bleeding, and such bleeding deserves the usual evaluation for cervical or endometrial pathology.

22. true p.785

IUD-related infection is now believed to be due to contamination of the endometrial cavity at the time of insertion. Infections that occur 3–4 months after insertion are believed to be due to acquired STDs, not the direct result of the IUD. The early, insertion-related infections, therefore, are polymicrobial, derived from the endogenous cervicovaginal flora, with a predominance of anaerobes.

23. true p.785

Asymptomatic IUD users whose cervical cultures show gonorrheal or chlamydia infection should be treated with the recommended drugs without removal of the IUD. If, however, there is evidence that an infection has ascended to the endometrium or fallopian tubes, treatment must be instituted and the IUD removed promptly. Bacterial vaginosis should be treated (metronidazole, 500 mg bid for 7 days), but the IUD need not be removed unless pelvic inflammation is present.

24. false p.786

For simple endometritis, in which uterine tenderness is the only physical finding, doxycycline (100 mg bid for 14 days) is adequate. If tubal infection is present, as evidenced by cervical motion tenderness, abdominal rebound tenderness, adnexal tenderness or masses, or elevated white blood count and sedimentation rate, parenteral treatment is indicated with removal of the IUD as soon as antibiotic serum levels are adequate. The previous presence of an IUD does not alter the treatment of PID.

25. false p.788

Fertility returns promptly and pregnancies after removal of an IUD occur sooner than after oral contraception, but later than after using the diaphragm. Pregnancy outcomes are within normal limits, and duration of use does not affect the return of fertility. If a patient wishes to continue use of an IUD, a new device can be placed immediately after removal of the old one. In this case, antibiotic prophylaxis is advised.

26. true p.788

When an IUD cannot be found, one has to consider, besides expulsion, perforation of the uterus into the abdominal cavity (a very rare event) or embedment into the myometrium. All IUDs are radiopaque, but localizing them radiographically requires 2–3 views, is time-consuming and expensive, and does not allow intrauterine direction of instruments. A quick, real-time sonographic scan in the office is the best method to locate a lost IUD, whether or not removal is desired.

27. A p.781

There are 3 basic types of IUDs. IUDs are either unmedicated (plastic or steel), wound with copper, or they release a progestin from a reservoir.

28. B p.782

The copper IUD releases free copper and copper salts which have both a biochemical and morphological impact on the endometrium. There is no measurable increase in the serum copper level. Copper has many specific actions, including the enhancement of prostaglandin production and the inhibition of various endometrial enzymes. Perhaps the overall inflammatory response is intensified.

The progestin-releasing IUDs add the endometrial action of the progestin to the foreign body reaction. The endometrium becomes decidualized with atrophy of the glands. The progesterone IUD probably has two mechanisms of action: inhibition of implantation and inhibition of sperm capacitation and survival. The levonorgestrel IUD also partially inhibits ovarian follicular development and ovulation. Finally, the progestin IUDs thicken the cervical mucus, creating a barrier to sperm penetration.

With the exception of the progestin-releasing IUDs, no major noncontraceptive benefits are associated with IUD use. The progestin IUDs decrease menstrual blood loss (about 40–50%) and dysmenorrhea. Average hemoglobin and iron levels increase over time compared to preinsertion values.

29. D p.783

The TCu-380A is approved for use in the United States for 10 years. The Multiload-375 should also be effective for 10 years. The progesterone-releasing IUD must be replaced every year because the reservoir of progesterone is depleted in 12–18 months. The levonorgestrel IUD can be used for at least 7 years, and probably 10. The Multiload-375 should also be effective for 10 years.

30. E p.783

In careful studies, with attention to technique and participation by motivated patients, the failure rate with the TCu-380A and the other newer copper IUDs is less than one per 100 women per year. The cumulative net pregnancy rate after 7 years of use is 1.5 per 100 woman-years. In developing countries, the failure rate with IUDs is less than that with oral contraception. Failure rates are slightly higher in younger (less than age 25), more fertile women.

31. E p.784

The lowest ectopic pregnancy rates are seen with the most effective IUDs, the newer copper devices (90% less likely compared to noncontraceptors). The rate is about one-tenth the ectopic pregnancy rate associated with the Lippes Loop or TCu-200. The progesterone-releasing IUD has a higher rate that, in fact, is about 50–80% greater than noncontraceptors. Very few ectopic pregnancies have been reported with the levonorgestrel IUD, presumably because it is associated with a partial suppression of gonadotropins with subsequent disruption of normal follicular growth and development and, in a significant number of cycles (20–30%), inhibition of ovulation.

The protection against ectopic pregnancy provided by the TCu-380A and the levonorgestrel IUD makes these IUDs acceptable choices for contraception in women with previous ectopic pregnancies.

32. A								p.784

The symptoms most often responsible for IUD discontinuation are increased uterine bleeding and increased menstrual pain. Because of a decidualizing, atrophic impact on the endometrium, amenorrhea can develop over time with the progestin-containing IUDs. For some women, the lack of periods is so disconcerting that they request removal. Sufficient progestin reaches the systemic circulation from the levonorgestrel-containing IUD so that androgenic side effects can occur such as acne and hirsutism. More extensive clinical studies are needed to assess the impact of this IUD on the lipoprotein profile; however, it is unlikely that the low dose of levonorgestrel has an important effect on cardiovascular risk.

Some women report an increased vaginal discharge while wearing an IUD. This complaint deserves examination for the presence of vaginal or cervical infection. Treatment can be provided with the IUD remaining in place.

33. E								p.786

Spontaneous abortion occurs more frequently among women who become pregnant with IUDs in place, a rate of approximately 50%. Because of this high rate of spontaneous abortion and the hazard of septic abortion, IUDs should always be removed if pregnancy is diagnosed and the string is visible. Use of instruments inside the uterus should be avoided if the pregnancy is desired, unless sonographic guidance can help avoid rupture of the membranes. After removal of an IUD with visible strings, the spontaneous abortion rate is approximately 30%. Combining ultrasonography guidance with carbon dioxide hysteroscopy, an IUD with a missing tail can be identified and removed during early pregnancy. If the IUD cannot be easily removed, the patient should be offered therapeutic abortion because the risk of life-threatening septic, spontaneous abortion in the second trimester is increased 20-fold if the pregnancy continues with the IUD in utero. Even if a patient plans to terminate a pregnancy that has occurred with an IUD in place, the IUD should be removed immediately rather than waiting until the time of the abortion, because septic abortion could ensue in the interval. If there is no evidence of infection, the IUD can safely be removed in a clinic or office.

34. A								p.787

Patient selection for successful IUD use requires attention to menstrual history and the risk for STDs. Age and parity are not the critical factors in selection; the risk factors for STDs are the most important consideration. In addition, there are other conditions that can compromise success. Women who have abnormalities of uterine anatomy (bicornuate uterus, submucous myoma, cervical stenosis) may not accommodate an IUD. The few individuals who have allergies to copper or have Wilson's disease (a prevalence of about 1 in 200,000) should not use copper IUDs. Immunosuppressed patients and patients at risk for endocarditis should not use IUDs. The IUD can be used by women with mitral valve prolapse, but prophylactic antibiotics are recommended at the time of insertion if mitral regurgitation is present. The IUD is a good choice for women with diabetes mellitus.

Preferably, the absence of cervical infection should be established before insertion. If this is not feasible, insertion should definitely be delayed if a mucopurulent discharge is present.

A careful speculum and bimanual examination is essential prior to IUD insertion. It is important to know the position of the uterus; undetected extreme posterior uterine position is the most common reason for perforation at the time of IUD insertion. A very small or large uterus, determined by examination and sounding, can preclude insertion. For successful IUD use, the uterus should not sound less than 6 cm or more than 10 cm.

25 Barrier Methods of Contraception

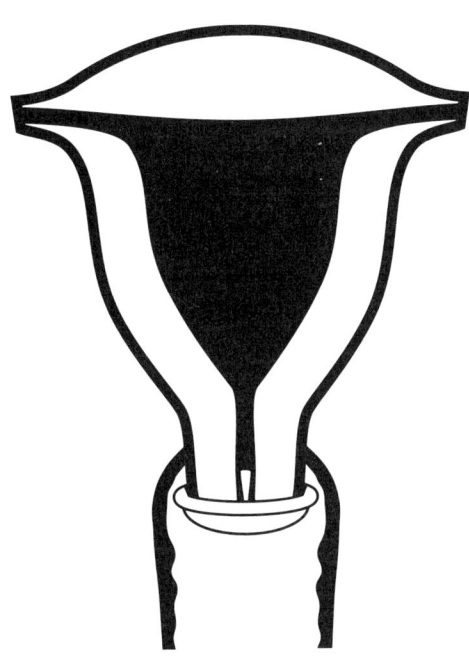

Learning Objectives

Be able to:

1. Describe the various barrier methods of contraception including their failure rates after one year of use as well as their various advantages and disadvantages.

2. Detail the noncontraceptive benefits of the various barrier methods.

Clinical Gynecologic Endocrinology and Infertility: Self Assessment and Study Guide

Pre-Test

A. Instructions: Fill in the blanks

1. _____ are approximately twice as common among diaphragm users as among women using oral contraception.

2. An infected man transmits gonorrhea to a susceptible woman about _____ of the time; while an infected woman transmits to a man about _____ of the time.

B. Instructions: True or False

3. The failure rate during the first year of use in the United States for the condom alone is less than that for the sponge, cervical cap or diaphragm and spermicides.

4. The efficacy of spermicides seems to depend more on the population studied than the agent used.

C. Instructions: For the following question choose:

A. if only 1, 2 and 3 are correct
B. if only 1 and 3 are correct
C. if only 2 and 4 are correct
D. if only 4 is correct
E. if all are correct

5. The diaphragm
   1. is discontinued in less than 1% of users due to vaginal irritation
   2. is associated with a greater frequency of UTIs than are oral contraceptives
   3. should be removed within 24 hours of use to minimize the risk of toxic shock
   4. reduces the incidence of cervical gonorrhea, pelvic inflammatory disease and tubal infertility

Post-Test

A. Instructions: Fill in the blanks

1. Barrier and spermicide methods provide protection and about a _____% reduction against sexually transmitted diseases and pelvic inflammatory disease.

2. Women who have never used barrier methods of contraception are almost _____ as likely to develop cancer of the cervix.

3. Patients who had _____ _____ syndrome are advised to avoid barrier methods.

4. Most women use diaphragm sizes between _____ and _____ mm.

5. The vaginal contraceptive sponge is a sustained release system for the spermicide, _____.

346

6. The chance of HIV infection after a single sexual exposure ranges from one in 1,000 to one in _____.

7. Condom failure is more likely due to _____ use than defective products.

B. Instructions: True or False

8. Many women find it difficult to place the posterior edge of flat diaphragms into the posterior cul-de-sac and over the cervix.

9. Additional spermicide should be placed in the vagina after initial placement of diaphragm with spermicide before each additional episode of sexual intercourse while the diaphragm stays in place.

10. The cervical cap is not approved by the FDA.

11. The diaphragm and cervical cap must be in place a minimum of 4 hours following coitus.

12. Spermicides require application 5 minutes prior to intercourse.

13. Postcoital douching may be an effective contraceptive if done using nonoxynol-9.

14. There is an increased incidence of congenital abnormalities and spontaneous abortions among users of spermicides than in the general population using no contraceptives.

15. Spermicides are absorbed through the vaginal mucosa in concentrations high enough to have systemic effects.

C. Instructions: For each of the following questions choose:

A. if only 1, 2 and 3 are correct
B. if only 1 and 3 are correct
C. if only 2 and 4 are correct
D. if only 4 is correct
E. if all are correct

16. The diaphragm fitting should be reassessed
    1. if weight loss occurs
    2. following a vaginal delivery
    3. if weight gain occurs
    4. following a C-section

17. The cervical cap has several advantages over the diaphragm
    1. it can be left in place for a longer time
    2. it can be more early fitted in 90% of women
    3. it does not require use with a spermicide
    4. it is associated with less foul-smelling discharge

18. The contraceptive sponge
    1. is a good choice of contraception for the parous females
    2. must be thoroughly moistened with water to activate the spermicide
    3. is associated with an increase incidence of toxic shock syndrome
    4. provides continuous protection for 24 hours regardless of frequency of coitus

19. Spermicides currently use
    1. octoxynol-9
    2. nonoxynol-9
    3. menfegol
    4. quinine sulfite

20. Spermicides
    1. are effective against STDs
    2. are effective against HIV
    3. are most effective against STDs when combined with condoms
    4. are effective against trichomoniasis

21. Condoms
    1. are made of latex and Lamb's intestine
    2. made of latex are thicker than the diameter of sperm
    3. made of latex are more protective of HIV than condoms made of Lamb's intestine
    4. probably do not protect against HPV

22. Proper wearing of a condom includes
    1. prior to unrolling the condom to the base of the penis, air should be squeezed out of the tip
    2. the tip of the condom should extend beyond the end of the penis
    3. the avoidance of oil based lubricants
    4. holding the condom at the base while the erect penis is withdrawn

---

Answers for Chapter 25 — Pre-Test Questions

1. Urinary tract infections p.797
Urinary tract infections are approximately twice as common among diaphragm users as among women using oral contraception. Possibly the rim of the diaphragm presses against the urethra and causes irritation which is perceived as infectious in origin, or true infection may result from touching the perineal area or incomplete emptying of the bladder. Studies also indicate that spermicide use can increase the risk of bacteriuria with *E coli*, perhaps due to an alteration in the normal vaginal flora. Clinical experience suggests that voiding after sexual intercourse is helpful, and if necessary, a single postcoital dose of a prophylactic antibiotic can be recommended.

2. 2/3; 1/3 p.803
Condom breakage is a greater problem for couples at risk for STDs. An infected man transmits gonorrhea to a susceptible woman about two-thirds of the time. If the woman is infected, transmission to the man occurs one-third of the time.

3. true p.797
(See table on page 349 in this Study Guide)

4. true p.801
Only periodic abstinence demonstrates as wide a range of efficacy in different studies as do the studies of spermicides. Efficacy seems to depend more on the population studied than the agent used. Efficacy ranges from less than 1% to nearly one-third in the first year of use. Failure rates of approximately 20% during a year's use are most typical. There are no comparative studies to indicate which preparations, if any, are better or worse.

5. E p.797,798,799
The diaphragm is a safe method of contraception that rarely causes even minor side effects. Occasionally women report vaginal irritation due to the latex rubber or the spermicidal jelly or cream used with the diaphragm. Less than 1%

Failure Rates During the First Year of Use, United States

Method	Percent of Women with Pregnancy	
	Lowest Expected	Typical
No method	85.0%	85.0%
Diaphragm and spermicides	6.0	18.0
Cervical cap	6.0	18.0
Sponge		
Parous women	9.0	28.0
Nulliparous women	6.0	18.0
Spermicides	3.0	21.0
Condom	2.0	12.0

discontinue diaphragm use for these reasons. Urinary tract infections are approximately twice as common among diaphragm users as among women using oral contraception. Diaphragm use reduces the incidence of cervical gonorrhea, pelvic inflammatory disease, and tubal infertility. This protection may be due in part to the simultaneous use of a spermicide. There are no data, as of yet, regarding the effect of diaphragm use on the transmission of the AIDS virus (HIV). An important advantage of the diaphragm is low cost. Diaphragms are durable and, with proper care, can last for several years.

Answers for Chapter 25 — Post-Test Questions

1. 50   p.796
Barrier and spermicide methods provide protection (about a 50% reduction) against sexually transmitted diseases and pelvic inflammatory disease. This includes chlamydia, gonorrhea, herpes simplex, cytomegalovirus, human papillomavirus, and human immunodeficiency virus (HIV). This protection has a beneficial impact on the risk of tubal infertility and ectopic pregnancy.

2. twice   p.796
Women who have never used barrier methods of contraception are almost twice as likely to develop cancer of the cervix.

3. toxic shock   p.796
The risk of toxic shock syndrome is increased with barrier methods, but the actual incidence is so rare that this is not a significant clinical consideration. Patients who have had toxic shock syndrome, however, should be advised to avoid barrier methods.

4. 65; 80   p.798
There are three types of diaphragms, and most manufacturers produce them in sizes ranging from 50 to 105 mm diameter, in increments of 2.5 to 5 mm. Most women use sizes between 65 and 80 mm.

5. nonoxynol-9   p.800
The vaginal contraceptive sponge is a sustained release system for the spermicide, Nonoxynol-9. The sponge also absorbs semen and blocks the entrance to the cervical canal. The "Today" sponge is a dimpled polyurethaned disc impregnated with one g of Nonoxynol-9. About 20% of the Nonoxynol-9 is released over the 24 hours the sponge is left in the vagina.

6. 10   p.803
The chance of HIV infection after a single sexual exposure ranges from one in 1,000 to one in 10.

7. non- or incorrect   p.803
Inconsistent use explains most condom failures. Incorrect use accounts for additional failures, and also, condoms sometimes break. Breakage rates range from 1–12 per 100 episodes of vaginal intercourse (and somewhat higher for anal intercourse). In a U.S. survey, one pregnancy resulted for every 3 condom breakages. Concomitant use of spermicides lowers failure rates in case of breakage.

8. true   p.799
The diaphragm made with a *flat metal spring* or a *coil spring* remains in a straight line when pinched at the edges. This type is suitable for women with good vaginal muscle tone and an adequate recess behind the pubic arch. However, many women find it difficult to place the posterior edge of these flat diaphragms into the posterior cul-de-sac and over the cervix.

9. true   p.799
About a teaspoonful of spermicidal cream or jelly, designated for use in conjunction with a diaphragm, should be placed in the dome of the diaphragm prior to insertion. Some of the spermicide should be spread around the rim with a finger. The diaphragm should be left in place for approximately 6 hours (but no more than 24 hours) after coitus. Additional spermicide (an applicatorful) should be placed in the vagina before each additional episode of sexual intercourse while the diaphragm is in place.

10. false   p.799
The cervical cap was popular in Europe long before its recent reintroduction into the United States. There are several types of cervical caps, but only the cavity rim (Prentif) cap is approved in the U.S. U.S. trials have demonstrated the cervical cap to be about as effective as the diaphragm but somewhat harder to fit (it comes in only four sizes) and more difficult to insert (it must be placed precisely over the cervix).

11. false   p.799
The diaphragm should be inserted no longer than 6 hours prior to sexual intercourse. The cap should be inserted at least 20 minutes and not more than 4 hours before intercourse. The diaphragm should be left in place for approximately 6 hours (but no more than 24 hours) after coitus.

12. false   p.801
Spermicides require application 10–30 minutes prior to sexual intercourse. Jellies, creams, and foams remain effective for as long as 8 hours, but tablets and suppositories are good for less than one hour. If ejaculation does not occur within the period of effectiveness, the spermicide should be reapplied. Reapplication should definitely take place for each coital episode.

13. false   p.801
Vaginal douches are ineffective contraceptives even if they contain spermicidal agents. Postcoital douching is too late to prevent the rapid ascent of sperm (within seconds) to the fallopian tubes.

14. false   p.801
No serious side effects or safety problems have arisen in all the years that spermicides have been used. The only serious question raised is that of a possible association between spermicide use and congenital abnormalities or spontaneous abortions. Epidemiologic analysis, including a meta-analysis, concludes that there is insufficient evidence to support these associations.

15. false   p.801
Spermicides are not absorbed through the vaginal mucosa in concentrations high enough to have systemic effects.

16. A   p.799
Weight loss, weight gain, vaginal delivery, and even sexual intercourse can change vaginal caliber. The fit of a

diaphragm should be assessed every year at the time of the regular examination.

17. B p.799

The cervical cap has several advantages over the diaphragm. It can be left in place for a longer time (up to 36 hours), and it need not be used with a spermicide. However, spermicide filling one-third of the dome before application is reported to prolong wearing time by decreasing the incidence of foul-smelling discharge (a common complaint after 24 hours). The cap should be inserted at least 20 minutes and not more than 4 hours before intercourse.

18. C p.800

The sponge must be thoroughly moistened with water to activate the spermicide. The sponge can be inserted immediately before sexual intercourse or up to 14 hours beforehand. There should always be a lapse of at least 6 hours after sexual intercourse before removal, even if the sponge has been in place for 24 hours before intercourse (maximal wear time, therefore, is 30 hours).

Obviously, the sponge is not a good choice for women with anatomical changes that make proper insertion and placement difficult. In most studies, the effectiveness of the sponge exceeds that of foam, jellies, and tablets, but it is lower than that associated with diaphragm or condom use. Some studies indicated higher failure rates (twice as high) in parous women, suggesting that one size may not fit all users.

Discontinuation rates are generally higher among sponge users, compared to diaphragm and spermicide use. For some women, however, the sponge is preferred because it provides continuous protection for 24 hours regardless of the frequency of coitus. In addition, it is easier to use and less messy.

Side effects associated with the sponge include allergic reactions in about 4% of users. Another 8% complain of vaginal dryness, soreness, or itching. There is no risk of toxic shock syndrome, and, in fact, the Nonoxynol-9 retards staphylococcal replication and toxin production.

19. A p.800

Various chemicals and a wide array of vehicles have been used vaginally as contraceptives for centuries. The first commercially available spermicidal pessaries were made in England in 1885 of cocoa butter and quinine sulfite. These or similar materials were used until the 1920s when effervescent tablets that released carbon dioxide and phenyl mercuric acetate were marketed. Modern spermicides, introduced in the 1950s, contain surface active agents that damage the sperm cell membranes (this same action occurs with bacteria and viruses, explaining the protection against STDs). The agents currently used are Nonoxynol-9, Octoxynol-9, and Menfegol. Most preparations contain 60–100 mg of these agents in each vaginal application.

20. A p.801

Spermicides provide protection against sexually transmitted diseases. In vitro studies have demonstrated that contraceptive spermicides kill or inactivate most STD pathogens, including HIV. However, there is no evidence as of yet that spermicides can prevent HIV infection. Clinical studies indicate reductions in the risk of gonorrhea, pelvic infections, and chlamydial infection. There is little difference in the incidence of trichomoniasis, candidiasis, or bacterial vaginosis among spermicide users. Spermicidal agents used in combination with condoms confer added protection against STDs.

21. A p.802

Two types of condoms are available. Most are made of latex. "Natural skin" (lamb's intestine) condoms are still obtainable (about 1% of sales). Latex condoms are 0.3–0.8 mm thick. Sperm which are 0.003 mm in diameter cannot penetrate condoms. The organisms that cause STDs and AIDS also do not penetrate latex condoms, but they can penetrate condoms made from intestine. Condom use (latex) also probably prevents transmission of human papillomavirus (HPV), the cause of condylomata acuminata. Because spermicides also provide significant protection against STDs, condoms and spermicides used together offer more protection than either method used alone.

22. E p.802

Prospective users need instructions if they are to avoid pregnancy and STDs. A condom must be placed on the penis before it touches a partner. Uncircumcised men must pull the foreskin back. Prior to unrolling the condom to the base of the penis, air should be squeezed out of the reservoir tip with a thumb and forefinger. The tip of the condom should extend beyond the end of the penis to provide a reservoir to collect the ejaculate (a half-inch of pinched tip). If lubricants are used, they must be water based. Oil based lubricants (such as Vaseline) will weaken the latex. Couples should understand that any vaginal medication can compromise condom integrity. After intercourse, the condom should be held at the base as the still erect penis is withdrawn. Semen must not be allowed to spill or leak. The condom should be handled gently as fingernails and rings can penetrate the latex and cause leakage. If there is evidence of spill or leakage, a spermicidal agent should be quickly inserted into the vagina.

26 Female Infertility

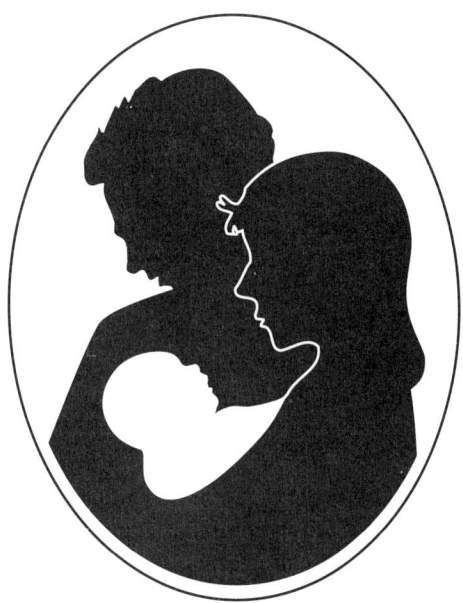

Learning Objectives

Be able to:

1. Describe the difference between fecundability and fecundity.

2. Understand the association of the changing demographics within the U.S. and its potential effect on women's fertility.

3. Discuss declining fecundity as a function of age and the importance of the oocyte versus a uterine factor.

4. Understand the limitations of the postcoital test.

5. Explain when prophylaxis for an HSG is indicated and when an HSG may be contraindicated.

6. Describe the use of hysteroscopy, outpatient canalization of the fallopian tube and laparoscopy in the infertility workup.

7. Discuss the disorders of ovulation associated with infertility and their potential treatment.

8. Discuss the prognosis for a couple with unexplained infertility with and without treatment.

Clinical Gynecologic Endocrinology and Infertility: Self Assessment and Study Guide

Pre-Test

A. Instructions: Fill in the blanks

1. A luteal phase defect can be found in up to _____% of isolated cycles of normal women.

2. Approximately _____% of couples with unexplained infertility of less than 3 years duration will become pregnant with 3 years of expectant management.

B. Instructions: True or False

3. Fecundity is the probability of achieving a pregnancy within one menstrual cycle.

4. 35% of couples who are never treated for infertility can expect to become pregnant.

C. Instructions: For each of the following questions choose:

A. if only 1, 2 and 3 are correct
B. if only 1 and 3 are correct
C. if only 2 and 4 are correct
D. if only 4 is correct
E. if all are correct

5. Declining male fertility with age is supported by
   1. the association of paternal age and an increase in the rate of nondisjunction
   2. well-designed cross-over studies involving old sperm inseminated into young recipients
   3. the association of new autosomal disease and an increase in the frequency of male gene mutations
   4. longitudinal data examining semen analysis as a function of age

6. The postcoital test suffers from
   1. poor validity
   2. a lack of standard methodology
   3. confusion over the definition of normality
   4. a lack of real clinical utility in a patient who is going to have superovulation combined with IUI

Post-Test

A. Instructions: Fill in the blanks

1. Infertility is defined as _____ year(s) of unprotected coitus without conception. It affects approximately _____% of couples in the reproductive age group.

2. The fecundability of a normal couple is about _____%.

3. The menstrual periods for 10–15 years before the menopause are regular, but there is a steady _____ in cycle length due to the _____ follicular phase.

4. About _____% of couples presenting after one year of infertility can be expected to become pregnant spontaneously in the following year.

5. Shaking movement of sperm in a postcoital test is a common finding in _____ infertility.

6. The appropriate therapy for a poor postcoital test is _____ without the need for ancillary superovulation.

7. Westrom's classic studies with laparoscopically confirmed pelvic inflammatory disease indicated that the incidence of subsequent tubal infertility is approximately ___% after one episode of pelvic infection, ___% after two episodes and _____% after three episodes.

8. The risk of ectopic pregnancy is increased _____ fold after pelvic infection.

9. Disorders of ovulation account for approximately _____% of all infertility problems in couples.

B. Instructions: True or False

10. After World War II, the U.S. total fertility rate reached a modern high of 3.8 births per woman.

11. The majority of early abortions after age 35 are due to autosomal trisomies.

12. Experience with donor oocyte programs argues, that the age-related decline in fecundity is primarily due to aging oocytes.

13. Despite the absence of pathology, as in unexplained infertility, couples with 3 years or more of infertility have a poor prognosis.

14. Exactly what constitutes a poor postcoital test in terms of sperm numbers is controversial.

15. Almost 50% of patients who are eventually found to have tubal damage and/or pelvic adhesions have no history of antecedent disease.

16. If there is a documented history of pelvic inflammatory disease the risk of a serious reinfection following HSG is too high, and it should be replaced by laparoscopy.

17. If anovulation is the only infertility factor, most couples will become pregnant within 2 months.

18. It is estimated that sperm retain the ability to fertilize 12 to 24 hours while the egg is fertilizable for 24 to 48 hours.

19. Culturing women for ureaplasma is not worthwhile in cases of unexplained infertility.

C. Instructions: For each of the following questions choose:

A. if only 1, 2 and 3 are correct
B. if only 1 and 3 are correct
C. if only 2 and 4 are correct
D. if only 4 is correct
E. if all are correct

20. Dramatic changes have taken place in infertility practice during the last 2 decades which include
    1. an increase in the proportion of couples considered infertile
    2. an increase in the number of infertile couples
    3. a decrease in public awareness regarding advanced assisted reproductive technologies
    4. an increase in the proportion of women over 35 seeking medical attention for infertility

21. The demographic change brought on by the post-war baby boom has had specific impacts on women which include
    1. a need for effective contraception
    2. the problem of achieving pregnancy later in life
    3. the problem of being pregnant later in life
    4. the need for effective counseling regarding the issues of menopause

22. Studies supporting the concept of declining fertility with age include data collected from
    1. the Hutterites
    2. donor insemination programs
    3. assisted reproductive technologies
    4. the Hite report

23. Evidence for the decline in fecundity with aging being primarily an oocyte factor as opposed to an uterine factor is supported by
    1. pregnancy rates from donor oocyte programs
    2. increased SAB rates among older women
    3. increased chromosomal anomalies associated with older women
    4. pregnancy rates from IVF-ET programs

24. Etiology of infertility is
    1. approximately 40% anovulatory
    2. approximately 40% due to tubal damage
    3. approximately 10% due to thyroid disease or anatomic abnormalities
    4. 40% due to endometriosis

25. Risk factors for the possibility of tubal damage includes a history of
    1. septic abortion
    2. ruptured appendix
    3. ectopic pregnancy
    4. tubal surgery

26. Outpatient tubal cannulation or balloon tuboplasty
    1. is usually of a similar level of discomfort as an HSG
    2. is successful in achieving patency in at least one tube in 80–90% of attempts
    3. is associated with a 30% pregnancy rate within 3–6 months following the procedure
    4. is more often performed at hysteroscopy than at fluoroscopy

27. Women at risk for a luteal phase defect include those
    1. with a history of recurrent spontaneous abortion
    2. taking clomiphene citrate for ovulation induction
    3. with short luteal phases demonstrated on BBT charts
    4. taking Pergonal for ovulation induction

28. Treatment of luteal phase defect includes
    1. clomiphene citrate
    2. Pergonal
    3. progesterone
    4. a dopamine antagonist in patients with hyperprolactinemia

29. Side effects of clomiphene include
    1. severe mood changes
    2. visual changes
    3. hot flushes
    4. risk of multiple births

30. Couples with unexplained infertility
    1. have an increase in monthly fecundity with clomiphene
    2. have an increase monthly fecundity rate of 10–15% with human menopausal gonadotropins
    3. should be offered superovulation or ART
    4. should be offered treatment with dopamine agonists

Answers for Chapter 26 — Pre-Test Questions

1. 30   p.827
A luteal phase defect, defined as a lag of more than two days in histologic development of the endometrium compared to day of the cycle (presumably due to inadequate progesterone secretion or action), can be found in up to 30% of isolated cycles of normal women, and only if the defect is found in 2 cycles is it thought to be a possible factor in infertility. Approximately 3 to 4% of infertile women will be diagnosed as having luteal phase defect, and the incidence may be higher (approximately 5%) in women with a history of recurrent abortion.

2. 60   p.831
The average monthly fecundity in normal couples is 25%; the monthly pregnancy rate in couples with unexplained infertility is 1.5–3%. After 3 years of infertility, the prospect of pregnancy decreases by 24% each year. Approximately 60% of couples with unexplained infertility of less than 3 years duration will become pregnant with 3 years of *expectant management*. Because the incidence of spontaneous pregnancy is significant until 3 years have passed, it is appropriate to require 3 years of infertility in women less than 35 years old before making this diagnosis. Further evaluation and therapy should not be deferred in older women.

3. false   p.809
Fecundability is the probability of *achieving a pregnancy* within one menstrual cycle (about 25% in normal couples); ***fecundity*** is the ability to *achieve a live birth* within one menstrual cycle.

4. true   p.814
There is an incidence of spontaneous pregnancy among infertile couples. In a life-table analysis of 58 untreated apparently normal infertile couples, 74% were pregnant by two years; however, normal couples achieve this rate in 9 months. Overall, approximately 40% of couples become pregnant after discontinuation of treatment, and 35% of couples never treated can expect to become pregnant.

5. B
p.812

The changes in the male with aging are modest, but significant. There are at least two reasons to believe that the quality of sperm decreases with aging. New autosomal disease can be attributed to an increase in the frequency of male gene mutations, and paternal age is related to the risk of trisomies, indicating an increase in nondisjunction in the male. It is possible, however, that the decrease in sperm in older men is not correlated with fecundability. To perform the appropriate study is probably impossible; the arrangements are forbidding (such as old sperm into young recipients).

6. E
p.820

The place of the postcoital test in the infertility investigation has recently been called into question. There has always been an undercurrent of discontent concerning standardization of the test, its interpretation, and most importantly, its prognostic significance. Griffith and Grimes reviewed the literature pertaining to the postcoital test and concluded that the sensitivity (the ability of the test to detect infertility) ranged from 0.09 to 0.71 (a value of 1.00 would represent the ability to detect all cases). The specificity (ability to identify fertility) ranged from 0.62 to 1.00 indicating that the test identified anywhere from 62% to 100% of fertile couples. They emphasized that the postcoital test suffers from poor validity, a lack of standard methodology, and confusion over the definition of normality. Others could find no difference in the subsequent pregnancy rates among groups having no sperm, no motile sperm, 1–5 motile sperm, 6–10 motile sperm, and 11 or more motile sperm. Another study indicated that there was a statistically significant increase in the percentage of pregnancies only when there were more than 20 sperm/HPF. Moreover, in a study of postcoital tests in *fertile* couples, 20% had either no sperm or less than one sperm/HPF.

A newer argument raised against use of the postcoital test is that widespread use of intrauterine inseminations (IUI) combined with superovulation has made the assessment of sperm-cervical mucus interactions merely an academic exercise. In this view, whether the postcoital test is normal or abnormal, the treatment is the same. An important underlying assumption is that combined IUI and superovulation is, in fact, effective therapy. Support for this as yet unproven premise may be forthcoming from the results of a prospective controlled trial now in progress.

Answers for Chapter 26 — Post-Test Questions

1. 1; 10–15
p.809

Infertility is defined as one year of unprotected coitus without conception. It affects approximately 10–15% of couples in the reproductive age group which makes it an important component of the practices of many physicians.

2. 25
p.817

Couples need to be aware that there is a normal time requirement to achieve pregnancy. In each ovulatory cycle normal couples have only about a 25% chance of becoming pregnant.

3. decrease; shortened
p.813

Prior to the menopause, there is a period with shorter follicular phases, with increased FSH levels, but normal luteinizing hormone (LH) levels and luteal phases. The menstrual periods for 10–15 years before the menopause are regular, but there is a steady decrease in cycle length due to the shortened follicular phase. Cycle lengths are the shortest (with the least variability) in the late 30s, a time when subtle but real increases in FSH and decreases in inhibin are occurring. For a period of several years (as much as 10 years in some women) prior to menopause, the cycles lengthen again.

4. 50
p.814

About one-half of couples presenting after one year of infertility can be expected to become pregnant spontaneously in the following year. In an English study, only 20% of women who had failed to have a birth within the first two years of marriage never had a child.

5. immunologic
p.819

In addition, sperm antibody testing is mandatory when, in a postcoital test with good mucus, the sperm are found shaking in place but not moving progressively. This shaking movement is a common finding in immunologic infertility.

6. IUI p.821

A postcoital test can guide treatment. *We believe that appropriate therapy for a poor postcoital test is IUI without the need for ancillary superovulation.* This decreases the risk of multiple births and hyperstimulation, and at a significantly lower expense.

7. 12; 23; 54 p.821

A history of pelvic inflammatory disease, septic abortion, ruptured appendix, tubal surgery, or ectopic pregnancy alerts the physician to the possibility of tubal damage. Pelvic inflammatory disease is unquestionably the major contributor to tubal infertility and ectopic pregnancies. Westrom's classic studies with laparoscopically confirmed pelvic inflammatory disease indicated that the incidence of subsequent tubal infertility is approximately 12% after one episode of pelvic infection, 23% after two episodes, and 54% after three episodes.

8. 6–7 p.821

The risk of ectopic pregnancy is increased 6–7-fold after pelvic infection.

9. 15 p.824

Disorders of ovulation account for approximately 15% of all infertility problems in couples. These may be anovulation or severe oligoovulation. In the latter cases, even though ovulation does occur, its relative infrequency decreases the woman's chances for pregnancy. If periods occur only every 3 or 4 months, for practical purposes it matters little whether these are ovulatory or anovulatory.

10. true p.810

After World War II, the U.S. total fertility rate reached a modern high of 3.8 births per woman. The last women born in this period won't be reaching their 45th birthday until around 2010. For approximately a 20-year period, therefore, there will be an unprecedented number of women in the later childbearing years.

11. true p.811

Age alone impacts on fertility. Certainly, aging of the reproductive system plays a role and spontaneous abortion provides another factor. The majority of early abortions after age 35 are due to autosomal trisomies, the incidence of which increases with maternal age. The risk of clinically recognized spontaneous abortion increases from about 10% until age 30, to 18% in the late 30s, and 34% in the early 40s. In addition, as women enter their 30s, there is a greater likelihood of being affected by a number of diseases, for example endometriosis, that can interfere with fertility. Cumulative exposures to occupational or environmental hazards also could lessen fertility as a woman ages. An additional factor that has contributed to infertility at all ages is the spread of sexually transmitted diseases with their damaging effect on the fallopian tubes.

12. true p.814

A pregnancy rate in older women of approximately 30% per cycle can be achieved in a donor oocyte program. In a large series, the rate of spontaneous abortion in recipients correlated with the age of the donors. The abortion rate increased from 14% in recipients who received oocytes from donors aged 20–24 years to 44.5% when the recipient received oocytes from donors older than age 35. These results further point out that the increased risks of spontaneous abortion and chromosomal anomalies associated with older age are also due primarily to aging oocytes. Pregnancy wastage directly correlates with the age of the woman who produces the oocytes.

13. true p.815

An often neglected goal is that of counseling a couple concerning the proper time to discontinue investigation and treatment. This is especially important in the 10–15% of couples with no known cause for their infertility. Despite the absence of pathology, couples with 3 years or more of infertility have a poor prognosis. Counseling must include consideration of assisted reproductive technologies.

14. true p.821

What constitutes a poor postcoital test in terms of sperm numbers is controversial. Intrauterine insemination has been reported to enhance the chances for pregnancy when there were 3 or fewer sperm/HPF in the postcoital test but not when there were 5 or more sperm/HPF. We continue to support a minimum level of one motile progressive sperm/HPF as compatible with normality. The finding of no sperm, all dead sperm or a large proportion of shaking sperm suggests a possible immunologic factor. These findings, specifically immotile or absent sperm, also should prompt inquiry concerning use of vaginal lubricants. Both Surgilube and KY Jelly can immobilize sperm and they should be avoided. If there are no motile sperm in the postcoital test, the pH of the mucus should be determined. Thus, whereas the usefulness of the postcoital test may be limited, it still has a place in the investigation of infertility.

15. true p.821

Almost one-half of patients who are eventually found to have tubal damage and/or pelvic adhesions, however, have no history of antecedent disease. Many of these women will have elevated anti-chlamydia antibodies, suggestive of prior infection. There have been a few reports of damaged tubes showing histologic evidence of viral infection which could explain the absence of traditional causes of tubal damage.

16. true p.821

Tubal disease is diagnosed by the hysterosalpingogram (HSG) and by laparoscopy. The HSG is performed 2 to 5 days after cessation of a menstrual flow. If there is a history suggestive of pelvic inflammatory disease, a sedimentation rate is obtained prior to the HSG and, if elevated, antibiotic therapy is given. The procedure is than postponed for a month when a repeat sedimentation rate is obtained. Only if this is normal is the HSG scheduled. If masses or tenderness are revealed by the pelvic examination at any time, the HSG should be bypassed and the pelvis evaluated by laparoscopy. If there is a documented history of pelvic inflammatory disease, the risk of a serious reinfection following HSG is too high, and it should be replaced by laparoscopy. If an HSG is performed in a patient who is at questionable risk for infection, a water-soluble rather than an oil dye should be used because of the faster absorption. The overall risk of infection with HSG is probably less than 1%, although in a high-risk population serious infection can occur in approximately 3% of cases. Clinically apparent infections were not present in 398 women who had nondilated tubes on HSG; however, 11% of those with dilated tubes developed pelvic inflammatory disease. Doxycycline, 200 mg after the procedure, can be administered if the tubes are dilated, followed by 100 mg bid for 5 days. Many clinicians routinely administer prophylactic antibiotics (doxycycline, 100 mg bid for 5 days, beginning 2 days before the procedure).

17. false p.824

Anovulatory or oligoovulatory women should be promptly treated with clomiphene citrate to increase the frequency of, or to initiate, ovulation, and the drug can be started immediately, even before other areas have been investigated. If anovulation is the only infertility factor, most couples will become pregnant within 3 months of ovulation induction.

18. false p.825

In discussing coital timing, the patient will usually want to know the fertilizable life of the sperm and the egg. The information on human gametes is speculative. Cases have been reported in which isolated coitus even up to 7 days prior to the rise in basal body temperature has resulted in pregnancy, but this probably represents the limits of biologic variation. It is estimated that sperm retain their ability to fertilize for 24 to 48 hours and that the human egg is fertilizable for 12 to 24 hours. However, immature human eggs aspirated from follicles for in vitro fertilization can be fertilized after incubation in vitro for even as long as 36 hours.

19. true p.830

A number of studies have established the widespread distribution of *ureaplasma urealyticum* in both fertile and infertile populations. Some have found higher colonization in infertile couples, whereas others have found no relationship between the organisms and infertility. In a study that received a great deal of media attention, it was reported that 60% of males who were culture positive for *ureaplasma urealyticum* and were cleared of infection by antibiotic treatment achieved a pregnancy. Failure to clear the infection resulted in a 5% pregnant rate. This study suffers from lack of clarity on the criteria for entry into treatment and from any mention of individuals lost to follow-up. The incidence of ureaplasma infection is only significantly higher in those women whose male partners have semen abnormalities.

It can be concluded that culturing for ureaplasma may be reasonable with male infertility but is not worthwhile in cases of unexplained infertility, and indiscriminate treatment with antibiotics is not warranted.

20. C
p.809–811

There have been 3 striking changes in infertility practice during the past 2 decades. First was the introduction of in vitro fertilization and other assisted reproductive technologies (ART) which have enlarged the possibilities for successful treatment and provided an opportunity to study basic reproductive processes. ART refers to all techniques involving direct retrieval of oocytes from the ovary. Second, and partially because of the media attention focused on ART, the public has become more aware of potential treatments, and this has generated a marked increase in patient visits for infertility. There has been no recent dramatic change in the proportion of couples considered infertile; however, there is an increasing number of infertile couples, due, in part, to the aging of the large post-World War II population boom generation. The third change is the increase in the proportion of women over 35 seeking medical attention for infertility. One of every five women in the United States is having a first child after 35, a marked increase over earlier figures. This reflects both a later age for marriage and postponement of pregnancy in marriage as women, by choice or by circumstances, commit to the workplace.

21. E
p.810

The aging of the World War II population boom is giving current times a greater number of women who are delaying marriage and childbirth. This demographic change has 3 specific impacts on couples.

1. A need for effective contraception.
2. The problem of achieving pregnancy later in life.
3. The problem of being pregnant later in life.

22. A
p.811, 812

The average age of the Hutterite women at the last pregnancy was 40.9 years, and there was a definite decrease in fertility with age. Eleven percent of the women bore no children after age 34; 33% of the women were infertile by age 40, and 87% were infertile at age 45. The French studied the pregnancy rate in a donor insemination program, including only women with azoospermic husbands. These women are less likely to have infertility factors than those women married to oligospermic males. A decrease in conception rate with age was noted. Below the age of 31 the pregnancy rate over one year was 74%. This decreased to 62% at ages 31 to 35 and to 54% when the women were older than 35. An American study with therapeutic insemination has demonstrated a similar relationship with age. Of note was the requirement for more treatment cycles to achieve pregnancy in older women, 9–10 cycles rather than the usual 6. In a donor insemination program in the Netherlands, the probability of having a healthy baby decreased 3.5% per year after age 30. A woman age 35 had 50% the chance of having a healthy baby compared to a woman age 25.

23. A
p.814

Experience has repeatedly demonstrated a reduction in in vitro fertilization pregnancy rates when the oocytes are of advanced age. When embryos from the same cohort of young donated oocytes were simultaneously transferred to young and older recipients, pregnancy rates were similar. The high rate of implantation and pregnancy in older women receiving donated younger oocytes has argued that uterine factors are not involved with the decline in fecundity with aging.

24. A
p.816

(See figure on page 362 in this Study Guide)

25. E
p.821

A history of pelvic inflammatory disease, septic abortion, ruptured appendix, tubal surgery, or ectopic pregnancy alerts the physician to the possibility of tubal damage.

26. A
p.824

Proximal tubal obstruction can be treated by outpatient tubal cannulation or balloon tuboplasty. Transcervical tuboplasty can be performed by either a fluoroscopic or hysteroscopic approach, although most of the experience thus far is with the fluoroscopic technique. The level of discomfort is similar to that with hysterosalpingography; intravenous sedation and a paracervical block are usually sufficient. Cannulation and balloon tuboplasty success is achieved in at least one tube in 80–90% of attempts. Approximately 30% of patients will become pregnant in the 3–6 months following the procedure. Further technical developments may eventually allow canalization of the tube to be

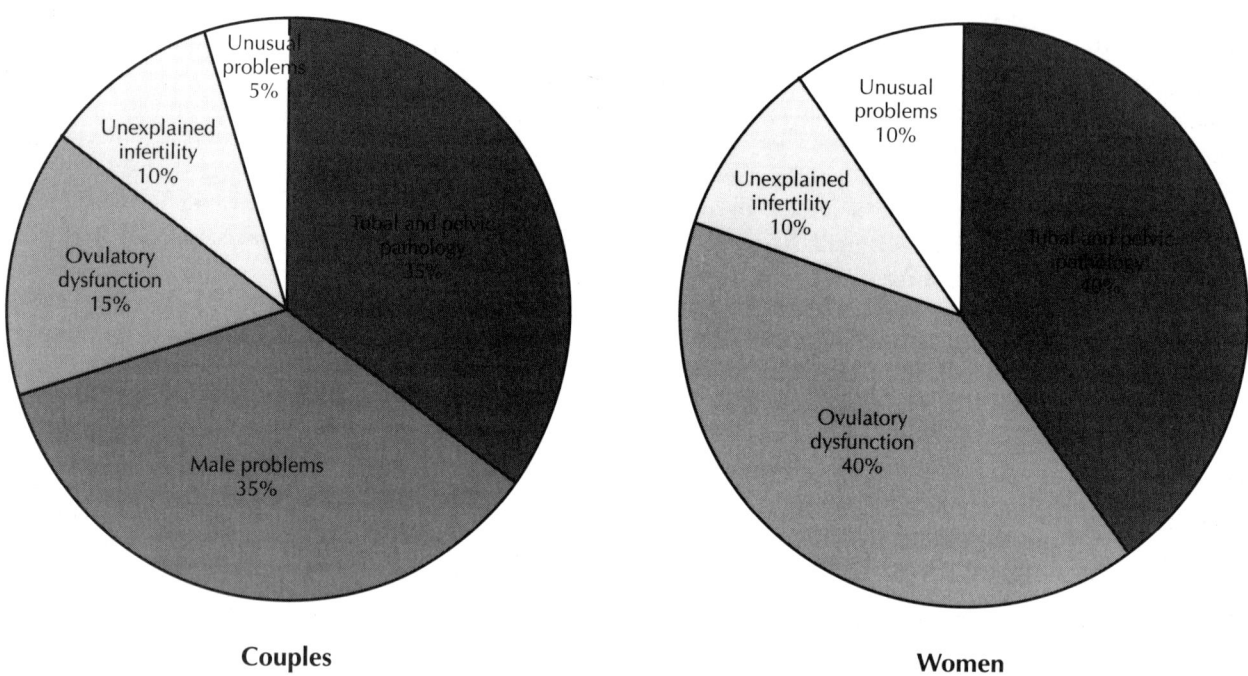

Causes of Infertility

Couples

Women

performed in the office, e.g., with ultrasonography. The advantage of these accomplishments is the avoidance of general anesthesia, surgery, and expensive hospitalization. Eventually, treatment of proximal tubal obstruction will immediately follow diagnosis.

27. A p.827

The diagnosis should be considered in women with normal cycles and unexplained infertility, women with short luteal phases demonstrated by basal body temperature charts, and women with a history of recurrent spontaneous abortion. Women taking clomiphene citrate for ovulation induction also are at risk.

28. A p.828,829

Based on findings that low FSH values prior to ovulation can be associated with luteal phase defect, it would seem reasonable, in selected cases, to use human menopausal gonadotropins or clomiphene citrate. Gonadotropin treatment has the potential for causing hyperstimulation of the ovaries, and it creates an increased risk of multiple births. Because of these effects, gonadotropin treatment is seldom used for this indication. Clomiphene citrate is the first choice of many physicians for the treatment of luteal phase defect. The only significant risk is a 5% (twice normal) chance of multiple births, essentially all twins. The initial dose is 50 mg a day for 5 days starting on day 3, 4, or 5 of the cycle.

Because there is a suspected deficiency of progesterone in luteal phase defect exogenous progesterone has been utilized. A vaginal suppository containing 25 mg of progesterone is inserted twice a day starting approximately 3 days after ovulation. Treatment is maintained until menstruation occurs or until a pregnancy is diagnosed. If the latter, a switch is made to weekly injections of 17-hydroxyprogesterone caproate (250 mg) through the 10th week of pregnancy. Using this therapy, success rates of approximately 50% have been achieved, but good control studies are lacking.

There is no difference in pregnancy rates in studies comparing clomiphene and progesterone treatment. In our view, this is an argument in favor of clomiphene because of a significant disadvantage associated with progesterone therapy. Progesterone supplementation prolongs the luteal phase and can delay the onset of menses. This is not a problem for the physician, but for the couple the disappointment at the time of delayed menses or a negative pregnancy test is even more profound.

Dopamine agonist treatment has been reported to correct luteal phase defect associated with hyperprolactinemia, but its value in women with normal prolactin levels has not been demonstrated. In a subgroup of patients with unexplained infertility, high normal prolactin levels, and expressible galactorrhea, treatment with bromocriptine enhanced fertility compared to similar women treated with pyridoxine. If galactorrhea is present, even if the prolactin is normal, ovulatory dysfunction responds well to dopamine agonist therapy. In the absence of galactorrhea, a prolactin elevation may be subtle (such as an increase in nocturnal peaks), and this could explain occasional good responses to dopamine agonist treatment. In evaluating any therapy it is important to keep in mind that pregnancies can occur without treatment in women who are diagnosed as having luteal phase defect.

Many physicians short circuit the diagnostic evaluation of hormone adequacy and automatically proceed to treatment of unexplained infertility with clomiphene citrate. They argue that there may be subtle hormonal abnormalities that cannot be diagnosed with current technology but which can be successfully treated by stimulating the ovaries. Moreover, there is a theoretical advantage in having more than one oocyte in the fallopian tube at the time of fertilization. Randomized placebo-controlled studies seem to support the efficacy of this approach. By contrast, some have not found a benefit for the use of clomiphene citrate in unexplained infertility.

29. E p.829

The drawbacks to clomiphene citrate use are the risk of multiple births, occasional hot flushes, and sometimes severe mood changes that some women experience. The most concerning side effects are visual changes which occur only rarely (and are always reversible) and usually with doses of 150 mg or higher. We do not object to the use of clomiphene for the empirical treatment of luteal phase defect, provided there is a clear understanding of the potential side effects and the uncertain efficacy of the medication.

30. A p.831

Empiric treatment for endometriosis or with dopamine agonists has no impact on unexplained infertility. However, the methods of assisted reproductive technology and superovulation with intrauterine insemination do increase the prospect of pregnancy (superovulation is probably the key factor and not intrauterine insemination). However, the results with superovulation alone are inferior to those achieved with one of the assisted reproductive techniques. The lower fertilization rate using in vitro fertilization, but a normal conception rate following embryo transfer, indicates that at least one subgroup of women with unexplained infertility has impaired oocytes.

A cumulative pregnancy rate of 40% can be achieved after 6 cycles of superovulation or 3 cycles of in vitro fertilization. In randomized, controlled clinical trials, the monthly pregnancy rates in couples with unexplained infertility is increased 3-fold (a monthly fecundity rate of 9%) with clomiphene treatment, and with human menopausal gonadotropins, the monthly fecundity rate is approximately 10–15%. Therefore couples with unexplained infertility should be offered superovulation or one of the assisted reproductive technologies.

27 Recurrent Early Pregnancy Losses

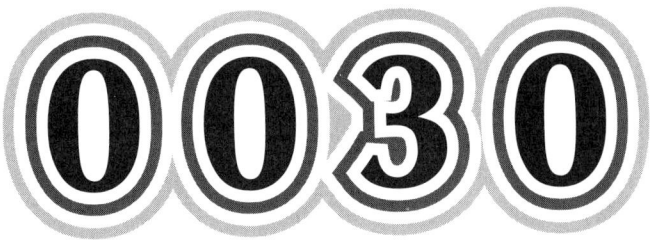

Learning Objectives

Be able to:

1. Describe the rate and etiologies of first and second trimester loss.

2. Discuss the causes of recurrent abortions.

3. Explain the workup for determining the cause of recurrent abortions.

4. Detail possible treatment options for each cause of recurrent abortion.

Pre-Test

A. Instructions: Fill in the blanks

1. The overall abortion risk (recognized and unrecognized) in women over age 40 is approximately ____%.

2. Treatment for significant titers of antiphospholipid antibodies consists of low dose _____ and low dose _____ as soon as the pregnancy is diagnosed.

B. Instructions: True or False

3. Translocations within families are usually associated with a mixed history of some normal pregnancies intermixed with recurrent abortions.

4. There is currently no hard evidence that bacterial or viral infections cause recurrent abortions.

C. Instructions: For each of the following questions choose:

   A. if only 1, 2 and 3 are correct
   B. if only 1 and 3 are correct
   C. if only 2 and 4 are correct
   D. if only 4 is correct
   E. if all are correct

5. Environmental factors associated with recurrent miscarriages include
   1. isotretinoin
   2. alcohol
   3. heavy coffee consumption
   4. video terminals

6. Antiphospholipid antibodies
   1. are directed against platelets and vascular endothelium
   2. block prostacyclin formation
   3. are associated with fetal growth retardation
   4. are associated with second trimester fetal death

Post-Test

A. Instructions: Fill in the blanks

1. Approximately _____% of all pregnancies between 4–20 weeks of gestation will undergo clinically recognized spontaneous abortions.

2. The true early pregnancy loss rate is _____% because of the high rate of unrecognized abortions in the 2–4 weeks immediately following conception.

3. Once a live embryo is detected by ultrasonography in normal women or women with infertility, the rate of fetal loss is _____%. However, in women with recurrent pregnancy loss, the rate of loss after detection of fetal cardiac activity is _____ times higher.

4. _____% of early spontaneous abortions are associated with fetal chromosomal abnormalities.

5. In addition to müllerian anomalies, another anatomic cause, although uncommon, of recurrent abortions is intrauterine _____.

6. Liveborn births occur eventually in ____% of those with recurrent abortions of unknown etiology without treatment.

7. _____% of women with histories of recurrent abortions have no identifiable abnormalities.

B. Instructions: True or False

8. The diagnostic and therapeutic response to a couple with pregnancy loss is dictated by the number of abortions.

9. About 50% of fertilized ova do not progress to a viable pregnancy.

10. Sensitive assays for human chorionic gonadotropin (HCG) suggest that up to 30% of pregnancies are lost between implantation and the 6th week.

11. The fetal chromosomal abnormalities in single spontaneous abortions are different than those in recurrent abortions.

12. Many patients with significant titers of antiphospholipid antibodies do not develop preeclampsia.

C. Instructions: For each of the following questions choose:

A. if only 1, 2 and 3 are correct
B. if only 1 and 3 are correct
C. if only 2 and 4 are correct
D. if only 4 is correct
E. if all are correct

13. The risk of pregnancy loss
    1. after 3 successive abortions is 30–45%
    2. after 3 consecutive abortions without a live birth is 40–45%
    3. after 3 consecutive abortions with a least one previous live birth is 30%
    4. after 3 consecutive abortions is 70%

14. A karyotype is useful in the workup of recurrent abortion
    1. as it will reveal an abnormality 10–15% of the time
    2. as it will reveal a balanced translocation as the most frequent genetic abnormality
    3. as it can determine single gene defects
    4. particularly when there has been a previously malformed or mentally retarded offspring

15. True statements regarding specific etiologies of recurrent miscarriage include
    1. a 90% healthy live birth rate after endocrine factors are corrected
    2. a 60% healthy live birth rate if known genetic factors are noted
    3. a 60–70% healthy live birth rate after corrected anatomic factors are made
    4. a 90% healthy live birth rate after correction of an immunologic problem

16. Uterine anomalies
    1. can result in impaired vascularization of a pregnancy and limited space for a fetus due to distortion of the uterine cavity
    2. are present in 12–15% of women with recurrent abortions
    3. are not always detailed sufficiently by HSG
    4. can be associated with recurrent miscarriages

17. Workup for autoimmunity as a cause of recurrent abortions include screening for
    1. lupus anticoagulant
    2. anticardiolipin antibodies
    3. partial thromboplastin time
    4. kaolin clotting time

18. Women with recurrent abortions who are more likely to have an immunologic cause
    1. have a history of previous spontaneous abortions
    2. are over 35 year old
    3. have aborted conceptus with a normal karyotype
    4. have no losses after the first trimester

Answers for Chapter 27 — Pre-Test Questions

1. 75   p.842
Approximately 80% of spontaneous abortions occur in the first 12 weeks of pregnancy, and nearly 70% of these abortions in early pregnancy are due to chromosomal anomalies. Clinically recognized abortion occurs in only 12% of women younger than age 20, but the incidence increases to 26% in women older than age 40. The overall abortion risk (recognized and unrecognized) in women over age 40 is approximately 75%! An appreciation for these statistics contributes significantly to a couple's ability to cope with a spontaneous abortion.

2. ASA; heparin   p.846
Our preferred treatment for significant titers of antiphsopholipid antibodies consists of the combination of low dose aspirin and low dose heparin as soon as pregnancy is diagnosed. Treatment is not always successful. Others advocate the addition of a glucocorticoid in a dose sufficient to restore the clotting studies to normal. The addition of glucocorticoids is not very effective in eliminating the anticardiolipin antibody.

3. true   p.843
Karyotyping is expensive. A factor that can help in decision-making is a positive family history for recurrent abortions. Translocations within families are usually associated with a mixed history: some normal pregnancies intermixed with recurrent abortions. Karyotyping is indicated when family members can be identified with multiple spontaneous abortions or the family has a malformed or mentally retarded child or a child with a known chromosomal abnormality. In any event, we recommend a karyotype when there is a history of 3 consecutive spontaneous early pregnancy losses and no previous normal liveborn.

4. true   p.845
Despite periodic reports that have implicated specific infectious agents as etiologic factors in recurrent spontaneous abortions, there currently is no hard evidence that bacterial or viral infections cause recurrent abortions. An impressive

incidence of antichlamydial antibody has been reported in women with 3 or more spontaneous abortions, but it is not certain whether this an association with *Chlamydia trachomatis* or whether this is a marker of a different immune response in women with recurrent abortions. Claims of effective antibiotic treatment have been derived without benefit of randomized studies. Perhaps an exception is infection with *Ureaplasma urealiticum.* Other organisms that have been implicated, but not substantiated, include *Toxoplasma gondii, Listeria monocytogenes, Mycoplasma hominis,* herpes virus, and cytomegalovirus. It is more cost-effective and time efficient to prescribe couples a course of doxycycline (100 mg bid for 14 days) or erythromycin (250 mg qid for 14 days) than to pursue multiple and repeated cultures.

5. A   p.844

Smoking, alcohol, and heavy coffee consumption are associated with an increased risk of recurrent abortions. The increase in risk is proportional to the number of cigarettes smoked. In these cases, the fetal chromosomes are normal. Anesthetic gases and tetrachloroethylene (used in dry cleaning) have been implicated as causative agents of abortion, but exposure to video terminals does not appear to be a factor. Exercise programs do not increase the risk of spontaneous abortion, and bed rest will not influence the risk of recurrent abortion. Isotretinoin (Accutane) is definitely associated with an increased incidence of spontaneous abortion.

6. E   p.846

In autoimmunity, a humoral or cellular response is directed against a specific component of the host. The lupus anticoagulant and anticardiolipin antibodies are antiphospholipid antibodies, which arise as the result of an autoimmune disease. The lupus anticoagulant is present in a variety of clinical conditions, not just with lupus erythematosus. The antiphospholipid antibodies are directed against platelets and the vascular endothelium and cause thrombosis, spontaneous abortion, and fetal wastage. These antibodies block prostacyclin formation, which results in unbalanced thromboxane activity, leading to vasoconstriction and thrombosis. In several series, 10–16% of women with recurrent abortions have had antiphospholipid antibodies. These antibodies are also associated with fetal growth retardation and fetal death in addition to recurrent abortion, and when present, there is a high rate of second trimester fetal deaths. The mechanism of pregnancy loss is probably decidual and placental insufficiency due to the thrombotic tendency.

Answers for Chapter 27 — Post-Test Questions

1. 15   p.841

Early pregnancy loss (abortion) is defined as the termination of pregnancy before 20 weeks of gestation (dated from the last menstrual period) or below a fetal weight of 500 g. Approximately 15% of all pregnancies between 4–20 weeks of gestation will undergo clinically recognized spontaneous abortions.

2. 50   p.841

The true early pregnancy loss rate is closer to 50% because of the high rate of unrecognized abortions in the 2–4 weeks immediately following conception. The majority of these very early cases are caused by chromosomal abnormalities in the sperm or the egg.

3. 5; 4–5   p.842

Once a live embryo is detected by ultrasonography in normal women or in women with infertility, the rate of fetal loss is 5%. However, in women with recurrent pregnancy loss, the rate of loss after detection of fetal cardiac activity is 4–5 times higher.

4. 70%   p.843

Approximately 70% of early spontaneous abortions are associated with fetal chromsomal abnormalities. In addition, 30% of second trimester abortions and 3% of stillbirths have abnormal chromosomes. In most cases, the couple is chromosomally normal and the fetal chromosomal abnormality is a random event. The abnormalities include maternal and paternal accidents in gametogenesis, as well as miscues after fertilization.

5. synechiae (Asherman's syndrome)   p.845

In addition to müllerian anomalies, another anatomic cause, although uncommon, of recurrent abortions is intrauterine synechiae (Asherman's syndrome). If an appropriate predisposing factor, such as uterine curettage or a severe uterine infection, can be identified, diagnostic hysterosalpingography or hysteroscopy should be performed.

6. 70   p.848

It should be emphasized that continued attempts at conception are rewarded with success in the majority of women (70–75%) labeled as recurrent aborters and who have no identifiable cause.

7. 40–50   p.848

Except in the case of a second trimester loss which is associated with a poor prognosis in the subsequent pregnancy with increased risks for preterm delivery, stillbirth, and neonatal death, approximately 40–50% of women with histories of recurrent abortions have no identifiable abnormalities and do well in their next pregnancies. All subsequent pregnancies should be closely monitored because there is a higher rate of ectopic pregnancies in women with recurrent abortions.

8. false   p.842

The diagnostic and therapeutic response to a couple with pregnancy loss is not dictated by the number of abortions. The response is significantly influenced by the woman's age, the couple's level of anxiety, and factors readily identified in the family and medical history. The degree of response will range from an educational discussion to a full diagnostic evaluation with appropriate treatment.

9. true   p.842

The reproductive loss between conception and clinically recognizable pregnancy is significant; about 50% of fertilized ova do not progress to a viable pregnancy.

10. true   p.842

The use of sensitive assays for human chorionic gonadotropin (HCG) suggests that up to 30% of pregnancies are lost between implantation and the 6th week. It is important for physicians and their patients to be aware of the high degree of reproductive loss, especially in older women due in part to the increasing frequency of trisomies with advancing age. However, the frequency of both euploid (normal) and aneuploid (abnormal) abortuses increases with maternal age.

11. true   p.843

The fetal chromsomal abnormalities in single spontaneous abortions are different than those in recurrent abortions. Autosomal trisomy is the most frequent anomaly (about 50% of early pregnancy abortions), due to nondisjunction or translocation. Trisomies of chromosomes 13, 16, 18, 21, and 22 are the most common. The next most common anomaly (about 25%) is 45,X which is responsible for Turner syndrome when the fetus survives. Of the remaining anomalies, most are polyploidies.

12. false   p.846

Many of these patients develop preeclampsia, often very severe, but approximately 75% of patients with antiphospholipid antibodies will deliver a viable infant in a treated pregnancy.

13. A   p.842

(See table on page 371 in this Study Guide)

14. C   p.843,844

A recognized cause of the problem is a genetic abnormality, and karyotyping of couples will reveal that 3–8% have some abnormality, most frequently a balanced chromosomal rearrangement, a translocation. Other abnormalities usually encountered include sex chromosome mosaicism, chromosome inversions, and ring chromosomes. It is important to emphasize that karyotyping uncovers only a percentage of those pregnancies lost due to genetic abnormalities. There may be single gene defects that are not manifested by chromosomal abnormalities, and it is very likely that a percentage of those patients now considered to have unexplained repetitive pregnancy loss have this type

The Risk of Recurrent Early Pregnancy Loss

	Number of Prior Losses	% Risk of Loss in Next Pregnancy
Women who have had at least one liveborn infant:	0	12%
	1	24%
	2	26%
	3	32%
	4	26%
Women who have not had at least one liveborn infant:	2 or more	40–45%

of genetic defect. In addition, karyotyping of blood cells misses abnormalities of meiosis, which can be found in sperm cell lines.

15. B   p.843

According to McDonough, treatment of endocrine factors yields a 90% normal child rate; correction of anatomic factors yields a 60–70% rate, but known genetic factors are associated with only a 32% expectation for a normal child.

16. E   p.845

Uterine abnormalities can result in impaired vascularization of a pregnancy and limited space for a fetus due to distortion of the uterine cavity. Approximately 12–15% of women with recurrent abortion have a uterine malformation, and this can be best diagnosed by vaginal ultrasonography, confirmed by magnetic resonance imaging. Hysterosalpingography is relatively inaccurate and decisions should not be based upon hysterosalpingography alone. The various uterine anomalies, including leiomyomata and diethylstilbestrol (DES) exposure. Surgical repair of these defects, often by hysteroscopy, is rewarded with delivery rates in the 70–80% range; however, this high rate of success must be tempered by the realization that it is not derived from randomized clinical trials. The septate uterus is the most frequent anatomic abnormality associated with recurrent early spontaneous abortions, and the results with hysteroscopic repair have been impressive. Repeat procedures are occasionally necessary; the surgical result should be evaluated several weeks postoperatively by hysterosalpingography (which is sufficiently accurate for this purpose) or office hysteroscopy. Surgery is unlikely to make a difference in a patient who has successfully delivered a liveborn term infant. The prophylactic use of cervical cerclage has not been supported by results from randomized trials. However, when there is nothing else to offer, cervical cerclage is worthwhile, e.g., in patients with late losses and müllerian anomalies such as a bicornuate or unicornuate uterus and in DES-exposed women with a hypoplastic cervix.

17. E   p.846

Despite activating thrombosis, the antiphospholipid antibodies prolong the prothrombin time and the partial thromboplastin time. The activated partial thromboplastin time is a relatively sensitive screening test, but we also obtain a kaolin clotting time. The anticardiolipin antibody can be identified and titered by specific immunoassays. The antiphospholipid antibodies all produce the same clinical impact and have identical effects on clotting tests. Although the prevalence is uncertain, patients with recurrent abortions should be screened with the activated partial thromboplastin time, a kaolin clotting time, and the anticardiolipin antibody.

18. B p.847

Women whose recurrent abortions are more likely to have an immunologic cause have the following characteristics:

   1. Many previous spontaneous abortions.
   2. No recent full term pregnancies.
   3. Less than 35 years old.
   4. Aborted conceptus with a normal karyotype.
   5. Usually at least one loss after the first trimester.

28 Endometriosis

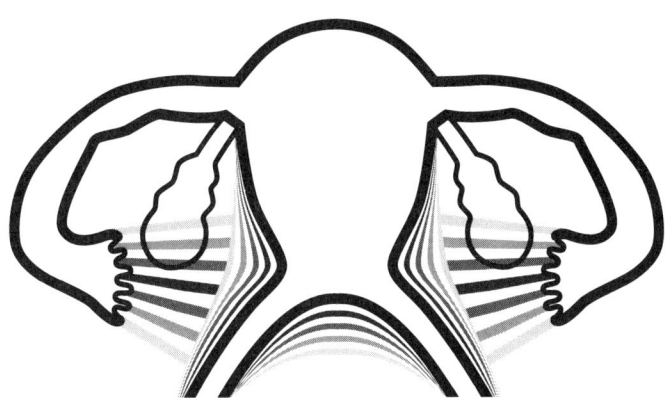

Learning Objectives

Be able to:

1. Discuss the theories which possibly explain the etiology of endometriosis.

2. Describe the utility and limitations of various diagnostic modalities in diagnosing endometriosis.

3. Detail the various medical and surgical options for treatment of endometriosis as well as their associated success rates for symptomatic relief, pregnancy and recurrence rates.

4. Understand the risks and benefits of each treatment option available for endometriosis.

Pre-Test

A. Instructions: Fill in the blanks

1. Many studies examining the issue of infertility and minimal or mild endometriosis are flawed by lack of _____ and failure to use _____ table analysis.

2. Hormone treatment for endometriosis must be viewed as _____ rather than curative.

B. Instructions: True or False

3. Although, hormonal therapy of infertility associated with endometriosis is not of proven value, medical therapy for dysmenorrhea, dyspareunia and pelvic pain associated with endometriosis is successful.

4. Danazol is no more effective than other medications used to treat endometriosis.

C. Instructions: For the following question choose:

A. if only 1, 2 and 3 are correct
B. if only 1 and 3 are correct
C. if only 2 and 4 are correct
D. if only 4 is correct
E. if all are correct

5. Support for the theory that endometriosis is due to coelomic metaplasia includes
   1. endometriosis occurring in adolescent girls in the absence of müllerian anomalies
   2. endometriosis having been reported in a prepubertal girl
   3. endometriosis having been reported in women who never menstruated
   4. endometriosis occurring in men

Post-Test

A. Instructions: Fill in the blanks

1. Endometriosis is a term indicating _____ endometrial glands and _____ (outside the uterus).

2. _____% of women in the reproductive age group and _____% of infertile women have endometriosis.

3. CA-125 is a cell surface _____ found on derivatives of the coelomic epithelium and is a useful marker in monitoring women with _____ ovarian carcinoma.

4. The appearance of endometriosis is _____.

5. A presacral neurectomy is only indicated in patients with pain limited to the _____ area.

6. _____ surgery for endometriosis indicates that reproductive function is maintained.

7. Hormone therapy in the treatment of endometriosis is designed to interrupt the cycle of _____ and _____.

8. The effects of danazol produce a _____ androgen, _____ estrogen environment that does not support the growth of endometriosis.

9. Both oral and injectable medroxyprogesterone acetate have been effective in treating endometriosis by causing _____ and subsequent _____ of endometrial tissue.

10. A long-acting GnRH agonist can create a _____ for the treatment of endometriosis.

11. The recurrence rate of endometriosis following medical therapy is _____ than that following conservative surgical excision.

B. Instructions: True or False

12. Endometriosis can occur in almost every organ of the body.

13. Endometriosis only occurs in goal-oriented women over the age of 30.

14. Endometriosis should be suspected in any women complaining of infertility.

15. Prophylactic uterine suspension is recommended to women with retroflexed uteri to avoid endometriosis.

16. Endometriosis lesions can be red, black, blue or white and nonpigmented.

17. Existing classification systems for staging endometriosis suffer from inherent weaknesses in their methodology.

18. Medical treatment of minimal to mild endometriosis has not been effective in improving fertility rates.

19. Women with endometriosis have higher levels of prostanoids in peritoneal fluid compared to other infertile women.

20. Luteinized unruptured follicle syndrome is secondary to endometriosis and causes infertility.

21. Based on monthly fecundity rates and life table analysis, no study has shown an advantage for conservative surgery as opposed to expectant management in the treatment of minimal or mild endometriosis.

22. Endometriotic tissue displays histologic and biochemical differences, including enzyme activity and receptor levels which differ in concentration and response compared to normal endometrium.

23. Danazol has been associated with the development of in utero female pseudohermaphroditism.

C. Instructions: For each of the following questions choose:

A. if only 1, 2 and 3 are correct
B. if only 1 and 3 are correct
C. if only 2 and 4 are correct
D. if only 4 is correct
E. if all are correct

24. Support for the theory that endometriosis is due to retrograde flow of endometrial tissue through the fallopian tubes is supported by
    1. endometriosis is most commonly found in dependent portions of the pelvis
    2. endometrial fragments from menstrual flow can grow in tissue culture
    3. a higher incidence of endometriosis is observed in women who have obstruction to the outward flow of menses
    4. the risk of endometriosis is increased in women with shorter menstrual cycles and longer menstrual flows

25. Theories explaining the etiology of endometriosis include
    1. retrograde flow of endometrial tissue
    2. vascular or lymphatic transport
    3. coelomic metaplasia
    4. chromosomal deletion

26. Dysmenorrhea
    1. is present in every woman with endometriosis
    2. is suggestive of endometriosis if it begins after 4 years of relatively pain-free menses
    3. which is associated with endometriosis is diffuse as opposed to being localized in the majority of cases
    4. when noted to be very severe is often associated with deeply infiltrating endometriosis

27. The serum CA-125 assay
    1. is often elevated in patients with endometriosis
    2. has a high degree of sensitivity
    3. often correlates with the severity of disease
    4. is not elevated in early pregnancy or women with acute pelvic inflammatory disease

28. Surgical treatment of endometriosis
    1. is useful when associated with adhesive disease or large endometriomas
    2. has the goal of restoring normal anatomical relationships and to excise or fulgurate as much of the endometriosis as possible
    3. may involve removal of severely diseased adnexa when the other side is more normal in appearance
    4. involves presacral neurectomy in order to enhance fertility

29. Success of surgical treatment of endometriosis
    1. is directly related to the severity of the disease
    2. is associated with the highest pregnancy rates in the first 3 years following treatment
    3. is a 60% pregnancy rate in patients with moderate disease and 35% pregnancy rate in those with severe disease
    4. is likely to be achieved even when second surgeries are necessary for treatment

30. Medical treatment options for endometriosis include
    1. DES
    2. oral contraceptives
    3. methyltestosterone
    4. medroxyprogesterone

31. Danazol's mechanisms of action in treating endometriosis include
    1. inhibition of pituitary gonadotropins midcycle surges
    2. altering basal gonadotropin concentrations
    3. inhibition of steroidogenesis
    4. decreasing sex hormone binding globulin production

32. The side effects of danazol include
    1. fluid retention
    2. atrophic vaginitis
    3. muscle cramps
    4. hot flushes

33. Metabolic side effects related to danazol include
    1. elevated renal function tests
    2. elevated liver function tests
    3. decreased white count
    4. increased cholesterol and LDL with decreased HDL

34. Treatment of endometriosis with a progestational agent can be associated with the following side effects
    1. fluid retention
    2. breakthrough bleeding
    3. weight gain
    4. depression

35. Progestational agents in the treatment of endometriosis
    1. can include megestrol acetate or medroxyprogesterone
    2. are not associated with breakthrough bleeding
    3. may relieve symptoms of endometriosis but not be effective in treating infertility
    4. are more effective than placebo in improving pregnancy rates following treatment

36. GnRH
    1. has a short half-life because it is rapidly cleaved between amino acids 5-6, 6-7 and 9-10
    2. agonist can achieve the best therapeutic effect by lowering estrogen levels to 40–60 pg/ml
    3. agonists have been produced by substituting the amino acid at the number 6 position
    4. agonist show superior results in terms of reduction of disease and pregnancy rates

37. Advantages of GnRH agonist over danocrine in the treatment of endometriosis include avoidance of
    1. hypoestrogenism
    2. adverse impact on serum lipids and lipoproteins
    3. risk of osteoporosis
    4. androgenic side effects

38. Curative surgery for severe endometriosis includes
    1. conservative surgery
    2. bilateral salpingo-oophorectomy
    3. resection of endometriosis
    4. abdominal hysterectomy and bilateral salpingo-oophorectomy with resection of all endometriosis

39. Moderate endometriosis incidentally found at surgery in a young woman without immediate interest in pregnancy may include 6 months of long-term therapy with
    1. a GnRH agonist
    2. danazol
    3. medroxyprogesterone acetate
    4. any of the above followed by continuous oral contraceptives

40. Superovulation with intrauterine insemination as a treatment for endometriosis
    1. is associated with increased fecundity rates
    2. is associated with improved cumulative pregnancy rates
    3. is not associated with improved cumulative pregnancy rates
    4. is not associated with increased fecundity rates

Answers for Chapter 28 – Pre-Test Questions

1. controls; life table   p.857

The question of how minimal or mild endometriosis can affect fertility now has been superseded by the question of whether there is *any* effect of mild endometriosis on fertility. More importantly, should endometriosis be treated if the complaint is infertility and not pain? Many articles purporting to show that therapy overcomes endometriosis-associated infertility are flawed by lack of control groups and the failure to use life table analyses. Moreover, expectant management of mild endometriosis is rewarded with reasonable pregnancy rates that are comparable to those obtained with treatment. A cumulative pregnancy rate after 5 years of 90% has been reported in women not treated for minimal or mild endometriosis.

2. suppressive   p.859

Until the late 1970s the most important alternative to conservative surgery was the use of combination oral contraceptives taken in a continuous fashion. It seems to matter little which low dose monophasic product is used to accomplish the conversion of endometrial implants into decidualized cells associated with a few inactive endometrial glands. At this time the efficacy of the multiphasic formulations is unknown. The usual dose of the combined oral contraceptive is one pill per day continuously for 6–12 months. Estrogen (conjugated estrogens 1.25 mg or estradiol 2.0 mg daily for 1 week) is added if breakthrough bleeding occurs. The treatment with oral contraceptives was called pseudopregnancy because of the amenorrhea and the decidualization of the endometrial tissue induced by the estrogen-progestin combination. It also reflected the commonly held belief that pregnancy can improve endometriosis, a belief that has been disputed. The side effects of treatment are those associated with oral contraceptives. Pregnancy rates after stopping medication are reported to be in the 40–50% range. Whereas published recurrence rates are not excessive, this therapy, as with all hormone treatment for endometriosis, must be viewed as suppressive rather than curative.

3. true   p.859

Although hormonal therapy of infertility associated with endometriosis is not of proven value, medical therapy for dysmenorrhea, dyspareunia, and pelvic pain associated with endometriosis is very successful (although relief may be short-term). The various agents used are comparable in terms of efficacy. Implants of endometriosis react to steroid hormones in a manner somewhat, but not exactly, similar to normally stimulated endometrium. However, endometriotic tissue displays histologic differences and biochemical differences, including enzyme activity and receptor levels which differ in concentration and response compared to normal endometrium. Nevertheless, estrogen stimulates growth of the implants. For this reason, endometriosis usually regresses following menopause and is usually not found prior to menarche unless there is a blockage of the outflow tract.

4. true   p.860

The golden age for danazol has passed. Although its expense and side effects seemed a reasonable tradeoff for an effective treatment, it is now apparent that danazol is no more effective than the other medications used to treat endometriosis.

5. E   p.854

The following arguments can be used to defend the coelomic metaplasia theory:

1. Endometriosis occurs in adolescent girls in the absence of müllerian anomalies, and it can be discovered a few years after menarche before many menstrual cycles have been experienced.
2. Endometriosis has been reported in a prepubertal girl.

3. Endometriosis has been encountered in women who never menstruated.
4. Endometiosis in unusual sites such as thumb, thigh, or knee can be explained by the fact that mesenchymal limb buds develop adjacent to coelomic epithelium during early embyrogenesis.
5. Although usually associated with high dose estrogen treatment, endometriosis does occur in men.

Answers for Chapter 28 – Post-Test Questions

1. ectopic; stroma p.853

Endometriosis is a term indicating ectopic endometrial glands and stroma (outside the uterus), and in its clinical manifestations it is a progressive disease that is a vexing problem for both patient and clinician. However, clinical studies over the past decade have provided information for a better understanding of the disease and better decision-making regarding management options.

2. 3–10%; 25–35% p.855

Widely varying figures for the prevalence of endometriosis have been published, and a rough estimate is that 3–10% of women in the reproductive age group and 25–35% of infertile women have endometriosis. About 4 per 1,000 women age 15–64 are hospitalized with endometriosis each year, slightly more than those admitted with breast cancer.

3. antigen; epithelial p.855

CA-125 is a cell surface antigen found on derivatives of the coelomic epithelium (which includes endometrium), and it is a useful marker in the monitoring of women with epithelial ovarian carcinoma. In addition, serum CA-125 levels are often elevated in patients with endometriosis and correlate with both the degree of disease and the response to treatment. The sensitivity of this assay is too low to use it as a screening test, but it can be a marker of response to treatment and for recurrence; however, elevated levels which suppress during medical treatment often promptly return to pretreatment concentrations immediately after cessation of therapy, limiting its clinical usefulness. Serum CA-125 determinations may be able to differentiate endometriotic from nonendometriotic benign adnexal cysts. Note that CA-125 levels can be elevated by early pregnancy, acute pelvic inflammatory disease, leiomyomata, and menstruation.

4. varied p.856

The appearance of endometriosis is quite varied. All too often the clinician fails to observe endometrial lesions because of a preconceived expectation limited to the classic blue or black powder burn appearance. Lesions can be red, black, blue, or white and nonpigmented. Biopsies from visibly normal peritoneum can contain endometriosis in 6–13% of infertile women; however, the clinical significance of this presence is uncertain (and, in our view, unlikely to be important). Adhesions, peritoneal defects, and tan, creamy, fresh-appearing endometrium also can be observed. The dark pigmented lesions are later consequences of tissue bleeding responses to cyclic hormones. The ovary is the most common site for both implants and adhesions, followed by widespread distribution, anteriorly and posteriorly, over the broad ligament and cul-de-sac.

5. midline p.858

Presacral neurectomy does not enhance fertility, although many surgeons advocate it to alleviate dysmenorrhea. This may be less compelling now that prostaglandin inhibitors are available to accomplish the same purpose. A careful study of presacral neurectomy concluded that this procedure is only indicated in patients with pain limited to the midline area.

6. Conservative p.858

The type of surgery that we have been discussing is labeled "conservative" to indicate that reproductive function is maintained. When endometriomas are removed a vigorous attempt should be made to leave behind any normal ovarian tissue. Even one-tenth of an ovary can be enough to preserve function and fertility. Conservative surgery can be accomplished by laparoscopy which decreases costs and morbidity, yet provides results that are as efficacious in all stages of disease as laparotomy.

7. stimulation; bleeding　　　　　　　　　　　　　　　　　　　　　　　　　　　　p.859

Hormonal therapy is designed to interrupt the cycle of stimulation and bleeding. The various agents used are comparable in terms of efficacy. Implants of endometriosis react to steroid hormones in a manner somewhat, but not exactly, similar to normally stimulated endometrium. However, endometriotic tissue displays histologic differences and biochemical differences, including enzyme activity and receptor levels which differ in concentration and response compared to normal endometrium. Nevertheless, estrogen stimulates growth of the implants. For this reason, endometriosis usually regresses following menopause and is usually not found prior to menarche unless there is a blockage of the outflow tract.

8. high; low　　　　　　　　　　　　　　　　　　　　　　　　　　　　　　　　p.861

The multiple effects of danazol produce a high androgen, low estrogen environment that does not support the growth of endometriosis, and the amenorrhea that is produced prevents new seeding from the uterus into the peritoneal cavity.

9. decidualization; atrophy　　　　　　　　　　　　　　　　　　　　　　　　　　p.862

Both oral and injectable medroxyprogesterone acetate have been effective in treating endometriosis by causing decidualization and subsequent atrophy of endometrial tissue. Medroxyprogesterone acetate in an oral dose of 30 mg daily has been demonstrated to be as effective as danazol in treating endometriosis. Similar results have been obtained with higher doses. For this reason and because it is more cost-effective and there are fewer side effects, medroxyprogesterone acetate is often the first choice for medical treatment of endometriosis. High doses of medroxyprogesterone can adversely affect the lipoprotein profile; there is no reason to use a dose greater than 30 mg/day. Megestrol acetate has been administered in a dose of 40 mg daily with good results.

10. pseudomenopause　　　　　　　　　　　　　　　　　　　　　　　　　　　　p.862

A long-acting GnRH agonist can create a pseudomenopause for the treatment of endometriosis. At the end of 2–4 weeks of daily administration of the agonist, estrogen levels will decrease to those found in oophorectomized women. Dosage can be adjusted by monitoring serum estradiol levels; the best therapeutic effect is associated with a range of 20–40 pg/mL (75–150 pmol/L). Thus, the "medical oophorectomy" caused by the continuous use of a GnRH agonist has provided a new approach to the treatment of endometriosis. Excellent, large, well-designed studies (with advanced disease in nearly 50% of the patients) have compared GnRH agonist therapy (with various agents) with danazol. The results in terms of reduction of disease (as demonstrated by post-treatment laparoscopies) and pregnancy rates have been the same with either treatment. However, GnRH agonist treatment does not have an adverse impact on serum lipids and lipoproteins compared to that observed with danazol. An experimental comparison of agonist and progestin treatment in monkeys concluded that the progestin was just as effective as the agonist.

11. greater　　　　　　　　　　　　　　　　　　　　　　　　　　　　　　　　　p.864

Endometriosis tends to recur unless definitive surgery is performed. The recurrence rate is approximately 5–20% per year (reaching a cumulative rate at 5 years as much as 40%). The recurrence rates 5 years after women were treated with various GnRH agonists were 37% for minimal disease and 74% for severe disease. After 7 years, 56% of all treated women had a recurrence. In women treated for pelvic pain, the symptoms usually return rather quickly after cessation of therapy. For a period of time after medical treatment, however, the intensity of symptoms is less severe. The recurrence rates after treatment with GnRH agonists are similar to those after danazol, and both are greater than that obtained with surgical excision.

12. true　　　　　　　　　　　　　　　　　　　　　　　　　　　　　　　　　　p.854

Endometriosis can occur in almost every organ of the body. For example, pulmonary endometriosis occurs and can be manifested by asymptomatic nodules or as pneumothorax, hemothorax, or hemoptysis during menses. Urologic endometriosis is of importance because of the possiblity for ureteral obstruction.

13. false　　　　　　　　　　　　　　　　　　　　　　　　　　　　　　　　　　p.855

The common perceptions that endometriosis only occurs in goal-oriented women over the age of 30 and is not found often in black women have now been discredited. Whereas endometriosis essentially does not occur before menarche, there are increasing reports of its occurrence in the teen years. A number of these cases involve anatomic abnormalities that obstruct the outflow tract.

14. true   p.855
Endometriosis is not confined to nulliparous women, and physicians should be alert to the presence of endometriosis in cases of secondary infertility.

15. false   p.856
The uterus is often in fixed retroversion and the ovaries may be enlarged. However, retroversion of the uterus is not an etiologic factor, and prophylactic uterine suspension is no longer recommended. Nodularity (which is usually tender) of the uterosacral ligaments and cul-de-sac can be found in one-third of patients with endometriosis. The diagnosis almost always should be confirmed by laparoscopy before treatment is initiated. Minimal findings such as slight beading and tenderness of the uterosacral ligaments in the young, asymptomatic patient can be treated, however, with combined, low dose oral contraceptives.

16. true   p.856
The appearance of endometriosis is quite varied. All too often the clinician fails to observe endometrial lesions because of a preconceived expectation limited to the classic blue or black powder burn appearance. Lesions can be red, black, blue, or white and nonpigmented. Biopsies from visibly normal peritoneum can contain endometriosis in 6–13% of infertile women; however, the clinical significance of this presence is uncertain (and, in our view, unlikely to be important). Adhesions, peritoneal defects, and tan, creamy, fresh-appearing endometrium also can be observed. The dark pigmented lesions are later consequences of tissue bleeding responses to cyclic hormones. The ovary is the most common site for both implants and adhesions, followed by widespread distribution, anteriorly and posteriorly, over the broad ligament and cul-de-sac.

17. true   p.856
Because both treatment and prognosis are determined to some extent by the severity of the disease, it is desirable to have a uniform system of classification that takes into account both the extent and severity of the disease. A uniform classification is also crucial for comparing the results of different treatments. The American Fertility Society developed a classification system based on findings at laparoscopy or laparotomy, and forms are available from the Society. However, there were weaknesses in the classification system, especially the fact that it was based upon the arbitrary impressions of the clinician. A second form was produced to standardize the documentation of findings in patients who have pelvic pain and endometriosis. There can be a high intraobserver and interobserver variability in the evaluation of endometriosis using a classification system. Therefore, efforts must continue to provide a useful method for staging.

18. true   p.856
When endometriosis involves the ovaries and causes adhesions that block tubal motility and pickup of the egg, there is no question of its role in causing mechanical interference with fertility. Less secure is the information on the role of peritoneal endometriosis on fertility. Many physicians believe that even minimal endometriosis can cause infertility. This argument has been weakened by a failure to find benefit from medical treatment of infertility associated with minimal to mild endometriosis.

19. false   p.857
Another mediator could be prostaglandins produced by the implants, which could, in turn, affect tubal motility, or folliculogenesis and corpus luteum function. Patients with endometriosis have been reported to have an increase in both the volume of peritoneal fluid and the concentration of thromboxane B_2 and 6-keto-prostaglandin $F_1 a$ in the fluid. Others, however, found neither an increase in peritoneal fluid nor an increase in concentration of peritoneal fluid prostaglandin E_2, prostaglandin $F_{2\alpha}$, 15-keto-13,14-dihydroprostaglandin $F_{2\alpha}$, and thromboxane B_2.

20. false   p.857
Luteinized unruptured follicle syndrome (LUF) in which the oocyte is not released at the time of follicle rupture (or there is a failure of the follicle to rupture) has been suggested as a cause of both unexplained infertility and infertility secondary to endometriosis. Although an unruptured follicle can occur in women, there currently is no impressive evidence that this syndrome is secondary to endometriosis or is even a cause of infertility.

21. true   p.858

It should be emphasized that based on monthly fecundity rates and life table analyses, no study has shown an advantage for conservative surgery as opposed to expectant management.

22. true   p.859

Endometriotic tissue displays histologic differences and biochemical differences, including enzyme activity and receptor levels which differ in concentration and response compared to normal endometrium. Nevertheless, estrogen stimulates growth of the implants. For this reason, endometriosis usually regresses following menopause and is usually not found prior to menarche unless there is a blockage of the outflow tract.

23. true   p.861

Because danazol has been associated with the development *in utero* of female pseudohermaphroditism, it should not be given if there is the possibility of pregnancy. The androgenic action of danazol can irreversibly deepen the voice. It is worth enquiring whether singing is an important part of your patient's life.

24. E   p.853,854

The conclusions of Sampson have been validated by the following observations:

1. During laparoscopy, flow of blood from the fimbriated end of the tube has been observed in virtually all menstruating women.
2. Endometriosis is most commonly found in dependent portions of the pelvis, most frequently on the ovaries, the anterior and posterior cul-de-sac, and the uterosacral ligaments, followed by the posterior uterus and posterior broad ligaments.
3. Endometrial fragments from the menstrual flow can grow both in tissue culture and following injection beneath the abdominal skin, and can be retrieved from the peritoneal fluid of most menstruating women.
4. Endometriosis developed when the cervices of monkeys were transposed so that menstruation occurred into the peritoneal cavity.
5. A higher incidence of endometriosis is observed in women who have obstructions to the outward flow of the menstrual effluvium.
6. The risk of endometriosis is increased in women with shorter menstrual cycles and longer flows, characteristics that give greater opportunity for ectopic endometrial implantation.

25. A   p.853,854

Endometriosis at sites distant from the pelvis may be due to vascular or lymphatic transport of endometrial fragments. Even the common occurrence of endometriosis on the ovaries can be explained by lymphatic flow from the uterus to the ovary. There are case reports of endometriosis in men who received treatment with estrogen, and therefore, another possible cause of endometriosis is the transformation of coelomic epithelium into endometrial-type glands as a result of unspecified stimuli. Because many women have reflux seeding of menstrual debris into the peritoneal cavity, and not all develop endometriosis, there may be genetic or immunologic factors that influence the susceptibility of a woman to the disease.

A consideration of the etiologic theories regarding endometriosis leads to the conclusion that all of these mechanisms may contribute to the clinical problem in an individual patient, and the degree of contribution for each probably varies from patient to patient. Endometrial cells can be spread by mechanical means, or perhaps can arise by metaplasia, and progression of the disease is influenced by the individual's immune mechanisms.

26. C   p.855

Dysmenorrhea is even more suggestive of endometriosis if it begins after years of relatively pain-free menses. It should be recognized, however, that many women who have endometriosis are asymptomatic. A common observation is that some women with extensive endometriosis have little or no pain, whereas others with only minimal endometriosis complain of severe pain. Very severe pain, however, is associated with deeply infiltrating endometriosis. Pain can be diffuse in the pelvis or it can be more localized, often in the area of the rectum. Symptoms also can arise from rectal, ureteral, or bladder involvement with endometriosis, and can be present throughout the month. Blockage of the ureter can occur, and urinary tract symptoms should be investigated with urologic and radiologic techniques. Low back pain, too, may be due to endometriosis. An association of endometriosis and premenstrual spotting has been suggested, but in most cases menstrual dysfunction is not increased with endometriosis. An association between galactorrhea and endometriosis has been claimed, but baseline elevations of prolactin are not higher in patients with endometriosis compared to normal women.

27. B   p.855,856

CA-125 is a cell surface antigen found on derivatives of the coelomic epithelium (which includes endometrium), and it is a useful marker in the monitoring of women with epithelial ovarian carcinoma. In addition, serum CA-125 levels are often elevated in patients with endometriosis and correlate with both the degree of disease and the response to treatment. The sensitivity of this assay is too low to use it as a screening test, but it can be a marker of response to treatment and for recurrence; however, elevated levels which suppress during medical treatment often promptly return to pretreatment concentrations immediately after cessation of therapy, limiting its clinical usefulness. Serum CA-125 determinations may be able to differentiate endometriotic from nonendometriotic benign adnexal cysts. Note that CA-125 levels can be elevated by early pregnancy, acute pelvic inflammatory disease, leiomyomata, and menstruation.

28. A   p.858

In contrast to the dispute over the proper treatment of mild endometriosis, there is little doubt that adhesive disease associated with endometriosis, or large (>2 cm) endometriomas, is best treated by surgery. The object of surgery should be to restore normal anatomical relationships and to excise or fulgurate as much of the endometriosis as possible. Removal of severely diseased adnexa when the other side is more normal produces better results than attempts to do major repairs. Presacral neurectomy does not enhance fertility, although many surgeons advocate it to alleviate dysmenorrhea. This may be less compelling now that prostaglandin inhibitors are available to accomplish the same purpose. A careful study of presacral neurectomy concluded that this procedure is only indicated in patients with pain limited to the midline area.

29. B   p.858

The success of surgery in relieving infertility is directly related to the severity of endometriosis. Patients with moderate disease can expect a pregnancy success of approximately 60%, whereas the comparable figure is 35% in those with severe disease. There is no convincing evidence that surgical treatment of early endometriosis enhances fertility. There is support for selective use of danazol for 2–3 months following laparoscopy and prior to conservative surgery, especially in patients with pain due to major disease. Similar favorable effects should result from the preoperative treatment with a progestin or a gonadotropin releasing hormone agonist. Preoperative treatment aids surgery by softening endometrial implants. Postoperative use of hormones has been the subject of greater controversy. The highest pregnancy rates following conservative surgery occur in the first year after surgery, and most physicians have been reluctant to use hormones that prevent pregnancy even for a few months. If pregnancy does not occur within 2 years of surgery for endometriosis, the chances are poor that pregnancy will occur. The recurrence rates reported for endometriosis after surgery are usually below 20%, but when it does recur, second surgeries to aid fertility have only a limited chance for success.

30. C   p.859,862

Hormonal therapy is designed to interrupt the cycle of stimulation and bleeding. An early approach was the use of massive doses of diethylstilbestrol (DES), which, because of variable success, the risk of affecting the fetus, and side effects of severe bleeding and nausea, is now of only historical interest. Treatment with androgens (methyltestosterone linguets 5–10 mg/day) can provide only transient relief of the pain of endometriosis, and its effect on infertility appears to be negligible. In addition, ovulation can occur while on treatment, and there is a risk of exposure of the fetus to the androgen.

Until the late 1970s the most important alternative to conservative surgery was the use of combination oral contraceptives taken in a continuous fashion. It seems to matter little which low dose monophasic product is used to accomplish the conversion of endometrial implants into decidualized cells associated with a few inactive endometrial glands. At this time the efficacy of the multiphasic formulations is unknown.

31. E p.860
The multiple actions of danazol include:

1. Binding to androgen, progesterone, and glucocorticoid receptors, producing both agonistic and antagonistic actions.
2. No binding to intracellular estrogen receptors.
3. Binding to sex hormone binding globulin (displacing testosterone and thus increasing free testosterone) and to corticosteroid binding globulin (with a small increase in free cortisol).
4. Decrease in sex hormone binding globulin production by the liver as well as an increase in a host of other liver proteins.
5. Prevention of the midcycle surge of FSH and LH, but no significant suppression of basal FSH or LH (mainly an androgen agonistic action).
6. No effect on aromatization.
7. Inhibition of the following enzymes involved in steroidogenesis:
   cholesterol side chain cleavage enzyme (P450scc)
   3β-hydroxysteroid dehydrogenase
   17β-hydroxysteroid dehydrogenase
   17-hydroxylase, 17,20-lyase (P450c17)
   11β-hydroxylase (P450c11)
   21-hydroxylase (P450c21)

32. E p.861
The side effects of danazol are related both to the hypoestrogenic environment it creates and to its androgenic properties. The most common side effects are weight gain, fluid retention, fatigue, decreased breast size, acne, oily skin, growth of facial hair, atrophic vaginitis, hot flushes, muscle cramps, and emotional lability. Some of these side effects occur in approximately 80% of women who are taking danazol, but less than 10% find the side effects sufficiently troublesome to warrant discontinuation of the drug.

33. C p.861
Danazol is metabolized largely in the liver, and in some patients it causes hepatocellular damage. Its use, therefore, is contraindicated in women with liver disease. Furthermore, liver enzymes should be monitored during treatment with danazol. The fluid retention that is often associated with danazol makes it dangerous to use when there is severe hypertension, congestive heart failure, or impaired renal function. It can produce increased cholesterol and low-density lipoprotein levels and decreased levels of high-density lipoprotein. It is unlikely that these short-term effects on lipids and lipoproteins are clinically important. The drug has been used to treat autoimmune disease, but it is not known if this action plays a role in its effects on endometriosis.

34. E p.862
Side effects of progestational agents include weight gain, fluid retention, and breakthrough bleeding. Breakthrough bleeding is a common occurrence although it is usually cleared by short-term (7 days) administration of estrogen. Depression is a significant problem, and both patient and physician should be alert for its development. The usefulness of depo-medroxyprogesterone acetate (150 mg im every 3 months) in infertile patients is limited by the varying length of time it takes for ovulation to resume after discontinuation of therapy. This is not a problem with oral administration.

35. B p.862
Both oral and injectable medroxyprogesterone acetate have been effective in treating endometriosis by causing decidualization and subsequent atrophy of endometrial tissue. Medroxyprogesterone acetate in an oral dose of 30 mg daily has been demonstrated to be as effective as danazol in treating endometriosis. Similar results have been obtained with higher doses. For this reason and because it is more cost-effective and there are fewer side effects, medroxyprogesterone acetate is often the first choice for medical treatment of endometriosis. High doses of medroxyprogesterone can adversely affect the lipoprotein profile; there is no reason to use a dose greater than 30 mg/day. Megestrol acetate has been administered in a dose of 40 mg daily with good results.

Medroxyprogesterone acetate, like danazol, can relieve the symptoms of endometriosis, but it is not effective in treating infertility. In a prospective, randomized clinical trial, there was no difference in pregnancy rates following treatment with medroxyprogesterone acetate (100 mg/day) or placebo.

36. B   p.862,863

Gonadotropin releasing hormone has a short half-life because it is rapidly cleaved between amino acids 5–6, 6–7, and 9–10. Analogues of GnRH have been produced by altering the amino acids at these positions. Substitutions of amino acids at the 6 position and/or replacement of the C-terminal glycine-amide (inhibiting degradation) produce agonists. The GnRH agonists are administered intramuscularly, subcutaneously, or by intranasal absorption. After an initial agonistic action (the so-called flare response), down-regulation and desensitization of the pituitary produce a hypogonadotropic, hypogonad state. The depot formulation of leuprolide is administered intramuscularly and monthly. Goserelin consists of a small biodegradable cylinder which is inserted subcutaneously and monthly using a prepackaged syringe.

A long-acting GnRH agonist can create a pseudomenopause for the treatment of endometriosis. At the end of 2–4 weeks of daily administration of the agonist, estrogen levels will decrease to those found in oophorectomized women. Dosage can be adjusted by monitoring serum estradiol levels; the best therapeutic effect is associated with a range of 20–40 pg/mL (75–150 pmol/L). Thus, the "medical oophorectomy" caused by the continuous use of a GnRH agonist has provided a new approach to the treatment of endometriosis. Excellent, large, well-designed studies (with advanced disease in nearly 50% of the patients) have compared GnRH agonist therapy (with various agents) with danazol. The results in terms of reduction of disease (as demonstrated by post-treatment laparoscopies) and pregnancy rates have been the same with either treatment.

37. C   p.863,864

GnRH agonist treatment does not have an adverse impact on serum lipids and lipoproteins compared to that observed with danazol. An experimental comparison of agonist and progestin treatment in monkeys concluded that the progestin was just as effective as the agonist.

As with all other drug therapies of endometriosis, the GnRH agonist provides suppression rather than cure of the disease. The long-term consequences of the hypoestrogenic state on calcium metabolism and bone are of concern. Therefore, treatment is usually limited to 6 months to avoid bone loss, although even during this time period there can be a 6–8% decrease in trabecular bone density. This short-term bone loss is reversed after cessation of therapy; however, many patients as much as one year later have not regained the bone that was lost. Long-term therapy, therefore, carries with it the concern over a lasting impact on the risk of osteoporosis. The addition of a progestational agent as add-back treatment can be effective in decreasing bone loss. A postmenopausal estrogen-progestin program can be utilized (conjugated estrogens 0.625 mg daily and medroxyprogesterone acetate 2.5 mg daily). This combined add-back treatment is effective for endometriosis and prevents the hypoestrogenic symptoms (especially hot flushes and vaginal dryness) associated with GnRH agonist therapy, including loss of bone. Endometriosis by itself is not a cause of accelerated bone loss.

38. D   p.864

Definitive surgery for severe endometriosis, which includes abdominal hysterectomy and bilateral salpingo-oophorectomy as well as resection of all endometriosis, is the only cure for the disease. If oophorectomy is performed, estrogen-progestin therapy at usual doses can be started immediately postoperatively with an essentially negligible risk of inciting growth of residual endometriosis. The addition of a progestational agent is strongly recommended because of reported cases of adenocarcinoma in endometriosis tissue in women treated with unopposed estrogen.

39. E   p.865

A common clinical problem is the incidental finding at surgery of mild endometriosis in a young woman who has no immediate interest in pregnancy. Cyclic combination oral contraceptives to prevent further seeding are appropriate for treatment of very mild disease, for example a few implants in the cul-de-sac. More advanced disease should be treated with 6 months of medroxyprogesterone acetate, a GnRH agonist, or danazol, followed by cyclic oral contraceptives to decrease the risks of progression of the disease. Although not well documented, clinical experience has suggested that continuous oral contraceptives are more effective as prophylaxis than the usual cyclic regimen. Indeed, we favor the continuous regimen without a break for this purpose.

40. B p.865

The use of superovulation with intrauterine insemination has been reported to increase fecundity rates in women with infertility associated with endometriosis. However, although superovulation raised fecundity rates, it did not raise cumulative pregnancy rates. This treatment may accelerate the occurrence of pregnancy without changing overall fertility.

Individuals with mild to moderate endometriosis do as well in in vitro fertilization programs as those with tubal disease. Although results with severe endometriosis have been poor in the past, more recent experience (perhaps reflecting improved technique and technology) has yielded good pregnancy rates.

29 Male Infertility

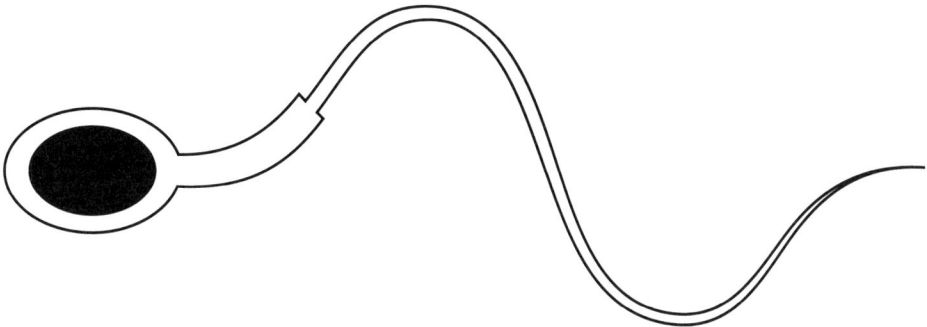

Learning Objectives

Be able to:

1. Explain the basic anatomy and physiology of the male reproductive system.

2. Describe the components of a semen analysis and the possible reasons each parameter is abnormal.

3. Detail the methods and principles of the sperm penetration assay (SPA) and the immunobead assay.

4. Discuss the arguments in favor and against varicocele repair.

5. Understand the possible benefits and side effects associated with gonadotropin superovulation and intrauterine insemination.

Pre-Test

A. Instructions: Fill in the blanks

1. It can take _____ months for the testes to recover from an insult and thus, it is reasonable to space semen specimens over time.

2. On the basis of the available literature, currently the 2 best tests for assaying fertility potential for in vitro fertilization are the evaluation of sperm morphology by _____ _____ and the human _____ _____ assay.

B. Instructions: True or False

3. Over the last 40 years there is evidence which points to a decreasing sperm count in men.

4. A fundamental problem in most studies of the efficacy of drug therapy in male infertility is the lack of a control group for comparison.

C. Instructions: For each of the following questions choose:

A. if only 1, 2 and 3 are correct
B. if only 1 and 3 are correct
C. if only 2 and 4 are correct
D. if only 4 is correct
E. if all are correct

5. The sperm penetration assay (SPA)
   1. involves the removal of the zona from superovulated hamster oocytes
   2. is positive when the presence of a swollen sperm head is noted in the egg cytoplasm
   3. involves culturing denuded oocytes with human sperm for 2–3 hours
   4. can be reported as the percentage of eggs penetrated compared to the percent penetrated by a known fertile sperm specimen

6. The immunobead test
   1. is a test of sperm function
   2. provides identification of the class of antibodies on the sperm
   3. will be positive in any sperm sample showing agglutination
   4. provides the site on the sperm where the beads are adherent

Post-Test

A. Instructions: Fill in the blanks

1. _____% of infertility is wholly or in part due to a male factor.

2. The testes have 2 distinct components, the seminiferous tubules (site of _____) and the Leydig cells (source of _____).

3. _____ at normal levels stimulates testosterone secretion, whereas hypersecretion of _____ leads to reduced testosterone secretion.

4. The Sertoli cells are controlled by 2 hormones, _____ and _____.

5. Spermatogenesis requires a very high local concentration of _____ and _____.

6. _____ is synthesized in the Sertoli cells in response to FSH and specifically inhibits _____ secretion in the pituitary.

7. The seminiferous tubules and the intraluminal environment are controlled by the _____ cells. Tight junctions between the _____ cells effectively seal off the tubules, creating the blood-testis barrier. The _____ cells are in the connective tissue between the seminiferous tubules.

8. The _____ _____ of the oocyte is impervious to foreign sperm and prevents polyspermia under normal circumstances.

B. Instructions: True or False

9. In men virtually all the estrone and estradiol present is derived from androstenedione and testosterone.

10. Testosterone binds to Sertoli cells and stimulates the production of the androgen binding protein (ABP).

11. There is no age-related decline in spermatogenesis that results in some decline in male fertility.

12. Increasing ejaculatory frequency more than every 2–3 days reduces the volume and count but has no significant impact on morphology and motility.

13. Semen liquefaction which occurs 20–30 minutes after ejaculation, is a necessary prerequisite for doing an accurate analysis.

14. At least 2 or 3 samples must be screened before an individual can be categorized as potentially fertile or infertile.

15. Computer-associated semen analysis (CASA) is the most accurate means of performing a sperm count.

16. It is important that any infection in the genitourinary tract be treated because white cells in the seminal plasma can significantly reduce sperm motility and egg penetration.

17. Hormone treatment of infertile males who do not have an endocrine disorder is sometimes useful.

C. Instructions: For each of the following questions choose:

   A. if only 1, 2 and 3 are correct
   B. if only 1 and 3 are correct
   C. if only 2 and 4 are correct
   D. if only 4 is correct
   E. if all are correct

18. Spermatozoa
    1. require 74 days for production
    2. reside in the seminiferous tubule for 50 days
    3. after leaving the testes take up to 3 weeks to travel the epididymis and appear in the ejaculate
    4. are haploid

19. The semen is composed of secretions which are contributed by
    1. prostate
    2. contents of the distal vas deferens
    3. seminal vesicle secretions
    4. corpus cavernosum

20. The most recent WHO criteria (1992) for semen analysis suggests normal values which include
    1. a normal morphology of 40% or more
    2. 50% or more with forward progression
    3. fewer than 40% spermatozoa with adherent particles on an immunobead test
    4. a sperm concentration of 20 million/ml or more

21. Kruger's "strict criteria" of semen analysis
    1. shift many sperm out of the traditional normal category
    2. are not subject to interobserver differences
    3. have been shown to be associated with fertilization rates in IVF programs
    4. have been shown to be associated with pregnancy rates in superovulation-IUI programs

22. Limitations of the sperm penetration assay (SPA) include
    1. its lack of standardization
    2. its prognostic value
    3. its variability within an individual over time
    4. its discomfort to the patient

23. The human zona binding assay
    1. has limited variability between laboratories
    2. evaluates the ability of sperm to bind to the zona
    3. is currently the gold standard for assessing fertilization potential
    4. depends on the limited availability of zonae in order to perform the test

24. Tests of sperm function commonly used in clinical practice include
    1. the hypoosmotic swelling test
    2. measurement of adenosine triphosphate
    3. measurement of the acrosome reaction
    4. sperm penetration assay

Chapter 29 Male Infertility

25. Sperm antibodies can form following
    1. vasectomy
    2. disruption of the blood-testis barrier
    3. testicular torsion
    4. infection

26. Contemporary treatment of sperm antibodies may include
    1. corticosteroids
    2. condoms
    3. intrauterine insemination of washed sperm
    4. aspirin

27. If the semen analysis is abnormal, inquiry should be made regarding the presence of the following factors
    1. history of heavy marijuana use
    2. history of cocaine
    3. coital frequency
    4. heat

28. A workup for obstruction or absence of the vas deferens may involve
    1. testing for the presence of fructose in the semen
    2. cystoscopy
    3. testicular biopsy
    4. retrograde ureterogram

29. An endocrine workup for male infertility may involve testing for
    1. gonadotropins
    2. prolactin
    3. testosterone
    4. thyroid function

30. Varicocele
    1. repair has been subject to a randomized study
    2. is present in 25–30% of infertile males
    3. ligation results in a 70–80% pregnancy rate
    4. is present in 10–15% of males in the general population

31. Potential complications associated with superovulation-IUI using gonadotropins include a 20%
    1. pelvic inflammatory disease rate
    2. multiple pregnancy rate
    3. severe ovarian hyperstimulation rate
    4. spontaneous miscarriage rate

32. Donor inseminations
    1. are associated with a 70% success rate over 5–6 cycles using fresh semen
    2. are associated with a higher success rate using fresh rather than frozen sperm
    3. are associated with the same background congenital anomaly rate of 4–5% following intercourse
    4. use sperm which have been cryopreserved and quarantined for at least 6 months

Answers for Chapter 29 — Pre-Test Questions

1. 2.5   p.877

To add to the difficulties of diagnosing male infertility is the variability in count and motility that can be seen in successive semen specimens from the same individual. This leads to one truism: at least two or preferably three samples must be screened before an individual can be categorized as potentially fertile, subfertile, or infertile (azoospermia). Because it can take 2.5 months for the testes to recover from an insult, it is reasonable to space the specimens over a longer period of time.

2. strict criteria; zona binding   p.880

On the basis of the available literature, currently the 2 best tests for assaying fertility potential for in vitro fertilization are the evaluation of sperm morphology by strict criteria and the human zona binding assay. However, both require standardization and some skills beyond the qualifications of most clinical laboratories, and thus they will not be universally applicable. The use of computer-driven assessments of sperm morphology may provide the information and universal availability needed to make this test a gold standard for evaluating the male. However, past experience suggests that no one test will ever be sufficient to test all the qualities of the sperm that are necessary for successful fertilization.

3. true   p.877

There is reason to believe that sperm counts are decreasing. In MacLeod's 1951 report, 5% of fertile men had counts below 20 million, while today 20–25% of fertile men have counts below 20 million. The mean sperm count in Denmark in 1990 was 66 million/mL compared to 113 million/mL in 1940. An argument can be made for an impact due to increased toxins in our environment. Despite suggestions that there is a decrease in sperm counts, the percent of American married couples who were infertile did not change significantly between 1962 and 1988. Thus, the apparent decrease in sperm count is not reflected in a parallel change in the rate of infertility.

4. true   p.886

A fundamental problem in most studies of the efficacy of drug therapy in male fertility is the lack of a control group for comparison. Investigators make the erroneous assumption that the spontaneous cure rate of male infertility is zero and that any pregnancy that occurs during or following treatment is due solely to that treatment. A number of studies, however, have attested to the spontaneous cure rate of male infertility. In one study approximately one-third of males with counts below 10 million/mL who were not treated successfully impregnated their partners. In summary, hormone treatment of infertile males who do not have an endocrine disorder is almost always unrewarding, and it does not improve fertility beyond what occurs by chance.

5. E   p.879

The zona pellucida of most mammalian species presents not only a block to polyspermia but also a barrier to fertilization of an egg by sperm of a different species. However, if the zona is removed by gentle enzyme digestion, foreign sperm can fuse with and penetrate an egg. In the sperm penetration assay, eggs are collected from superovulated golden hamsters; the zonae are removed by enzymes, and the denuded eggs are cultured for 2–3 hours with human sperm that have been washed and incubated overnight in culture media. Presence of a swollen sperm head in the egg cytoplasm is evidence of successful penetration. Most laboratories report the percentage of eggs penetrated and compare this figure to the percent penetrated by a known fertile sperm specimen (some laboratories use the criterion of number of sperm penetrations per egg with 2 or more considered normal). Whereas the concept of the SPA as a measure of sperm fertilizing ability is an attractive one, the practical aspects of the test have hindered its standardization. For example, the source of the albumin used as the protein supplement in the media can influence the result as can use of resuspended compared to swimup sperm. Moreover, an individual's results in the SPA can vary over time. In addition, different laboratories utilize different cutoff points for the lower limit of normal penetration with the most common points being 0, 10, 14, and 20%.

6. C   p.882

The immunobead test has beads labeled with anti-IgG, anti-IgA, or anti-IgM and thus it provides identification of the class of antibodies on the sperm. The site on the sperm where the beads are adherent also can be noted. Anti-IgA localizes to the tail and anti-IgG to the head of the sperm. Antibody localized only to the tip of the tail usually is not significant, whereas antibody on the rest of the tail may interfere with sperm motility. Antibodies on the head of the sperm can cause failure of fusion with the egg.

Answers for Chapter 29 — Post-Test Questions

1. 40%   p.873

The perception of the degree of male involvement in infertility has undergone a number of revisions during the past 50 years. Initially, infertility was considered primarily a female problem. This notion gave way to the realization that 40% of infertility is wholly or in part due to a male factor. More recently, there have been attempts to redefine, in a downward direction, the lower limit of "normal" for a sperm count. Thus, many men who in the past would have been categorized as subfertile now are considered normal, and the focus has returned to their female partners.

2. spermatogenesis; testosterone   p.873

The testes have 2 distinct components, the seminiferous tubules (site of spermatogenesis) and the Leydig cells (source of testosterone). The function of these 2 components requires both pituitary gonadotropins, follicle-stimulating hormone (FSH) and luteinizing hormone (LH). The primary effect of LH is to stimulate the synthesis and secretion of testosterone by Leydig cells (about 5–10 mg per day), an effect that is enhanced by FSH, which also binds to Leydig cells and increases the number of LH receptors on the cells. Increasing levels of testosterone, in turn, inhibit LH secretion, acutely through the hypothalamus and chronically at the pituitary level. This negative feedback action does not require aromatization to estrogen.

3. Prolactin; prolactin   p.874

Leydig cells contain receptors for prolactin. Prolactin at normal levels stimulates testosterone secretion, whereas hypersecretion of prolactin leads to reduced testosterone secretion. Although studies suggest that prolactin synergizes with LH and testosterone in the testes, a role for prolactin has not been established for normal testicular function.

4. FSH; testosterone   p.874

FSH, in conjunction with testosterone, acts on the seminiferous tubules to stimulate spermatogenesis. This effect may be mediated by activation of Sertoli cell function. The Sertoli cells are controlled by 2 hormones, FSH and testosterone.

5. testosterone; dihydrotestosterone   p.874

Spermatogenesis requires a very high local concentration of testosterone and dihydrotestosterone, 50 times higher than that present in the circulation and greater than can be administered exogenously. The ABP is secreted into the tubule lumen and binds testosterone and dihydrotestosterone as they diffuse into the lumen, concentrating the androgens in the seminiferous epithelium for spermatogenesis and in the epididymis for sperm maturation.

6. Inhibin; FSH   p.875

In contrast to the effects of testosterone on LH, steroid hormones at physiologic levels do not suppress FSH secretion. Orchiectomy is followed, however, by a rise in FSH levels. This phenomenon led to the discovery of inhibin. Inhibin is synthesized in the Sertoli cells in response to FSH and specifically inhibits FSH secretion in the pituitary. Inhibin has been found in seminal fluid, spermatozoa, and Sertoli cells. The story is more complicated in that inhibin is also found in Leydig cells, and its secretion is further modulated by LH, human chorionic gonadotropin (HCG), and testosterone. UndoubtedLy, autocrine/paracrine regulation by growth factors and local peptides is involved in a system analogous to the complex interaction in the ovarian follicle.

7. Sertoli; Sertoli; Leydig   p.875

The seminiferous tubules and the intraluminal environment are controlled by the Sertoli cells. Tight junctions between the Sertoli cells effectively seal off the tubules, creating the blood-testis barrier. The seminiferous tubules, therefore, are essentially avascular, and regulatory substances must enter by diffusion. The blood-testis barrier protects the germ cells from antigens, antibodies, and environmental toxins. The Leydig cells are in the connective tissue between the seminiferous tubules.

8. zona pellucida　　p.880

Whereas the SPA tests the ability of sperm to penetrate or to be engulfed by the egg, it does not test the critical ability to pass through the zona pellucida. The zonae are, of course, removed in preparation for the SPA because they are, with rare exceptions, impervious to foreign sperm. Thus, to test zona penetrating or zona binding ability of human sperm requires the use of human zonae.

9. true　　　p.873

In men virtually all the estrone and estradiol present is derived from androstenedione and testosterone; there is essentially no direct secretion of estrogen.

10. false　　p.874

FSH binds to Sertoli cells and stimulates the production of several proteins, chief of which is ABP, the androgen binding protein.

11. false　　p.876

There is an age-related decline in spermatogenesis that results in some decline in male fertility. Precise estimates of the magnitude of this decline are not available because this issue has not been studied. There is no doubt, however, that many elderly men continue to have the ability to produce pregnancies.

12. true　　　p.876

An abstinence period of 2–3 days prior to semen collection is adequate, although some urologists favor 5 days. Increasing the ejaculatory frequency reduces the volume and count but has no significant impact on quality (morphology and motility).

13. true　　　p.876

Semen liquefication, which occurs 20–30 minutes after ejaculation, is a necessary prerequisite for doing an accurate analysis. On occasion, a specimen does not undergo normal liquefication or is abnormally viscid, and, if this is associated with a poor postcoital test, it may be a factor in infertility. Techniques used to break up a viscid specimen in preparation for doing a sperm count or for artificial insemination include mechanically dispersing the gel by running the semen repeatedly through a number 19 needle, collecting the semen as a split ejaculate because the first part may be less viscid or treating the semen with proteolytic enzymes. If the postcoital test is normal, however, high viscosity probably is not an infertility factor.

14. true　　　p.877

To add to the difficulties of diagnosing male infertility is the variability in count and motility that can be seen in successive semen specimens from the same individual. This leads to one truism: at least two or preferably three samples must be screened before an individual can be categorized as potentially fertile, subfertile, or infertile (azoospermia).

15. false　　p.877

Confidence in any figure is limited by the inaccuracies inherent in the methods used for counting sperm. When a group of technicians and pathologists used a counting chamber to do a semen analysis on the same pooled specimen, the mean sperm count was 46.7 million/mL with a range of values lying between 10 and 98 million/mL giving a coefficient of variation of 37.8%. These inconsistent results are not necessarily remedied even with computer-assisted semen analysis (CASA). Significant errors can still occur with CASA, especially with specimens containing low numbers where other cells can be miscounted as sperm. Perhaps this is one reason it has been difficult to establish a prognostic value for the sperm count. A similar, albeit somewhat lesser, uncertainty surrounds assessments of sperm motility.

16. true　　　p.885

It is important that any infection in the genitourinary tract, including those caused by mycoplasma and chlamydia, be treated because white cells in the seminal plasma can significantly reduce sperm motility and egg penetration.

17. false   p.886

Hormone treatment of infertile males who do not have an endocrine disorder is almost always unrewarding, and it does not improve fertility beyond what occurs by chance.

18. E   p.875,876

Developing sperm are enveloped by Sertoli cells that influence the sequential process of spermatogenesis. Spermatogonia undergo mitotic division to form the primary spermatocytes, which in turn form the haploid (23 chromosomes) secondary spermatocytes by meiotic division. The secondary spermatocytes proceed through a maturation process to the spermatid stage, ultimately becoming the spermatozoa. In female somatic cells, one X chromosome is inactivated; however, in the oocyte both X chromosomes are genetically active. The opposite situation prevails in the male where the single X chromosome is genetically active in somatic cells but inactive in spermatogenesis. Normal spermatogenesis is directed by the genes on the Y chromosome, although many required regulating proteins are derived from autosomal chromosomes.

Most of the testis is composed of the tightly coiled seminiferous tubule, which, if uncoiled, would reach a length of 70 cm. Approximately 74 days are required to produce spermatozoa, about 50 days of which are spent in the tubule. After leaving the testes, sperm take 12–21 days to travel the epididymis (which is 5–6 meters long) and appear in the ejaculate. The vas deferens is 30–35 cm in length, begins at the cauda epididymis and terminates in the ejaculatory duct near the prostate. Because of the long development and transit times the semen analysis can reflect events which occurred days or weeks earlier.

19. A   p.876

The semen is composed of secretions contributed in a sequential fashion, first the prostatic fluid and contents of the distal vas deferens, followed by seminal vesicle secretions.

20. C   p.878

The World Health Organization (WHO) suggests the following for normal values, but these should be viewed as rough guidelines only.

Volume	2.0 mL or more
Sperm concentration	20 million/mL or more
Motility	50% or more with forward progression, or 25% or more with rapid progression within 60 minutes of ejaculation
Morphology	30% or more normal forms
White blood cells	fewer than 1 million/mL

21. B   p.878

Kruger and coworkers, in a series of articles, championed morphology as the best prognostic indicator for subsequent successful fertilization with in vitro fertilization. They utilize "strict criteria" that shift many sperm out of the normal category by including as abnormal, sperm with even minor abnormalities as well as those with abnormalities of the acrosome (in addition to the usual head and tail abnormalities).

Using these strict criteria males with greater than 14% normal forms have normal rates of fertilization with in vitro fertilization, whereas those with less than 4% normal forms have fertilization rates of only 7–8%. Values between 4% and 14% normal forms are associated with intermediate rates of fertilization. Technicians well trained in using strict criteria can provide highly reproducible results, but the standardization may not be possible on a more widespread scale. Interobserver differences in assessing sperm morphology could be eliminated if newly developed computer-assisted morphometric evaluations prove to be workable.

22. A   p.879,880

Equally important has been a continuing controversy over the prognostic value of the test. A meta-analysis concluded that the test was not of value. Other authors, however, have found correlations with eventual fertility. An SPA result of greater than 19% was associated with a pregnancy rate of 48%, whereas below 20% eggs penetrated was associated with a pregnancy rate of 20%. However, even with an SPA of 0% the pregnancy rate in this series was 16%. This has been a common finding. Failure of the sperm to penetrate the hamster egg is not an absolute indication that the sperm cannot penetrate the human egg. Because of this limitation of the SPA, attempts have been made to optimize the test with a goal of eliminating these false negative results. Strategies to eliminate or to lower the number of false negative tests include treatment of sperm with follicular fluid, test yolk buffer, calcium ionophore, miniaturizing the test, and adjusting the concentration of albumin or the ions in the culture media. With any of these maneuvers an SPA showing no or low penetration should be a more accurate harbinger of poor results in human in vitro fertilization (IVF). Although the tests are still not 100% accurate, if an optimized SPA has zero penetration, the couple should be given the option of considering use of donor sperm. In contrast to the problems with low SPAs, normal levels of sperm penetration correlate quite well, although not absolutely, with human fertilization in vivo and in vitro.

23. C   p.880

The limited availability of zonae will restrict the overall utilization of this test. Moreover, variability in test results between laboratories can be anticipated, which means that each laboratory must establish its own range of normal values. In the future, development of materials that mimic the properties of the zona should allow widespread application of this attractive test.

Both the human zona binding assay and evaluation of sperm morphology by strict criteria require standardization and some skills beyond the qualifications of most clinical laboratories, and thus they will not be universally applicable. The use of computer-driven assessments of sperm morphology may provide the information and universal availability needed to make this test a gold standard for evaluating the male. However, past experience suggests that no one test will ever be sufficient to test all the qualities of the sperm that are necessary for successful fertilization.

24. D   p.879–882

Tests used occasionally in clinical practice include the human zona binding asay, in vitro tests of sperm penetration into mucus, assessments of sperm motility, and measurement of sperm velocity. Tests that are probably not clinically useful include the hypo-osmotic swelling test, measurement of adenosine triphosphate, measurement of the acrosome reaction, and measurement of acrosin.

25. E   p.882

Sperm are very antigenic and are normally isolated by the blood-testis barrier. Disruption of this anatomic and functional barrier in the seminiferous tubules can lead to antibody formation; hence antibodies can follow vasectomy, testicular torsion, infections, or trauma. In addition, there are women who have allergic reactions to semen manifested by reactions as diverse as irritation of the vagina and cardiovascular collapse following intercourse. The basic question for the infertility physician is whether more subtle immunologic reactions can occur that interfere with fertility.

26. B   p.883,884

Use of condoms to avoid contact between sperm and the female with antibodies has been abandoned because of lack of efficacy. The current office treatments for sperm antibodies in the male are the use of steroids or ejaculation into media containing protein combined with intrauterine inseminations. We have encountered antibody positive men with poor to zero performance on sperm penetration assays who have improved sperm penetration and achieved pregnancy with treatment consisting of prednisone, 5 mg tid for at least 3 months. Similar corticosteroid treatment in the female has not been aggressively investigated or used.

The most popular therapy involves intrauterine insemination of washed spermatozoa in conjunction with gonadotropin treatment of the female. Determination of the efficacy of this treatment has been hindered by difficulties in deciding what constitutes a positive sperm antibody test in the female and reports that lumped together patients who were antibody positive with others who may not have been afflicted with antibodies but who had poor postcoital tests.

Use of in vitro fertilization, with placement of sperm near the oocyte, is a reasonable final approach to the treatment of sperm antibodies in both the male and the female. If antibody is hampering sperm transport, IVF is a means of overcoming this problem.

27. E   p.884,885

If the semen analysis is abnormal, inquiry should be made concerning the presence of the following factors, any of which can produce abnormal sperm quality and quantity.

1. History of testicular injury, surgery, or mumps.
2. Heat. A small rise in scrotal temperature can adversely affect spermatogenesis and a febrile illness may produce striking changes in sperm count and motility. The effect of the illness can be seen in the sperm count and motility even 2–3 months later. This reflects the 74 days required for a spermatozoon to be generated from a primary germ cell. Environmental sources of heat, such as the use of jockey shorts instead of boxer shorts, excessively hot baths, hot tubs, or occupations that require long hours of sitting, e.g., long distance truck driving, may all decrease fertility potential; however, none of these factors has ever been substantiated by clinical study.
3. Severe allergic reactions.
4. Exposure to radiation or to industrial or environmental toxins This area has received increasing attention, highlighted by studies suggesting a deterioration of semen quality over the past decades. One hypothesis is that industrial pollution may be responsible, and a study from Scandinavia did show lower sperm counts in males from an urban area compared to males in rural areas. More direct evidence of a deleterious effect of environmental hazards is difficult to obtain because there is a reluctance of workers to produce the serial semen specimens that would be required for a thorough industrial study. In any case, the physician should determine if a male with an abnormal semen specimen has had exposure to industrial or environmental toxins.
5. Heavy marijuana and alcohol use can depress sperm counts and testosterone levels, and there is evidence that cigarette smoking can depress sperm motility. Cocaine use within 2 years is associated with an increased risk of lower sperm counts. Certain drugs, including cimetidine, spironolactone, nitrofurans, sulfasalazine, erythromycin, tetracyclines, anabolic steroids, and chemotherapeutic agents, depress sperm quantity and quality. Cephalosporins, penicillins, quinolones, and the combination of sulfamethoxazole and trimethoprim are relatively safe to use when there is concern about effects on sperm. Neurologic ejaculatory dysfunction can be caused by α-blockers, phentolamine, methyldopa, guanethidine, and reserpine.
6. Coital frequency. Counts at the lower levels of the normal range may be depressed to below normal levels by ejaculations occurring daily or more frequently. Conversely, abstinence for 10–14 days or more to save up sperm may be counterproductive because the gain in numbers can be offset by the lower motility produced by the increased proportion of older sperm. For most couples, coitus every 36 hours around the time of ovulation will give the optimal chance for pregnancy.
7. Exposure to diethylstilbestrol in utero has been suggested, but not proven, as a cause of male infertility.

28. B p.885

Obstruction or absence of the vas deferens is a relatively uncommon cause of male infertility; however more aggressive evaluation (including vasography) may detect obstructions that can be surgically corrected. If the ducts are congenitally absent, fructose which is produced in the seminal vesicles will be absent from the semen. Testicular biopsy can differentiate between a block in the outflow tract or primary damage to the testes. In the latter case, if the biopsy reveals hyalinization and fibrosis of the seminiferous tubules, there is very little chance for fertility. Testicular damage or maldevelopment can be found following mumps orchitis, cryptorchidism, or in association with Klinefelter's syndrome. Males with the latter genetic abnormality (XXY) usually have small testes and azoospermia. With blockage of the vas, sperm can be aspirated from the epididymis and vasa efferentia. Successful fertilization in vitro can result in pregnancy.

29. E p.886

Although endocrine disorders are an uncommon cause for infertility, testing for thyroid, gonadotropins, prolactin, and testosterone may uncover unsuspected abnormalities. FSH levels are elevated with germ cell aplasia, and testosterone levels are decreased in men who are hypogonadotropic. Hyperprolactinemia is commonly associated with impotence, and in the absence of impotence, measuring a prolactin level is unlikely to aid in the diagnosis. Azospermia has been reported in a man with a mutation that caused a substitution of arginine for glutamine in the beta-subunit of LH; this man presented with hypogonadism, a normal FSH level, and an elevated immunoactive (but biologically inactive) LH level.

30. C   p.886

A varicocele is an abnormal tortuosity and dilatation of the veins of the pampiniform plexus within the spermatic cord. Approximately 25–30% of infertile males have a varicocele, usually on the left side because of the direct insertion of the spermatic vein into the renal vein. Varicoceles, in all likelihood, exert their effects by raising testicular temperature, an effect mediated by increased arterial blood flow.

Approximately 10–15% of males in a general population have a varicocele on physical examination, but there is no evidence that males with normal semen characteristics need treatment even if a varicocele is present. They should be checked periodically, however, to be sure that there is no deterioration in their semen characteristics.

Ligation of varicoceles results in a 30–50% pregnancy rate. Although the beneficial effects of treatment of varicocele have been disputed by some investigators who found equal results without treatment, current clinical practice supports the utilization of varicocele ligation in those males who have infertility and an impaired semen specimen. Nevertheless, there has not been a randomized study of varicocele repair. However, varicocele is more commonly found in men with abnormal semen, and there is evidence that a varicocele may exert an increasingly deleterious effect over time.

31. C   p.889

Prior down-regulation with GnRH agonist treatment does not seem to enhance results with gonadotropin/IUI. Similarly, intraperitoneal or intratubal inseminations of sperm, although conceptually attractive, have no proven advantage over intrauterine insemination. Moreover, intratubal transfer probably increases the risk of infection. Infection with IUI is rare, probably in the range of 1 in 500. Multiple pregnancies occur in approximately 20% of cases of gonadotropin/IUI, and the pregnancy loss rate is approximately 20%. Hyperstimulation can be minimized, but not eliminated, by monitoring of ovarian follicle numbers and growth by ultrasound, and by monitoring estrogen levels.

32. E   p.889,890

Donor inseminations do not guarantee pregnancy. The success rate with fresh semen is about 70% over 5–6 cycles. The use of frozen semen lowers the success rate. The fecundibility (chance of getting pregnant per cycle) has been reported to be 18.9% with fresh semen and only 5.0% with frozen semen. However, with exceptionally good frozen specimens success can approach that achieved with fresh specimens. Over 80% of pregnancies that will occur do so within 6 months with fresh semen and within 12 months with frozen semen. In a summary of nearly 3,000 treatment cycles with frozen sperm, the cumulative pregnancy rates were 21% at 3 months, 40% at 6 months, and 62% at 12 months for women less than 30 years old. For women over the age of 30, the pregnancy rates were 17%, 26%, and 44%, respectively. Because of the risk of acquired immunodeficiency syndrome (AIDS), use of frozen sperm that has been quarantined for 6 months is now accepted clinical practice. However, preparation of washed, swim-up sperm for intrauterine insemination appears to effectively remove human immunodeficiency virus (HIV)-infected cells and avoids HIV seroconversion, providing a safer method to achieve a healthy pregnancy and child for these couples. Because of the importance and seriousness of this situation, these results require corroboration.

The couple needs to give some thought to their feelings should the child be born with a congenital anomaly. This will occur in perhaps 4–5% of all pregnancies, irrespective of whether they follow intercourse or therapeutic donor insemination.

30 Induction of Ovulation

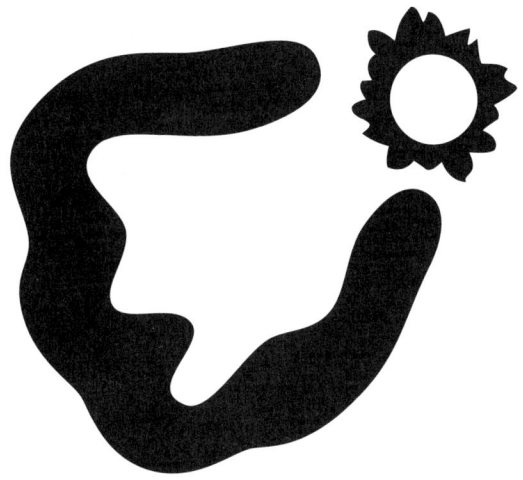

Learning Objectives

Be able to:

1. Describe the mechanism of action, half-life, indications, possible side effects and complications associated with clomiphene citrate and human menopausal gonadotropins (HMG).

2. Discuss the probability for ovulation, conception rate, multiple pregnancies and ovarian hyperstimulation syndrome associated with clomiphene citrate and HMG.

3. Detail the indications, possible complications and success rate associated with selective multifetal pregnancy reduction.

4. Understand the pathophysiology, signs, symptoms, management and possible complications associated with ovarian hyperstimulation syndrome.

5. Discuss the availability and potential uses of purified FSH, bromocriptine and gonadotropin releasing hormone in the induction of ovulation.

6. Explain the principles and possible indications for laparoscopic ovarian multiple cystotomy.

Pre-Test

A. Instructions: Fill in the blanks

1. The antiestrogen action of clomiphene is reflected by a _____% incidence of poor cervical mucus on postcoital test.

2. Approximately ____% of patients treated with doses of 150–250 mg of clomiphene will become pregnant.

B. Instructions: True or False

3. Hyperprolactinemia has no adverse effect on response to human menopausal gonadotropins in patients who cannot tolerate bromocriptine.

4. A cumulative conception rate of 90% after 6 treatment cycles can be achieved in women with hypothalamic amenorrhea who undergo ovulation induction with HMG.

C. Instructions: For the following questions choose:

A. if only 1, 2 and 3 are correct
B. if only 1 and 3 are correct
C. if only 2 and 4 are correct
D. if only 4 is correct
E. if all are correct

5. Side effects from clomiphene
   1. are dose-related
   2. include blurring vision and/or scotoma
   3. include breast discomfort more commonly than vasomotor flushes
   4. include significant ovarian enlargement about 5% of the time

6. Complications as a result of using HMG for ovulation induction include
   1. no increased risks of spontaneous abortions
   2. a 1–2% risk of serious ovarian hyperstimulation
   3. a 25% risk of developing ovarian cancer
   4. a 10–40% multiple pregnancy rate

Post-Test

A. Instructions: Fill in the blanks

1. Clomiphene citrate was approved for clinical use in the U.S. in _____.

2. Clomiphene citrate is an orally active nonsteroidal agent structurally related to _____.

3. It is the physician's responsibility to rule out disorders of _____, _____, and _____ origin before initiating clomiphene therapy.

4. ____% of pregnancies occur during the first 3 treatment cycles of clomiphene.

5. Human menopausal gonadotropins (HMG) consist of a purified preparation of gonadotropins extracted from the _____ of _____ women. HMG is inactive orally and therefore must be given by _____ route.

6. The risk of ectopic pregnancy is _____ with ovulation induction.

7. HCG disappears from the blood with an initial component having a half-life of about _____ hours and a second, slower, component with a half-life of about _____ hours.

8. The HCG concentrations after the ovulation injection should be less than 50–100 IU/L by day _____ after the injection.

9. In a patient who is pregnant ovarian hyperstimulation syndrome will cover a period of approximately _____ days in contrast to _____ days in a patient who is pregnant.

B. Instructions: True or False

10. Clomiphene acts primarily as an antiestrogen in the uterus, cervix and vagina.

11. Clomiphene has progestational but no corticotropic, androgenic, or antiandrogenic effects.

12. The half-life of oral clomiphene is 10 days.

13. There is no convincing evidence that clomiphene is teratogenic in humans.

14. Cases of ovarian failure are unresponsive to any form of ovulation induction.

15. Clomiphene has been demonstrated to be superior to progesterone in the treatment of luteal phase defect.

16. At the present time there is no clinical or laboratory parameter that can predict the dose of clomiphene necessary to achieve ovulation.

17. Prior to initiating human menopausal gonadotropins for ovulation induction a thorough infertility investigation must be performed.

18. Ultrasonographic surveillance of ovaries reveals that mittelschmerz is associated with follicular rupture.

19. Ovulation can be successfully induced with HCG administration when the follicular diameter reaches 18–20 mm when taking clomiphene but, 15–18 mm when taking HMG.

20. Ultrasound monitoring during ovulation induction will eliminate the risks of multiple gestation and hyperstimulation.

21. Selective reduction of monochorionic pregnancies is not advisable because of shared vasculature and the high risk of losing all fetuses.

22. The clomiphene challenge test is designed to be a bioassay of estradiol response.

C. Match each definition of ovulatory deficiency with each condition

  A. hypothalamic-pituitary failure (Group I)
  B. hypothalamic-pituitary dysfunction (Group II)
  C. ovarian failure (Group III)

23. hypergonadotropic hypogonadism
24. anorexia nervosa
25. polycystic ovary syndrome
26. stress-related amenorrhea
27. Kallman's syndrome

D. Instructions: For the following questions choose:

  A. if only 1, 2 and 3 are correct
  B. if only 1 and 3 are correct
  C. if only 2 and 4 are correct
  D. if only 4 is correct
  E. if all are correct

28. Clomiphene citrate
    1. exerts only a weak biologic estrogenic effect
    2. modifies hypothalamic activity by affecting the concentration of the intracellular estrogen receptors
    3. when administered to normally cycling women, FSH and LH pulse frequency is increased
    4. directly stimulates ovulation

29. Prior to beginning clomiphene a work-up should include
    1. documentation of absent ovulation in women with infrequent periods
    2. an endometrial biopsy in women who have been anovulatory for a long period of time
    3. a HSG in women without previous medical or surgical problems
    4. a serum prolactin

30. To accurately rule out hypergonadotropic hypogonadism
    1. obtain a serum FSH
    2. perform a ovarian biopsy
    3. initiate a progestational challenge test
    4. initiate a clomiphene challenge test

31. Indications for clomiphene citrate include
    1. unexplained infertility
    2. hyperprolactinemia
    3. oligoovulation
    4. hypoestrogenism

32. The dosage of clomiphene
    1. is usually initiated at 100 mg daily
    2. may be reduced to 25 mg daily in the patient who is exceptionally sensitive and still achieve pregnancy
    3. should be increased initially when given to obese women
    4. is increased in a staircase fashion by 50 mg increments to a maximum of 200–250 mg daily for 5 days when ovulation and a normal luteal phase are not achieved in a cycle

33. Results of properly selected patients given clomiphene include
    1. an 80% ovulation rate
    2. a 40% pregnancy rate
    3. a 5% multiple pregnancy rate
    4. a 20–25% pregnancy per induced ovulatory cycle rate

34. Those who fail to become pregnant with clomiphene up to the highest dose have options which include
    1. the addition of dexamethasone to clomiphene in patients with hirsutism and elevated androgens
    2. extended clomiphene treatment
    3. pretreatment suppression followed by clomiphene
    4. the addition of bromocriptine to clomiphene

35. If HMG stimulation is excessive during superovulation and intrauterine insemination there are several options which include
    1. avoiding HCG administration and cancelling the cycle
    2. aspirating most of the ovarian follicles with ultrasound guidance
    3. proceeding with in vitro fertilization
    4. giving 5,000 units instead of 10,000 units of HCG

36. Proper monitoring for ovulation induction while using gonadotropins includes
    1. serum estradiol levels
    2. serum progesterone levels
    3. ultrasound monitoring
    4. serum LH levels

37. Multiple pregnancies following HMG used for ovulation induction are
    1. increased for monozygotic twinning
    2. secondary to multiple ovulations
    3. at increased risk for fetal loss
    4. due to significantly higher amounts of HMG than single pregnancies

38. Multifetal pregnancy reduction
    1. if performed transvaginally should be performed between 8 and 9 weeks of gestation
    2. occurs spontaneously in approximately 5% following fetal heartbeat identification
    3. if performed transabdominally should be performed between 11 and 12 weeks of gestation
    4. is associated with a 10% loss of the pregnancy

39. Ovarian hyperstimulation syndrome
    1. occurs in its moderate to severe forms in 1–2% of cases
    2. can be avoided by withholding the administration of HCG
    3. is most likely to occur in women with polycystic ovaries
    4. can be avoided by using a GnRH agonist in combined therapy

40. Potential complications of ovarian hyperstimulation include
    1. decreased renal perfusion
    2. severe acidosis
    3. increased coagulability
    4. encephalopathy

41. Tests which may be useful in predicting a woman's response to ovulation induction include
    1. a midluteal progesterone
    2. day 3 serum FSH
    3. a preovulatory progesterone
    4. clomiphene challenge test

42. GnRH agonist added to HMG
    1. can decrease premature LH surges
    2. will prevent hyperstimulation from occurring
    3. can result in a "flare" response particularly if given in the follicular phase
    4. does not require additional luteal phase support

43. Destruction of ovarian tissue at multiple sites for the purpose of achieving spontaneous ovulation or increased sensitivity to clomiphene
    1. results in lowering intraovarian androgens and inhibin
    2. may be achieved by either cautery, diathermy or laser by laparoscopy
    3. may potentially result in a problem with adhesion formation
    4. is appropriate to offer to an individual suspected of having polycystic ovary disease who has not tried clomiphene before

Answers for Chapter 30 — Pre-Test Questions

1. 15   p.901
Despite the antiestrogen action of clomiphene the incidence of poor cervical mucus on the postcoital test is only 15%. In the past, estrogen (0.625 to 2.5 mg conjugated estrogens daily) was administered from day 10 to day 16 (for 1 week starting the day after the last day of clomiphene administration) in an effort to improve mucus production. Although high doses of estrogen do not interfere with the gonadotropin response, ovulation, or the pregnancy rate, there is reason to believe that estrogen treatment is ineffective. Another alternative, the one we prefer, is to proceed with intrauterine inseminations of prepared sperm, bypassing the cervix.

2. 15   p.905
With additional treatment cycles, the pregnancy rate decreases, although the ovulatory rate remains high. Approximately 15% of patients treated with the higher doses of 150–250 mg will become pregnant.

3. true   p.909
Because some patients cannot tolerate bromocriptine, it is important to know that hyperprolactinemia has no adverse effect on response to HMG.

4. true   p.913
The most significant aspect of this method of treatment is that it does achieve pregnancy in otherwise untreatable situations. A cumulative conception rate of 90% after 6 treatment cycles can be achieved in women with hypothalamic amenorrhea (this rate exceeds that observed in spontaneously ovulating women), with a 23% rate of spontaneous abortion.

5. C   p.905
Side effects do not appear to be dose-related, occurring more frequently at the 50 mg dose. Patients requiring the high doses are probably less sensitive to the drug. The most common problems are vasomotor flushes (10%), abdominal distention, bloating, pain, or soreness (5.5%), breast discomfort (2%), nausea and vomiting (2.2%), visual symptoms (1.5%), headache (1.3%), and dryness or loss of hair (0.3%). Patients who are extremely sensitive to the side effects of clomiphene can be sucessfully treated with half a tablet (25 mg) daily for 5 days, and even with half a tablet daily for 3 days.

6. C   p.913,914
A slightly higher rate of spontaneous abortion reflects the combination of better detection of early pregnancy loss, advanced maternal age, and the increased incidence of multiple pregnancies. As with clomiphene, there is a normal incidence of congenital malformations, and the children have a normal postnatal development.

The likelihood of ovulation is dose related, and complications are likewise dose related. The rate of serious hyperstimulation has been 1–2%. Prior to the present era of more careful monitoring, the multiple pregnancy rate was reported as approximately 30% (triplets or more, 5%). Currently, the multiple pregnancy rate can be as low as 10% with careful monitoring and good medical judgment; however, rates as high as 40% are reported.

Answers for Chapter 30 — Post-Test Questions

1. 1967   p.898
Clomiphene citrate was first synthesized in 1956, introduced for clinical trials in 1960, and approved for clinical use in the United States in 1967. Clomiphene citrate is an orally active nonsteroidal agent distantly related to diethylstilbestrol. Its chemical name is 2-[p-(2-chloro-1,2-diphenylvinyl)phenoxy]triethylamine dihydrogen citrate. Clomiphene is a racemic mixture of its 2 stereochemical isomers, originally described as the cis and trans isomers. This designation is now recognized to have been inaccurate, and the isomers have been relabeled as zuclomiphene and enclomiphene citrate. Clomiphene is available in 50 mg tablets, under the trade names of Clomid and Serophene, which contain 38% of the active zuclomiphene form.

2. estrogen   p.898,899
The similarity of clomiphene's structure to an estrogenic substance is the clue to its mechanism of action. Clomiphene exerts only a very weak biologic estrogenic effect. The structural similarity to estrogen is sufficient to achieve uptake and binding by estrogen receptors; however, there are several important different characteristics. Perhaps most importantly, clomiphene occupies the nuclear receptor for long periods of time, for weeks rather than hours.

3. pituitary, adrenal, thyroid   p.900
Absent or infrequent ovulation is the chief indication for clomiphene therapy. It is the physician's responsibility to rule out disorders of pituitary, adrenal, and thyroid origin requiring specific treatment before initiating clomiphene therapy. A complete history and physical examination are mandatory, but only a minimum of laboratory procedures is necessary. Liver function evaluation should precede clomiphene therapy if history and physical examination findings suggest liver disease. The vast majority of patients are healthy women suffering only from infertility secondary to oligoovulation or anovulation.

4. 75   p.900
Because approximately 75% of pregnancies occur during the first 3 treatment cycles, the infertility workup is pursued only after the patient has responded with 3 months of ovulatory cycles and has not become pregnant. This is appropriate because clomiphene is simple, safe, and cost-effective.

5. urine; postmenopausal; intramuscular   p.908
Human menopausal gonadotropins consist of a purified preparation of gonadotropins extracted from the urine of postmenopausal women. The generic name is menotropins. The commercial preparation is available with either 75 units of FSH and 75 units of LH per ampule, or in an ampule with twice the amount, 150 units. The potency is expressed in terms of international units based on an international reference preparation. A significant factor in the use of HMG is its high cost. Treatment may cost from $1,000 to $1,500/cycle for the drug alone. HMG is inactive orally and, therefore, must be given by intramuscular injections.

6. increased   p.913
The risk of ectopic pregnancy is increased with ovulation induction, a consequence of multiple oocytes and high hormone levels. These patients should be closely monitored in the early weeks of their pregnancies.

7. 6; 24   p.914
HCG disappears from the blood with an initial component having a half-life of about 6 hours and a second, slower, component with a half-life of about 24 hours. It is this relatively slow half-life that enables a single injection of 10,000 IU to maintain the corpus luteum until pregnancy takes over.

8. 14   p.914

The HCG concentration after the ovulation injection should be less than 50–100 IU/L by day 14 after the injection. A β-subunit assay of HCG at this time or one of the urine assays performed 2–4 weeks after the HCG injection are reliable tests for pregnancy. Additional HCG (during the luteal phase) does not improve pregnancy rates. Luteal supplementation is required only with concurrent treatment with a GnRH agonist.

9. 7; 10–20   p.916

The key point is that the hyperstimulation syndrome will undergo gradual resolution with time. In a patient who is not pregnant, the syndrome will cover a period of approximately 7 days. In a patient who is pregnant and in whom the ovaries are restimulated by the emerging endogenous HCG production, the syndrome will last 10–20 days.

10. true   p.899

In the absence of estrogen, clomiphene is an estrogen agonist, directly enhancing FSH stimulation of LH receptors in granulosa cells. In an important contrast, in the uterus, cervix, and vagina, clomiphene acts primarily as an antiestrogen.

11. false   p.900

Clomiphene has no progestational, corticotropic, androgenic, or antiandrogenic effects. Clomiphene does not interfere with adrenal or thyroid function.

12. false   p.900

Although the effect of the drug is brief, only 51% of the oral dose is excreted after 5 days, and radioactivity from labeled clomiphene appears in the feces up to 6 weeks after administration. Significant plasma concentrations of the active zu isomer can be detected up to 1 month after treatment with a single dose of 50 mg.

13. true   p.900

In rats and rabbits, a dose-dependent increase in the incidence of fetal malformations is seen when clomiphene is given during the period of organogenesis. Clomiphene has been found to cause disruptions of the organization of the uterine mesenchyme and tubal epithelium in human fetal reproductive tissue transplanted to athymic nude mice. Extremely high doses inhibit fetal development. In these experiments, exposure took place at later periods of gestation than those associated with clomiphene exposure when the drug is taken for the induction of ovulation. Although clomiphene therapy should be withheld if there is any possibility of pregnancy, there is no good evidence that clomiphene is teratogenic in humans. Furthermore, infant survival and performance after delivery are normal.

14. true   p.901

Cases of ovarian failure are unresponsive to any form of ovulation induction. Therefore, the presence of ovarian tissue capable of responding to gonadotropins must be documented. This is only a problem in the patient with amenorrhea, since the presence of menstrual bleeding confirms the function (although perhaps limited) of the hypothalamic-pituitary-ovarian axis.

15. false   p.901

If the mechanism of an inadequate corpus luteum is inadequate FSH stimulation during the follicular phase, it makes sense to treat this condition with clomiphene, and a good response has been observed by ourselves and others. Two randomized trials comparing clomiphene to progesterone treatment for inadequate luteal phases demonstrated equal pregnancy rates with each treatment. Clomiphene does not prolong the luteal phase (as progesterone supplementation does). This is an important advantage, avoiding the anxiety and heightened monthly emotional response of infertile couples.

16. true   p.904

At the present time there is no clinical or laboratory parameter that can predict the dose of clomiphene necessary to achieve ovulation. Androgen and estrogen levels do not show any correlation with the dose of clomiphene that proves successful.

17. true   p.909

Not only because of its expense but because of its greater complication rate, patients should not receive HMG without a very careful evaluation. An absolute requirement is the demonstration of ovarian competence. A thorough infertility investigation must be performed. In addition to the demonstration of ovarian competence, tubal and uterine pathology should be ruled out, anovulation documented, and semen analysis obtained. Nongynecologic endocrine problems must be treated. Hypogonadotropic function (low serum gonadotropins), including galactorrhea syndromes, requires evaluation for an intracranial lesion, with appropriate imaging and measurement of prolactin levels. It is imperative to take all steps necessary to exclude treatable pathology to which anovulation is secondary.

18. false   p.912

During the 5 days preceding ovum expulsion, the dominant follicle exhibits a linear growth pattern of approximately 2 to 3 mm per day, followed by rapid exponential growth during the last 24 hours prior to ovulation. *Ultrasonographic surveillance of ovaries reveals that mittelschmerz is associated not with follicular rupture but with the rapid expansion of the dominant follicle, thus the pain precedes follicular rupture.*

19. true   p.912

In response to clomiphene treatment, follicles pursue a linear but generally accelerated rate of growth compared to spontaneous cycles. The maximal diameter of clomiphene-induced preovulatory follicles is similar to that seen with spontaneous cycles, 20–24 mm, but ovulation can be successfully induced with HCG administration when the diameter reaches 18–20 mm (by the time of ovulation, the follicle will have grown another 2–3 mm). With HMG, the maximal follicular diameter (15–18 mm) is smaller than that seen during spontaneous and clomiphene-induced cycles. When follicles reach this size, ovulation will occur approximately 36 hours after HCG is administered.

20. false   p.912

Ultrasound monitoring does not eliminate the risks of multiple gestation and hyperstimulation. It is claimed that a higher pregnancy rate can be achieved when ultrasound is combined with estrogen monitoring. The guiding principle has been to administer HCG when mature follicles correlate with an estrogen level of 400 pg per follicle.

21. true   p.914

Reduction of a monochorionic pregnancy is not advisable because of shared vasculature and the high risk of losing all fetuses.

22. false   p.918

Navot and colleagues developed the clomiphene challenge test as a bioassay of FSH response (which in turn probably reflects ovarian follicular inhibin capability). Clomiphene is administered in a dose of 100 mg/day on days 5–9. The levels of FSH on days 9–11 are compared to the baseline levels on days 2–3. An exaggerated FSH response of 26 IU/L or more is 2 standard deviations above the control values, and this increase in FSH is associated with a significant prospect for failure to achieve pregnancy. There is a high incidence of abnormal responses in women over 35; 85% of women with increased FSH levels respond poorly to ovarian stimulation, and long-term pregnancy rates are drastically reduced.

23. C   p.898

24. A   p.898

25. B   p.898

26. A   p.898

27. A   p.898

1. **Group I: Hypothalamic-Pituitary Failure.** This classfication includes patients diagnosed as hypothalamic amenorrhea, and includes stress-related amenorrhea, anorexia nervosa and its variants, Kallmann's syndrome, and isolated gonadotropin deficiency. These patients display hypogonadotropic hypogonadism with low FSH and estrogen levels, normal prolactin concentrations, and a failure to bleed after the administration of a progestational agent (the progestational challenge).
2. **Group II: Hypothalamic-Pituitary Dysfunction.** This classification includes normogonadotropic,

normoestrogenic, anovulatory, oligoamenorrheic women. The classic anovulatory polycystic ovary syndrome is in this category.

3. **Group III: Ovarian Failure.** Patients in this classification are hypergonadotropic hypogonadal individuals with low estrogen levels. All variants of ovarian failure and ovarian resistance are in this category.

28. A p.899

When exposed to clomiphene, the hypothalamic-pituitary axis is blind to the endogenous estrogen level in the circulation. Because receptor capacity is reduced and the true estrogen signal falsely lowered, negative feedback is diminished and the neuroendocrine mechanism for GnRH secretion is activated. When clomiphene is administered to normally cycling women, FSH and luteinizing hormone (LH) pulse frequency (but not amplitude) is increased, suggesting an increase in GnRH pulse frequency. Anovulatory women, however, respond in a different fashion. Clomiphene stimulates an increase in gonadotropin pulse amplitude, presumably because GnRH pulses are already operating at maximal frequency in anovulatory women with polycystic ovaries. Nevertheless, the experimental data indicate that the primary site of action is the hypothalamus.

During clomiphene administration, circulating levels of FSH and LH rise. The subsequent ovulation that occurs after clomiphene therapy is a manifestation of the hormone and morphologic changes produced by the growing follicles. Clomiphene therapy does not directly stimulate ovulation, but it retrieves and magnifies the sequence of events that are the physiologic features of a normal cycle.

29. C p.900

A complete history and physical examination are mandatory, but only a minimum of laboratory procedures is necessary. Liver function evaluation should precede clomiphene therapy if history and physical examination findings suggest liver disease. The vast majority of patients are healthy women suffering only from infertility secondary to oligoovulation or anovulation.

If periods are infrequent, it is not absolutely necessary to document infrequent or absent ovulation by basal body temperature records and endometrial biopsy. An endometrial biopsy is a wise precaution in a patient who has been anovulatory for a long period of time because of the tendency for these patients to develop hyperplasia and even carcinoma of the endometrium. It is also wise to precede therapy with an evaluation of the semen, to avoid an unnecessary waste of time and effort in the presence of azoospermia. A dedicated effort must be made to detect galactorrhea, and the prolactin level must be measured. Galactorrhea or hyperprolactinemia dictates a different therapeutic approach: bromocriptine. The remainder of the infertility workup in a patient with no previous medical or surgical problems is deferred until after a trial of clomiphene therapy

30. B p.901

The patient with amenorrhea who fails to produce a withdrawal bleed after a course of a progestational agent (medroxyprogesterone acetate, 10 mg daily for 5 days) must be further evaluated. A case has been made by others for the usefulness of an ovarian biopsy, perhaps via the laparoscope, to establish the presence of competent ovarian tissue. It is our practice, however, to rely on the immunoassay of gonadotropin levels and the response to a progestin, thus avoiding unnecessary surgical and anesthetic risks, to accurately rule out hypergonadotropic hypogonadism (ovarian failure). Attempts at medical induction of ovulation in these patients would be a waste of time and money.

31. B p.901,902

Any otherwise medically uncomplicated patient with infertility secondary to lack of ovulation is a candidate for clomiphene therapy unless galactorrhea or hyperprolactinemia is present. Hypoestrogenic women respond so rarely, however, that it is appropriate to omit treatment with clomiphene and move to other more productive options.

In addition to anovulation, treatment with clomiphene is indicated to improve the timing and frequency of ovulation and to enhance the possibilities of conception in the patient who ovulates only occasionally. Clomiphene is also useful to regulate the timing of ovulation in women undergoing insemination.

Clomiphene is used for the treatment of unexplained infertility, i.e., women who have prolonged (>3 years) infertility but who ovulate spontaneously and repeatedly by all available measures and do not have other abnormalities.

32. C   p.902,903

A program of clomiphene therapy is begun on the 5th day of a cycle following either spontaneous or induced bleeding. It has not been established that a progestin withdrawal bleed is necessary before starting clomiphene treatment; we often omit this step if we are certain that the patient is not pregnant. The initial dose is 50 mg daily for 5 days. There is no advantage to beginning with a higher dose for the following two reasons: 1) in a random distribution of our patients begun with initial doses of either 50 mg or 100 mg daily, the pregnancy rate was identical; and 2) the highest incidence of side effects in our experience occurs at the 50 mg dose; however, at 100 mg, patients may develop more serious reactions. About 50% of patients conceive at the 50 mg dose, and another 20% at 100 mg. An occasional patient will be exceptionally sensitive to clomiphene and can achieve pregnancy at the reduced dose of 25 mg.

Beginning clomiphene on the 5th day is a method arrived at empirically; however, we can now offer a rational explanation based on current physiology. The clomiphene-induced increase in gonadotropins during days 5–9 occurs at a time when the dominant follicle is being selected. Beginning clomiphene earlier can be expected to stimulate multiple follicular maturation resulting in a greater incidence of multiple gestation. Indeed, clomiphene is administered earlier in in vitro fertilization programs in order to obtain more than one oocyte. However, in standard ovulation induction protocols, no differences have been observed in the rates of ovulation, pregnancy, or spontaneous abortion whether clomiphene was started on day 2, 3, 4, or 5.

If ovulation is not achieved in the very first cycle of treatment, dosage is increased to 100 mg. Thereafter, if ovulation and a normal luteal phase are not achieved in any cycle, dosage is increased in a staircase fashion by 50 mg increments to a maximum of 200–250 mg daily for 5 days. The highest dose is pursued for 3–4 months before considering the patient to be a clomiphene failure. The quantity of drug and the number of cycles go beyond those recommended by manufacturers. However, in our experience those recommendations are inappropriately limiting. We have achieved a 15% pregnancy rate at the 150 mg and 200 mg dose levels.

33. E   p.905

In properly selected patients, 80% can be expected to ovulate, and approximately 40% become pregnant. The percent of pregnancies per induced ovulatory cycle is about 20–25%. The multiple pregnancy rate is approximately 5%, almost entirely twins; there have been rare cases of quintuplet and sextuplet births. In our own experience, with standardization of therapy, the incidence of twins has decreased.

34. E   p.907

There are several options available for the 10–20% of women who fail to become pregnant with clomiphene up to the highest dose. Knowledge gained from experience with in vitro fertilization provides us with several explanations for failure to respond to clomiphene. These include the effects of excessive LH in the follicular phase, the dysfunctional effects of an untimely LH surge, and excess local concentrations of androgens. These mechanisms may yield impaired folliculogenesis, increased atresia, poor oocyte quality, precocious or impaired oocyte maturation, low fertilization rates, variable implantation rates, and deficient corpus luteum function. Strategies have developed to mitigate or avoid many of these detrimental effects: the supplemental use of dexamethasone (to reduce androgen burden), GnRH agonists (to eliminate endogenous LH intrusion), pulsatile GnRH therapy (to preserve physiologic interactive feedback mechanisms), "pure" FSH (to diminish excessive LH in the follicular phase), and, finally, the use of human menopausal gonadotropins. We are also seeing the return of modified ovarian wedge resection by laparoscopic multiple ovarian tissue destruction by cautery or laser techniques.

35. A   p.910

The incidence of multiple births and ovarian hyperstimulation is higher with this empiric treatment. Patients and clinicians undertaking empiric superovulation should have ready recourse to in vitro fertilization. *If HMG stimulation is excessive, several choices are available: avoiding HCG administration and canceling the cycle, aspirating most of the ovarian follicles with ultrasound guidance, or proceeding with in vitro ferilization.*

36. B   p.911,912

The use of estrogen measurements is necessary to choose the correct moment for administering the ovulatory dose of

HCG in order to prevent hyperstimulation. Ultrasound assessment of the growth and development of the ovarian follicle indicates the degree of follicular maturity and capability.

37. A
p.914

Currently, the multiple pregnancy rate can be as low as 10% with careful monitoring and good medical judgment; however, rates as high as 40% are reported. The multiple pregnancies are secondary to multiple ovulations, and therefore the siblings are not identical. The rate of spontaneous occurrence of twins is only about 1% and that of triplets 0.010–0.017% of the pregnant population. Dizygotic twinning varies among different populations and is inherited through the mother. The monozygotic twinning rate is about 0.3–0.4%, fairly constant, and uninfluenced by heredity. Surprisingly, induction of ovulation increases the frequency of monozygotic twinning 3-fold. It is not known whether the multiple pregnancy rate with HMG is significantly affected by a maternal history of twinning.

Maternal complications and fetal loss caused by prematurity in the multiple pregnancies have been serious problems. In addition, the abortion rate with HMG is somewhat higher (25%) than normal, probably a combination of the effect of age, multiple pregnancies, and recognition of early abortions.

38. E
p.914

Under ultrasound guidance, a gestational sac can be aspirated or a cardiotoxic drug (potassium chloride) can be injected into, or adjacent to, the fetal heart. The transvaginal procedure is best performed between the 8th and 9th weeks of gestation and the transabdominal procedure between the 11th and 12th weeks. A later procedure is worthwhile because there is an incidence of spontaneous disappearance of one or more gestational sacs in multiple gestations, approximately 5% after fetal heartbeats have been identified. Selection of which gestational sac to be terminated is based solely on technical considerations, such as accessibility. The subsequent risk of losing one or more of the remaining fetuses is 4–9%, and of losing the pregnancy, 10% by experienced clinicians and higher with less experience.

39. A
p.915

The incidence of clinically important hyperstimulation is striking. Although it might be expected that the mild type would be relatively common, the moderate to severe form appears at an impressive rate (1–2%). Two-thirds of cases occur early in a conception cycle, the remainder in nonconception cycles. For purposes of one of the methods of assisted reproduction, the ovaries are stimulated at an even greater rate than for conventional ovulation induction; however, the incidence of hyperstimulation is no greater. For this reason, it has been suggested that follicular aspiration offers partial protection against the hyperstimulation syndrome. Some reports have indicated a higher incidence of hyperstimulation in in vitro fertilization protocols using the combination of HMG and a GnRH agonist. Because support during the luteal phase is required when GnRH agonist treatment is used, the additional HCG administered is responsible for greater stimulation. The use of progesterone for luteal support is probably safer, and therefore, when estradiol levels are high (>2,500 pg/mL [9,200 pmol/L]) and when the follicle number is greater than 15, intravaginal or intramuscular progesterone is recommeded instead of HCG.

Anovulatory women with polycystic ovaries are at greatest risk for the hyperstimulation syndrome. The use of a GnRH agonist in combined therapy does not eliminate this risk. These patients should be treated slowly with careful titration of dose, and therapy should be started at a dose of 75 units per day.

40. B
p.915

The loss of fluid and protein into the abdominal cavity accounts for the hypovolemia and hemoconcentration. This in turn results in low blood pressure and decreased central venous pressure. The major clinical complications are increased coagulability and decreased renal perfusion. Blood loss as the cause of the clinical picture can be easily ruled out since a hematocrit will reveal hemoconcentration. The decreased renal perfusion leads to increased salt and water reabsorption in the proximal tubule, producing oliguria and low urinary sodium excretion. With less sodium being presented to the distal tubule, there is a decrease in the exchange of hydrogen and potassium for sodium, resulting in hyperkalemic acidosis. A rise in the blood urea nitrogen (BUN) is due to decreased perfusion and increased urea reabsorption. Because it is only filtered, creatinine does not increase as much as the BUN. Thus, the patient is hypovolemic, azotemic, and hyperkalemic. In response to these changes, aldosterone, plasma renin activity, and antidiuretic hormone levels are all elevated.

41. C   p.918

Regardless of age, women with elevated day 3 FSH levels and/or abnormal responses to the clomiphene challenge test should consider in vitro fertilization with young, donated oocytes.

42. B   p.918,919

Premature LH effects on the follicle and the burden of excess local androgen can be diminished and an improved therapeutic response achieved. There is reason to believe that women with anovulatory polycystic ovaries have a higher incidence of spontaneous abortion following induction of ovulation with HMG; combining the GnRH agonist with HMG not only yields a greater pregnancy rate, but also reduces the abortion rate. Furthermore, premature LH release is believed to contribute to the risk of ovarian hyperstimulation in women with polycystic ovaries. Combining a GnRH agonist with HMG treatment could reduce (although not eliminate) the risk of this serious complication.

The administration of a GnRH agonist to a woman who has menstrual function will initially produce a stimulatory response, known as the "flare." The magnitude of the flare response depends upon when in the cycle the agonist is administered. During the follicular phase or in anovulatory women, the flare is greater, and enlarged follicular cysts can occur. This response can be minimized by beginning therapy during the midluteal phase or by administering a progestational agent (e.g., 10 mg medroxyprogesterone acetate daily for 10 days) and beginning GnRH agonist treatment after 3 days of progestin.

43. A   p.922

The purpose of wedge resection of the ovaries is to remove a significant amount of hormone-producing tissue. Documentation of hormone changes following wedge resection indicates that an important change is a sustained reduction in testosterone levels. This suggests that the barrier to ovulation is the intraovarian, atresia-promoting effects of the high testosterone production. Removal of androgen-producing tissue effectively lowers this barrier, and ovulatory cycles can ensue. Another contributing factor is a reduction in circulating levels of inhibin which follows the loss of ovarian tissue. A rise in FSH occurs in the days after wedge resection; successful ovulation reflects the combined effects of increased FSH and the removal of the local androgen obstruction to the emergence of a dominant follicle.

The response to ovarian wedge resection is variable. Some patients resume ovulation permanently. However, most patients return to their anovulatory state. Some patients fail to respond at all. Furthermore, the surgical procedure carries with it the potential problem of postoperative adhesion formation.

The operative risk, the variable response, and the possibility of postoperative adhesion formation are the liabilities of wedge resection. These must be weighed against the excellent results obtained with medical induction of ovulation (approximating the normal conception rate when anovulation is the only fertility problem present). It should truly be a rare patient in whom wedge resection of the ovaries is necessary.

Today, a new type of "wedge resection" is available. Using either cautery, diathermy, or laser vaporization by means of the laparoscope, destruction of ovarian tissue at multiple sites (15–20 per ovary) can achieve spontaneous ovulations or an increased sensitivity to clomiphene. These procedures are associated with the same decrease in androgens and inhibin as observed with wedge resection. When clomiphene is reinstituted, 70–80% of patients will ovulate, and approximately 60% will achieve pregnancy. Adhesion formation remains a problem, but perhaps it is less profound than in the traditional surgery. Second look laparoscopy with lysis of adhesions is indicated if pregnancy does not follow successful ovulations. This therapy can be performed at the time of a planned diagnostic laparoscopy in a patient with known anovulation and polycystic ovaries. These procedures are worth considering by patients who are reluctant to pursue the more expensive and difficult methods of the assisted reproductive technologies.

31 Assisted Reproduction

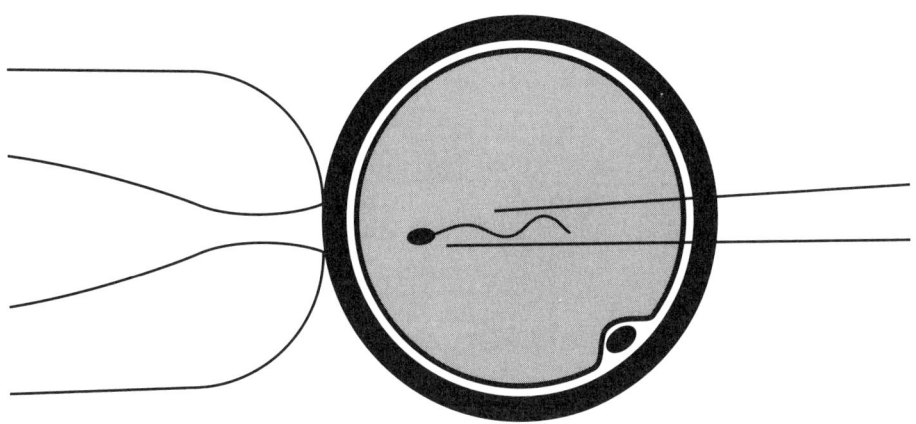

Learning Objectives

Be able to:

1. Define the various techniques available for assisted reproduction.

2. Describe the use of assisted reproductive technologies (ART) in the treatment of nontubal disease.

3. Discuss the prognostic factors for success in a couple undergoing ART.

4. Describe the common ovulation induction protocols, monitoring and timing of triggering an IVF cycle.

5. Explain the various ways success rates could be reported from IVF programs.

6. Detail the most recent advances in treating male factor infertility using ART.

Pre-Test

A. Instructions: Fill in the blanks

1. Inspection of the oocyte for the presence of 2 _____ confirms that fertilization has taken place.

2. In experienced hands the risk of losing the entire pregnancy from selective fetal reduction is less than ___%.

B. Instructions: True or False

3. All discussions pertaining to specific hormone levels must take into account that specific cutoff values depend upon the particular assay system being used.

4. The use of FSH as opposed to HMG in women with polycystic ovaries is protective against hyperstimulation.

C. Instructions: For each of the following questions choose:

A. is only 1, 2 and 3 are correct
B. if only 1 and 3 are correct
C. if only 2 and 4 are correct
D. if only 4 is correct
E. if all are correct

5. The addition of GnRH agonists to ovulation induction protocols in preparation for ART have resulted in
   1. decreased cancellation rates
   2. increased oocyte yields
   3. increased pregnancy rates
   4. decreased expense of a cycle

6. Methods of preimplantation genetic diagnosis include
   1. removal of first polar body
   2. biopsy of cells destined to become placenta
   3. blastomere biopsy
   4. pronuclear biopsy

Post-Test

A. Instructions: Fill in the blanks

1. Elevated FSH levels, indicative of decreased ovarian response result from a failure of aging ovaries to produce _____.

2. The clomiphene challenge test is a bioassay of _____ response.

3. Natural cycle in vitro fertilization has a delivery rate per retrieval of approximately _____%.

4. In the late 1980's _____ were introduced as a means of down-regulating the pituitary to prevent premature ovulation which in the past had necessitated canceling approximately _____% of IVF cycles.

5. Most IVF programs use both measurements of serum _____ and _____ of ovarian follicles to monitor the ovarian response to stimulation.

6. Risks of hyperstimulation can be decreased by lowering the dose of _____ used to initiate the cycle.

7. Oocytes have a higher chance for fertilization if insemination follows retrieval by _____ hours.

8. Assisted hatching consists of making an opening in the _____ to help the embryo emerge.

9. Only _____% of normal women who attempt pregnancy in a given cycle are successful.

B. Instructions: True of False

10. It takes 3 natural cycles to achieve the pregnancy rate achieved in one stimulated cycle of IVF.

11. The majority of IVF programs presently use a combination of a GnRH agonist plus HMG controlled hyperstimulation with exogenous HCG to trigger ovulation.

12. Ovulation induction regimens including mostly FSH with only a small amount of LH offer a distinct advantage over the equal mixture of FSH and LH.

13. Oocyte retrieval is usually performed transvaginally using ultrasound approximately 24 hours after HCG injection.

14. About 90% of the embryos cryopreserved survive the freezing-thaw process.

15. IVF success rates should be reported in terms of the number of live births per retrieval.

C. Match each acronym with the appropriate description

A. ZIFT　　　C. POST　　　E. ICSI
B. TET　　　D. SUZI

16. peritoneal oocyte and sperm transfer
17. tubal embryo transfer
18. subzonal insertion of sperm by microinjection
19. intracytoplasmic sperm injection
20. zygote intrafallopian transfer

D. Instructions: For each of the following questions choose:
   A. is only 1, 2 and 3 are correct
   B. if only 1 and 3 are correct
   C. if only 2 and 4 are correct
   D. if only 4 is correct
   E. if all are correct

21. Although it is reasonable to recommend tubal surgery in young women with mild distal tubal disease, IVF is the treatment of choice for patients
    1. with more severe tubal disease
    2. with proximal obstruction
    3. who have failed to achieve pregnancy within 2 years after tubal surgery
    4. with moderate endometriosis

22. Which of the following diagnostic tests can provide information for discussing with patients their expectations for success with IVF
    1. day 3 serum FSH
    2. day 21 luteal progesterone
    3. clomiphene challenge test
    4. basal DHEAS

23. Maturity of the oocyte is determined by
    1. the width of the zona pellucida
    2. the morphology of the surrounding cumulus-corona cell complex
    3. its color and contour
    4. the presence or absence of the germinal vesicle and the first polar body

24. Cryopreservation of embryos
    1. can occur at the 2 pronuclei stage
    2. increases the cost of IVF
    3. adds significantly to the success rate
    4. can store embryos safely up to only 3 years

25. Embryo transfer
    1. usually occurs between the 4 and 10 cell stage
    2. occurs approximately 48–80 hours after retrieval
    3. usually includes no more than 4 or 5 embryos
    4. of more than one embryo results in a multiple pregnancy rate of approximately 30%

26. Choice of a particular method of assisted reproductive technology depends upon
    1. the basis of the infertility
    2. chance for success
    3. cost
    4. risk

27. Preimplantation genetic diagnosis has been successful in detecting single gene defects in disorders including
    1. Duchene's muscular dystrophy
    2. Sickle cell disease
    3. Hemophilia
    4. Tay-Sachs disease

28. Success rates of IVF are impacted by
   1. the ages of the women treated
   2. the degree of tubal factor disease
   3. the presence or absence of male factor
   4. the presence or absence of endometriosis

29. Pregnancies resulting from IVF
   1. can be ectopic in 5% of cases
   2. can be heterotopic on rare occasion
   3. can be multiple in 30% cases
   4. have an increased incidence of congenital anomalies

30. Possible treatments of severe male factor using assisted reproductive technologies include
   1. GIFT
   2. SUZI
   3. TET
   4. ICSI

Answers for Chapter 31 — Pre-Test Questions

1. pronuclei p.937

Approximately 50,000–100,000 motile sperm (and much higher for male factor cases) are added to each dish containing an oocyte. The day after insemination, cumulus cells that remain attached to the zona pellucida are removed, and the egg is examined for evidence of fertilization (the presence of 2 pronuclei).

2. 10 p.937

The ability to use fetal reduction to limit the number of continuing fetuses has lessened slightly the concern over multiple births. In experienced hands the risk of losing the entire pregnancy from selective fetal reduction is less than 10%.

3. true p.932

Three distinct populations have been identified on the basis of the cycle day three FSH. With FSH values less than 15 IU/L, the pregnancy rate with IVF was 24%, whereas when the FSH values were 15 to 24.9 IU/L, the pregnancy rate was 13.6%. When the FSH was 25 IU/L or higher the pregnancy rate was 10.7%. However, the ongoing pregnancy rate in this latter group was only 3.6%. A common experience is that successful pregnancy is rare when the FSH is above 25 IU/L. Remember in all discussions pertaining to specific hormone levels that these may vary widely, even in the same sample, depending on which assay system is used. Thus, a figure cited as abnormal in one laboratory may not be abnormal in another.

4. false p.935

Cancellation and avoidance of HCG injections should also be considered if the ovaries are markedly hyperstimulated (greater than 25 follicles) or the total estradiol is greater than 5,000 pg/mL (18,500 pmol/L). Again, the specific values may not be valid with other assays, and each program must establish which estradiol level is its warning sign. The use of FSH as opposed to HMG in women with polycystic ovaries is not protective; with all stimulation protocols, the key is careful use of appropriate doses. An important protection which can be accorded if the women proceed to retrieval is to use progesterone rather than HCG injections to support the luteal phase. Retrieval itself, with aspiration of follicular fluid and granulosa cells, is somewhat but not absolutely protective against hyperstimulation.

5. A p.933

The down-regulating effects of GnRH agonists, as opposed to the stimulatory effects of GnRH, are related to the frequency of administration and the prolonged occupation of GnRH receptors by the agonists. Since their introduction, pregnancy rates have increased because of the opportunity to retrieve cycles that would have been lost to early ovulation and because of the increase in the number of oocytes obtained in GnRH agonist cycles. However, use of an agonist increases the amount of gonadotropins needed to stimulate follicular growth, and thus, it also increases the expense.

6. A p.941

Diagnosing genetic disorders before implantation provides couples with the option of foregoing the attempt to establish a pregnancy. This avoids the difficult decision whether or not to continue an affected pregnancy when the diagnosis is made at amniocentesis or by chorionic villus biopsy. There are 3 possible approaches for preimplantation diagnosis. The first is the removal of the first polar body. The polar body contains only one copy of the gene, but if the copy is found to be normal, it can be presumed that the oocyte contains the abnormal copy. However, this method is technically very difficult and subject to error if crossing-over occurs and both copies are present in the polar body. A second method is to biopsy cells which are destined to become placenta. This requires opening the zona pellucida in the 5–6 day embryo. The disadvantage is the lower pregnancy rate when the embryo is transferred at this later stage. The third method is the removal of a single cell from the 6–8 cell embryo (blastomere biopsy) for DNA amplification and analysis. The biopsy procedure does not affect development and implantation, and the diagnostic testing is rapid; the biopsy and DNA analysis are accomplished within 8 hours.

Answers for Chapter 31 — Post-Test Questions

1. inhibin p.932

In successful IVF programs, where take-home baby rates can be in the 35% range for women 36 and younger, for women over 39 the figure is in the 10% range. Beyond the simple effect of age, there also may be a negative influence on IVF success from decreased ovarian responsiveness. This can be manifested by poor response to exogenous gonadotropin stimulation and by abnormal hormone profiles. The exact definition of a poor responder is uncertain but it encompasses those who respond to stimulation with the development of 4 or less follicles or with depressed estrogen levels. Pretreatment diagnosis of these individuals can be achieved by measuring basal FSH and estradiol levels. Elevated FSH levels, indicative of decreased ovarian reserve, result from a failure of aging ovaries to produce inhibin.

2. FSH p.932

Further attempts to gain prospective information on ovarian responsiveness has centered on provocative tests to stimulate FSH and estradiol. Navot and colleagues developed the clomiphene challenge test as a bioassay of FSH response.

3. 6 p.933

Nonstimulated cycles are still used as a means of decreasing expenses, but the delivery rate per retrieval is approximately 6%. The very low success rate associated with this approach led to the use of clomiphene citrate and human menopausal gonadotropins (HMG) to stimulate the development of multiple ovarian follicles. Injections of human chorionic gonadotropin (HCG), whose biologic activity mimics that of LH, were utilized to allow more certain timing of oocyte retrieval.

4. GnRH agonists; 15 p.933

In the late 1980's gonadotropin releasing hormone agonists (GnRH agonists) were introduced as a means of down-regulating the pituitary to prevent premature ovulation which in the past had necessitated canceling approximately 15% of IVF cycles.

5. estradiol; ultrasound p.935

Most programs use both measurements of serum estradiol and ultrasound imaging of ovarian follicles to monitor the ovarian response to stimulation. The minimum goal of stimulation is to achieve the growth of a lead follicle to at least 17 mm diameter, and at least 3 or 4 other follicles with diameters of 14 mm or greater, combined with estradiol levels of approximately 200 pg/mL (740 pmol/L) per large (14 mm or greater) follicle.

6. HMG   p.935

Risks of hyperstimulation can be decreased by lowering the dose of HMG used to initiate the cycle.

7. 4–6   p.936

One of the major breakthroughs in IVF was the discovery that sperm should not be added to the eggs immediately after retrieval; oocytes have a higher chance for fertilization if insemination follows retrieval by 4 to 6 hours.

8. zona   p.937

Assisted hatching consists of making an opening in the zona pellucida to help the embryo emerge. Assisted hatching is associated with an increased implantation rate, especially in older women.

9. 25   p.938

Many programs have now achieved delivery/retrieval pregnancy rates of more than 25%.

10. true   P.933

It is still possible to reduce costs and the risks of multiple pregnancy by retrieval of a single oocyte from a natural menstrual cycle; however, it requires 3 natural cycles to achieve the pregnancy rate achieved in one stimulated cycle (eventually about one-half the cumulative pregnancy rate).

11. true   p.933

The combination of GnRH agonist and HMG controlled hyperstimulation of the ovary and substitution of exogenous HCG for the endogenous LH surge is now utilized by most IVF programs. This approach has another beneficial attribute; it allows more flexible scheduling of the necessary interventions.

12. false   p.934

Use of a preparation which contains mostly FSH with only a small amount of LH does not seem to offer any striking advantages. It is thought to be of some value for ovulation induction in women with polycystic ovarian disease where endogenous baseline LH levels are elevated and when high doses (450–600 IU) of HMG are used. One of the goals in limiting the dose of LH is to decrease stimulation of the androgenic component of the ovarian response. A newer, purer preparation of FSH, which can be given subcutaneously, will replace the HMG and FSH preparations currently on the market. Eliminating the sometimes painful intramuscular injections will be a major benefit.

13. false   p.936

Ultrasonically guided vaginal oocyte retrieval is performed approximately 34–36 hours after the HCG injection, but as late as 39 hours with the combined use of a GnRH agonist and HMG. The HCG injection allows for confidence in this precise timing.

14. false   p.937

Extra embryos can be cryopreserved at the 2 pronuclei stage. There is no known limit on duration of cryopreserved embryo storage. About two-thirds of embryos survive the process. The transfer of cryopreserved embryos adds significantly to success rates with IVF and lowers the cost.

15. true   p.938

To avoid confusion, only those pregnancies that contain identifiable products of conception, an amniotic sac, or a fetus with a heartbeat on ultrasound examination should be considered a pregnancy for reporting purposes. The most important statistic, which is the number of live births per retrieval, should be the one used for comparison.

16. C   p.931

17. B   p.931

18. D   p.931

19. E   p.931

20. A   p.931

    IVF — In Vitro Fertilization: extraction of oocytes, fertilization in the laboratory, transcervical transfer of embryos into the uterus.
    GIFT — Gamete Intrafallopian Transfer: the placement of oocytes and sperm into the fallopian tube.
    ZIFT — Zygote Intrafallopian Transfer: the placement of fertilized oocytes into the fallopian tube.
    TET — Tubal Embryo Transfer: the placement of cleaving embryos into the fallopian tube.
    POST — Peritoneal Oocyte and Sperm Transfer: the placement of oocytes and sperm into the pelvic cavity.
    SUZI — Subzonal insertion of sperm by microinjection.
    ICSI — Intracytoplasmic sperm injection (of a single spermatozoon).

21. A   p.932

Although it is reasonable to recommend tubal surgery in young women with mild distal tubal disease, IVF is the treatment of choice for patients with more severe distal disease, proximal obstruction (especially after 6 months have elapsed following cannulation or balloon tuboplasty), and for patients who have failed to achieve pregnancy within 2 years after tubal surgery or when tubal obstruction persists after surgery.

22. B   p.934

Whatever protocol is used there is a 10–30% cancellation rate because of inadequate follicular response. Measurements of basal FSH and estradiol and the clomiphene challenge test can provide information for discussing with patients the expectations for success.

23. C   p.936

Maturity of the oocyte is determined by the morphology of the surrounding cumulus-corona cell complex or by the presence or absence of the germinal vesicle and the first polar body.

24. B   p.937

Extra embryos can be cryopreserved at the 2 pronuclei stage. There is no known limit on duration of cryopreserved embryo storage. About two-thirds of embryos survive the process. The transfer of cryopreserved embryos adds significantly to success rates with IVF and lowers the cost. Increasing age is associated with a decrease in pregnancy rates because of a reduction in pre-embryo quality; cycle day 3 FSH levels greater than 15 IU/L are also associated with decreased pregnancy rates, in this case because of fewer embryos available for cryopreservation. Neither age nor basal FSH levels, however, predict failure to survive cryopreservation and thawing.

25. E   p.937

Embryos have been transferred successfully at any stage from the pronuclear to the blastocyst, although most commonly, they are transferred when development is between the 4 and 10 cell stage, approximately 48–80 hours after retrieval. Transfer of more than one embryo increases the chances for pregnancy, but in general no more than 4 or 5 embryos are transferred to limit the risks of multiple births. The multiple pregnancy rate with transfers of more than one embryo is approximately 30%. This risk decreases with advancing age. Thus, in women 40 or older it is reasonable to place higher numbers of embryos.

26. E   p.941

The choice of methods, IVF, GIFT, ZIFT, can be made on the basis of infertility factors, chance for success, cost, and risk. If the problem is male infertility then it is important to know if fertilization can occur, and therefore GIFT would not be an appropriate choice. If there is tubal damage, then GIFT or ZIFT would be unwise. In rare instances where there is scarring of the cervix one of the intratubal techniques would be preferable. The additional cost of GIFT or ZIFT because of the need for anesthesia and operating room time may be a deterrent for many individuals. Moreover, anesthesia entails an additional risk that is usually not associated with IVF. Also important in terms of choosing a technique is consideration of which one the program is most comfortable with and with which it has achieved the best results. These individual results are more important than countrywide statistics. Both GIFT and ZIFT can be accomplished by transcervical cannulation of the fallopian tube with injection of gametes or embryos into the tube. Despite the attractiveness of these cannulation techniques because they do not require anesthesia, they have not provided an increase in pregnancy rates over that achieved with IVF.

27. E   p.941
Preimplantation genetic diagnosis has successfully detected single gene defects in disorders such as Duchene's muscular dystrophy, sickle cell disease, hemophilia, Tay-Sachs disease, and Lesch-Nyhan syndrome. These methods can also be used to predict the sex of embryos from couples who are at risk for transmitting X-linked disorders.

28. B   p.938
Success rates are impacted by the ages of the women treated by the programs and the presence or absence of male factors.

29. A   p.938
Surprisingly, 4–5% of pregnancies achieved through IVF are ectopic, emphasizing the need for close ultrasonographic and HCG titer surveillance. Pregnancies occurring simultaneously in different body sites (heterotropic pregnancies) are a rare condition, occurring in 1 of 30,000 spontaneous pregnancies. The incidence of combined pregnancy among patients who have undergone one of the assisted reproduction procedures is much higher, closer to 1 in 100 pregnancies. A case-control study has concluded that the risk of ectopic pregnancy with assisted reproduction is due to the multiple ovulations and high hormone levels secondary to the stimulation protocols. Twenty percent of clinical pregnancies result in spontaneous abortions because that is close to the rate in infertility populations; there is no increase in the rate of congenital malformations. The multiple pregnancy rate is approximately 30% (25% twins and 5% triplets or more).

30. C   p.939,940
IVF provides the ability to visualize the results of sperm and egg interaction and thus to quickly determine if specific manipulations of the sperm can affect fertilization. A variety of sperm treatments have been attempted. One approach is to increase the number of sperm in the dish with the hope that even with abnormal specimens there will be a few normal sperm that can achieve fertilization. By increasing the numbers in each dish there will be more normal sperm per egg. A second approach is to isolate the best sperm from the specimen, not from the standard swim-up technique, but by using Percoll gradients. In some hands this has provided increased fertilization rates, but others have not found it to be a significant advantage. Similar contradictory results have been reported with drug treatment of the semen; the most popular such treatment has utilized pentoxifylline which acts by increasing cyclic AMP in cells. The drug must be washed out from the sperm specimen before incubation with the egg because it may have adverse effects on the latter. Another treatment that has been used to enhance sperm is incubation in follicular fluid. In men with sperm autoantibodies, in vitro fertilization is correlated with the extent the sperm are covered with antibodies, but if fertilization occurs, pregnancy follows at the usual rates.

Micromanipulation
Many of these techniques now have been overshadowed by the use of sperm micromanipulation. Initially, a microneedle was used to make a small puncture in the zona pellucida (partial zona dissection) with the presumption that sperm would be able to breach the opening and proceed on to the egg membrane. Limited success with this technique led to the development of subzonal insertion of sperm (SUZI) by microinjection. In this technique 5 to 10 sperm are injected into the perivitelline space. More than one sperm are injected because not all are physiologically prepared for membrane fusion. Injection of more than one sperm under the zona does increase somewhat the risk of forming triploid embryos.

The most startling of the microneedle approaches has been the direct injection of one sperm into the egg cytoplasm. Van Steirtenghen and his coworkers in Belgium pioneered the technique for intracytoplasmic sperm injection (ICSI) of a single spermatozoon and have reported it to be superior to subzonal insemination (SUZI). Fifty-three percent of oocytes injected into the cytoplasm with a single sperm had two pronuclei compared to 17% with SUZI. The clinical pregnancy rate with ICSI was 26% per cycle. With ICSI, in vivo protective mechanisms against abnormal sperm are bypassed. However, it is reassuring that Van Steirtenghen reported that 151 normal karyotypes were obtained by prenatal diagnosis from his patients, and that follow-up of 119 children born following ICSI did not reveal an increase in major congenital anomalies. An alternative has been suggested, using "heavy insemination" (effective concentrations of 1 to 5 million sperm per mL in a microdroplet under oil) of individual oocytes. These techniques have achieved pregnancies with sperm counts less than 100,000/mL and with zero motile spermatozoa and no normal forms. Thus, the andrologist and the embryologist now have a variety of techniques to call on to overcome that most difficult of problems — male infertility.

32 Ectopic Pregnancy

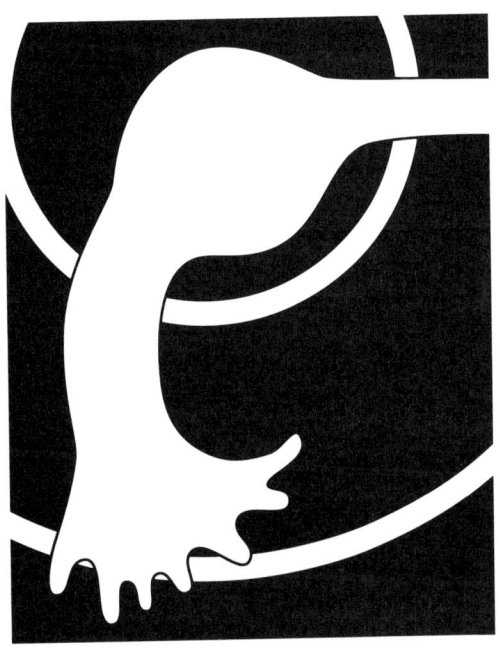

Learning Objectives

Be able to:

1. Describe the known risk factors and suspected etiologies of ectopic pregnancy.

2. Discuss the methods of early diagnosis of an ectopic pregnancy.

3. Detail treatment options available for both medical and surgical resolution of ectopic pregnancy.

4. Discuss what is known regarding the diagnosis and treatment of persistent trophoblast tissue.

Pre-Test

A. Instructions: Fill in the blanks

1. A progesterone value of _____ng/ml or more is 98% of the time associated with a normal intrauterine pregnancy, while a value of less than _____ ng/ml identifies a nonviable pregnancy, regardless of location.

2. The most common complication following laparoscopic salpingostomy for treatment of an unruptured ectopic is _____ trophoblast tissue.

B. Instructions: True or False

3. Although the number of ectopic pregnancies in the U.S. has stabilized since 1987, the fatality rate has decreased 90%.

4. The risk of ectopic pregnancy is reduced with all methods of contraception.

C. Instructions: For the following questions choose:

A. if only 1, 2 and 3 are correct
B. if only 1 and 3 are correct
C. if only 2 and 4 are correct
D. if only 4 is correct
E. if all are correct

5. In the surgical management of an ectopic pregnancy radical (salpingectomy) may be preferred to conservative surgery in the setting of
   1. a second ectopic in the same tube
   2. childbearing has not been completed
   3. uncontrolled bleeding
   4. a normal appearing contralateral tube

6. Results following laparoscopic salpingostomy for ectopic pregnancy includes
   1. success in 95% of cases
   2. 70% subsequent intrauterine pregnancy rate
   3. 12% subsequent ectopic pregnancy rate
   4. 15% subsequent persistent trophoblast rate

Post-Test

A. Instructions: Fill in the blanks

1. Today management intervention occurs prior to tubal rupture in more than ____% of cases.

2. The incidence of a heterotopic pregnancy following assisted reproductive technologies is _____% of pregnancies.

3. The maternal circulating HCG concentrate is approximately _____ IU/L at the time of the expected but missed menses.

4. From 2 to 4 weeks after ovulation HCG titers double every _____ days until the titer is greater than _____.

5. Approximately _____% of women presenting with ectopic pregnancy can be managed expectantly and _____% of this select group of patients will avoid surgery and have successful outcomes.

6. Baseline laboratories required prior to administering methotrexate for ectopic pregnancy include _____ and _____ function tests, complete blood and platelet counts.

7. An ectopic pregnancy after a previous tubal ligation is usually located in the segment of tube containing the _____.

8. Rhogam should be administered to any patient who is Rh negative with an ectopic of greater than _____ weeks of gestation.

B. Instructions: True or False

9. In the last 20 years the treatment of ectopic pregnancy has shifted from the saving of lives to the preservation of fertility.

10. In 1970, there were 17,800 ectopic pregnancies reported in the U.S. by 1987 the number had increased to 88,000, a rate increase of 4.5 to 16.8 ectopic pregnancies per 1,000 pregnancies.

11. Ectopic pregnancies do occur in totally normal tubes.

12. The classic triad of delayed menses, irregular vaginal bleeding and abdominal pain is most commonly encountered in the setting of an ectopic pregnancy.

13. Most patients presenting with an ectopic pregnancy have a recognized risk factor.

14. Pregnancies following tubal surgery or treatment with a method of assisted reproduction should, ideally, be diagnosed immediately.

15. The modern copper-bearing IUDs do not increase the risk of ectopic pregnancy.

16. If pregnancy occurs while a woman is using Norplant one must rule out ectopic pregnancy as soon as possible.

17. Contrary to the experience with tubal pregnancy recurrence in nontubal sites is rare.

18. With multiple gestation, a gestational sac will not be apparent until the HCG titer is a little higher than that expected for a singleton pregnancy (i.e., 1500 IU/L).

19. Expectant management of an ectopic pregnancy can be attempted in a woman with plateauing HCG titers.

C. Instructions: For the following questions choose:

- A. if only 1, 2 and 3 are correct
- B. if only 1 and 3 are correct
- C. if only 2 and 4 are correct
- D. if only 4 is correct
- E. if all are correct

20. Contributing factors to the increase in incidence of ectopic pregnancy are due to increases in
    1. sexually transmitted diseases
    2. tubal surgery
    3. assisted reproductive technologies
    4. earlier, more accurate diagnosis

21. A woman with a history of previous pelvic inflammatory disease
    1. has a four-fold increased risk of ectopic pregnancy
    2. increases her risk for an ectopic with each inflammatory episode
    3. may have damage of the endosalpinx with agglutination of the mucosal folds
    4. does not have circulating antibodies to chlamydia

22. Women with specific types of tubal surgery have an increased risk of ectopic pregnancy. Specific types include
    1. prior conservative surgery for ectopic pregnancy
    2. fimbrioplasty
    3. interval tubal sterilization
    4. tubal anastomosis

23. Medical treatment of ectopic pregnancy with methotrexate
    1. can involve single or multiple dose methods
    2. can be associated with stomatitis, gastritis, diarrhea and/or abdominal cramping
    3. can be associated with a persistent mass on ultrasound despite negative HCG titers following treatment
    4. has been compared for short- and long-term success to laparoscopic salpingostomy in a randomized, controlled study

24. The preference of methotrexate to surgery is particularly suited for ectopics located
    1. in the abdomen
    2. in the cornua
    3. in the omentum
    4. in the cervix

25. Salpingocentesis as a treatment for ectopic pregnancy
    1. is as effective as systemic medical therapy
    2. is as effective as surgical therapy
    3. is as effective as expectant management
    4. is limited because the efficacy, safety and long-term reproductive outcome are unknown

26. Persistent trophoblastic tissue
    1. occurs rarely following laparoscopic salpingostomy
    2. is more common following laparoscopic salpingostomy than salpingostomy by laparotomy
    3. commonly becomes choriocarcinoma
    4. stresses the importance of following HCG titers to undetectable levels following salpingostomy

Answers for Chapter 32 — Pre-Test Questions

1. 25; 5 p.955

Serum progesterone levels have a wide spectrum with considerable overlap between normal and ectopic pregnancies. This measurement must be viewed as an adjunct to HCG levels and ultrasonography. The concentration of the serum progesterone is usually lower in ectopic pregnancies. A value of 25 ng/mL (80 nmol/L) or more is 98% of the time associated with a normal intrauterine pregnancy, while a value of less than 5 ng/mL (16 nmol/L) identifies a nonviable pregnancy, regardless of location. The value of the serum progesterone is to help make a decision regarding the viability of a possible intrauterine pregnancy prior to curettage. In most cases, however, this is a decision easily made by the combined results of the clinical presentation, the HCG titers, and ultrasonography. The great majority of patients will have a progesterone level between 10 and 20 ng/mL (30 and 60 nmol/L) at presentation, significantly limiting the clinical usefulness of progesterone measurement. The value of 25 ng/mL as an indicator of a normal intrauterine pregnancy was established in women with spontaneous ovulations and pregnancies. The appropriate number for women receiving medication for the induction of ovulation is probably higher, and in these cases, the use of the progesterone level is even more limited.

2. persistent p.961

The risk of a persistent ectopic pregnancy with conservative surgery by laparotomy is 5%. Laparoscopic salpingostomy is associated with a higher rate of persistent trophoblastic tissue; approximately 15% of patients will require further treatment.

3. true p.948

Since 1987, the number of ectopic pregnancies in the United States has stabilized. *However, at the same time, the fatality rate decreased from 35.5 to 3.8 per 10,000 ectopic pregnancies, a decrease of 90%.*

4. false p.950

The risk of ectopic pregnancy is reduced with all methods of contraception except the progesterone-containing intrauterine device.

5. B p.960

Indications for Salpingectomy
    Childbearing completed.
    Second ectopic pregnancy in the same tube.
    Uncontrolled bleeding.
    Severely damaged tube.

6. E p.961

Results with Laparoscopic Surgery

Successful	95%
Subsequent intrauterine pregnancy	70%
Subsequent tubal patency	84%
Subsequent ectopic pregnancy	12%
Persistent trophoblast	15%

Answers for Chapter 32 — Post-Test Questions

1. 80
p.948

Today management intervention occurs prior to tubal rupture in more than 80% of cases. This can be attributed directly to three diagnostic advances: a highly specific and sensitive immunoassay for human chorionic gonadotropin (HCG), ultrasonography, and the use of laparoscopy.

2. 1
p.950

Pregnancies occurring *simultaneously* in different body sites *(heterotopic pregnancies)* are a rare condition, occurring in 1 of 30,000 spontaneous pregnancies. The incidence of combined pregnancy among patients who have undergone one of the assisted reproduction procedures (in vitro fertilization, gamete intrafallopian transfer, and even superovulation) is much higher, closer to 1 in 100 pregnancies.

3. 100
p.952

HCG is secreted by the syncytiotrophoblast and reaches a maximal level of 50,000–100,000 IU/L at 8–10 weeks of gestation. The maternal circulating HCG concentration is approximately 100 IU/L at the time of the expected but missed menses.

4. 2; 10,000
p.952

A landmark observation was reported in 1981, documenting that HCG levels approximately double every 2 days in early, normal intrauterine pregnancies, and that a lesser increase is associated with ectopic pregnancies and spontaneous abortions. In the first 6 weeks of normal pregnancy, the concentration of HCG in the maternal blood follows a well-recognized pattern. The rate of increase is nonlinear, changing with advancing gestational age and increasing HCG concentrations. However, during the time period when the diagnosis of ectopic pregnancy is most important, from 2 to 4 weeks after ovulation, the relationship between HCG titers and gestational age is linear, approximately doubling every 2 days until the titer is greater than 10,000. Use of the HCG titer requires medical judgment. Some ectopic pregnancies will display a normal rise in titer (at least for awhile), and some normal pregnancies (about 10%) will have an abnormal doubling time.

5. 25; 70
p.956

Part of the increased incidence of ectopic pregnancy is due to earlier diagnosis detecting ectopic pregnancies which previously resolved and remained clinically undiagnosed. Not all tubal pregnancies progress to clinical manifestations, and therefore expectant management of ectopic pregnancies diagnosed very early is an appropriate choice. Expectant management includes the monitoring of clinical symptoms, HCG titers, and ultrasonography findings. Approximately one-fourth of women presenting with ectopic pregnancy can be managed expectantly, and 70% of this select group of patients will avoid surgery and experience successful outcomes. The long-term outcome (subsequent intrauterine and ectopic pregnancies) is similar to that with active treatment interventions.

6. liver; renal
p.957

Prior to Methotrexate Treatment
1. Administer Rhogam if patient is Rh negative and greater than 8 weeks gestation.
2. Obtain baseline liver and renal function tests, complete blood and platelet counts.
3. Consider uterine curettage.

7. fimbria
p.961

An ectopic pregnancy after a previous tubal ligation is usually located in the segment of tube containing the fimbria. The pregnancy occurs because of small channel recannulation through the ligation site, allowing sperm to migrate toward the oocyte. A prophylactic procedure should be highly considered. Removing both fimbrial segments and fulgurating the proximal segments (either by laparoscopy or laparotomy) will prevent the recurrence of another ectopic pregnancy.

8. 8
p.961

Despite underutilization of Rhogam in Rh-negative women, no apparent increase in sensitization has been observed. This indicates that ectopic pregnancies do not contain sufficiently large quantities of fetal red blood cells. The use of

Rhogam should be considered only for ectopic pregnancies that are older than 8 weeks gestation.

9. true p.948

Asepsis, anesthesia, and antibiotics (and blood transfusions) combined to save the lives of many women. But diagnosis was still difficult, and surgical intervention was relatively late. Even in the first half of the 20th century, the maternal mortality rate in the United States ranged from 200 to 400 per 10,000 cases of ectopic pregnancies. As dramatic as the contribution of immediate salpingectomy coupled with simultaneous blood transfusion was, progress in the last 20 years has been even more impressive. Treatment has shifted from the saving of lives to the preservation of fertility.

10. true p.948

The Centers for Disease Control first began to report the incidence of ectopic pregnancies in the U.S. in 1970. In 1970, there were 17,800 ectopic pregnancies, and by 1987, the number had increased to 88,000, a rate increase of 4.5 to 16.8 ectopic pregnancies per 1,000 pregnancies.

11. true p.948

The increase in ectopic pregnancies has not been paralleled by a similar increase in sexually transmitted diseases (STDs), and therefore, the increased incidence of ectopic pregnancies is not due to STDs alone. Ectopic pregnancies do occur in totally normal tubes, suggesting that abnormalities of the conceptus or maternal hormonal changes can function as etiologic factors.

12. false p.949

Ectopic pregnancy is the great masquerader. The clinical presentation can vary from vaginal spotting to vasomotor shock with hematoperitoneum. The classic triad of delayed menses, irregular vaginal bleeding, and abdominal pain is most commonly *not* encountered. The exact frequency of clinical symptoms and signs is hard to assess. Standard descriptions in texts are based upon older reports and, thus, older methods of diagnosis.

Patients with normal intrauterine pregnancies can present with the same symptoms encountered in patients with unruptured ectopic pregnancies. The best way to diagnose ectopic pregnancy is to be highly suspicious and sensitive to its possibility, and to utilize the new tools of diagnosis: the quantitative measurement of HCG and ultrasonography. Laparoscopy is necessary only when the diagnosis is in doubt, or when laparoscopy is the technique selected for surgical treatment. (See figure on page 430 in this Study Guide)

13. false p.949

Relevant factors in a patient's medical history include previous pelvic inflammatory disease, prior tubal surgery, the use of assisted reproductive technology, exposure to diethylstilbestrol (DES), and the method of contraception. However, most patients presenting with an ectopic pregnancy do not have a recognized risk factor, suggesting dysfunctional problems in tubal transport or impaired implantation due to some abnormality in the conceptus.

14. true p.949

Pregnancies following tubal surgery or treatment with one of the methods of assisted reproduction should, ideally, be diagnosed immediately and followed closely with HCG titers and ultrasonography.

15. true p.950

The IUD has been traditionally listed as a risk factor for ectopic pregnancy. It should be emphasized that the modern copper-bearing IUDs do *NOT* increase the risk of ectopic pregnancy and, in fact, offer considerable protection. The largest study, a World Health Organization multicenter study, concluded that IUD users were 50% less likely to have an ectopic pregnancy when compared to women using no contraception. However, if an IUD user becomes pregnant, the pregnancy is more likely to be ectopic. About 3–4% of IUD pregnancies have been ectopic, making the actual occurrence a rare event. The protection against ectopic pregnancy provided by the copper and levonorgestrel IUDs makes these IUDs acceptable choices for contraception in women with previous ectopic pregnancies.

16. true p.950

The risk of an ectopic pregnancy during use of Norplant is lower than the general rate. However, because of the impressive contraceptive efficacy of Norplant, when pregnancy does occur, ectopic pregnancy should be suspected.

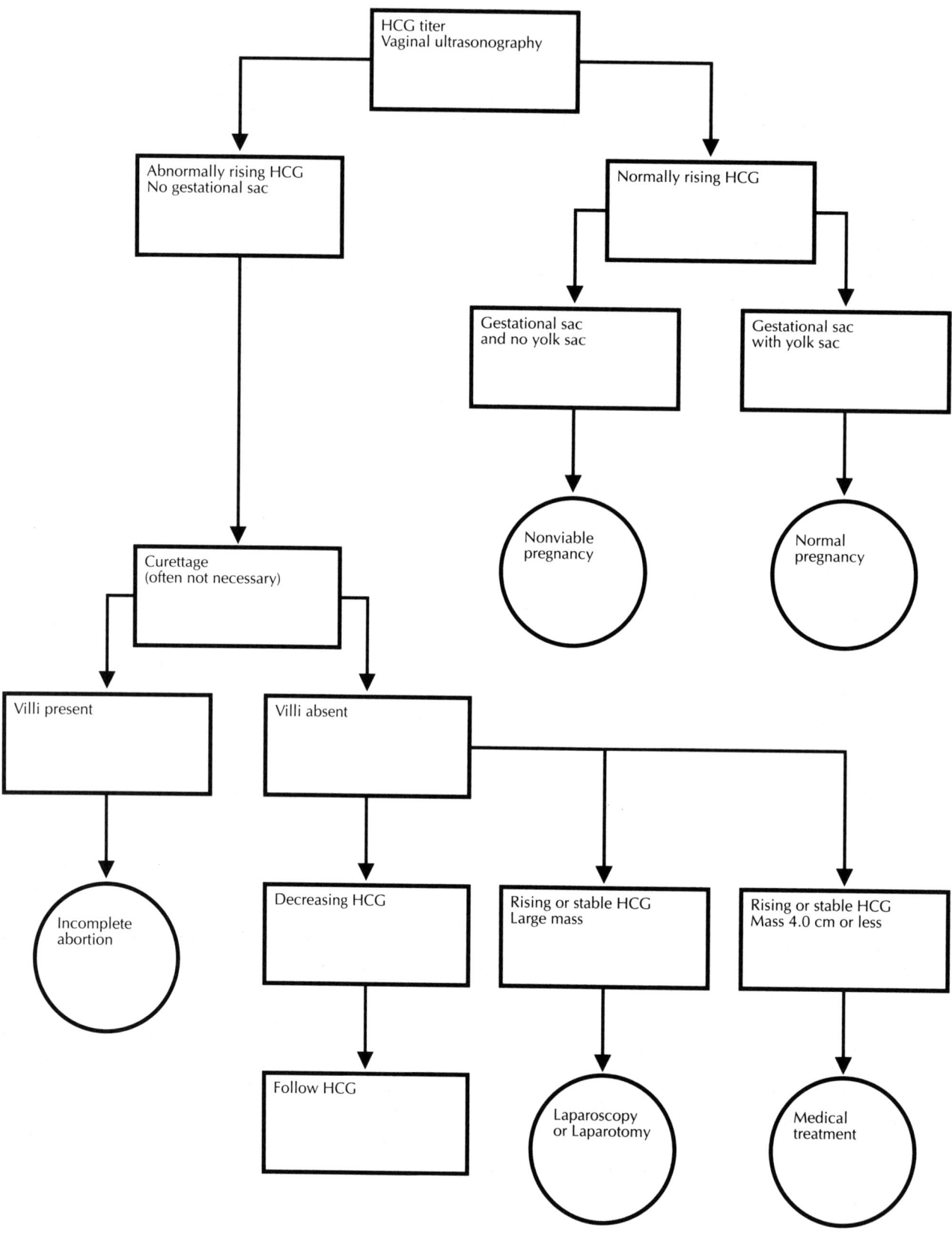

With the progestin-only minipill, ectopic pregnancy is not prevented as effectively as intrauterine pregnancy. Although the overall incidence is not increased, the situation is similar to that with Norplant. When pregnancy occurs, an ectopic gestation must be suspected.

17. true p.951

Almost all ectopic pregnancies are located in the tube. Although relatively uncommon, ectopic pregnancies in nontubal sites are very susceptible to complications, especially hemorrhage. For example, abdominal pregnancies are often misdiagnosed, and the mortality rate is 17 times greater compared to the overall ectopic rate. Contrary to the experience with tubal pregnancy, recurrence in nontubal sites is rare.

18. true p.952

When the titer exceeds 1,000–1,500 IU/L, vaginal ultrasonography should identify the presence of an intrauterine gestation. With multiple gestation, a gestational sac will not be apparent until the titer is a little higher. In an asymptomatic patient, repeat ultrasonography 2–3 days later is warranted.

19. false p.956

Criteria for Expectant Management
1. Falling HCG titer.
2. Ectopic pregnancy definitely in the tube.
3. No significant bleeding.
4. No evidence of rupture.
5. Ectopic mass not larger than 4 cm in greatest diameter.

20. E p.948,949

The important contributing factors to an increase in ectopic pregnancies are STDs, reconstructive tubal surgery, assisted reproductive technologies, and most importantly, earlier and more accurate diagnosis.

21. A p.949

In Westrom's classic report, women with a history of salpingitis (verified by laparoscopy) had a four-fold increased risk of ectopic pregnancy. The one predisposing factor identified most often is previous pelvic inflammatory disease, either by history or histologic evidence in removed tubal tissue. Salpingitis damages the endosalpinx, resulting in agglutination of the mucosal folds and adhesion formation. The risk of an ectopic pregnancy increases with each inflammatory episode. Evidence of chlamydial infection (circulating antibodies) is associated with a greater than two-fold increased risk of ectopic pregnancy. A similar increased risk is associated with douching, but the presence of infection may be the reason for the douching.

22. E p.949,950

Women with tubal surgery have an increased risk of ectopic pregnancy. High risk surgery includes any infertility surgery on the tube, but not abdominal or pelvic surgery that avoids the tubes. Women with an ectopic pregnancy treated by conservative surgery have a ten-fold increased risk of a subsequent ectopic. Ectopic pregnancies occur after tubal occlusion procedures for sterilization that are not performed immediately postpartum (interval sterilization); the risk with postpartum sterilization is very low, comparable to that observed in oral contraceptive users. With interval sterilization, bipolar tubal coagulation is more likely to result in ectopic pregnancy than is mechanical occlusion. This is attributed to fistula formation that allows sperm passage, and this may explain the difference in ectopic pregnancy rates between interval and postpartum sterilization because postpartum procedures are mostly by the Pomeroy method. Ectopic pregnancies following tubal ligation usually occur two or more years after the sterilization, rather than immediately after. In the first year after sterilization, about 6% of sterilization failures will be ectopic pregnancies, but the majority of pregnancies that occur 2–3 years after occlusion will be ectopic. Overall, the ectopic risk in women with interval sterilizations is 80% less than that in nonsterilized women; however, the relative risk is 3.7 times that of women using oral contraception and 2.8 times that with barrier methods of contraception.

23. A p.957,958

The initial protocols for treatment utilized multiple doses of methotrexate together with citrovorum factor (folinic acid) to minimize side effects. Treatment with this method has been 95% successful. Failures have been more common with

HCG levels greater than 5,000 IU/mL, and thus the presence of fetal cardiac activity is generally a contraindication. Side effects (in 3–4% of patients) include mild stomatitis, gastritis, diarrhea, and transient elevations in liver enzymes. Significant reactions (bone marrow suppression, dermatitis, pleuritis) have been very rare. The incidence of non-responders and/or tubal rupture is 3–4%.

In terms of subsequent fertility, methotrexate compares favorably with conservative laparoscopic surgery. In Stovall's experience, of those attempting pregnancy, 62.5% became pregnant with a recurrent ectopic rate of 10.8%. The mean time to return of menses was 26 days (usually within the first month). These results match well with the 67% intrauterine pregnancy rate and 12% recurrent ectopic rate with laparoscopic surgery.

The ultrasonographic picture of a mass persists after HCG titers become negative. The time for resolution of the mass is variable, and often it takes several months. Thus, the persistence of a mass should not be interpreted as a treatment failure.

Experience with the multiple dose method indicated that a significant number of patients responded promptly and did not require several doses. With lesser dosing, fewer side effects could be anticipated, and the use of citrovorum factor could be abandoned. The initial results with a single dose have been very encouraging, even with very high HCG titers and the presence of fetal cardiac activity. The HCG titers usually keep rising for 3 days after treatment but by day 7 are declining. Full resolution requires 3 to as much as 6 weeks. Serious side effects are virtually absent. If there is less than a 15% decline on day 7 (the usual assay variation), the treatment protocol is repeated (necessary in approximately 3% of patients). In a prospective series of 120 patients, 87.2% achieved a subsequent intrauterine gestation, whereas 12.8% experienced a subsequent ectopic pregnancy.

24. C p.959

Treatment with methotrexate is especially useful when the pregnancy is located in a site (cervix, ovary, or cornua) where surgical treatment carries significant risk. Methotrexate treatment is an attractive option when an ectopic pregnancy is in the interstitial portion of the tube, growing in the wall of the uterus (diagnosed by ultrasonography).

25. D p.959

Salpingocentesis is the injection of a substance directly into the gestational sac within the tube, either at laparoscopy or under ultrasound guidance. Various substances have been used, including methotrexate, potassium chloride, prostaglandins, and hyperosmotic glucose. The efficacy, safety, and the long-term impact on fertility have not been established. Thus far local injections have been associated with inconsistent results; at least one clinical trial was discontinued because of poor results with tubal injection of methotrexate while another claimed excellent results, especially when the HCG level was under 5,000 IU/L. Circulating levels of methotrexate are similar when gestational sac injection is compared to intramuscular injection. Thus, local treatment with methotrexate offers no obvious advantage over systemic treatment. Hyperosmotic glucose (a 50% solution) appears to be safe and effective when the HCG titers are less than 2,500 IU/L.

26. C p.961

Laparoscopic salpingostomy is associated with a higher rate of persistent trophoblastic tissue; approximately 15% of patients will require further treatment. Persistence of ectopic trophoblastic tissue can be associated with hemorrhage and tubal rupture (usually within 2 weeks); however, regression without clinical sequelae is the general rule. For this reason, **weekly HCG measurements are necessary following conservative surgery.** The incidence of persistent trophoblastic tissue is greater (not surprising) with higher HCG titers, and relatively rare with a titer less than 3,000 IU/L. The risk of persistent trophoblastic tissue is very significant with a hematosalpinx greater than 6 cm in diameter, an HCG titer greater than 20,000 IU/L, and a hematoperitoneum greater than 2,000 mL. Rupture is unlikely for an ampullary pregnancy with an HCG level of 100 or less, but not so for an isthmic pregnancy.

The average time for HCG levels to become undetectable is 4 weeks, but it can take 6 weeks. The need for treatment of persistent trophoblastic tissue can emerge in a few days or not until 1 month later. Although reoperation is always a treatment option, the use of methotrexate in one of the above protocols is preferable. Even lower doses (15 mg im) have been successfully used. Low and declining HCG levels warrant only close surveillance; only persistent or rising titers require treatment (a small minority of patients). Symptomatic patients, of course, usually demand surgical therapy.

33 Clinical Assays

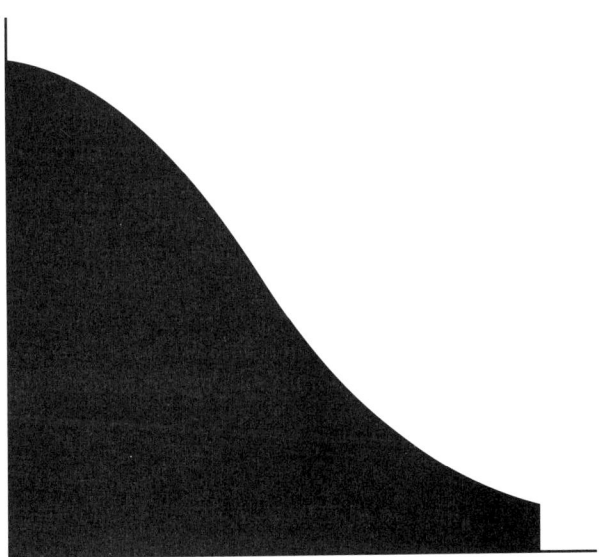

Learning Objectives

Be able to:

1. Discuss the basic principles of IRMAs, the production of monoclonal antibodies, ELISA and RIAs.

2. Describe the standards used for HCG assays.

3. Detail examples and the logistics of performing diagnostic adrenal testing.

Clinical Gynecologic Endocrinology and Infertility: Self Assessment and Study Guide

Pre-Test

A. Instructions: Fill in the blanks

1. The immunoassay of _____ has replaced the measurement of urinary 17-ketosteroids for the routine evaluation of adrenal androgen production.

2. The most widely used current standard for HCG is the First _____ _____ _____.

B. Instructions: True or False

3. Progesterone levels during pregnancy plateau in the second trimester and do not exceed 100 ng/ml for the remainder of the gestation.

4. Pregnanediol is the main urinary metabolite of estradiol.

C. Instructions: For the following questions choose:

A. if only 1, 2 and 3 are correct
B. if only 1 and 3 are correct
C. if only 2 and 4 are correct
D. if only 4 is correct
E. if all are correct

5. Examples of different methods which use the saturation analysis principle include
   1. RIA
   2. IRMA
   3. monoclonal antibodies
   4. ELISA

6. HCG
   1. peak levels of 100,000 IU/L occur at 8–10 weeks of gestation
   2. concentration is 50 IU/L about the date of expected menses
   3. levels decline to 10 to 20,000 IU/L by 12–14 weeks
   4. levels double every 2 days above 6,000 IU/L

Post-Test

A. Instructions: Fill in the blanks

1. The conversion from conventional to System International (SI) units represents the change in the expression of concentration from mass per volume to _____ per volume.

2. The conversion from conventional units to SI units is based on the _____ weight of the analyte.

3. Reactions in saturation analysis follow the law of _____ _____.

4. The initial step in measuring a substance is to obtain a pure sample by performing an _____ process which removes compounds that may interfere with a planned assay.

5. Since steroid compounds are not _____, the production of a specific antiserum depends upon the linkage of a steroid to a _____ protein molecule.

6. Serum FSH and LH values less than _____ IU/L are consistent with a hypogonadotropic state.

7. _____ is the urinary metabolite of 17-hydroxyprogesterone.

8. At 8 PM the level of serum cortisol is about _____ the morning concentration.

B. Instructions: True or False

9. The need for radioisotopes in saturation analysis can be replaced by the use of chemiluminescence, fluroimmunoassays, or enzyme linked assays.

10. In immunoradiometric assays (IRMAs) the antibody is labeled instead of the hormone.

11. Over-the-counter LH kits are available to detect the LH midcycle surge in urine utilizing enzyme immunoassays with monoclonal antibodies.

12. The immunoassay of 17-hydroxyprogesterone has replaced measurement of the urinary pregnanetriol level for the diagnosis of adrenal enzyme deficiency.

13. Serum DHAS decreases with age.

14. 2 units of the Second International Standard are approximately equivalent to 1 unit of the International Reference Preparation.

15. It is wise to obtain a urinary creatinine as a check of the validity of a 24 hour urine specimen.

16. Blood levels of ACTH and cortisol are highest in the early morning and lowest in the evening.

C. Match each SI prefix with the correct log expression in grams

A. pico
B. micro
C. nano
D. femto

17. 10^{-9}
18. 10^{-12}
19. 10^{-15}

D. Instructions: For the following questions choose:

- A. if only 1, 2 and 3 are correct
- B. if only 1 and 3 are correct
- C. if only 2 and 4 are correct
- D. if only 4 is correct
- E. if all are correct

20. Traditionally hormones were measured in blood by bioassays. However, bioassays had various limitations which included
    1. imprecision
    2. nonspecificity
    3. expensive
    4. labor intensive

21. The ELISA method
    1. does not require a radioactive tracer
    2. uses two monoclonal antibodies for the measurement of HCG, LH or TSH
    3. is utilized for most over-the-counter LH tests and pregnancy tests
    4. usually takes more time to perform than an RIA

22. The accuracy of results from various methods of saturation analysis depends upon
    1. the specificity of the antibody
    2. the purity and specificity of the radiolabeled tracer
    3. the purity and availability of the standard reference hormone
    4. the sensitivity and precision of the assay

23. Routine assessment of adrenal androgen production
    1. utilizes an immunoassay for DHAS
    2. requires a fasting sample
    3. does not utilize urinary 17-ketosteroids
    4. must correct for body weight

24. The ACTH stimulation test
    1. is administered as synthetic ACTH injected as a bolus of 0.50 mg
    2. is a test for adrenal reserve
    3. is an expensive test
    4. should result in an increase of at least 2 times over baseline at 30 and 60 minutes

25. The metyrapone test
    1. is a test of ACTH reserve
    2. is a test of ovarian reserve
    3. is administered as a 250 mg every 4 hours for 6 doses
    4. is a commonly used test in reproductive endocrinology

Answers for Chapter 33 — Pre-Test Questions

1. DHAS
   p.976

The immunoassay of dehydroepiandrosterone sulfate (DHAS) has replaced the measurement of urinary 17-ketosteroids for the routine evaluation of adrenal androgen production. A random sample is sufficient, needing no corrections for body weight, creatinine excretion, or random variation. Variations are minimized because of its high circulating concentration and its long half-life. It is a direct measure of adrenal androgen activity correlating clinically with the urinary 17-ketosteroids.

2. International Reference Preparation p.978

The most widely used current standard is the First International Reference Preparation provided by the World Health Organization. The 1st IRP succeeded the Second International Standard; 2 units of the 1st IRP are approximately equivalent to 1 unit of the 2nd IS. A third standard is appearing, the 3rd International Standard. Care must be taken in comparing values obtained in different assays with different standards.

3. false p.975

	Estradiol	**Progesterone**	**Testosterone**
Follicular phase	25–75 pg/mL	Less than 1 ng/mL	20–80 ng/dL
Midcycle peak	200–600 pg/mL		20–80 ng/dL
Luteal phase	100–300 pg/mL	5–20 ng/mL	20–80 ng/dL
Pregnancy: 1st trimester	1–5 ng/mL	20–30 ng/mL	
Pregnancy: 2nd trimester	5–15 ng/mL	50–100 ng/mL	
Pregnancy: 3rd trimester	10–40 ng/mL	100–400 ng/mL	
Postmenopause	5–25 pg/mL	Less than 1 ng/mL	10–40 ng/dL

4. false p.977

Pregnanediol is the main urinary metabolite of progesterone, although it accounts for only 7–20% of total progesterone production. Measurement of pregnanediol in a 24-hour urine sample has been used in the past to document pregnancy and especially the well-being of an early pregnancy. However, with the advent of the measurement of plasma progesterone, the use of urinary pregnanediol has waned.

5. E p.970–72

In immunoradiometric assays (IRMAs), the antibody is labeled instead of the hormone. The advantage is the greater stability in iodinated immunoglobulins compared to iodinated hormones. Monoclonal antibodies are homogeneous, eliminating the heterogeneity and variability associated with antiserum obtained by the regular immunization process (polyclonal antibodies). ELISA stands for enzyme-linked immunosorbent assay, also known as the sandwiched technique. This method does not require a radioactive tracer.

6. B p.978

Peak levels of HCG (mean values of 50,000 to 100,000 IU/L and a range of 20,000 to 200,000 IU/L) occur at 8–10 weeks of gestation, declining and remaining at approximately 10,000–20,000 IU/L by 12–14 weeks. Evaluation of a patient following a spontaneous or therapeutic abortion is occasionally a difficult problem. The urinary pregnancy test will be negative 3 weeks after abortion. The HCG level increases at different rates in normal and ectopic pregnancies. In a normal pregnancy the HCG should approximately double every 2 days in the 2–4 weeks after ovulation. When the HCG titer exceeds 1,000–1,500 IU/L, vaginal ultrasonograpy will identify the presence of an intrauterine gestation. When the HCG titer is below 1,500 IU/L and ultrasound examination fails to identify an intrauterine pregnancy, a patient may be managed expectantly if the HCG titer doubles in 2 days. If the titer does not double, an ectopic pregnancy must be suspected.

In clinical practice, these guidelines are not always so clear and definitive. The rate of HCG increase changes with advancing gestational age and increasing HCG concentrations. While the HCG level approximately doubles every 2 days below a level of 1,200 IU/L, from 1,200–6,000 IU/L, it takes nearly 3 days to double, and above 6,000 IU/L, about 4 days. In addition the zone at which a gestational sac is seen by ultrasound varies for different assays and different reference preparations. One should be sure that the discriminatory zone of 1,000–1,500 IU/mL applies to your local assay.

Answers for Chapter 33 — Post-Test Questions

1. amount p.967

The International System of Units (SI units — Systeme International) has been adopted throughout the world in all areas of science and industry. In medicine, the major change is the expression of concentration as amount per volume (moles per liter) instead of mass per volume (milligrams per deciliter).

2. molecular p.967

Because the conversion from conventional units to SI units is based on the molecular weight of the analyte, a conversion factor can be derived and utilized; to convert from conventional to SI units, multiply by the conversion factor; to convert from SI to conventional units, divide by the conversion factor.

3. mass action p.970

The methods of saturation analysis yield greater simplicity, sensitivity, and precision. Reactions in saturation analysis follow the law of mass action. A protein or antibody (R) is mixed with a substance (S) for which it has specific binding sites, forming a complex, RS. The radioactive form of the substance (S*) also forms a complex, RS*. Since the number of binding sites on the protein or antibody are limited, the labeled and unlabeled compound, S and S*, will compete for binding sites in proportion to their concentrations. Since the binding reagent, R (protein or antibody), is kept constant, increasing the unlabeled compound, S, will displace more and more labeled tracer, S*. Plotting the change in either bound or unbound (free) tracer, S*, against the amount of unlabeled compound, S, added will produce a standard curve. The amount of radioactivity bound or free in the presence of an unknown level of compound will reveal the concentration of the compound when compared to the standard curve.

4. extraction p.971

A purified, labeled amount of the substance to be measured is added to the biologic sample (e.g., plasma) to be assayed. The radioactive tracer equilibrates with the unlabeled and unknown amount of compound in the sample. The sample is now mixed with an appropriate solvent to extract the desired compound and tracer. The extraction process usually removes several compounds that may interfere with the assay, and separation (purification) of the desired substance is frequently necessary. A chromatographic separation utilizing thin layer chromatography or column chromatography was used for most steroid assays, but solid phase systems and even magnetic separation of bound and free fractions are currently utilized. Direct assays on untreated serum are less accurate.

5. antigenic; large p.971

Since steroid compounds are not antigenic, the production of a specific antiserum depends upon the linkage of a steroid to a large protein molecule. The protein molecule is antigenic in itself, but when combined with a steroid, the steroid-protein complex (hapten) stimulates a variety of antibodies, some of which recognize and are specific for the steroid. Thus, when the steroid-protein complex is injected into an animal the antiserum formed may be utilized as a reagent (R) for measurement of the steroid (S) in the technique of saturation analysis.

6. 5 p.975

(See table on page 439 in this Study Guide)

7. Pregnanetriol p.977

Pregnanetriol is the urinary metabolite of 17-hydroxyprogesterone, and was used for the diagnosis of adrenal hyperplasia (the adrenogenital syndrome). Very little pregnanetriol is found in the urine of normal adults, but with the increased production of 17-hydroxyprogesterone due to an enzyme deficiency in the adrenal gland, increased urinary excretion of pregnanetriol will occur.

Clinical State	Serum FSH	Serum LH
Normal adult female	5–30 IU/L, with the ovulatory midcycle peak about 2 times the base level	5–20 IU/L, with the ovulatory midcycle peak about 3 times the base level
Hypogonadotropic state: Prepubertal, hypothalamic and pituitary dysfunction	Less than 5 IU/L	Less than 5 IU/L
Hypergonadotropic state: Postmenopausal, castrate and ovarian failure	Greater than 30 IU/L	Greater than 40 IU/L

8. half p.988,989

ACTH is secreted in a pulsatile fashion with the pulses being more frequent and of greater magnitude in the early morning hours, shortly before waking. A nadir in secretion is reached in the evening. Blood levels of ACTH and cortisol are highest in the early morning and lowest in the evening. When the sleep-awake cycle is altered, the diurnal rhythm shifts over about a week's time to resume the same sleep-awake pattern. A 8 AM, the normal plasma cortisol concentration ranges from 10 to 25 mg/dL. At 8 PM, the level is about half the morning concentration, and at 10 PM the level is usually less than 12 mg/dL.

9. true p.970

The requirements for saturation analysis are, therefore, either a suitable binding protein, or an antibody, and a labeled pure form of the compound to be measured. The need for radioisotopes can be eliminated by the use bioluminescence, chemiluminescence, fluoroimmunoassays, and enzyme-linked assays.

10. true p.971

In immunoradiometric assays (IRMAs), the antibody is labeled instead of the hormone. The advantage is the greater stability in iodinated immunoglobulins compared to iodinated hormones.

11. true p.974

Over-the-counter LH kits are readily available to detect the LH midcycle surge in urine, utilizing enzyme immunoassays with monoclonal antibodies. The enzymes linked to the antibodies produce a color change in tubes, strips, or absorbent pads. The tests will detect the presence of LH in the urine 24–40 hours before ovulation, and thus provide a means to time conception. Intercourse or insemination is recommended the day after a positive test. Clinicians should keep in mind that this is not a test for ovulation. A midcycle surge in LH does not guarantee that ovulation and a normal luteal phase will follow.

12. true p.975

The immunoassay of 17-hydroxyprogesterone has replaced measurement of the urinary pregnanetriol level for the diagnosis of adrenal enzyme deficiency. Dramatic differences exist between normal individuals and patients with adrenal hyperplasia. Levels from 5 to 2,000 times greater than normal have been observed.

13. true p.976

As with urinary 17-ketosteroids, aging is associated with a decrease in DHAS, accelerating after menopause with DHAS becoming almost undetectable after age 70.

14. false p.978

The 1st IRP succeeded the Second International Standard; 2 units of the 1st IRP are approximately equivalent to 1 unit of the 2nd IS. A third standard is appearing, the 3rd International Standard.

15. true   p.979

A 24-hour urine specimen is required to avoid the variations in steroid excretion which occur throughout a day. Refrigeration is essential to avoid degradation of metabolites. It is wise to obtain a urinary creatinine as a check of the validity of the 24-hour collection. Urinary creatinine excretion is a reflection of body muscle mass and remains relatively constant, approximately 1,000 mg/24 hours.

16. true   p.988

Blood levels of ACTH and cortisol are highest in the early morning and lowest in the evening. When the sleep-awake cycle is altered, the diurnal rhythm shifts over about a week's time to resume the same sleep-awake pattern.

17. C   p.968

18. A   p.968

19. D   p.968

SI Prefixes and Their Symbols

10^{9}	giga	G
10^{6}	mega	M
10^{3}	kilo	k
10^{2}	hecto	h
10^{1}	deka	da
10^{-1}	deci	d
10^{-2}	centi	c
10^{-3}	milli	m
10^{-6}	micro	μ
10^{-9}	nano	n
10^{-12}	pico	p
10^{-15}	femto	f
10^{-18}	alto	a

20. E   p.967

Classically, hormones were measured in blood by bioassays, i.e., dose-response measurements based upon organ responses in animals. Some of the principles fundamental to endocrinology were established by such methods. However, bioassay methods, although adequate for qualitative statements, were relatively imprecise, nonspecific, time-consuming, expensive, and required too large an amount of the biologic sample in order to meet the quantitative requirements of modern research and clinical practice.

21. A   p.972

ELISA stands for enzyme-linked immunosorbent assay, also known as the sandwiched technique. This method does not require a radioactive tracer. A monoclonal antibody is coupled to an enzyme, e.g., horseradish peroxidase, that provides a color endpoint which can be measured by spectrophotometry. For the measurement of the glycopeptides (HCG, LH, TSH), this technique uses two monoclonal antibodies, one against the alpha-subunit and coupled to a bead or a plastic tube, and the other antibody against the beta-subunit is coupled to the enzyme. The antibody to the alpha-subunit binds the intact glycoprotein molecule; the beta-subunit antibody and the enzyme then sandwich the intact molecule by binding to the exposed beta-subunit. The result is obtained by comparing the enzyme reading on the spectrophotometer to a standard curve. Antibodies can be attached to other active substances that produce luminescence. ELISA technology is utilized for most over-the-counter LH tests and pregnancy tests.

22. E p.973

The accuracy of the results depends upon the following:

1. Specificity of the antibody or protein for the hormone to be measured, and therefore, the degree of interference or cross-reaction with other substances.
2. Purity and specificity of the radiolabeled tracer.
3. Purity and availability of the standard reference hormone.
4. *Sensitivity* (the smallest amount that can be measured) of the assay.
5. *Precision,* the variation observed when multiple measurements are obtained with the same sample, expressed as the coefficient of variation for intraassay precision and interassay precision.

23. B p.976

The immunoassay of dehydroepiandrosterone sulfate (DHAS) has replaced the measurement of urinary 17-ketosteroids for the routine evaluation of adrenal androgen production.

24. C p.989

This is a test for adrenal reserve. Adrenal glands not exposed to ACTH over a long period of time will not have a normal response. Synthetic ACTH is injected in a bolus of 0.25 mg. The plasma cortisol should increase 2–3 times over baseline at 30 and 60 minutes.

25. B p.989

This is a test for hypothalamic-pituitary-adrenal function (a test of ACTH reserve). Metyrapone blocks 11β-hydroxylase enzyme activity in the adrenal gland, thus interfering with cortisol production. After a baseline 24-hour urinary 17-hydroxycorticosteroid or plasma 11-deoxycortisol is obtained, metyrapone is given orally, 250 mg every 4 hours for 6 doses. The 17-OHC should at least double during the 24 hours of metyrapone administration or the next day. A plasma 11-deoxycortisol at 8 AM, 4 hours after the last dose of metyrapone, should exceed 7 mg/dL.